Coronary Heart Disease

Coronary Heart Disease

A Medical-Surgical Symposium
Sponsored by the American College of Cardiology and
St. Barnabas Hospital, New York City

Edited by

HENRY I. RUSSEK, M.D.

*Senior Attending Cardiologist, St. Barnabas Hospital,
New York, New York and Visiting Professor in
Cardiovascular Disease, Hahnemann Medical College
and Hospital, Philadelphia, Pennsylvania*

and

BURTON L. ZOHMAN, M.D.

*Clinical Professor of Medicine, State University of
New York Downstate Medical Center College of Medicine,
Brooklyn, New York and Senior Attending Cardiologist,
St. Barnabas Hospital, New York, New York*

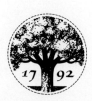

J. B. Lippincott Company
PHILADELPHIA · TORONTO

Distributed in Great Britain by
Blackwell Scientific Publications, Oxford and Edinburgh

Library of Congress Catalog Card Number 79-109952

Printed in the United States of America

1 3 2

Dedication

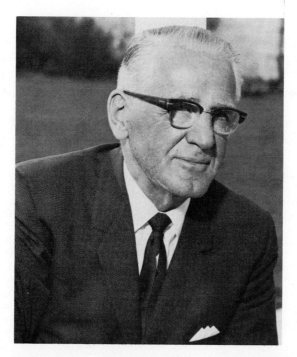

It is a privilege and honor to write this page dedicating this volume to George Griffith. I have followed his career with great interest and admiration since we first met many years ago and have marvelled at his accomplishments many times in the face of odds that would have discouraged and defeated the average man. His robust and optimistic personality and leadership, not only in medicine but in every aspect of his life, have established for him an unsurpassed position in this country and abroad and I salute him.

His heart attack, which unhappily descended upon him recently, has been borne with his customary courage and patience and I send to him my best wishes, reinforced by his dramatic recovery, as well as my affection and esteem.

George Griffith's dedication to the American College of Cardiology and his promotion of its purposes and programs have been outstanding, and it is indeed a pleasure to acknowledge this in the page of dedication.

PAUL DUDLEY WHITE, M.D.
Boston, Massachusetts

Contributors

William B. Abrams, M.D., F.A.C.C.
Director of Clinical Pharmacology, Hoffman-LaRoche Inc., Nutley, N.J.

Ezra A. Amsterdam, M.D.
Assistant Professor of Medicine, University of California, Davis

Charles P. Bailey, M.D., F.A.C.C.
Director of Thoracic Cardiovascular Surgery, St. Barnabas Hospital, New York, N.Y.

Richard J. Bing, M.D., F.A.C.C.
Professor of Medicine, University of Southern California; Research Associate, California Institute of Technology; Director of Cardiology and Intramural Medicine, Huntington Memorial Hospital.

Louis F. Bishop, M.D., F.A.C.C.
Senior Attending Cardiologist, St. Barnabas Hospital, New York, N.Y.

Dedo Boettcher, M.D.,
Research Associate, Department of Cardiology, University of Hanover

John F. Briggs, M.D., F.A.C.C.
Clinical Professor of Medicine, The University of Minnesota Medical School, St. Paul, Minn.

George E. Burch, M.D., F.A.C.C., M.A.C.P.
Henderson Professor and Chairman, Department of Medicine, Tulane University School of Medicine, New Orleans, La.

William P. Castelli
Research Associate, Heart Disease Epidemiology Study, Framingham, Mass.

Theodore Cooper, M.D., F.A.C.C.
Director, National Heart and Lung Institute, National Institutes of Health, Bethesda, Md.

Eliot Corday, M.D., F.A.C.C.
Clinical Professor of Medicine, University of California, Los Angeles School of Medicine, Los Angeles, Calif.

Giancarlo Corsini, M.D.
Assistant Professor of Medicine, University of Naples, Naples, Italy

Simon Dack, M.D., F.A.C.C.
Clinical Professor of Medicine, Mt. Sinai School of Medicine of the City University of New York, New York, N.Y.; Attending Physician for Cardiology, Mt. Sinai Hospital, New York, N.Y.

Peter J. Dempsey, M.D.
Research Associate, National Heart and Lung Institute, National Institutes of Health, Bethesda, Md.

E. Grey Dimond, M.D., F.A.C.C.
First Distinguished Professor of Medicine, The University of Missouri School of Medicine, Columbia, Mo.

Ephraim Donoso, M.D.
Associate Professor of Medicine, Mt. Sinai School of Medicine of the City University of New York, New York, N.Y.

James Flynn
Assistant Instructor and Senior Resident, Department of Medicine, Hahnemann Medical College and Hospital, Phila., Pa.

Charles K. Friedberg, M.D.
Clinical Professor of Medicine, Mt. Sinai School of Medicine of the City University of New York, New York, N.Y.

Meyer Friedman, M.D.
Director, Harold Brunn Institute, Mount Zion Hospital and Medical Center, San Francisco, Calif.

Zane N. Gaut
Research Assistant, Department of Clinical Pharmacology, Hoffman-LaRoche Inc., Nutley, N.J.

Nora Goldschlager
Senior Cardiac Fellow, Department of Cardiology, Presbyterian Medical Center, San Francisco, Calif.

Richard Gorlin, M.D.
Associate Professor of Medicine, Harvard Medical School; Director, Cardiovascular Unit, Peter Bent Brigham Hospital

William J. Grace, M.D., F.A.C.P.
Director, Department of Medicine, St. Vincent's Hospital and Medical Center, New York, N.Y.; Professor of Clinical Medicine, New York University, Bellevue Medical Center

Donald E. Gregg, Ph.D., M.D., F.A.C.C.
Chief, Department of Cardiorespiratory Diseases, Walter Reed Army Institute of Research, Washington, D.C.

George C. Griffith, M.D., F.A.C.C., D.Sc. (Hon.)
Emeritus Professor of Medicine (Cardiology), The University of Southern California School of Medicine, Los Angeles, Calif.

Sigmundur Gudbjarnason, Ph.D.
Professor of Biochemistry, University of Iceland.

Teruo Hirose, M.D., F.A.C.C.
Senior Attending in Thoracic and Cardiovascular Surgery and Director of the Cardiovascular Laboratory, St. Barnabas Hospital, New York, N.Y.

J. Campbell Howard, M.D., F.A.C.C.
Medical Director, Schering Laboratories, Union, N.J.

William B. Kannel, M.D.
Medical Director, Heart Disease Epidemiology Study, Framingham, Mass.; Lecturer in Preventive Medicine, Harvard Medical School.

Adrian Kantrowitz, M.D., F.A.C.C.
Chief of Surgery, Sinai Hospital of Detroit, Detroit, Mich.

Arnold M. Katz, M.D., F.A.C.C.
Director, Division of Cardiology, Mount Sinai Hospital; Philip J. and Harriet L. Goodhart, Professor of Medicine (Cardiology), Mount Sinai School of Medicine of the City University of New York, New York, N.Y.

Harvey G. Kemp, M.D.
Cardiovascular Unit, Department of Medicine, Peter Bent Brigham Hospital, Boston, Mass.

Richard J. Kennedy, M.D., F.A.C.P.
Associate Director of Medicine, Chief, Cardiology, St. Vincent's Hospital, New York, N.Y.; Clinical Professor of Medicine, New York University, Bellevue Medical Center.

Ancel Keys, Ph.D., F.A.C.C.
Director, School of Public Health, The University of Minnesota, Minneapolis, Minn.

Thomas Killip III, M.D.
Roland Harriman Professor of Medicine and Chief, Division of Cardiology, Cornell University Medical College, New York, N.Y.

Leslie A. Kuhn, M.D., F.A.C.C.
Associate Professor of Medicine, Mt. Sinai School of Medicine of the City University of New York, New York, N.Y.; Director, Coronary Care Unit, Mt. Sinai Hospital, New York, N.Y.

John S. LaDue, M.D., F.A.C.C.
Associate Professor of Clinical Medicine, Cornell University Medical College, New York, N.Y.

Tzu-Wang Lang, M.D.
Senior Research Scientist, Cedars-Sinai Medical Center, Los Angeles, Calif.

Maurice Lev, M.D., F.A.C.C.
Director, Congenital Heart Disease Research and Training Center, Chicago, Ill.

William Likoff, M.D., F.A.C.C.
Clinical Professor of Medicine, Hahnemann Medical College and Hospital, Phila., Pa.

C. Walton Lillehei, M.D., F.A.C.C.
Lewis Atterbury Stimson Professor of Surgery, Department of Surgery, Cornell University Medical College, New York, N.Y.

Patricia M. McNamara
Biostatistician, Heart Disease Epidemiology Study, Framingham, Mass.

Arthur M. Master, M.D., F.A.C.C.
Consulting Cardiologist, Mt. Sinai Hospital, New York, N.Y.

Campbell Moses, M.D.
Medical Director, American Heart Association, New York, N.Y.

John H. Moyer, M.D., F.A.C.C., F.A.C.P.
Professor of Medicine, Chairman, Department of Medicine, Hahnemann Medical College and Hospital, Phila., Pa.

Wilhelm Raab, M.D., F.A.C.C.*
Emeritus Professor of Experimental Medicine, The University of Vermont College of Medicine and Director, Cardiovascular Unit, Medical Center Hospital of Vermont, De Goesbriand Unit, Burlington, Vt.

Dr. Ray H. Rosenman, M.D.
Assistant Director, Harold Brunn Institute and Associate Chief, Department of Medicine, Mount Zion Hospital and Medical Center, San Francisco, Calif.

Eduardo Rosselot, M.D.
Hospital J. J. Aguirre, Universidad de Chile, Santiago, Chile.

Henry I. Russek, M.D., F.A.C.C.
Senior Attending Cardiologist, St. Barnabas Hospital, New York, N.Y.; Visiting Professor in Cardiovascular Disease, Hahnemann Medical College and Hospital, Phila., Pa.

David Scherf, M.D., F.A.C.C.
Emeritus Professor of Clinical Medicine, New York Medical College, New York, N.Y.

Herbert Shubin, M.D., F.A.C.P., F.A.C.C.
Associate Director, Center for the Critically Ill and the Shock Research Unit, University of Southern California School of Medicine, Los Angeles, Calif.

F. Mason Sones, Jr., M.D., F.A.C.C.
Head, Department of Cardiovascular Disease and the Cardiac Laboratory, Cleveland Clinic Foundation, Cleveland, Ohio

Meyer Texon, M.D., F.A.C.C.
Associate Professor of Forensic Medicine, New York University School of Medicine, New York, N.Y.

Jerome S. Tobis, M.D.
Professor and Chairman, Department of Physical Medicine and Rehabilitation, University of California, Irvine, Calif.

*Deceased September 12, 1970.

Arthur M. Vineberg, M.D., F.A.C.C.
Professor of Surgery, Royal
Victoria Hospital, Montreal,
Canada

John K. Vyden, M.B., B.S.
Associate Director Peripheral
Vascular Laboratory, Cedars-
Sinai Medical Center, Los
Angeles, Calif.

**Max Harry Weil, M.D., Ph.D.,
F.A.C.P., F.A.C.C.**
Associate Professor of Medi-
cine, Director, Center for the
Critically Ill and the Shock Re-
search Unit, University of
Southern California School of
Medicine, Los Angeles, Calif.

Raymond E. Weston, M.D., Ph.D.
Associate Clinical Professor of
Medicine, Loma Linda Univer-
sity School of Medicine, Loma
Linda, Calif.

Paul Dudley White, M.D., F.A.C.C.
Emeritus Clinical Professor of
Medicine, Harvard Medical
School and Consultant in Medi-
cine, Massachusetts General
Hospital, Boston, Mass.

Steven Wolfson, M.D.
Assistant Professor of Medicine,
Director, Cardiac Catheteriza-
tion Laboratory, Yale University
School of Medicine, New
Haven, Conn.

**Irving S. Wright, M.D., F.R.C.P.
(Lond.), F.A.C.C.**
Emeritus Clinical Professor of
Medicine, Cornell University
Medical College, New York,
N.Y.

Burton L. Zohman, M.D., F.A.C.C.
Clinical Professor of Medicine,
State University of New York
Downstate Medical Center Col-
lege of Medicine, Brooklyn,
N.Y.; Senior Attending Cardi-
ologist, St. Barnabas Hospital,
New York, N.Y.

Lenore R. Zohman, M.D.
Director, Work Physiology
Unit, Division of Rehabilitation
Medicine, Montefiore Hospital
and Medical Center, New
York, N.Y.

Preface

Coronary heart disease may well be termed "the black plague" of the twentieth century. Although inroads against its ravages have been discernible during the past few decades, the malady continues to remain the primary health problem of our time. It appears incongruous that, in an era which has seen the development of nuclear energy, antibiotics, radar, the electronic computer and rocketry, no form of therapy has yet emerged to alter the appalling death rate attributable to ischemic heart disease.

On the positive side, the accumulation of considerable knowledge gained from epidemiologic studies offers hope for primary prevention in coronary-prone subjects. In addition, as the physician has become more acutely aware of the magnitude of the problem, his diagnostic skill has materially improved and, with increasing success, he is continuing to devise techniques to salvage patients acutely afflicted with the complications of the disease. New and effective medicinal therapy, based on the synergistic effects of a combination of propranolol and certain nitrates has markedly reduced the incidence of "intractability" in angina pectoris. The surgeon has persevered in devising ingenious methods for revascularization of the myocardium and has succeeded, at least technically, in transplanting the human heart. These advances have evolved not only from a close alliance and constructive interaction between internist and surgeon but also from the prudent application of fundamental researches in physiology, anatomy, pathology, and biochemistry.

This publication, for the most part, represents the renewed, revised and edited proceedings of the American College of Cardiology-St. Barnabas Hospital Symposium on "Advances in Coronary Heart Disease" which was held at the Plaza Hotel in New York City, December 13–15, 1968. As one of the courses in the Program for Continuing Medical Education of the American College of Cardiology, this offering was so greatly over-subscribed and evoked so much interest among physicians that it was decided to make the authors' contributions available to an even wider audience. Many of the participants in this symposium have been responsible not only for where we are, at present, but also for the direction in which we are moving in the cardiovascular field. The sharing of scientific knowledge has always been in the highest tradition of the medical profession and it is in the fulfillment of this ideal that the historical continuity of all medical progress is brought into clear focus. The contributors to this volume have endeavored to place new concepts and techniques in historical perspective, to survey horizons for future achievement, and to define with candor the bounds of present-day knowledge.

The American College of Cardiology and St. Barnabas Hospital wish to express their sincere thanks to the members of the faculty of this Symposium who not only gave of their time without remuneration but cooperated in providing manuscripts of their work so that this volume might come into being.

We wish to express our deep appreciation to Dr. George Griffith, Chairman of the National Program Committee for Continuing Medical Education of the American College of Cardiology for his guidance, cooperation and encouragement and to Dr. Charles P. Bailey, Director of Thoracic Cardiovascular Surgery, St. Barnabas Hospital, New York, for valuable suggestions and advice in the formulation of the scientific program.

The success of this Symposium was in no small measure the result of the excellent administrative management provided by Mr. William D. Nelligan, Executive Director of the American College of Cardiology and his able associates, Anne Crossette and Mary Anne McInerny who gave unstintingly of their time, energy, and experience. To them we extend our warm thanks for a job superbly done.

Finally, we wish to express our appreciation to the following organizations for educational grants in partial support of this program:

Warner-Lambert Research Institute
Geigy Pharmaceuticals
Ives Laboratories
Kenwood Laboratories, Inc.
Ayerst Laboratories

Merck Sharp and Dohme
William S. Merrell Company
Schering Corporation
Smith Kline and French Laboratories
Upjohn Company

Abbott Laboratories
Burroughs Wellcome and Company, Inc.
Ciba Pharmaceutical Products, Inc.
Hoechst Pharmaceuticals

Eli Lilly and Company
McNeil Laboratories
Mead Johnson Laboratories
Wallace Laboratories

Their assistance in this endeavor has served the public interest in helping to improve the quality of medical care in this country.

Henry I. Russek
Burton L. Zohman

Contents

DIAGNOSIS OF ISCHEMIC HEART DISEASE. Part One.
Chairman: Burton L. Zohman

Part Two. *Chairman: Louis F. Bishop*

LONG-TERM MANAGEMENT OF ISCHEMIC HEART DISEASE. *Chairman: George E. Burch*

Introduction

Chairman

Henry I. Russek, M.D.

Coronary Artery Disease: Looking Back

George C. Griffith, M.D.

Coronary Artery Disease: Looking Back

George C. Griffith

INTRODUCTION

Dr. Russek, you, your associates and the registrants honor the American College of Cardiology Continuing Educational Program.

This paper is a recital by date, author, and contribution of the advances in knowledge of the anatomy and function of the coronary arteries. In 1922 at Jefferson Medical College, professor Thomas Mc-Crae of Osler and McCrae fame did not lecture on the subject of coronary artery disease. We studied the coronary arteries as nutrient vessels to the heart and considered the pathologic changes in the arteries as having been brought about by the aging process. Today, 46 years later, 800 of us will spend three days in studying the coronary arteries and the disease to which they are prone. Therefore, it is my purpose to relate the outstanding bits of knowledge chronologically.

3000 B.C.: In the Edwin Smith papyrus papers reference is made to the circulation as found in the heart. (W. W. Harburger, Am. Heart J., March, 1939)

2500 B.C.: The earliest record of sudden death due to coronary occlusion. (Walter L. Bruetsch, Circulation, 1959)

460 B.C.: Hippocrates refers to the heart as a "firm, thick mass so richly supplied with fluid that it does not suffer pain." (Vierodt, Herman, Op. Cit., P. 831)

130 A.D.: Galen applied the term "coronary" to the arteries of the heart.

1452 A.D.: Leonardo da Vinci sketched the coronary vessels. (The Anatomist by McMurrick, 1930)

1543 A.D.: Vesalius further defined the coronary arteries and veins.

1628 A.D.: William Harvey described the capillary divisions of the coronary circulation in his "De Motus Cordis."

1628 and 1694 A.D.: Malpighi and Leewenbrock further described the myocardial capillaries. (Charles Ricket, 1926)

1654–1720: Giovanni Lancisi reported aneurysmal changes in the heart muscle due to calcific coronary artery occlusion as found in his treatise "De Motus Cordis et de Aneurysmatibus."

1706: Lancisi wrote about sudden death in another treatise titled "De Subitaneis Moribus duo Libri."

1749: Jean Baptiste Senac recognized the fact that "ossification of the coronary arteries caused a thinning out of the heart muscle wall."

1761: Giovanni Battista Morgagni, a pathologist, attributed heart block to the ossification of the coronary arteries as noted in superb reports published under the title of "De Sedibus et Causus Morborum."

1768: William Heberden in "Some Account of a Disorder of the Breast" gave the name of angina pectoris, but had no idea that this clinical syndrome had a direct relationship to the heart and even less to the coronary arteries. An admirable account of William Heberden was written in 1959 by Leroy Crummer.

1728–1793: The great John Hunter autopsied John Fothergill's patients who died of angina pectoris and found that "the two coronary arteries from their origin to many of their ramifications became a piece of bone," and that "the heart was of ligamentous consistency and many parts of the left ventricle were white and hard."

1793: Edward Jenner autopsied John Hunter's heart. Hunter had Heberden's angina pectoris and predicted that his own coronary vessels would show ossifications. Jenner found Hunter's "coronary arteries to be extensively ossified."

1799: Caleb Hillier, Parry and Jenner were the original proponents of the belief that coronary artery disease and thrombosis caused angina pectoris. (Parry: Syncope anginosa)

1809: Allan Burns reported that "angina pectoris is due to relative ischemia of the heart muscle."

1842: John Ericksen ligated coronary arteries of dogs and noted sudden loss of heart action.

1850: Sir Richard Quain recognized coronary artery ossification and occlusion as a cause of angina pectoris.

1852: Karl Rokitansky wrote in his pathologic anatomy text that "arteriosclerosis is due to minute thromboses."

1867: Sir Thomas Brunton writing in Lancet described the use of amyl nitrite for relief of angina pectoris.

1878: Adam Hammer (Wein) diagnosed a "Case of Thrombotic Occlusion of a Coronary Artery," thus becoming the first physician to make a premortem diagnosis.

1879: William Murrell first used nitroglycerin for relief of angina pectoris.

1881: Julius Cohnheim wrote: "Obstruction of a large coronary artery causes sudden death while gradual obstruction causes myocardial fibrosis."

1884: Ernest Von Leyden described 4 types of coronary artery sclerosis: (a) symptomless coronary sclerosis, (b) acute coronary thrombosis, (c) diffuse fibrosis, (d) and diffuse fibrosis plus acute thrombosis.

At this point in time, why did physicians ignore the writings of the pathologists? I believe that the axiom "A heart without murmurs is a normal heart" is the answer.

1892: Ludvig Hektoen writing in Medical News stated: "Sudden death is due to embolic obstruction of the left coronary artery."

1896: George Dock, the father of our contemporary William Dock, reported 4 cases of acute coronary thrombosis with symptoms and postmortem findings in the Medical and Surgical Reporter, Philadelphia, July, 1896. In one case, he reported the premortem diagnosis accurately.

1910: Sir William Osler in his Lumleian lecture did not relate angina pectoris to coronary artery disease.

1910: Obrastzow and Straschesko in Zeitschrift reported 3 cases of "The Recognition of Thrombosis of the Coronary Arteries."

1912: J. B. Herrick writing in J.A.M.A. became the first American physician to clearly describe the "Clinical Features of Sudden Obstruction of the Coronary Arteries."

1913: Sir James MacKenzie wrote that angina pectoris is due to "exhaustion of the heart muscle."

1915: Sir Clifford Albutt in rebuttal wrote, "Angina is due to disease of the aorta and death is due to vagal inhibition."

1916: McLean and Howell discovered and used heparin as an antithrombin agent.

1918: Guy Blonsfield reported the electrocardiographic changes caused by an acute coronary occlusion.

1920: Sir James MacKenzie wrote that angina pectoris is due to insufficient blood supply to the heart muscle and that sudden death is due to ventricular fibrillation.

1920: Harold Pardee made a similar observation.

1926: Isaac Starr described the ballistocardiographic changes brought about by coronary artery disease.

1928: Harold Feil made a similar observation.

1929: Werner T. Forsmann passed a catheter into his own right heart.

1930 through 1954: C. S. Beck maintained the concept that "hearts are too good to die" and that the zone of myocardial ischemia is the zone of hyperirritability.

1933: H. L. Blumgart advocated total ablation of the thyroid function by thyroidectomy as a treatment for angina pectoris.

1934–1948: J. D. White advocated and performed cervical sympathectomy for relief of angina pectoris.

1935: A. J. Quick developed one-stage prothrombin test.

1935: George E. Fahn introduced the concept of a true vector and recognized the relationshid of bundle branch block patterns to coronary artery disease.

1936: Frank Wilson in the U.S.A. and Fritz Schellong in Germany separately used the principle of the central terminal electrode and the cathode ray oscilloscope to detect and localize a myocardial injury.

1936: L. O'Shaughnesy implanted the omentum to the ischemic myocardium.

1936: Robert Levy introduced the concept of using nitrous oxide in the recognition of coronary artery insufficiency.

1937 to 1955: C. Bailey and J. Jones resected myocardial aneurysms.

1938: H. Mann developed vectorcardiographic concepts related to coronary artery disease.

1941: A. M. Master, R. Gubner, and S. Dack introduced the two step test for recognition of coronary artery insufficiency.

1941: Andie F. Cournand established cardiac catheterization and gave the study of coronary flow great impetus.

1941: Link discovered bishydroxycoumarin in spoiled sweet clover.

1946: Irving Wright made the first statistical study of the value of the oral anticoagulants.

1946: A. M. Vineberg developed the technic of implantation of the left internal mammary artery, later added the omental graft and the bilateral internal mammary artery implantation.

1949: P. W. Duchosal added to the vectorcardiographic concepts.

1951: P. P. Grant made further additions to the concepts of vectorcardiographic changes.

1952: C. M. Agress, A. Karman, J. La Due, and F. Wroblewski related the myocardial enzyme serum changes, the SGOT, LDH, SHBD and CPK to acute myocardial injury.

1952: E. Grey Dimond made significant advances in vectorcardiographic concepts.

1952: Lawrence E. Lamb further clarified vector-cardiographic concepts of changes due to coronary artery disease.

1953: A. A. Luisado described the use of fluoroscan.

1954: E. Frank described newer concepts in vector-cardiography.

1955: H. L. Blumgart introduced the I-131 technic for thyroid ablation therapy.

1955: E. Corday described the use of radiosodium.

1955: C. T. Dotter and I. Steinberg developed the angiocardiographic concept.

1956: J. A. Abildskow described a "linear time scale for spatial vectorcardiography." (Circulation, 1956)

1956 to present: G. E. Burch, R. P. Grant, R. McFee, and T. Winsor have added further concepts in the recognition of vectorcardio-graphic changes in coronary artery disease.

1956 to 1958: F. M. Sones described cine coronary arteriography in dogs.

1957: C. T. Dotter and associates developed the balloon obstruction of the ascending aorta with flush fill of the coronary arteries.

1958: F. M. Sones described selective cine coronary arteriography in man.

1958: R. Glover and J. R. Kitchell introduced the ligation of the internal mammary artery technic for relief of angina pectoris.

1958 to 1966: A. Kattus, Charles Bailey, W. Lon-guine introduced the technic of coronary endarterectomy.

1960: E. Grey Dimond and F. Kittle did the Sham operation for ligation of the internal mammary artery.

1960: E. Corday and J. L. Jaffe used I-131 therapy in small increments to reduce but not totally ablate the thyroid function.

1963: A. Benchimol and E. Grey Dimond made significant observations related to coronary artery disease utilizing the special technic of apex cardiography.

1963: D. F. Effler introduced the tunnel technic for internal mammary artery implantation.

1963: E. Lepeschkin introduced the QX-QT quotient as of significance in coronary artery disease.

1964: E. Tafur, L. S. Cohen, and H. D. Levine related the apex cardiogram to electrical, acoustic and mechanical events.

1965: E. Craige, E. E. Edleman, and T. Kobayashi related kinetocardiography to coronary artery disease.

Newer studies in establishing the role of diet, hypertension, diabetes, hyperuricemia, obesity, tobacco and lack of exercise are suggested as accelerating factors in the etiology of coronary artery disease.

I trust this paper dealing with dates and names will stimulate an interest in the voluminous literature containing these facts.

Anatomy

The Anatomy of the Coronary Arteries and Its Functional Import

Maurice Lev, M. D.

Obstructive Disease of the Coronary Circulation: New Concepts

Harvey G. Kemp, M.D.

The Anatomy of the Coronary Arteries and Its Functional Import

Maurice Lev

This paper deals with (1) the coronary artery distribution and the blood supply to the ventricles, atria, and the conduction system, (2) the question of anastomoses, and (3) the functional import of these anatomic considerations. The statements made are based on several thousand dissections at autopsy and the work of Gross,[1] James,[2] Baroldi and Scomazzoni,[3] and Lascano.[4]

CORONARY DISTRIBUTION (FIG. 1)

The right coronary (right circumflex) artery arises from the right aortic sinus of Valsalva. It gives off the sino-atrial or SA nodal artery (ramus ostii cavae superioris) in about 60 per cent of the cases, the right conal artery in about 35 per cent of cases, the right atrial arteries, the anterior right ventricular artery, the acute marginal artery, the posterior right ventricular artery, the AV nodal artery (ramus septi fibrosi), and the posterior descending artery. In the majority of cases it terminates by branches to the posterior wall of the left ventricle. In about 10 per cent of the cases it terminates on the acute margin or between the acute margin and the posterior interventricular groove. In about 15 per cent of cases, it terminates as the obtuse marginal artery. In about 65 per cent of cases, the right conal artery is given off independently from the right sinus of Valsalva.

The left coronary artery arises from the left aortic sinus of Valsalva. There are usually no branches from the left main coronary artery. Occasionally it gives rise to an anterior left atrial artery, and a left adipose artery. After a distance varying from a few millimeters to 4 cm., it divides into the anterior descending and left circumflex. The anterior descending in its distal sojourn may divide into two equal branches. In the majority of cases the anterior descending gives rise to the left conal artery. It may also give rise to the left anterior ventricular (left diagonal). For a varying distance it may be intramyocardial. The left circumflex gives off the SA nodal

artery (ramus ostii cavae superioris) in about 40 per cent of cases; the left atrial arteries, the anterior left ventricular artery (in some cases), terminate in this manner in about 15 per cent of cases. In about 75 per cent of cases it terminates as the obtuse marginal artery, or after giving off this vessel ends between the obtuse margin and the posterior interventricular groove. In about 10 per cent of cases it continues on to form the posterior descending, and in some cases gives off the right posterior ventricular artery. In a small percentage of cases, instead of following the left AV groove, the left circumflex descends obliquely over the surface of the left ventricle terminating at the distal one half of the posterior interventricular groove.

In general it may thus be stated that there are three patterns of distribution of the coronary arteries. What may be called the balanced circulation occurs in about 75 per cent of cases. Here the right coronary artery gives off the posterior descending and terminates in a variable pattern on the posterior wall of the left ventricle. What is called the dominant left type occurs in about 10 per cent of cases. Here the left coronary artery gives off the posterior descending, and may even be more extensive terminating in variable patterns on the posterior wall of the left ventricle. What is called the dominant right coronary artery occurs in about 15 per cent of the cases. Here the right coronary artery terminates in the obtuse marginal artery. Sometimes there are two posterior descending arteries, one from the right and one from the left. This may be considered a balanced type.

BLOOD SUPPLY OF THE VENTRICLES

From the above it can be deduced that in the balanced type of circulation, the right coronary artery supplies most of the anterior wall of the right ventricle, the entire posterior wall of the right ventricle, the posterior third of the ventricular septum,

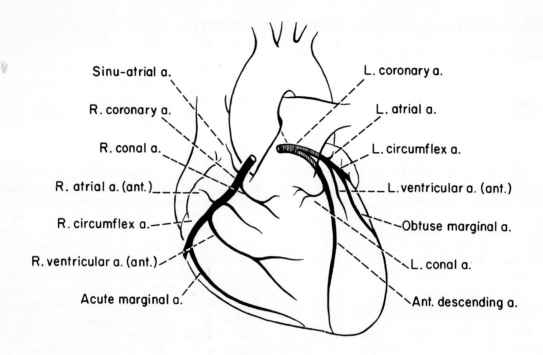

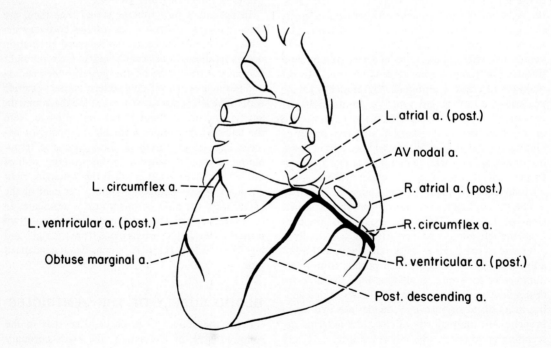

Fig. 1.   The balanced type of coronary circulation in the human heart. (*Top*) Anterior view. (*Bottom*) Posterior view.

with the exception in some cases of its most apical portion, and contributes to the supply of the posterior wall of the left ventricle. In this type of circulation, the left coronary artery supplies all of the anterior wall of the left ventricle, contributes to the supply of the anterior wall of the right ventricle, and posterior wall of the left ventricle, and supplies the anterior two thirds of the septum and most of the apical portion of the septum. In the dominant left type, the left coronary artery takes over the entire supply of the septum, and contributes to the supply of the posterior wall of the right ventricle. In the dominant right type, the right coronary artery takes over the entire supply of the posterior wall of the left ventricle.

The concept of dominance does not imply that more blood is going through the dominant artery as compared to its fellow. The terms used simply indicate a preponderant type as compared to an average which for convenience is called "balanced."

BLOOD SUPPLY OF THE ATRIA

The left atrium is supplied by branches from the left circumflex and the right atrium by branches from the right circumflex. Because of varying origin of the SA nodal artery (ramus ostii cavae superioris), the roof of the atria may be supplied mostly by either the left or right circumflex.

BLOOD SUPPLY OF THE CONDUCTION SYSTEM

The SA node is supplied by the SA nodal artery (ramus ostii cavae superioris) which, as pointed out above, may be a branch of the right or left circumflex. The AV node and bundle are supplied by the AV nodal artery (ramus septi fibrosi). The first part of the right bundle branch is supplied by the AV nodal artery, the ramus septi ventriculorum superior, and the ramus cristae, all of which emerge from the right coronary, and from the first two anterior perforating branches of the anterior descending. The second part of the right bundle branch is supplied by the ramus limbi dextri coming from a branch of the anterior descending and by anterior and posterior perforating arteries originating from both the anterior and posterior descending. The third part of the right bundle branch is supplied by the same arteries that nourish the surrounding septum. The first part of the left bundle branch is supplied by the terminal portion of the AV nodal artery. The ramus septi ventriculorum superior, and the ramus cristae, all coming from the right coronary artery reinforced by some branches from the left anterior descending.

ANASTOMOSES

There are both intracardiac and extracardiac anastomoses present normally.

INTRACARDIAC

From birth on there are anastomotic channels between the branches of the same coronary artery (homoanastomoses) or between branches of different coronary arteries (intercoronary anastomoses) in all normal hearts. This means that the coronary arteries are not end arteries. The diameter and length of these anastomoses increase with age and reach normal size at 18–20 years. There is no difference in the presence of anastomoses between male and female. These are present in the interatrial and interventricular septa, most of the ventricular and atrial walls, and in the apex and crux. Under the influence of ischemia there is an increase in number and size of the anastomoses. It is not known whether these constitute enlargement of existing anastomoses or a production of new anastomoses.

EXTRACARDIAC

There are probably anastomoses between the coronaries and the vasa vasorum of the aorta, pulmonary trunk and superior and inferior vena cava. With advancing age, anastomoses also develop between adipose branches of the coronary arteries and epicardial branches.

FUNCTIONAL IMPORT OF THE ANATOMY

The type of circulation that is present in any one case is of importance. The narrowing or occlusion of a dominant vessel is of greater importance than the narrowing of an average or less dominant one. However there is no evidence that atherosclerosis, thrombosis, or hemorrhage is more common in any one type of circulation.

The presence of anastomoses is of great importance in narrowing or occlusive phenomena. Since they are normally present at birth and are more numerous and increase in size with ischemia, which is in general a function of time, it follows that the blood supply of a region should be considered to be constituted by both its main and its collateral one. In younger people, these collaterals are not yet well developed, and hence an occlusion of the main blood supply may produce infarction. However, with advancing age and the ubiquitous ischemia, and the concomitant increase in number and size of collaterals, it is necessary to occlude both the main and collateral blood supply to produce infarction. Thus in older people at autopsy, the presence of a myocardial infarct is associated with at least the occlusion of two coronary arteries supplying an area. Likewise the speed with which the narrowings are produced may be considered a factor in the pathogenesis of infarction. Thus in some people, the presence of a myocardial infarct may be associated with one occlusion by a recent thrombus. Also hearts may be found at autopsy with multiple narrowings and no infarcts.

REFERENCES

1. Gross, L.: The Blood Supply to the Heart in its Anatomical and Clinical Aspects. New York, Paul B. Hoeber, 1921.
2. James, T. N.: Anatomy of the Coronary Arteries. New York, Paul B. Hoeber, 1961.
3. Baroldi, G. and Scomazzoni, G.: Coronary Circulation in the Normal and the Pathologic Heart. Office of the Surgeon General, Department of the Army, Washington, D. C., 1967.
4. Lascano, E. F.: Irrigacion normal del nodulo de Tawara, haz de His y sus ramas. Rev. argent. cardiol. *10*:23, 1943.

Obstructive Disease of the Coronary Circulation: New Concepts*

Harvey G. Kemp

Although earlier investigators had noted the relationship between the clinical syndrome of angina pectoris and the presence of coronary atherosclerosis,[1] the constancy of this relationship was emphasized by the careful postmortem studies of the 1940's and early 1950's.[2,3] It has subsequently become axiomatic that a history of pain in the anterior chest that is precipitated by exertion and relieved by rest indicates atherosclerotic involvement of the coronary vessels which is usually extensive. The increasingly widespread use of coronary arteriography over the past ten years has reopened this issue. In our laboratory, 9 per cent of patients referred because of the anginal syndrome as defined above do not have arteriographically demonstrable intraluminal coronary obstruction. This group correlates well with other larger series.[4] This report is intended to review our experience with this interesting group of patients who have the anginal syndrome associated with normal coronary arteriograms.

A total of 37 subjects with this syndrome have been in our laboratory and the results of these studies have been reported in detail elsewhere.[5] In contrast to some other series,[6] men as well as women were found to have this syndrome, though women outnumbered men by nearly 2:1. Ages ranged from 28 to 60 and duration of symptoms from 5 months to 25 years.

The history in each instance was taken by a member of our department. Though the exertional component of the pain was all that was required to satisfy the criteria for inclusion, there was a high incidence of typical radiation of pain into the arms and rapid relief with nitroglycerin. In fact, no historical clue could be detected in the response of these patients to the usual precipitating factors which would distinguish them from patients with extensive coronary atherosclerosis.

* Supported by USPHS Grants 1-P01-HE11306 and 5-R01-HE08591 and a grant from Women's Aid for Heart Research, Boston, Massachusetts.

Metabolic factors which might predispose to premature atherosclerotic disease were routinely sought. Thirty-four per cent of the patients had either overt diabetes, or an abnormal intravenous glucose tolerance defined as a K value of less than 1.0. Fourteen per cent had a lipid abnormality, defined as a fasting serum cholesterol of over 300 mg. per 100 cc., triglycerides of 150 mg. per 100 cc. or a distinctly abnormal pattern on lipoprotein electrophoresis.

Extracardiac sources of pain were carefully excluded. Upper GI series, cholecystograms, and films of the cervicodorsal spine were available on over 90 per cent of these patients and failed to reveal any likely sources of chest pain.

Resting electrocardiograms showed some abnormality in over 60 per cent of the patients. By far the commonest abnormality was relatively minor, stable ST-T abnormalities in leads II, III, aVF, and V 4–6. Other abnormalities rarely noted were right and left bundle branch block and left ventricular hypertrophy.

Standard double Master's exercise electrocardiography was available in 80 per cent of the patients studied. An ischemic response was defined as a 0.5 mm. segmental RS-T depression in any lead, and 20 per cent of the total group showed such an ischemic response.

Standard hemodynamic parameters including cardiac output, central aortic and left ventricular pressures as well as left ventriculography were normal in all patients. This was in part due to definition, because patients with cardiomegaly and evidence of left ventricular dysfunction were classified as primary myocardial disease, which can, of course, be accompanied by anginal pain. No patients with valvular heart disease were included. Tests of coronary hemodynamics were available in 22 subjects at rest and 13 subjects during isoproterenol infusion. Coronary blood flow, oxygen extraction and coronary venous oxygen content were normal both at rest and following isoproterenol stress.

Paired arterial-coronary sinus blood samples were obtained at rest and after isoproterenol stress in 31 subjects and were analyzed for lactate concentration. Lactate is normally removed from the arterial blood by the heart and used as a metabolic substrate. In ischemia, however, an imbalance may occur between anaerobic glycolysis and oxidative metabolism such that lactate is actually liberated by the ischemic tissue. Animal studies have shown that relatively profound hypoxia is necessary to cause lactate production by the heart.[7] Experience with normal subjects without chest pain in this laboratory has shown that lactate is consistently extracted by the myocardium at rest and with isoproterenol stress.[8] Ten of the 31 subjects in the present study had abnormal lactate production by the myocardium during isoproterenol stress.

We have no evidence to suggest that this group of patients is a homogeneous one. It seems likely, in fact, that several underlying mechanisms may be at work. In those subjects in whom no objective evidence of ischemic heart disease is present, psychiatric illness may be the primary disorder. This is extremely difficult to include or exclude on an objective basis, although we are currently making an attempt at psychiatric evaluation.

A number of these patients, however, do have objective evidence of organic heart disease, despite their normal coronary arteriograms: 80 per cent have some abnormality of their resting electrocardiograms, 20 per cent have an ischemic electrocardiographic response to exercise, and 30 per cent have abnormal myocardial lactate production. Approximately 15 per cent have the combination of ischemic electrocardiographic response and lactate production. It seems unlikely that these abnormalities can be explained on the basis of psychiatric disease alone.

Is it possible that atherosclerotic disease was present that was not visualized by arteriography? Coronary atherosclerosis is a disease almost exclusively of the large epicardial coronary vessels. When coronary vessels dip into the myocardium, the atherosclerotic process usually follows for only a few millimeters.[9] These large vessels are well revealed by coronary arteriography. A recent study performed in our laboratory indicated that coronary arteriography could predict with great precision the atherosclerotic lesions later found at postmortem examination.[10] Therefore, it seems unlikely that underestimation of atherosclerosis by coronary arteriography plays a significant role in the etiology of this syndrome.

One mechanism that has been postulated is an abnormality of oxygen-hemoglobin dissociation so that despite normal arterial oxygen saturation, reduced amounts of oxygen are available for tissue metabolic needs.[11] If this were the case, one would expect to find elevated resting coronary blood flow, diminished oxygen extraction, and high coronary sinus oxygen content. Our findings of normal coronary hemodynamics would argue strongly against this hypothesis.

Perhaps one of the most appealing possible causes is small vessel disease of the myocardium. James has described such a microangiopathy in a variety of diseases including Friedreich's ataxia, progressive muscular dystrophy and primary pulmonary hypertension.[12] The collagen vascular diseases, particularly polyarteritis nodosa and rheumatoid arthritis, may show small vessel disease. Two patients in our small series have subsequently developed typical acute rheumatoid arthritis. Further follow-up with the eventual availability of pathologic material may help establish the presence or absence of small vessel disease.

How should these patients be managed? Because no deaths have occurred in our patients, nor have they been reported elsewhere, we have tended to reassure our patients concerning longevity. We have continued the use of nitroglycerin if it gives symptomatic relief. Propranolol has proved helpful in only about 20 per cent of these patients in contrast to over 80 per cent benefit in the atherosclerotic group, but if it is beneficial in a blind trial, we continue it. Graded exercise, weight reduction, cessation of smoking and other general measures have proved useful, as well as simple encouragement from an interested, sympathetic physician. More specific measures must await a better understanding of the underlying pathophysiology of this syndrome.

REFERENCES

1. MacKenzie, Sir James: Angina Pectoris, London, Henry Frowde and Hodder and Stoughton, 1923.
2. Blumgart, H. L., Schlesinger, M. J., and Davis, D.: Studies on the relation of the clinical manifestations of angina pectoris, coronary thrombosis and myocardial infarction to the pathological findings, Am. Heart J. *19*:1, 1940.
3. Zoll, P. M., Wessler, S., and Blumgart, H. L.: Angina pectoris, a clinical and pathologic correlation, Am. J. Med. *11*:331, 1951.
4. Proudfit, W. L., Shirey, E. K., and Sones, F. M., Jr.: Selective cine coronary arteriography, correlation with clinical findings in 1000 patients, Circulation *33*:901, 1966.
5. Kemp, H. G., Elliott, W. C., and Gorlin, R.: The anginal syndrome with normal coronary arteriography, Trans. Assn. Am. Phys. *80*:59, 1967.
6. Likoff, W., Segal, B. L., and Kasparian, H.: Normal selective coronary arteriograms in coronary heart disease, New Eng. J. Med. *276*:1063, 1967.

7. Shea, T. M., Watson, R. M., Piotrowski, F., Dermksian, G., and Case, R. B.: Anaerobic myocardial metabolism, Am. J. Physiol. *203*:463, 1962.

8. Cohen, L. S., Elliott, W. C., Klein, M. D., and Gorlin, R.: Coronary heart disease, clinical, cine arteriographic and metabolic correlations, Am. J. Card. *17*:153, 1965.

9. Osborn, G. R.: Incubation Period of Coronary Thrombosis, London, Butterworth & Co., Ltd., 1963.

10. Kemp, H. G., Evans, H., Elliott, W. C., and Gorlin, R.: Diagnostic accuracy of selective coronary cine arteriography, Circulation *36*:526, 1967.

11. Eliot, R. S., and Mizukami, H.: Oxygen affinity of hemoglobin in persons with acute myocardial infarction and in smokers, Circulation *34*:331, 1966.

12. James, T. N.: Pathology of small coronary arteries, Am. J. Card. *20*:679, 1967.

Pathophysiology and Pathogenesis

Physiologic Factors Which Determine Coronary Blood Flow
Donald E. Gregg, Ph.D., M.D.

Technics for Measurement of the Coronary Circulation: Determination of Total and Nutritional Coronary Blood Flow Using Coincidence Counting
Giancarlo Corsini, M.D.
Dedo Boettcher, M.D.
Nora Goldschlager, M.D.
Richard J. Bing, M.D.

Neurohumoral Control of the Coronary Circulation
Harvey G. Kemp, M.D.

Cardiac Innervation: Anatomic and Pharmacologic Relationships
Peter J. Dempsey, M.D.
Theodore Cooper, Ph.D., M.D.

Effects of Ischemia and Hypoxia Upon the Myocardium
Arnold M. Katz, M.D

Physiologic Factors Which Determine Coronary Blood Flow

Donald E. Gregg

I should like to consider two experimental models that have been developed in our laboratory over the past few years for the study of the coronary circulation of the dog as it naturally exists. The first model was developed for the study of the normal coronary circulation. The second model was developed for the study of the coronary circulation in the presence of coronary insufficiency and myocardial infarction. A number of individuals are responsible for these models, especially Mr. Khouri, Dr. Elliot, Dr. Granata, Dr. Olsson, Dr. Pitt and, more recently, Dr. Pasyk.

In the model for study of the normal coronary circulation,[1-4] implantations were then made of special electromagnetic flowmeters on the ascending aorta and the descending and circumflex branches of the left coronary artery; placement was also made of small pneumatic cuffs on the coronary branches just beyond the flow transducers to obtain temporary coronary flow zeros, and of tubes in the aorta for

sampling pressure and in the coronary sinus for estimating metabolic changes across the myocardium. In some dogs, one or more of three additional technics were also used. A small tube was implanted in the circumflex coronary branch for injection of drugs. To obviate the effects of changing heart rate, the atrioventricular node was interrupted and the heart paced at a rate of 70 to 100 per minute. Finally, to test the role of the central nervous system in the control of the coronary circulation, the autonomic nerve supply to the heart was interrupted by a stripping technic at time of flowmeter implantation.[5] The animals were studied for 1 to 4 months after recovery from operation.

RESTING CORONARY FLOW

Figure 1 shows basic data and the pressure curve from the aorta and flow curves from the main left coronary artery and the ascending aorta obtained 28

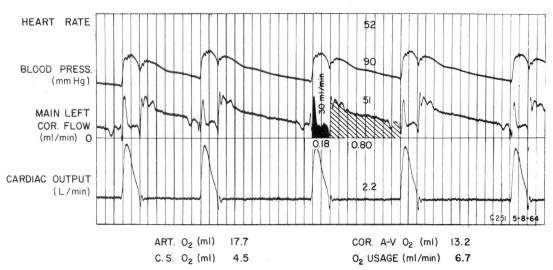

| ART. O$_2$ (ml) | 17.7 | COR. A-V O$_2$ (ml) | 13.2 |
| C.S. O$_2$ (ml) | 4.5 | O$_2$ USAGE (ml/min) | 6.7 |

FIG 1. Record showing phasic aortic pressure and phasic flow in the main left coronary artery and ascending aorta obtained by means of a strain gauge and electromagnetic flowmeters. Black area is systolic flow; lined area is diastolic flow. Vertical lines 0.1 sec. Modified from Gregg, et al.[1]

19

days postoperatively in a dog lying at rest and in a semibasal state.[1] Here the coronary inflow per 100 gm. of myocardium is 51 ml., and the oxygen extraction by the myocardium is about 75 per cent, leaving 4.5 vol. per cent in the coronary sinus blood. Since this main left coronary inflow supplies about 80 per cent of the coronary flow to the whole heart, total coronary flow is about 64 ml./min. This is a surprisingly low value and is at most 3 per cent of the cardiac output of 2.2 L.

Older teachings have indicated that there is essentially no flow into the left coronary artery during systole and that increased coronary flow during stress states results from a combination of more heart beats per minute and a decrease in coronary flow per heart beat. Neither appears to be true. As indicated in Figure 1, the main left coronary flow pattern has a forward movement of blood, a smaller one in systole during the period of ejection (represented by the solid area), and a larger one in diastole (represented by the lined area). The systolic flow component is of particular interest. In late systole, the flow rate is 30 ml./min. Under resting conditions in different dogs, this varies from 20–40 ml./min. The volume flow during systole is 0.18 ml. or about 25 per cent of the volume flow during diastole. This percentage can vary from 15 to 45 per cent, being lowest the closer the dog is to the basal state.

Obviously, some of this systolic flow must go to radially expand the epicardial arteries. Since in some stress states the late systolic flow rate can rise to 200 ml./min., and the systolic volume flow can equal the diastolic volume flow, it is our view without quite certain proof that much of it must penetrate deeply into the myocardium during its contraction. Unfortunately, as yet no methods are available to estimate the volume concerned or the depth to which it penetrates.

CORONARY CIRCULATION IN EXERCISE AND EXCITEMENT

Let us now consider typical patterns of response of the left coronary circulation to the natural stress of exercise.[6] Figure 2 shows the response to heavy exercise in which the dog was first at standing rest on a treadmill and then ran at 16 km./hr. at a 10° grade. The early systemic responses at 6 seconds are large increases in heart rate and cardiac output, both reaching a maximum within 20 seconds, after which

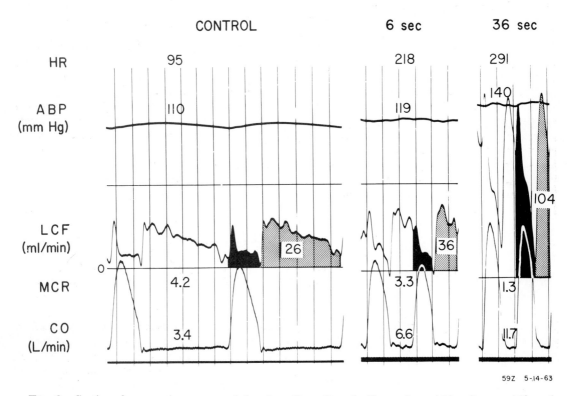

FIG. 2.   Sections from continuous record showing effect of treadmill exercise at 16 km./hr. at a 10° grade on heart rate (HR), mean aortic blood pressure (ABP), phasic circumflex coronary flow (LCF), mean coronary resistance (MCR), and cardiac output (CO). Time lines 0.1 sec. Modified from Khouri, et al.[6]

they are maintained. Mean blood pressure rises more slowly and only mildly, and thus leads to a marked decrease in peripheral resistance. Stroke cardiac output generally increases mildly after an initial transient sizable decrease. The coronary flow increases from 26 to 104 ml./min. About two-thirds of the increase is caused by more heart beats per minute; about one-third comes from an increased volume of coronary flow for each heart beat. At low to moderate levels of physical exertion, however, the increase in coronary flow arises entirely from the acceleration of the heart with no change or even a small decrease in the volume of coronary flow for each heart beat. In either case, there is a marked redistribution of flow during the cardiac cycle; in this record, the systolic flow increases largely to approximate the diastolic flow which is unchanged. At the same time, the rate of late systolic flow rises greatly from 21 ml./min. to 105 ml./min. Thus, the maintenance and augmentation of the coronary flow per heart beat is almost entirely through adjustments of the systolic flow. Without this systolic flow component which occupies more than 60 per cent of the cardiac cycle time, the heart would surely perish. Again, it is felt that much of this must penetrate deeply into the myocardium. Finally, coronary resistance to flow or the ratio of aortic pressure to coronary flow is reduced greatly, for despite a 70 per cent decrease in duration of a heart beat, coronary flow for each heart beat increases 37 per cent with only a mild elevation in blood pressure.

In this heart, oxygen usage increases from 3.5 to 14.0 ml./min. but not all the extra oxygen used by the myocardium is made available through increased coronary flow. The oxygen supply can be augmented by an additional 30 per cent through a markedly increased extraction of oxygen lowering the coronary sinus oxygen from 4.5 to about 1.5 volumes per cent. This phenomenon developed in this experiment after sustained exercise.

The responses of the systemic and coronary circulations to excitement induced by noise, fright, olfactory and thermal stimuli are generally similar to those occurring in muscular activity, although the increase in stroke coronary flow can be larger, at times rising by as much as 100 per cent.[7] There is, however, one fundamental difference. The oxygen extraction falls instead of rising and the coronary sinus oxygen saturation can increase up to 50 per cent.

REACTIVE HYPEREMIA

Although various stress states lead to massive coronary dilatation with increased blood pressure

and heart rate, the magnitude of this dilatation is much less than the maximum dilatation obtainable without change in blood pressure and heart rate. The most important index of this ability is the peak flow response obtained 5–6 seconds after release of a temporary occlusion of a coronary artery.[8] This is called "reactive hyperemia." In different dogs, this varies from 300 to 700 per cent of the control flow. Although reactive hyperemia is regarded as the most characteristic and important response of the coronary vascular bed, the underlying mechanism is not known. Presumably, it occurs with every heart beat following ventricular contraction. Reactive hyperemia taken almost simultaneously from different branches of the left coronary artery can vary considerably; it is not affected by chronic denervation of the heart or by pharmacologic elimination of coronary artery constrictor tone with agents such as Dibenzyline and Dibenamine; it can be decreased or eliminated by massive dilatation of the coronary bed or by inducing coronary insufficiency by means of chronic constriction of a coronary artery.

VARIATIONS IN CORONARY FLOW PATTERN AND STROKE CORONARY FLOW UNDER DIFFERENT CONDITIONS

The preceding indicates that the coronary circulation responds to natural stress with a relatively fixed flow pattern. Actually, under some circumstances, the pattern can be greatly altered. For example, stimulation of the left stellate ganglion, on which a bipolar electrode has been previously implanted, can cause almost complete disappearance of the systolic flow in the presence of massive coronary dilatation and greatly increases diastolic flow.[8] On the other hand, late in irreversible hemorrhagic shock, the systolic flow can become dominant and the flow curve resembles a systemic pressure curve.

THE SEPARATE CONTROLS OF THE CORONARY CIRCULATION

The mechanisms of control of such massive dilatation as just described are difficult to establish. The responses could be related to the generally associated large increases in heart rate; they could arise from catecholamine release and action of the sympathetic nervous system on the heart or they could be entirely controlled locally within the myocardium. Although there is no final answer, I should like to consider now the preliminary explorations we have made in this fascinating area.

The fact that the coronary circulation responds

quite well in the presence of a fixed heart rate suggests that it is not the prime regulator of this circulation. If changes in heart rate are prevented during exercise and excitement, stroke coronary flow can increase 100 to 300 per cent. This is massive dilatation, for the blood pressure is unchanged while both systolic and diastolic flows per heart beat are greatly increased. Thus, the large increase in heart rate which usually accompanies stress states obscures the large increase in stroke coronary flow which would have occurred if the heart rate had been slower. Since these hearts do perform quite well, it raises the question of the desirability of the naturally occurring very large cardiac acceleration in these situations.

The experiments on nervous control of the coronary circulation have been concerned with: (1) the existence in the coronary vasculature and myocardium of adrenergic receptors that can be activated by catecholamine administration or by circulating catecholamines; (2) the possible importance of these receptors during natural stress states; and (3) func-

however, draw attention to the fact that both beta (vasodilator) and alpha (vasoconstrictor) adrenergic receptor activity can be demonstrated in the coronary arteries of the unanesthetized dog.[12]

In Figure 3, isoproterenol was injected into the left circumflex coronary branch of a dog with an intact conducting system. Beta receptor activity is indicated by the marked increase in coronary blood flow from 22 to 58 ml./min. at 7 seconds, and the decrease in coronary resistance without any alteration in systemic dynamics. Later, myocardial effects become noticeable and at 25 seconds are manifested by a decrease in the systolic ejection period and an increase in peak ventricular ejection rate. After beta adrenergic blockade with intravenous propranolol, isoproterenol did not increase coronary blood flow or change systemic hemodynamics.

Intracoronary injection of epinephrine also invariably causes primary coronary vessel dilatation. The response to norepinephrine can be similar or, at times, its injection causes coronary vasoconstriction indicating the response of a predominance of alpha

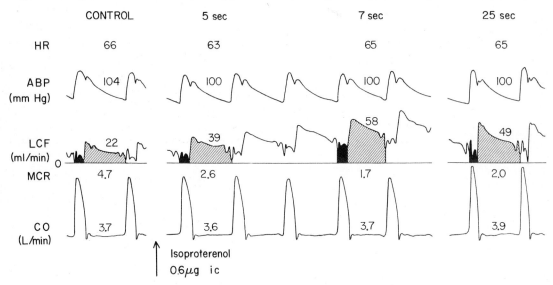

FIG. 3.   Hemodynamic effects of intracoronary injection of isoproterenol in dog with normal conducting system. Ordinate symbols as in Fig. 2. Vertical lines 0.1 sec. Modified from Pitt, et al.[12]

tioning of the coronary circulation in the denervated heart in which the sympathetic and parasympathetic connections to the heart are cut and the catecholamine content of the heart muscle is essentially zero.

First of all, there is general agreement that the myocardium contains adrenergic receptors whose stimulation by cardiac sympathetic nerves or by circulating catecholamines results in a marked increase in myocardial contractility, cardiac activity and coronary flow. I shall not discuss this. I would,

adrenergic receptors.

Alpha coronary vessel receptor activity causing coronary vasoconstriction can also be demonstrated in a number of ways. Intravenous injections of phenylephrine in a dog with a fixed heart rate decreases left coronary flow and increases coronary resistance despite an increase in aortic blood pressure. In addition, after beta adrenergic blockade, intravenous epinephrine which normally increases coronary flow now decreases the flow in the presence of an elevated blood pressure.

Although both alpha and beta adrenergic receptors can be demonstrated in the coronary system, their usefulness or function can only be told by observations during stress states. Actually, the hemodynamic and coronary flow responses to excitement are reduced but not eliminated by pharmacologic blockade. Similarly, the dog can achieve the same level of submaximal exercise after blockade as before it but this is accomplished with marked attenuation of the increases in cardiac work and coronary flow.[12]

Thus, these experiments indicate that adrenergic receptors exist and function in the coronary arteries of the normal dog heart but that they are not necessary for submaximal heart performance under various stress states.

Finally, the functioning of the coronary circulation after cardiac neural ablation by the stripping technic has been followed in five dogs for many weeks.[5] These hearts are believed to have been completely denervated at the time of operation and to have remained so as evidenced by their failure to respond to large intravenous doses of Tyramine and atropine, their failure at time of sacrifice to respond to stellate ganglion and cardiac sympathetic nerve stimulation and the almost total loss of catecholamines from their myocardiums.

The dog with the denervated heart appears entirely normal. Apparently, however, its coronary flow and oxygen usage are considerably lower than those of the heart with nerves intact. The average and range of values for the systemic, coronary, and metabolic data have been compiled from five denervated dogs during a 30 day postoperative period extending from the 15th to 45th day. These are compared with the values from seven normal dogs of comparable weight (40–45 lb.) and training and whose cardiac nerves were intact. With roughly comparable heart rate, blood pressure and cardiac output prevailing in the two groups, the average circumflex flow of 19 ml./min. and the oxygen usage of 2.3 ml./min. in the dogs with denervated hearts are only about half the average values in the dogs with normal hearts. Other than the preceding, the response of the denervated heart to various stresses does not appear to be fundamentally different from that of the heart with intact nerves.

What I have considered is only a progress report on the beginning of work in this field and in our understanding of the normal coronary circulation. It considers only the entrance flow and tells us nothing of events within the walls of the myocardium. Consideration of this microcirculation and its local control is, of course, far more important but a much more difficult task. It involves as an irreducible minimum, the availability of technic to estimate nutritional flow or the portion of entrance flow having to do with capillary exchange, and secondly, to estimate the extent of homogeneity of coronary flow and other coronary phenomena at different depths within the myocardium of the normal heart. Since such methodology and information is largely nonexistent, final consideration of the role of local control of the coronary circulation must await further experimentation.

REFERENCES

1. Gregg, D. E., Khouri, E. M., and Rayford, C. R.: Systemic and coronary energetics in the resting unanesthetized dog, Circulation Res. *16*:102, 1965.
2. Khouri, E. M., and Gregg, D. E.: An inflatable cuff for zero determination in blood flow studies, J. Appl. Physiol. *23*:395, 1967.
3. Elliot, E. C., Jones, E. L., Bloor, C. M., Leon, A. S., and Gregg, D. E.: Day-to-day changes in coronary hemodynamics secondary to coronary artery constriction in dogs, Circulation Res. *22*:237, 1968.
4. Pitt, B., and Gregg, D. E.: Coronary hemodynamic effects of increasing ventricular rate in the unanesthetized dog, Circulation Res. *22*:753, 1968.
5. Gregg, D. E., Khouri, E. M., Donald, D. E., Pasyk, S., and Lowensohn, H.: The coronary circulation in the conscious dog with cardiac neural ablation, Circulation *38*:vi-88, 1968.
6. Khouri, E. M., Gregg, D. E., and Rayford, C. R.: Effect of exercise on cardiac output, left coronary flow and myocardial metabolism in the unanesthetized dog, Circulation Res. *17*:427, 1965.
7. Rayford, C. R., Khouri, E. M., and Gregg, D. E.: Effect of excitement on coronary and systemic energetics in unanesthetized dogs, Am. J. Physiol. *209*: 680, 1965.
8. Olsson, R. A., and Gregg, D. E.: Myocardial reactive hyperemia in the unanesthetized dog, Am. J. Physiol. *208*: 224, 1965.
9. Granata, L., Olsson, R. A., Huvos, A., and Gregg, D. E.: Coronary inflow and oxygen usage following cardiac sympathetic nerve stimulation in unanesthetized dogs, Circulation Res. *16*:114, 1965.
10. Granata, L.: Coronary circulation during hemorrhagic shock. In Coronary Circulation and Energetics of the Myocardium, International Symposium in Milan, 1966, Basel, Karger, 1967, p. 78.
11. Pitt, B., Elliot, E. C., Khouri, E. M., and Gregg, D. E.: Effect of adrenergic blockade on the coronary hemodynamic response to excitement at fixed ventricular rate in the unanesthetized dog, Physiologist *9*: 267, 1966.
12. Pitt, B., Elliot, E. C., and Gregg, D. E.: Adrenergic receptor activity in the coronary arteries of the unanesthetized dog, Circulation Res. *21*:75, 1967.

Technics for Measurement of the Coronary Circulation: Determination of Total and Nutritional Coronary Blood Flow Using Coincidence Counting*

Giancarlo Corsini, Dedo Boettcher, Nora Goldschlager, and Richard J. Bing

Organ blood flow has been differentiated into total and nutritional circulation.[1-3] The latter is the circulation that is involved in the metabolic exchange with the tissues.[4] Differential organ blood flow can be determined by means of intravascular nondiffusible substances (RISA-131, Diodrast-131),[5,6] highly diffusible inert gases (N_2O, Kr, Xe),[7-11] or diffusible substances which actively enter the cell (K^{42}, Rb^{86}, Rb^{84}).[12-16]

Rubidium is a substance which is metabolically similar to potassium.[12,17] The isotope Rb^{84} decays by positron emission 19 per cent of the time and produces two gamma photons of 0.51 million electron volts (M.E.V.) directed 180° apart, or back to back.[16]

The detection system† used in our laboratory for measuring myocardial clearance of Rb^{84} consists of pairs of coincidence counting crystals placed anteriorly and posteriorly to the chest 180° apart, and has been described in detail in previous publications.[16,18] The major advantage of the double coincidence counting technic is that without elaborate collimation it is possible to define the radiation from the heart muscle independent of surrounding structures. Other advantages of the double coincidence counting system and Rb^{84} are that (a) the field of view of a detection system is precisely defined; (b) background activity from natural radioactivity, cosmic ray activity and radioactive contaminants in the room is negligible; and (c) for equal injected activities of rubidium and identical detector fields of view, the coincidence method using Rb^{84} gives five times the counting rate that Rb^{86} would yield using the standard single technic.[18]

*This work was supported by U.S. Public Health Service Grant No. HE-05043, Michigan Heart Association, Detroit General Hospital Research Corporation, United Foundation of Detroit and The John A. Hartford Foundation.

†CO-INSITRON: American Science and Engineering, Inc., Cambridge, Massachusetts.

This communication represents an effort to assess the difference between total and nutritional flow of the heart of closed chest anesthetized dogs, using the coincidence counting system and Rb^{84} clearance. Total flow was determined by the Fick principle and nutritional circulation was evaluated by Rb^{84} clearance after a single slug injection. Additional experiments were carried out to evaluate the effects of adrenergic drugs, of hyperkalemia, and of hypoxia on the nutritional circulation of the heart.

MATERIAL AND METHODS

Mongrel dogs weighing from 10 to 25 Kg. were anesthetized with sodium pentobarbital (30 mg./Kg.), anticoagulated with heparin (2 mg./Kg.) and ventilated with room air through endotracheal tubes by means of a respiratory pump (Harvard respirator). The animals were placed in the left lateral position so that the outline of the heart (previously drawn on the chest wall during fluoroscopy) could be positioned between the 4 inch pair of coincidence counting detectors. Prior to all injections of Rb^{84}, background activity was determined. In all experiments, aortic pressure and electrocardiograms were continuously monitored.

Measurements of total coronary blood flow and myocardial clearance were made under control conditions, and after administration of adrenergic agents, potassium infusion or the induction of hypoxemia. In each instance, the bolus of Rb^{84} (0.4 μc./lb.) was injected into the inferior vena cava through a catheter inserted into a femoral vein. Myocardial radioactivity was recorded for a period of 4 1/2 minutes following each injection; however, only the precordial activity between 90 and 270 seconds was used for determination of myocardial uptake (Fig. 1). As demonstrated previously,[19] the initial distribution of Rb^{84} in the heart is complete at 90 seconds following injection; therefore, after 90 seconds, while the output of the detectors remains constant, it is possible to measure the accumulated myocardial activity from the bolus injection. This activity represents myocardial uptake of the tracer and is used in the formulas for flow and clearance (see below). Precordial counts were summated at 3-second intervals and recorded as a direct printout, and the sum of these counts from 90 to 270 seconds (3 minutes) was converted to average activity per minute.

Arterial blood was withdrawn from the descending aorta through a catheter introduced through a femoral artery. This blood was circulated through a radicoil in a well counter and reinfused into the distal femoral artery by means of a roller-pump* at a constant flow of 40 cc./min. The activity of the

arterial blood detected in the well counter was printed at 3-second intervals by the same counting apparatus. For the determination of the total organ blood flow according to the Fick principle, the integrated arterial concentration of Rb^{84} over a period of two minutes following injection was used; this time period was chosen because in this interval arterial and venous activity approached constant values, permitting the determination of the arteriovenous difference following the slug injection of Rb^{84} (Fig. 1).

In order to determine coronary venous activity of Rb^{84}, a catheter was directed, under fluoroscopic control, from the external jugular vein into the coronary sinus. Coronary sinus blood was collected at a constant rate during the same two-minute period in which arterial activity was determined. Three samples of 1 cc. each were then pipetted from the collection flask into test tubes, and the activity in each aliquot was later determined in the same well counter used to register activity in arterial blood. The values obtained were corrected for the geometric difference of the test tube as compared to the radicoil by means of a conversion factor. The conversion factor was obtained by relating activity of an aqueous solution of Rb^{84} in the test tube to that in the radicoil.[18,19]

To obtain the integrated arterial activity. during the first circulation for the myocardial clearance of Rb^{84} (Fig. 1), the arterial concentrations were summated from the onset of the appearance of the tracer to the beginning of recirculation. The downslope was plotted on semilog paper and the area under the curve was calculated. Another conversion factor was used to relate the activity obtained from the well counter to precordial counts, the heart size as compared to the size of the detector crystal, and the radioactivity transmitted by the entire body. The determination of this coefficient has been previously described.[18] The reproducibility of the method has been tested previously and the results have been published.[19]

Isoproterenol (1μg./Kg./min.) and norepinephrine (0.25, 0.5 and 1.0 μg./Kg./min.) were infused intravenously in experiments designed to determine the relation between total flow and clearance as influenced by adrenergic agents.

The effect of changes in intracellular concentration of potassium on total and nutritional coronary blood flow was studied in five animals by infusion of 1.5 per cent KCl at a speed of 4 cc./min. Total and nutritional flows were determined when the electrocardiogram showed the typical changes of hyper-

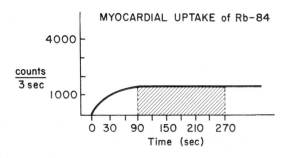

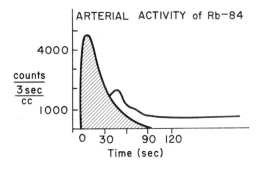

FIG. 1. Presented on linear scale, the curves illustrating the radioactivity over the heart (myocardial uptake)and during the first arterial circulation (A_1) of Rb^{84}. Shaded areas represent period of constant myocardial uptake and A_1, respectively.

Myocardial uptake of the tracer is determined from 90 to 270 seconds after the bolus injection, during which time detector output is constant. This is given as $U_H(t)$ (counts/min.), and is the height of the myocardial uptake curve.

The downslope of the arterial curve is extrapolated on semilog paper to zero and the area under it represents the integrated arterial concentration of the isotope. This is expressed as $\int_0^t A_1(t)dt$ (see text).

*Sarns Low-Flow Pump, Model No. 3500; Sarns, Inc., Ann Arbor, Michigan.

kalemia (flattening of P-wave, widening of QRS and increase in voltage of T-wave). In a second series of five dogs, in order to avoid possible distortion of radioactive background introduced by the control injection of Rb[84], flows were determined only during the infusion of 1.5 per cent KCl. Open-chest dogs were used to ascertain the direct effect of potassium infusion on the myocardial uptake of Rb[84]. After thoracotomy and pericardiotomy, a single slug of Rb[84] (0.5 μc./Kg.) was injected intravenously. A first cardiac biopsy was performed 3 minutes later. Following this, an infusion of 1.5 per cent KCl at a speed of 4 cc./min. was started and a second biopsy was performed 25 minutes later, at a time when electrocardiographic changes were observed. A third biopsy was taken after onset of cardiac arrhythmias. Biopsies were obtained according to a method previously published.[20] The samples obtained were digested overnight in a 2N solution of KOH, and the solution was then counted directly in the well counter. In all experiments, the concentration of potassium in the serum was determined before and after potassium infusion.

The effect of hypoxia on total and nutritional myocardial blood flow was studied in 12 animals. After control measurements were obtained and arterial oxygen saturation measured, the animals were administered a mixture of 90 per cent nitrogen and 10 per cent oxygen through an endotracheal tube by means of a respiratory pump (Harvard respirator). When an arterial oxygen saturation of approximately 70 per cent had been reached, total and nutritional blood flow were again determined.

Clearance of a tracer such as rubidium from a tissue (washout) or blood (uptake) is related to the capillary blood flow rate, the permeability of the capillary and cell membranes, and the capillary surface area.[1,21,22] Therefore, clearance is a measure of effective capillary blood flow (nutritional blood flow) when permeability is not a limiting factor. This concept is further discussed in a subsequent paragraph.

Based on the findings of Sapirstein,[14] who, using the principle of fractional distribution of isotopes, suggested that organ extraction ratio of rubidium must equal the total body extraction ratio, it follows that myocardial uptake of the tracer is related to body uptake (the total amount of injected rubidium) as nutritional myocardial blood flow is related to cardiac output.

1. $\dfrac{U_H(t)}{U_B(t)} = \dfrac{NBF}{CO}$

$U_H(t)$ represents myocardial uptake of Rb[84] (counts/min.), measured 90–270 seconds following the injection.

$U_B(t)$ represents the total body uptake of Rb[84] following injection (counts/min.). This equals the amount of Rb[84] injected.

NBF equals nutritional myocardial blood flow (cc./min.) and CO equals cardiac output (cc./min.).

It is assumed that this expression (Formula 1) is true under both control and experimental conditions. Solving for nutritional blood flow:

2. $NBF = \dfrac{U_H(t) \times CO}{U_B(t)}$

Cardiac output is calculated by the Stewart-Hamilton formula[23]:

3. $CO = \dfrac{U_B(t)}{\displaystyle\int_0^\infty A_1(t)dt}$

where $\displaystyle\int_0^\infty A_1(t)dt$ represents the integrated concentration of Rb[84] during the primary arterial circulation (counts/cc.).

Substituting Equation 3 for cardiac output in Equation 2:

4. Nutritional Blood Flow (NBF) $= \dfrac{U_H(t)}{\displaystyle\int_0^\infty A_1(t)dt}$

This expression is henceforth referred to as myocardial Rb[84] clearance (MCl).

Consequently, NBF equals myocardial uptake of Rb[84] divided by the integrated arterial concentration prior to recirculation (cc./min./whole heart).

The validity of this assumption can now be tested by comparing NBF as defined by Equation 4 to total myocardial blood flow as determined by the Fick principle[24] (Equation 5):

5. Total Blood Flow (TBF) $= \dfrac{U_H(t)}{\displaystyle\int_0^t A_1(t)dt - \int_0^t V(t)dt}$

$\displaystyle\int_0^t A_1(t)dt$ represents the integrated arterial concentration of Rb[84] during a defined period of time in counts/cc.

$\displaystyle\int_0^t V(t)dt$ represents the integrated concentration of Rb[84] in coronary sinus blood and determined for the same period of time and expressed in counts/cc.

Nutritional flow was calculated from the formula:

$$NBF \, \dfrac{U_H(t)}{\displaystyle\int_0^t A_1(t)dt}$$

where $\displaystyle\int_0^t A_1(t)dt$ represents the integrated concentration of Rb[84] during the primary arterial circulation (counts/cc.). It is not necessary to obtain heart weight as the radioactivity over the entire heart is counted by the 4 inch crystals. Solving equations for TBF and NBF, it is apparent that these values are expressed as cc./min./whole heart.

RESULTS

The data obtained in 60 anesthetized closed chest dogs under control conditions are shown in Figure 2, which is constructed from the average values of total and nutritional coronary blood flow. It can be seen that total coronary blood flow and nutritional flow (myocardial clearance) are closely related. The mean difference between nutritional and total flow is 5.0 cc./min., or 4.3 per cent, which is not statistically significant (p > 0.1) (Fig. 2). This is in contradistinction to a previous report from this laboratory,[19] which suggested that this difference was statistically

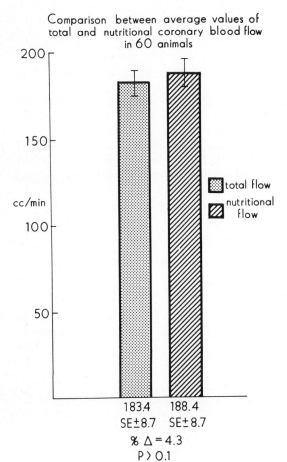

Comparison between average values of total and nutritional coronary blood flow in 60 animals

FIG. 2. The bars represent the average total and nutritional coronary flow in 60 anesthetized dogs.

significant (p < 0.02); however, in this previous publication the total number of experiments was smaller.

Table 1 shows the effect of norepinephrine and isoproterenol on total and nutritional blood flow. The original data have been previously presented in detail;[19] therefore, Table 1 contains only average values. It is seen that norepinephrine produces a marked increase in total coronary blood flow, but that nutritional flow is not increased proportionally. Table 1 also shows that the increase in total and nutritional blood flow produced by isoproterenol is proportional.

Tables 2, 3 and 4 show the values for total and nutritional flow during potassium infusion when serum potassium ranged from 5.8 to 9.1 mEq./1. A total of 15 dogs was studied. Measurements were made in five dogs before and during infusion (Table 3). The myocardial uptake of Rb[84] in an additional five dogs was determined directly by counting aliquots of digested heart muscle in a well counter (Table 4). It is seen that in four out of ten dogs in which uptake was measured by means of the external counter (Tables 2 and 3), total flow rates were increased to improbable levels; e.g. > 390 and > 4600 cc./min./whole heart. Data obtained by direct counting of digested myocardial samples (Table 4) show that the number of counts decreases in every case, indicating a gradual diminution of the initial uptake of rubidium by the myocardium. This finding is surprising in view of previous reports which demonstrate that the uptake of rubidium remains constant for a long period of time following intravenous injection of the isotope.[12,14,19,25,26] It is possible that potassium displaces rubidium from its intracellular location and that therefore a steady state of myocardial uptake of the radionuclide does not exist. Lack of a steady state would invalidate measurements of total blood flow and myocardial clearance under these conditions.

Table 5 illustrates data obtained during periods of hypoxia. It is seen that total blood flow increases in every case, whereas nutritional flow of Rb[84] does not change. The difference between total and nutritional flow becomes statistically significant during hypoxia.

DISCUSSION

This report utilizes the diffusible isotope rubidium[84], a positron emitter, in measuring nutritional and total coronary blood flow. The Fick principle, which measures flow through both arteriovenous shunts and nutrient channels, is applied in the measurement of total flow.[27] Clearance of diffusible substances, such as Rb[84], which actively enter the

TABLE 1

*Average Values Obtained During Infusion of Norepinephrine and Isoproterenol ***

	Flow (cc./min.)	Clearance (cc./min.)	Clearance—Flow △	%△	Mean Aortic Pressure (mm. Hg)	Heart Rate (beat/min.)	Change in % of Control			
							Flow	Clearance	Pressure	Heart Rate
Control	169.7±22.0	179.1±23.5	9.4	6.9	84	159				
Norepinephrine							102.6	33.3	63.5	−21.9
During Infusion	324.7±62.3	222.5±20.5	101.9	−19.8	134	120				
Control	162.0±17.2	178.4±19.9	16.4	11.1	92	153				
Isoproterenol							93.0	79.9	−29.6	28.9
During Infusion	313.8±41.6	316.8±37.6	2.8	3.2	64	195				

*Summarized from previous tables published in Journal of Nuclear Medicine.

TABLE 2

Effect of Potassium Infusion on Values Obtained with the Fick Principle as Compared to Clearance Values

Experiment No.	Weight (Kg.)	Flow (cc./min.)	Clearance (cc./min.)	Before Infusion of KCl. Clearance-Flow △	%△	During Infusion of KCl. Flow (cc./min.)	Clearance (cc./min.)	Clearance-Flow △	%△	Plasma Level of K⁺ mEq./L. Bef-ore	Dur-ing	Mean Aortic Pressure (mm.Hg) Be-fore	Dur-ing	Heart Rate (beat/min.) Be-fore	Dur-ing
50	15.0	179.9	160.8	−19.9	−11.1	4621.4	171.6	−4445.7	−96.2	3.6	8.1	97	100	152	168
51	18.1	234.7	196.1	−38.5	−16.4	393.3	171.8	−221.5	−56.3	3.7	8.2	96	110	180	156
52	14.1	186.1	207.9	+21.8	+11.7	221.1	205.7	−15.4	−7.0	2.7	7.4	108	116	198	168
53	15.4	144.7	166.6	+21.9	+15.1	177.2	167.2	−10.0	−5.7	3.3	8.4	91	107	188	159
54	12.7	134.5	147.4	+12.8	+ 9.5	194.3	136.6	−57.6	−29.6	2.8	7.0	100	121	168	144
Average	15.1	176.0	175.8	−00.4	+ 1.8	1121.5	170.6	−950.0	−38.9	3.2	7.8	98	111	177.1	159

TABLE 3

Effect of Potassium Infusion on Values Obtained with the Fick Principle as Compared to Clearance Values

Experiment No.	Weight Kg.	During Infusion of KCl. Flow (cc./min.)	Clearance (cc./min.)	Clearance-Flow △	%△	Plasma Level of K⁺ mEq./L. Before	During	Mean Aortic Pressure (mm. Hg)	Heart Rate (beat/min.)
55	14.5	226.0	196.8	−29.2	−12.9	2.8	5.9	105	159
56	18.1	133.8	123.0	−10.8	− 8.0	2.8	7.1	95	164
57	13.6	234.4	163.0	−71.4	−30.4	2.6	9.0	98	148
58	19.5	332.3	262.4	−69.8	−21.0	3.0	5.8	102	172
59	17.9	936.3	271.0	−665.3	−71.0	3.5	6.5	88	180
Average	16.7	372.6	203.2	−169.3	−28.7	2.9	6.9	97.6	164.6

TABLE 4

Myocardial Uptake of Rb⁸⁴ Determined from Heart Muscle Directly During Infusion of KCl.

Experiment No.	Counts/mg./of myocardium 3rd min.	25th min.	30th min.	Plasma Level of K⁺ mEq./L. Before	During
1	39.5	23.2	30.8		
2	37.0	24.7	22.7	3.6	6.1
3	25.1	16.1	16.7	4.4	9.1
4	35.9	26.2	21.0	4.2	7.5
5	26.0	25.0	26.4	4.7	7.2
Average	32.7	23.0	23.5	4.2	7.5

cell, represents nutritional blood flow.[28-30] As this report deals with an attempt to differentiate nutritional from total coronary flow, a brief review of the methods of their evaluation appears to be in order.

Total coronary flow can be measured in animals with electromagnetic flowmeters implanted around the main coronary vessels; in man, an indirect method using lipid-soluble radioactive tracers, or nitrous oxide[31-35] is used. Total flow has also been measured with large nondiffusible molecules (RISA-131, Diodrast-131) by applying the indicator dilution principle of Stewart and Hamilton. [5,6] The Fick principle for measuring total coronary blood flow can be used if highly diffusible and lipid-soluble substances (inert gases, N_2O, Kr, Xe) are employed; in this procedure, the measured concentration of the substance in the venous channels is determined without permitting tissue exchange. The same diffusible substances (N_2O, Kr, Xe) can be used for measuring total flow with the washout technic[36] by direct injection into the coronary artery.[27]

When measuring total and nutritional blood flow with lipid-insoluble diffusible substances (potassium, rubidium), consideration must be given to the fact that there is active transport of the tracer across the cell membrane. Factors involved in the exchange of such substances between blood and tissue are the rate of flow, capillary surface area and permeability of the capillary and cell membranes.[15,27] When the blood-tissue permeability is great in comparison to blood flow, the exchange between blood and tissue is essentially a flow-limited process and the clearance of the substance can be used as an estimate of local nutrient circulation. Renkin[15,37] found that extraction of potassium and rubidium is influenced by the time spent by blood in the capillary (blood flow) and

the diffusional barrier of the capillary. He defined permeability capillary surface area product (PS) as the diffusional barrier of the capillary beds and of the cell membranes. At very high flows, clearance tends to approach a constant value equal to PS and represents the maximum capillary clearance possible for a given substance in a capillary bed of given permeability and surface area (limiting clearance).[15,37] When blood flow is less than one-half the limiting clearance, the observed clearance is equal to blood flow and transport is essentially blood-flow limited.[15] Clearance measures PS only at very high levels of flow, which must be kept constant; therefore, during *in vivo* experiments when blood flow is within physiologic ranges, it is not possible to measure limiting clearance or permeability surface area product. On the other hand, a measure of clearance will be a significant index of blood flow as long as blood flow remains below this limiting clearance.

The reasons potassium or rubidium can therefore be used in the measurement of organ clearance are: (1) extremely rapid transport across cell membranes,[15] thereby eliminating membrane transport as a rate-limiting factor, and (2) the amount of intracellular potassium in muscle is so great compared with that present in plasma that an almost "infinite sink"[15] is provided, thereby minimizing back-diffusion of rubidium. Thus, when flow is the limiting factor, myocardial clearance of potassium or rubidium is a measure of effective nutritive flow. Under certain circumstances, the usual relationship between total and nutritional flow is altered. Stimulation of the hypothalamic vasodilator center,[3,38] drugs,[30,39,40] reactive hyperemia,[10] and endogenous vasoactive substances[38] can produce a dichotomous effect on the nutritional and total circulation.

TABLE 5

Effect of Hypoxemia on Total Coronary and Nutritional Flow

Exp. No.	Weight Kg.	Arterial Control%	Saturation O_2 during Hypoxemia%	Flow (cc./min.)	Control Clearance (cc./min.)	Clearance-Flow $\triangle$	$\triangle\%$	During Flow (cc./min.)	Clearance (cc./min.)
60	14.98	93	73	177.0	179.5	2.5	1.4	287.2	203.4
61	20.43	96	76	151.9	117.0	−34.9	−23.0	209.6	151.8
62	20.43	94	79	280.8	263.9	−16.8	−6.0	436.7	324.0
63	18.60	96	48	223.8	239.9	16.1	7.2	298.5	228.8
64	15.00	96	77	95.5	109.1	13.6	14.2	126.6	159.8
65	14.10	95	61	193.5	154.0	−39.5	−20.4	436.6	156.9
66	23.60	91	57	250.8	230.2	−20.6	−8.2	301.1	249.1
67	29.1	92	67	262.6	202.2	−60.4	−23.0	218.2	155.2
68	15.0	95	72	456.9	455.9	− 1.0	−0.2	506.2	389.0
69	13.2	93	72	276.5	310.7	34.2	12.4	228.0	259.0
70	24.1	94	82	271.5	289.4	17.9	6.6	245.5	227.8
71	24.3	94	69	270.6	287.5	16.9	6.2	230.8	241.2
Average	19.4	94	69	242.7± 25.7	236.8± 27.8	−5.9± 8.2 NS	−2.7	293.8± 32.2	228.8± 20.9

Shunting of blood may alter the flow-clearance relation. Any pathway between an artery and vein that has a smaller extraction ratio than the average for the vascular bed may act as a type of shunt.[4,30] Despite the lack of morphologic evidence of arteriovenous shunts in skeletal muscle, experimental evidence suggests that physiologic shunts do indeed exist.[41-44] The presence of coronary arteriovenous anastomoses has been suggested;[45] therefore, physiologic shunts in the coronary system can be postulated.[46] Areas of high and low metabolic requirements in the myocardium have been described.[47] A drug might produce redistribution of blood to areas of high metabolic requirement and as a result clearance would increase without changing total flow.

We have compared total and nutritional coronary flow in closed chest anesthetized dogs and have shown that in control experiments, nutritional circulation in the heart is of the same magnitude as total flow (Fig. 1). The fact that in our experiments nutritional flow is slightly greater than total flow (4.3%) may be due to errors inherent in the method.[19]

During infusion of 1.0 μg./Kg./min. of isoproterenol (Table 1), total and nutritional coronary flows are increased proportionally, suggesting that a larger capillary bed, and therefore an increased capillary surface area, is available to accommodate the increase in flow. Isoproterenol may therefore act at the level of arterioles and precapillary sphincters, serving to dilate these vessels.

Norepinephrine increases total coronary flow without an equivalent increase in nutritional flow (Table 1), confirming the findings of Winbury.[48,49] This might be due to opening of physiologic shunts which have a smaller rate of exchange with the tissues than the average capillary bed. This divergent effect of isoproterenol and norepinephrine on the nutri-

tional circulation has been observed previously in skeletal muscle.[50,51] Our studies show that the same situation pertains to the myocardium and may be due to the different action of two drugs on the adrenergic receptors;[49] elucidation of the mechanisms involved awaits further study.

Tables 2 and 3 show that in a small number of experiments, potassium infusion increases the values for total flow beyond reasonable levels. Data obtained by direct counting of myocardial samples (Table 3) show that tracer uptake by the heart declines in every instance. If total flow in fact increases in hyperkalemia, the disparity between flow and clearance at the cellular level might be best explained by lack of a steady state, possibly due to competition between potassium and rubidium. Because normal cellular exchange of the tracer may be interfered with, the use of rubidium in determining nutritional and total flow is precluded under these conditions.

The observed increase in total blood flow as a result of hypoxemia (arterial O_2 saturation less than 70%) (Table 5) is in accord with the findings of many investigators.[52-54] Our studies show that myocardial clearance of Rb^{84} does not increase proportionally under these conditions; this is in contrast to the findings of Love,[54] who, in maintaining an arterial O_2 saturation above 75 per cent, found a proportional increase in both clearance and flow. Our findings can be explained in two ways. Anoxia interferes with the intracellular-extracellular distribution of potassium (and therefore possibly of rubidium) as evidenced by a change in the resting membrane potential[55]; under these conditions, transport of rubidium across the cell membrane rather than flow could become the rate-limiting factor. An alternative explanation is that hypoxemia, by causing vasodilatation, results in the opening

TABLE 5 *(Continued)*

Hypoxemia Clearance-Flow		Increase Flow %	Increase Clearance %	Mean Aortic Pressure			Heart Rate		
$\triangle$	%$\triangle$			Control	Hypoxia	Increase %	Control	Hypoxia	Increase %
−83.8	−29.2	62.3							
			13.3						
−57.8	−27.6	38.0	23.0						
−112.7	−25.8	55.5	22.8						
−69.7	−23.4	33.4	−4.6	125	171	36.8	175	220	25.7
33.2	26.2	32.6	46.5	92	87	−5.4	150	150	0
−279.7	−64.1	125.6	1.9	98	102	4.0	154	166	7.8
−52.1	−17.3	20.1	8.2	102	110	7.8	174	176	1.1
−63.0	−28.9	16.9	−23.4	131	131	0	186	174	−6.4
−117.2	−23.1	10.8	−14.7	110	89	−19.1	138	160	15.9
31.0	13.6	−17.5	−16.6	67	80	1.9	162	168	3.7
−17.7	−7.2	−9.6	−21.3	91	82	−1.0	174	168	−3.4
10.4	4.5	−15.0	−16.6	67	80	−1.2	174	138	−20.7
−64.9± 24.4	16.9	29.4	15.4	101	104	2.6	165	169	2.6

TABLE 6
Summarizing Table on the Effect of Potassium Infusion and Hypoxemia

		Flow (cc./min.)	Clearance (cc/.min.)	Clearance—Flow $\triangle$	Clearance—Flow $\%\triangle$	Mean Aortic Pressure (mm. Hg.)	Heart Rate (beat/min.)	Change in % of Control Flow	Change in % of Control Clearance	Change in % of Control Pressure	Change in % of Control Heart Rate
Potassium	Before	176.0	175.8	−0.4	−1.8	98	177				
	During	1121.5	170.6	−950.0	38.9	111	159	537.2	−2.9	13.2	−10.2
Hypoxemia	Before	242 7±25.7	236.8±27.8	−5.9	−2.7	101	165				
	During	293.8±32.2	228.8±20.9	−64.9	−16.9	104	169	29.4	−1.5	2.6	2.6

of physiologic shunts with a small extraction ratio.

The results of our studies indicate that, although in the control animal total and nutritional coronary flows are equal, the administration of certain pharmacologic agents results in changes compatible with the concept that not all the coronary flow is involved in metabolic exchange. Particular attention must be given to the condition under which the method is limited, as in hyperkalemia. See also Table 6.

SUMMARY

Total and nutritional flow to the heart was measured in closed chest anesthetized dogs after pentobarbital anesthesia, using Rb^{84} as the indicator and a double coincidence counting system. Total coronary flow was measured by applying the Fick principle, and nutritional flow by assessing myocardial clearance of the isotope. The difference between total and nutritional flows is not statistically significant under control conditions. Infusion of isoproterenol (1 μg./Kg./min.) does not affect the relation between total and nutritional flow, whereas norepinephrine (1 μg./Kg./min.) increases total flow to a greater extent than nutritional flow. Hyperkalemia (serum K^+ 7–8 mEq./L), possibly by altering cellular transport of rubidium, invalidates the method. Hypoxia (arterial O_2 saturation less than 70%) increases total flow without an equivalent increase in nutritional flow. Reasons for these circulatory responses are discussed.

REFERENCES

1. Kety, S. S.: Measurement of regional circulation by the local clearance of radioactive sodium, Am. Heart J. *38*:321, 1949.
2. Hyman, C.: Physiological implications of dual circulation in muscle, Angiologie *9*:25, 1957.
3. Hyman, C., Rosell, S., Rosen, A., Sonnenschein, R. R., and Uvnas, B.: Effects of alternations of total muscular blood flow on local tissue clearance of radio-iodide in the cat, Acta physiol. scandinav. *46*:358, 1959.
4. Robertson, J. S.: Mathematical treatment of uptake and release of indicator substances in relation to flow analysis in tissues and organs, *in* Handbook of Physiology, Section 2: Circulation, Vol. 1, Hamilton, W. F., and Dow, P., (eds.), pp. 617-644, American Physiological Society, Washington.
5. Fox, I. J.: Indicators and detectors for circulatory dilution studies and their application to organ or regional blood flow determination, Circulation Res. *10*:447, 1962.
6. Mnea, I., Kattus, A. A., Greenfield, M. A., and Bennett, L. R.: Effect of coronary blood flow on radioisotope dilution curves measured by precordial scintillation detection, Circulation Res. *9*:911, 1961.
7. Kety, S. S., and Schmidt, C. F.: The nitrous oxide method for the quantitative determination of cerebral blood flow in man: Theory, procedure and normal values, J. Clin. Invest. *27*:476, 1948.
8. Hansen, A. J., Haxholdt, B. F., Husfeldt, E., Lessen, N. A., Munck, O., Sorenson, H. R., and Winkler, K.: Measurement of coronary blood flow and cardiac efficiency in hypothermia by use of radioactive krypton-85, Scandinav. J. Clin. & Lab. Invest. *8*:182, 1956.
9. Lassen, N. A., and Munck, O.: The cerebral blood flow in man determined by the use of radioactive krypton, Acta physiol. scandinav. *33*:30, 1955.
10. Lassen, N. A., Lindbjerg, I. F., and Munck, O.: Measurement of blood flow through skeletal muscle by intramuscular injection of xenon-133, Lancet I:686, 1964.
11. Bernstein, L., Friesinger, G. C., Lichtlen, P. R., and Ross, R. S.: The effect of nitroglycerin on myocardial blood flow in man as measured with xenon-133, Circulation *33*:107, 1966.
12. Love, W. D., Romney, R. B., and Burch, G. E.: A comparison of the distribution of potassium and exchangeable rubidium in the organs of the dog, using rubidium[86], Circulation Res. *2*:112, 1954.
13. Sapirstein, L. A.: Fractionation of the cardiac output of rats with isotopic potassium, Circulation Res. *4*:689, 1956.
14. Sapirstein, L. A.: Regional blood flow by fractional distribution of indicators, Am. J. Physiol. *193*(1): 161, 1958.
15. Renkin, E. M.: Transport of potassium-42 from blood to tissue in isolated mammalian skeletal muscles, Am. J. Physiol. *197*:1205, 1959.
16. Bing, R. J., Bennish, A., Bluemchen, G., Cohen, A., Gallagher, J. P., and Zaleski, E. J.: The determination of coronary flow equivalent with coincidence counting technic, Circulation *29*:833, 1964.
17. Nolting, D., Mack, R., Luthy, E., Kirsch, M., and Hogancamp, G.: Measurement of coronary blood

flow and myocardial uptake with rubidium-86, J. Clin. Invest. *37*:921, 1958.

18. Cohen, A., Gallagher, J. P., Luebs, E.-D., Varga, Z., Yamanaka, J., Zaleski, E. J., Bluemchen, G., and Bing, R. J.: The quantitative determination of coronary flow with a positron emitter (rubidium-84), Circulation *32*:636, 1965.

19. Boettcher, D., Corsini, G., Daniels, C. G., Cowan, C., and Bing, R. J.: The determination of myocardial blood flow in the anesthetized dog following a slug injection of rubidium-84, J. Nuclear Med. (In press.)

20. Braasch, W., Gudbjarnason, S., Puri, P. S., Ravens, K. G., and Bing, R. J.: Early changes in energy metabolism in the myocardium following acute coronary artery occlusion in anesthetized dogs, Circulation Res. (In press.)

21. Gemmell, W., and Veall, N.: The factors influencing the clearance of radioactive sodium, Strahlentherapie Sonderbaende *35*:120, 1956.

22. Renkin, E. M.: Blood flow and transcapillary exchange in skeletal muscle, Fed. Proc. *24*:1092, 1965.

23. Hamilton, W. F., Moore, J. E., Kinsman, J. M., and Spurling, R. C.: Simultaneous determination of the greater and lesser circulation times of the mean velocity of blood flow through the heart and lungs, of the cardiac output and an approximation of the amount of blood actively circulating in the heart and lungs, Am. J. Physiol. *85*:377, 1928.

24. Fick, A.: Ueber die Messung des Blutquantums in den Herzventrikeln, Sitzung Physiol. Med. Ges. zu Wurtzburg. July, 1870, 16.

25. Levy, M. N., and Oliveira, J. M.: Regional distribution of myocardial blood flow in the dog as determined by Rb[86], Circulation Res. *9*:96, 1961.

26. McHenry, P. L., and Knoebel, S. B.: Measurement of coronary blood flow by coincidence counting and a bolus of Rb[84], Cl. J. Appl. Physiol. *22*:495, 1967.

27. Kety, S. S.: Theory of blood-tissue exchange and its application to measurement of blood flow, *in* Methods in Medical Research, Vol. 8, Bruner, H. D., (ed.), Chicago, The Year Book Publishers, Inc., pp. 223–227.

28. Conn, H. L., Jr.: Use of external counting technics in studies of the circulation, Circulation Res. *10*:505, 1962.

29. Love, W. D.: Isotope clearance and myocardial blood flow, Am. Heart J. *67*:579, 1964.

30. Winbury, M. M., and Gabel, L. P.: Effect of nitrates on nutritional circulation of heart and hindlimb, Am. J. Physiol. *212*:1062, 1967.

31. Bing, R. J.: Coronary circulation in health and disease as studied by coronary sinus catheterization, Bull. N.Y. Acad. Med. *27*:405, 1951.

32. Herd, J. A., Hollenberg, M., Thorburn, G. D., Kopald, H. H., and Barger, A. C.: Myocardial blood flow determined with krypton-85 in unanesthetized dogs, Am. J. Physiol. *203*:122, 1962.

33. Cohen, L. S., Elliott, W. C., and Gorlin, R.: Measurement of myocardial blood flow using krypton-85, Am. J. Physiol. *206*(5):997, 1964.

34. Hansen, A. J., Haxholdt, B. F., Husfeldt, E., Lessen, N. A., Munck, O., Sorenson, H. R., and Winkler, K.: Measurement of coronary blood flow and cardiac efficiency in hypothermia by the use of radioactive krypton-85, Scandinav. J. Clin. & Lab. Invest. *8*:182, 1956.

35. Ross, R. S., Ueda, K., Lichtlen, P. R., and Rees, J.R.: Measurement of myocardial blood flow in animals and man by selective injection of radioactive inert gas into the coronary arteries, Circulation Res. *15*:28, 1964.

36. Johansson, B., Linder, E., and Seeman, T.: Collateral blood flow in the myocardium of dogs measured with krypton-85, Acta physiol. scandinav. *62*:263, 1964.

37. Renkin, E. M.: Blood flow and transcapillary exchange in skeletal muscle, Fed. Proc. *24*:1092, 1965.

38. Clarke, N. P., and Rushmer, R. F.: Tissue uptake of Rb[86] with electrical stimulation of hypothalamus and midbrain, Am. J. Physiol. *213*(6):1439, 1967.

39. Renkin, E. M., and Rosell, S.: The influence of sympathetic adrenergic vasoconstrictor nerves on transport of diffusible solutes from blood to tissues in skeletal muscle, Acta physiol. scandinav. *54*:223, 1962.

40. Mellander, S.: Comparative effects of acetylcholine, butyl-norepinephrine (Vasculat), noradrenaline, and ethyladrianol (Effontil) on resistance, capacitance and precapillary sphincter vessels and capillary filtration in cat skeletal muscle, Angiologica *3*:77, 1966.

41. Renkin, E. M., Hudlicka, O., and Sheehan, R. M.: Influence of metabolic vasodilatation on blood-tissue diffusion in skeletal muscle, Am. J. Physiol. *211*:87, 1966.

42. Walder, D. N.: The relationship between blood flow, capillary surface area and sodium clearance in muscle, Clin. Sc. *14*:303, 1955.

43. Friedman, J. J.: Microvascular flow distribution and rubidium extraction, Fed. Proc. *24*:1099, 1965.

44. Friedman, J. J.: Total, non-nutritional, and nutritional blood volume in isolated dog hindlimb, Am. J. Physiol. *210*:151, 1966.

45. MacLean, L. D., Hedenstrom, P. H., and Kim, Y. S.: Distribution of blood flow to the canine heart, Proc. Soc. Exp. Biol. Med. *107*:786, 1961.

46. Winbury, M. M., Kissil, D., and Losada, M.: Functional organization of myocardial circulation: Effect of nitrites, Circulation *32*:220, 1965.

47. Barlow, T. E., Haigh, A. L., and Walder, D.N.: Evidence for two vascular pathways in skeletal muscle, Clin. Sc. *20*:367, 1961.

48. Winbury, M. M., Gabel, L., and Grandy, R. P.: Effect of vasoactive agents on myocardial Rb[86]-uptake in the dog using a double-isotope technique. Pharmacologist *4*:180, 1962.

49. Winbury, M. M., Kissil, D., and Losada, M.: Approaches to the study of nutritional blood flow-extraction of Rb[86] by the heart and hindlimb *in* Isotopes in Experimental Pharmacology, Roth, L. J. (ed.), Chicago and London, Univ. of Chicago Press, 1965, pp. 229–248.

50. Sheehan, R. M., and Renkin, E. M.: Influence of adrenergic drugs on blood-tissue diffusion, Pharmacologist *7*:178, 1965.

51. Gosselin, R. E.: Local effects of catecholamines on radioiodide clearance in skeletal muscle. Am. J. Physiol. *210*:885, 1966.

52. Berne, R. M.: Cardiac nucleotides in hypoxia: possible role in regulation of coronary blood flow, Am. J. Physiol. *204*(2):317, 1963.

53. Love, W. D., Tyler, M. D., Abraham, R. E., and Munford, R.S.: Effects of O_2, CO_2 and drugs on estimating coronary blood flow from Rb[86] clearance. Am. J. Physiol. *208*:1206, 1965.

54. Love, W. D., and Tyler, M. D.: Effect of hypoxemia and hypercapnia on regional distribution of myocardial blood flow, Am. J. Physiol. *208*:1211, 1965.

55. Kardesch, M., Hogancamp, C. E., Michal, G., and Bing, R. J.: The survival of excitability, energy production and energy utilization of the heart, Tr. A. Am. Physicians *71*:152, 1958.

The authors gratefully acknowledge the invaluable technical assistance of Miss Marlene Ranke.

Neurohumoral Control of the Coronary Circulation*

Harvey G. Kemp

Physiologists have long been interested in the neurohumoral control of the coronary circulation, but only recently has the clinician been drawn into the field. The introduction of potent beta-blocking agents has stimulated interest in this area and placed emphasis on adrenergic control mechanisms. Clinically, beta-blocking agents provide the most successful therapy for the management of angina pectoris since nitroglycerin. To the physiologist, they have provided a means for studying the relative effects of alpha and beta receptor stimulation. This review will be limited to recent advances in our knowledge of the effects of the catecholamines on the coronary vasculature with emphasis on clinical pertinence.

The concept of alpha and beta adrenergic receptors was first proposed by Ahlquist[1] studying the comparative actions of several catecholamines on a variety of effector systems (ileum, myometrium and various vascular beds). He found that either vasoconstriction or vasodilatation could be produced in the vascular beds studied depending on the particular catechol used. Also he found that there appeared to be an order of potency such that norepinephrine was the most potent vasoconstrictor and isoproterenol the most potent vasodilator. Because of the effects of catechols on intestinal and other nonvascular smooth muscle, simple terms such as constricting and dilating receptors would not be accurate, so the noncommittal terms alpha and beta were suggested and have come into wide use. Though the concept of alpha and beta receptors antedated the majority of receptor blocking agents, the latter have made possible our current understanding of adrenergic effects. This broad area has recently been reviewed in a symposium of the New York Academy of Sciences.[2]

It is a common misunderstanding that only beta receptors are present in the coronary circulation. This stems from the fact that the effect of catechols on contractility, rhythmicity and impulse conduction are mediated through beta receptors. It is clear, however, that both alpha and beta receptors are

present in the coronary vascular bed. Perhaps the most direct evidence is that of Zuberbuhler and Bohr[3] who have recently studied the effects of catechols on isolated coronary smooth muscle strips. The results of these experiments serve as useful background before considering the complexities of the intact heart.

Isoproterenol, norepinephrine and epinephrine uniformly cause relaxation of small coronary arteries (outside diameter 250–500μ). This dilating or relaxing effect of the catechols is specifically inhibited by the beta blocking agent propranolol, so that no vasodilating effect is seen after isoproterenol or norepinephrine, and slight constriction is seen after epinephrine. These findings have been interpreted as indicating that beta receptors are present in these small vessels, that they mediate coronary vasodilatation, and, further, that beta receptors predominate over alpha receptors in these small coronary vessels. Large coronary arteries are less consistent in response. They show either contraction followed by relaxation or only contraction in response to catechol stimulation. Contraction is inhibited by alpha blocking agents and relaxation by beta blocking agents. The authors conclude that there is a difference in the relative population of alpha and beta receptors in large and small coronary vessels, the ratio of alpha to beta receptors increasing the more proximal the section of coronary artery.

Caution must be exercised in applying these concepts to other models, for substantial differences have been seen in various organs and species, as well as in response to different doses of agonists and antagonists.

In the intact heart it is difficult to differentiate direct effects of catechols on the coronary vasculature from effects on the myocardium and the peripheral vasculature. The many factors affecting coronary blood flow have been reviewed by Berne.[4] Effects of catecholamines on myocardial oxygen requirements will secondarily alter coronary blood flow. The exact mechanism by which oxygen needs regulate coronary blood flow remains unclear, but is observed after such nonpharmacologic interventions

*Supported by USPHS Grants 1-P01-HE11306 and 5-R01-HE08591 and a grant from Women's Aid for Heart Research, Boston, Massachusetts.

as increasing heart rate by atrial pacing and constriction of the aorta. Catechols increase myocardial oxygen consumption by their effects on heart rate, contractility, and tension in the left ventricular wall.[5] To a lesser extent, changes in heart rate and myocardial wall tension affect coronary blood flow by lessening diastolic time available for flow and by changing extravascular resistance to blood flow. Also, changes in peripheral vascular resistance and central aortic pressure may secondarily affect coronary blood flow by increasing or decreasing the pressure gradient across the coronary vascular bed. All of these secondary effects serve to obscure a primary action of the catechols on the coronary vascular smooth muscle.

Two experimental methods have proven useful in measuring the direct vascular effects of catechols in the intact heart. The first has been to measure alterations in coronary blood flow (CBF) on coronary vascular resistance in the nonbeating heart after the administration of catechols. Berne,[6] utilizing a fibrillating heart preparation, observed that the intracoronary injection of epinephrine and norepinephrine caused a brief decrease in CBF followed by a prolonged increase above control levels. Myocardial oxygen consumption was increased approximately threefold during the period of increased coronary blood flow, and coronary sinus O_2 content fell. Berne's interpretation of these observations was that the primary effect of epinephrine and norepinephrine on the coronary vascular bed in the intact heart was constriction, with dilatation only secondary to increasing myocardial O_2 requirements. Klocke and co-workers[7] have recently reinvestigated this issue, utilizing the potassium-arrested dog heart and selecting isoproterenol, a potent beta receptor stimulator, as the antagonist. Interestingly, myocardial O_2 consumption did not change significantly in these experiments, yet there was a consistent dilatory response to isoproterenol as shown in a constant flow preparation by a decrease in coronary perfusion pressure. Beta blocking agents abolished this response.

These findings are not as inconsistent as they might first appear. Both alpha (constricting) and beta (dilating) activity can be demonstrated in the nonbeating heart, and appropriate blockade will abolish these responses. Further, these responses appear to follow the known relative alpha and beta stimulating properties of the drug involved. The nonbeating heart preparation is only useful to the extent that it eliminates the effect of catechols on myocardial O_2 consumption, and this issue remains unsettled. It seems likely that these effects are partially dose dependent, with higher doses of catechols causing an increase in resting oxidative metabolism, and that various catecholamines differ in this regard.

To determine direct catechol effects on coronary hemodynamics in the beating heart, investigators have focused on early alterations in CBF presumably occurring before effects on myocardial metabolism. In the open-chest animal, Berne[6] found a transient decrease in coronary blood flow after the intracoronary injection of epinephrine and norepinephrine. As with the fibrillating heart, he attributed subsequent coronary dilatation to an increase in myocardial oxygen consumption. Klocke and associates found a consistent decrease in coronary vascular resistance in the beating heart after intravenous[7] isoproterenol infusion. Peripheral effects were excluded by cannulation of the left main coronary artery, and infusion of blood by a constant pressure pump. The rise in coronary blood flow was apparent by the end of one minute. Coronary venous O_2 rose simultaneously, indicating diminished oxygen extraction by the myocardium, and suggesting a primary or "active" decrease in coronary vascular resistance. Pitt, Elliot, and Gregg,[8] studying the trained, closed-chest, unanesthetized dog, have observed only coronary vasodilatation immediately after the intracoronary injection of both isoproterenol and epinephrine. After beta adrenergic blockade with propranolol, epinephrine caused coronary vasoconstriction, and after alpha blockade with Dibenzyline, vasodilatation. All of these observations were made in the first few seconds, prior to any significant change in central aortic pressure, heart rate, ejection period or cardiac output.

It is of interest to note that Bohr[9] has observed biphasic responses to epinephrine in smooth muscle strips taken from large coronary vessels. Utilizing moderate doses of epinephrine, Bohr observed an initial contraction followed by relaxation, and suggested that there may be a different time course for activation of alpha and beta receptors. This observation might help to explain some of the inconsistencies in the data obtained from very early changes in coronary blood flow in the beating heart experiments.

The foregoing discussion illustrates the problem of investigating the direct action of the catechols on the coronary vasculature in man. Of the various technic available, for determining coronary blood flow none has been found which permits study of the very early transient changes measurable in canine preparations with electromagnetic flowmeters. Therefore, investigators have relied on alterations in patterns of oxygen extraction to differentiate primary from secondary changes in CBF. In man, as well as in the dog, increases in myocardial oxygen requirements are largely met by increases in coronary blood flow with little change in oxygen extraction or coronary sinus oxygen content. Such changes in coronary blood flow are considered to be passive or secondary to the change in myocardial oxygen consumption. If oxygen extraction by the myocardium diminishes, active or primary coronary vasodilatation has taken place, while if myocardial oxygen extraction increases, active vasoconstriction has taken place.

Gorlin and co-workers[10–12] have investigated the effects of intravenous isoproterenol, epinephrine and norepinephrine on coronary hemodynamics and oxygen consumption in man. Isoproterenol caused both an increase in myocardial oxygen consumption and in coronary blood flow; however, CBF rose in excess of the increase in oxygen consumption so that extraction ratio fell, and coronary sinus oxygen content rose. Norepinephrine, conversely, caused an increase in myocardial oxygen consumption while coronary blood flow rose little, if at all, and the increased oxygen need was met by increasing oxygen extraction, with an associated striking decrease in coronary sinus oxygen content. Infusion of epinephrine caused an increase in myocardial oxygen consumption which was met by a corresponding increase in CBF with no change in oxygen extraction.

These findings are broadly in agreement with the data from intact heart studies. Isoproterenol, because of the effects just described, is considered a primary vasodilator in man. Klocke and associates[7] have also shown vasodilatation following isoproterenol administration in both the intact beating and fibrillating dog heart, and Pitt et al.[8] has reported similar observations in the unanesthetized dog. Epinephrine does not alter myocardial oxygen extraction in man, though coronary blood flow and oxygen consumption rise. Because of this passive vasodilation, a primary vasodilating effect could be obscured. In the animal, epinephrine remains controversial, but Pitt et al. have found it to be a vasodilator in perhaps the most physiologic canine preparation. Norepinephrine in man appears to be a primary vasoconstrictor. Berne's data[6] shows primary vasoconstriction in the dog but Pitt et al. found varying responses after intravenous and intracoronary injections of norepinephrine.

Responses to catechols after adrenergic blockade have not been measured in man, though the effects of beta blockade alone have been studied and have yielded some interesting information on the influence of beta receptor activity on the resting vascular tone of the coronary bed. These studies have used propranolol as the beta receptor blocking agent.

Propranolol may have some direct action on the coronary vascular bed, shown in studies by Whitsett and Lucchesi[13] in the dog utilizing the d-isomer which has negligible beta receptor blocking activity. Nevertheless, it seems clear that the administration of propranolol to both dog and man will reduce both myocardial oxygen consumption and coronary blood flow. Because perfusion pressure varies little, calculated coronary vascular resistance rises. The problem again is whether flow decreases passively with decreasing oxygen requirements or whether there is an element of active constriction. McKenna et al.[14] using rather large doses of propranolol in the dog (2 mg./Kg.), found that coronary venous oxygen fell, supporting the primary constrictor concept, while Nayler et al.[15] found increasing coronary venous oxygen content after several doses of propranolol (0.15 to 5.0 mg./Kg.). Further investigation will be required to resolve this issue. In man, Wolfson and Gorlin[16] observed little change in myocardial oxygen extraction after 5 mg. of propranolol administered intravenously. Interestingly, there was a tendency for normal subjects to show a vasodilation pattern while subjects with angiographically demonstrated coronary heart disease showed a pattern of constriction. This finding would imply that beta receptor activity does not play an important role in coronary vascular tone in normal man at rest, but may play some role in disease states, in particular coronary artery disease.

Lest some clinicians stop using propranolol as a potential "constricting" agent in coronary disease, it should be added that arteriolar tone may play a relatively less important role in the determination of regional coronary blood flow in coronary artery disease than does the relatively fixed proximal resistance caused by an atherosclerotic stenosis. In this instance, reduction of myocardial oxygen needs by reduction in heart rate and contractile force may allow adequate oxygenation by reducing coronary flow requirements to levels that can be attained past fixed obstructive lesions.

SUMMARY

Both alpha and beta adrenergic receptors have been demonstrated in the coronary vascular bed and they subserve vasoconstriction and vasodilatation respectively. Appropriate blocking agents will accentuate the opposing effect. The direct effects of catechols on coronary smooth muscle are difficult to evaluate in the intact beating heart, because of secondary effects on myocardial oxygen consumption. Nevertheless, both dilating and constricting effects have been convincingly demonstrated. In man, isoproterenol has been shown to be a potent dilating agent, and norepinephrine a potent constricting agent. Beta blockade has little direct effect on resting coronary vascular tone in the animal or in man. The therapeutic effect of propranolol in angina pectoris is probably due to negative chronotropic and inotropic effects with secondary reduction in myocardial oxygen consumption.

REFERENCES

1. Ahlquist, R. P.: A study of the adrenergic receptors, Am. J. Physiol. *153*:586, 1948.
2. Moran, N. C. (Consulting Editor): New adrenergic blocking drugs: their pharmacological, biochemical and clinical actions, Ann. New York Acad. Sc., *193*:541, 1967.
3. Zuberbuhler, R. C., and Bohr, D. F.: Responses of coronary smooth muscle to catecholamines, Circulation Res. *16*:431, 1965.
4. Berne, R. M.: Regulation of coronary blood flow. Physiol. Rev. *44*:1,1964.
5. Braunwald, E., Ross, J., and Sonneblick, E. H.: Mechanisms of Contraction of the Normal and Failing Heart, Boston, Little, Brown and Co., 1967, Chapter 6.
6. Berne, R. M.: Effect of epinephrine and norepinephrine on coronary circulation, Circulation Res. *6*:644, 1958.
7. Klocke, F. J., Kaiser, G. A., Ross, J., Jr., and Braunwald, E.: An intrinsic adrenergic vasodilator mechanism in the coronary vascular bed of the dog, Circulation Res. *16*:376,1965.
8. Pitt, B., Elliot, E. C., and Gregg, D. E.: Adrenergic receptor activity in the coronary arteries of the unanesthetized dog, Circulation Res. *21*:75,1967.
9. Bohr, D. F.: Adrenergic receptors in coronary arteries, Ann. New York Acad. Sc. *139*:799, 1967.
10. Krasnow, N., Rolett, E. L., Yurchack, P. M., Hood, W. B., and Gorlin, R.: Isoproterenol and cardiovascular performance, Am. J. Med. *37*:180, 1964.
11. Sullivan, J. M., and Gorlin, R.: Effect of L-epinephrine on the coronary circulation in human subjects with and without coronary artery disease, Circulation Res. *21*:919, 1967.
12. Yurchak, P. M., Rolett, E. L., Cohen, L. S., and Gorlin, R.: Effects of norepinephrine on the coronary circulation in man, Circulation *30*:180,1964.
13. Whitsett, L. S., and Lucchesi, B. R.: Effects of propranolol and its stereoisomers upon coronary vascular resistance, Circulation Res. *21*:305,1967.
14. McKenna, D. H., Corliss, R. J., Sialer, S., Zarnstorff, W. C., Crumpton, C. W., and Rowe, G. G.: Effect of propranolol on systemic and coronary hemodynamics at rest and during simulated exercise, Circulation Res. *19*:520,1966.
15. Nayler, W. G., McInnes, I., Swann, J. B., Carson, V., and Lowe, T. E.: Effect of propranolol, a beta-adrenergic antagonist, on blood flows in the coronary and other vascular fields, Am. Heart J. *73*:207, 1967.
16. Wolfson, S., and Gorlin, R.: Submitted for publication.

Cardiac Innervation:
Anatomic and Pharmacologic Relationships

Peter J. Dempsey and Theodore Cooper

Unlike skeletal muscle which requires intact innervation for functional integrity, the heart continues to function quite well without any extrinsic innervation. Thus we must ask what the role of the extrinsic innervation of the heart is, how it differs from that of other striated muscle, and if the presence of nerves with their stores of catecholamine is essential for effective muscle cell performance.

Since function is always dependent, at least in some measure, upon anatomy, the way we shall approach this problem is to consider first the anatomy of the cardiac nerves, their relationship to the fine structure of the heart, and the pharmacologic processes involved in normal function. The consequences of an interruption of the normal cardiac

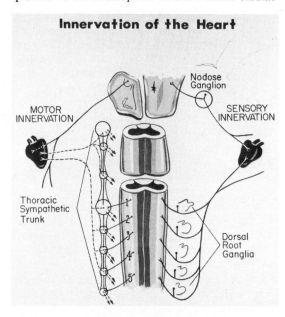

Innervation of the Heart

Nodose Ganglion

MOTOR INNERVATION

SENSORY INNERVATION

Thoracic Sympathetic Trunk

Dorsal Root Ganglia

FIG. 1. A schematic outline of the sensory and motor innervation of the heart. Sensory innervation is depicted on the right, while motor innervation is on the left. With regard to the motor component, preganglionic fibers are the solid lines, while the postganglionic fibers are the broken lines.

neural pathways will then be discussed.

There are three different types of nerve fiber found in the heart: afferent sensory fibers, efferent sympathetic fibers, and efferent parasympathetic fibers (Fig. 1). The sensory receptors are distributed universally in the heart, and the associated afferent fibers (with the exception of the superior cardiac branch) leave through the sympathetic and the parasympathetic nerves to traverse the autonomic ganglia without interruption. Their cell bodies, like those of the visceral afferent system in general, lie in one of the cerebrospinal ganglia. For the cardiac nerves this is the nodose ganglion of the tenth cranial nerve. There are also afferent fibers which go directly to cell bodies located in the dorsal root ganglia of the first five thoracic spinal cord segments. Both bulbar and spinal sensory cell bodies are involved in the reflexes concerned with alteration in the inotropic, dromotropic, and chronotropic state of the heart. It is currently believed that in the resting state, control of these parameters is mediated primarily through the vagal system, whereas adjustment to excitatory exogenous stimuli is mediated through the sympathetic system.[1,2] Sensory fibers also mediate the sensation of ischemic pain associated with angina pectoris. Since the most common termination for the afferent fibers carrying these pain sensations is in the first two thoracic segments of the cord, patients most commonly perceive this as pain referred to the cutaneous area supplied by these segments, namely the left shoulder region.

The sympathetic component of the visceral efferent innervation of the heart arises in the following way: The superior, middle and inferior cardiac nerves arise respectively from the superior, middle and inferior cervical sympathetic ganglia. In addition, direct branches to the deep cardiac plexus arise from the upper four or five thoracic sympathetic ganglia.[3]

In the parasympathetic system, each vagus nerve contributes to the cardiac plexus via the superior and inferior cervical nerves and a thoracic cardiac branch from each recurrent laryngeal nerve.

All of these sympathetic and parasympathetic fibers combine to form the so-called cardiac plexus in the region of the concavity of the aortic arch. This plexus may be subdivided into two parts, the smaller superficial cardiac plexus, located in a ventral position on the aortic arch to the right of the ligamentum arteriosum, and the larger deep cardiac plexus behind the arch in the tissue overlying the tracheal bifurcation.

The main sympathetic postganglionic fibers (in company with myelinated afferent fibers) enter the base of the heart anteriorly between the aorta and the pulmonary artery. Each trunk distributes branches to the ipsilateral ventricular myocardium but to a lesser extent to the corresponding atrium.

The vagal trunks approach the ipsilateral atria posteriorly forming the epicardial and myocardial plexuses of nerves associated with many ganglia. The cell bodies of these ganglia give rise to postganglionic fibers, presumably parasympathetic in nature.

A system of nerves with ganglia derived from the vagal plexuses of the atria enters the interatrial system near the level of the coronary sinus. These vagal fibers extend beyond the A-V node and continue into the ventricular system. Other nerves of the atrial vagal plexuses continue into the ventricular epicardium. These epicardial nerves occasionally enter the myocardium directly although they usually travel with the branches of the coronary arteries. These nerves branch dichotomously and are usually distributed in the heart in association with the arteries.[4]

Innumerable, sinuous, large and small fascicles of fibers, derived from the epicardial and intracardial nerves, extend universally through all of the cardiac tissues (Fig. 2). The fibers in these fascicles are bound together with collagen. The subdivisions of the fascicles extend parallel with aggregates of myocardium between the muscle bands. This fascicular form of axonal distribution effects a separation as well as a universal dispersion of the motor and sensory fibers. Finer fibrils branch from these bundles.[3] Beyond this, the terminal innervation of cardiac muscle presents an enigma.

At this point it should be stated that although it is known that the coronary arteries are autonomically innervated,[5] the functional significance of this innervation is unclear since it is extremely difficult to study the coronary arteries directly. In perfusion preparations, the coronary vasculature not only extracts drug from the available pool of drug molecules, but may also influence the distribution and rate of interaction between receptor and drug. Furthermore, the physical dimensions of the coronaries are largely effected by the state of myocardial

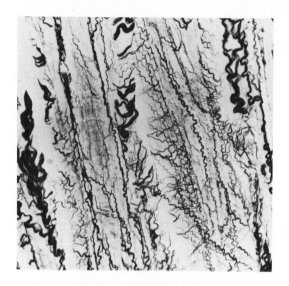

FIG. 2. Section of normal right ventricular myocardium taken from a cat and stained by a modified Bielschowski silver staining technic. Large argyrophilic axon bundles are seen running parallel to the myocardial cells with finer fibrils branching from these. (Courtesy Dr. E. F. Hirsch)

contraction and metabolism,[6,7] oftentimes in a regionally selective manner.[8] In actively contracting preparations uneven distribution of a positive inotropic substance may result in asynchronous and dystonic muscular activity, and the recording of such activity as a contractile event may differ quantitatively from a record of a preparation in which the units react synchronously and with homogeneous force.

From a pharmacologic standpoint, it must be remembered that ganglionic transmission from preganglionic to postganglionic fibers in both sympathetic and parasympathetic systems, as well as parasympathetic transmission from postganglionic fiber to effector cell is cholinergic in nature, that is to say, mediated by acetylcholine. In relation to the cholinergically mediated ganglionic transmission, Jacobowitz[9] has shown in excellent studies using a histofluorescence technic that the ganglion cells contained within the hearts of rats, mice, guinea pigs and cats are associated with adrenergic (sympathetic) terminals making synaptic contact with cell bodies. In addition, small cells with catecholamine fluorescence, resembling the chromaffin cells of the adrenal medulla, are localized in the vicinity of the cardiac ganglia. Most of these cells are innervated by acetylcholinesterase-staining nerve fibers. Some receive a postganglionic parasympathetic innervation from cholinergic ganglionic cells of the heart. He believes that this system of chromaffin cells and adrenergic fibers in what was believed to be cholinergic ganglia functions as a self-controlling, modifying, or inhibitory influence on ganglionic transmission.

The postganglionic sympathetic or adrenergic nerve terminal, on the other hand releases norepinephrine to effect its response. In contrast to preganglionic effects which are mediated by acetylcholine which in turn is inactivated by acetylcholinesterase, the inactivation of norepinephrine after receptor interaction is accomplished primarily by reuptake into the nerve terminals. This holds true for exogenously administered as well as endogenously released norepinephrine.[10]

The study of the effects of various adrenergic agents upon the heart is hampered by several "indirect effects" which these agents initiate. For example, a certain percentage of a given dose of drug may be diverted from receptor action by affinity for smooth muscle or postganglionic sympathetic nerve terminals. Uneven coronary flow may divert drug from one area to another resulting in uneven perfusion in whole heart preparations. In addition drug stimulation of a peripheral neural reflex (the aortic baroreceptor reflex, for example) may result in autonomic reaction masking the primary drug effect. Thus the complexity of the heart as a whole organ makes it an elusive subject for well controlled studies.

At this point, a brief look at striated muscle and a comparison between it and cardiac muscle may help to put these considerations in perspective.

The work of Birks, Katz, and Miledi[11] on frog sartorius muscle showed that the end-plate is seen by the electron microscope as a discrete, three layered structure comprised of the Schwann cell sheath, the axon terminal, and the junctional folds of the muscle. In the innervated skeletal muscle fiber the end-plate area is the main area which is sensitive to the acetylcholine released by the nerve ending.[12] When the normal skeletal muscle innervation is removed, a chain of anatomic and functional changes occurs as follows: the axon terminal degenerates between the third and fifth days leaving a two layered endplate remnant instead of the normal three layered structure. The muscle begins to atrophy, becoming supersensitive to its normal neurotransmitter, ACH,

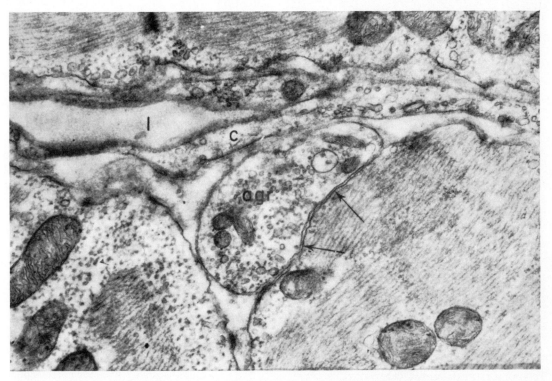

FIG. 3. Electronmicrograph taken from normal frog ventricle showing a nerve process (agr) containing agranular vesicles and some glycogen particles that is situated within the perivascular space where it is making intimate contact with the surface of the cardiac muscle cells (arrows). X30,000. C = Capillary; L = Lumen of capillary. (Courtesy Dr. J. C. Thaement)

owing to a well documented postjunctional change in which the chemosensitive membrane area (previously confined to the area of the end-plate) spreads, eventually covering the entire muscle surface.

Within 10 to 14 days after denervation, the entire muscle fiber is as sensitive as the end-plate region (which retains its original sensitivity). When tested experimentally, these newly formed acetylcholine receptors have properties similar to those at a normally innervated end-plate.[13]

In the heart on the other hand, there has never been an anatomic demonstration of an end-plate. In serial electron micrographs of frog ventricle, Thaemert[14] has shown areas where neural elements and myocardial cells are juxtaposed (Fig. 3). However, repeated histologic examination has failed to disclose any structure which might be interpreted as being a specialized area of neuromuscular transmission.

From a biochemical standpoint, cholinergic terminals (as in skeletal muscle) release acetylcholine, which effects its response and is immediately destroyed by acetylcholinesterase. The adrenergic terminals, on the other hand, release norepinephrine, most of which is taken up again by the nerve terminals after reaction with the receptor. Extrinsic cardiac denervation results in a degeneration of the adrenergic nerves, but it has been repeatedly shown that an intrinsic system of ganglia with their contained nerve cells and concomitant axons remains after denervation (Fig. 4).[4] This system is presumed to be of postganglionic parasympathetic nature, but as alluded to above, synaptic relation to the adrenergic system has not been conclusively ruled out.

A supersensitivity to the neurotransmitter norepinephrine does develop after denervation[15,16] (Fig. 5), but all experiments conducted in the past have indicated that this may be explained solely on the basis of a loss of binding (inactivation) sites for endogenous or exogenous norepinephrine. Thus a greater percentage of a given dose would be available for receptor interaction.

The question that still remains is whether or not there is a postjunctional change after cardiac denervation. Since an extrinsically denervated heart is not a heart without nerves, the role of the intrinsic system of cardiac nerves in maintaining the contractile integrity of the heart remains to be elucidated.

It is known that activation of the extrinsic adrenergic innervation results in a marked increase in the inotropic and chronotropic state of the heart. In striking contrast to skeletal muscle, an extrinsically denervated heart (though grossly appearing some-

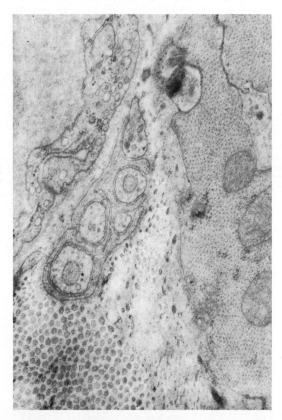

FIG. 4. Electronmicrograph taken from a right ventricular papillary muscle of a cat 41 days following extrinsic cardiac denervation. A neural element consisting of an enveloping Schwann cell sheath and several axons is seen here in cross section. A myocardial cell is seen on the right, and a capillary wall on the left.

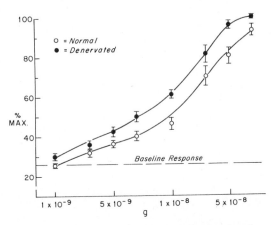

FIG. 5. Dose-response curves for norepinephrine in the normal vs. extrinsically denervated cat heart. Ordinate is the per cent of maximum response as plotted against dose in grams on the abscissa. Bars represent ±1 SE.

what enlarged) functions in a remarkably normal manner physiologically.[17,18] Thus the point is not only what role the normal innervation plays, but what effect basic cardiac-active drugs will have upon the extrinsically denervated heart. The most cogent example of such an agent is digitalis. It has been shown in chronically denervated dogs, for instance, that the mean increment in contractile force produced by ouabain is the same as that in a normally innervated animal.[19] In addition, isolated right ventricular papillary muscles from denervated cats exhibited normal force-velocity relationships and normal increases in isometric tension development in response to digitalis.[20]

One of the very interesting aspects of chronic vascular disease of the heart is the effect of the reduction of blood flow upon the integrity of the normal cardiac innervation. In other words, does interruption of the blood supply to the cardiac nerves, even in a partial way, significantly change their functional characteristics or capabilities? Could this area of investigation be a lead in the intriguing problem of arrhythmias following coronary artery occlusion? Thus the autonomic innervation of the heart may well play a significant, though currently poorly understood, role in the pathogenesis of coronary artery disease.

REFERENCES

1. Epstein, S. E., Robinson, B. F., Kahler, R. L., and Braunwald, E.: Effects of beta-adrenergic blockade on the cardiac response to maximal and submaximal exercise in man, J. Clin. Invest. *44*:1745, 1965.
2. Glick, G., and Braunwald, E.: Relative roles of the sympathetic and parasympathetic nervous systems in the reflex control of the heart, Circulation Res. *16*:363, 1965.
3. Barry, A., and Patten, B. M.: Structure of the adult heart, *in* Pathology of the Heart and Blood Vessels, S. E. Gould. (ed.), Springfield, Illinois, Charles C Thomas, 1968, p. 129.
4. Hirsch, E. F., Willman, V. L., Jellinek, M., and Cooper, T.: Terminal innervation of the heart I, A. M.A. Arch. Path. *76*:667, 1963.
5. Hirsch, E. F., and Borhgard Erdle, A. M.: The innervation of the human heart: I. The coronary arteries and the myocardium. A.M.A. Arch. Path. *71*:384, 1961.
6. Mayer, S. E.: Action of epinephrine on glucose uptake and glucose-6-phosphate in the dog heart in situ, Biochem. Pharmacol. *12*:193, 1963.
7. Mayer, S. E., Cotten, M. de V., and Moran, N. C.: Dissociation of the augmentation of cardiac contractile force from the activation of myocardial phosphorylase by catecholamines, J. Pharmacol. & Exper. Therap. *139*:275, 1963.
8. Cooper, T., Willman, V. L., and Hanlon, C. R.: Influence of cardiac innervation on the response of the heart to adrenergic agents, *in* Factors Influencing Myocardial Contractility, R.D. Tanz, F. Kavaler, and J. Roberts (eds.), New York, Academic Press, 1967, p. 465.
9. Jacobowitz, D.: Histochemical studies of the relationship of chromaffin cells and adrenergic nerve fibers to the cardiac ganglia of several species, J. Pharmacol. & Exper. Therap. *158*:227, 1967.
10. Potter, L.T.: Storage of norepinephrine in sympathetic nerves, Pharmacol. Rev. *18*:439, 1966.
11. Birks, R., Katz, B., and Miledi, R.: Physiological and structural changes at the amphibian myoneural junction, in the course of nerve degeneration, J. Physiol. *150*:145, 1960.
12. Miledi, R.: The acetylcholine sensitivity of frog muscle fibres after complete or partial denervation, J. Physiol. *151*:1, 1960.
13. Thesleff, S.: Effects of the motor innervation on the chemical sensitivity of skeletal muscle, Physiol. Rev. *40*:734, 1960.
14. Thaemert, J. C.: Ultrastructure of cardiac muscle and nerve contiguities, J. Cell. Biol. *29*:156, 1966.
15. Cooper, T.: Physiologic and pharmacologic effects of cardiac denervation, Fed. Proc. *24*:1428, 1965.
16. Dempsey, P. J., and Cooper, T.: Supersensitivity of the chronically denervated feline heart, Am. J. Physiol. *215*:1245, 1968.
17. Blinks, J. R., and Waud, D. R.: Effect of graded doses of reserpine on the response of myocardial contractility to sympathetic nerve stimulation, J. Pharmacol. & Exper. Therap. *131*:205, 1961.
18. Spann, J. F., Jr., Sonnenblick, E. H., Cooper, T., Chidsey, C. A., Willman, V. L., and Braunwald, E.: Cardiac norepinephrine stores and the contractile state of heart muscle, Circulation Res. *19*:317, 1966.
19. Morrow, D. H., Gaffney, T. G., and Braunwald, E.: Studies on digitalis. VIII. Effect of autonomic innervation and of myocardial catecholamine stores upon the cardiac action of ouabain, J. Pharmacol & Exper. Therap. *140*:236, 1963.
20. Spann, J. F., Jr., Sonnenblick, E. H., Cooper, T., Chidsey, C. A., Willman, V. L., and Braunwald, E.: Studies on digitalis. XIV. Influence of cardiac norepinephrine stores on the response of isolated heart muscle to digitalis, Circulation Res. *19*:326, 1966.

Effects of Ischemia and Hypoxia Upon the Myocardium*

Arnold M. Katz

Both ischemia and hypoxia have profound detrimental effects on the performance of the mammalian heart. Effective myocardial contraction ceases after only a few seconds of ischemia, and as little as 5 minutes of anoxia can damage the mechanisms of energy production so severely that recovery of the affected tissue is not complete when oxygen is resupplied. The mechanisms responsible for these effects of ischemia and hypoxia will be considered in this chapter.

In this discussion, myocardial ischemia and hypoxia will generally be considered together, although significant differences exist between their effects. In the ischemic heart, metabolites from the injured cells accumulate in the extracellular space, whereas such substances are washed away in the perfused hypoxic heart. Most important of these metabolites is potassium ion, which when present in high extracellular concentrations can itself arrest cardiac contraction by depolarizing the cell membrane. However, most biochemical sequelae of myocardial ischemia to be considered here are due to cellular hypoxia.†

MYOCARDIAL FUNCTION

Interruption of coronary blood flow, whether by ligation of a coronary artery[1] or by microsphere injection into the coronary vessel[2], is quickly followed by a decrease in blood pressure and cardiac output. The myocardium rapidly becomes cyanotic[3] and deterioration in myocardial function is evidenced by flattening of the ventricular pressure pulse and depression of the rate of intraventricular pressure rise.[4] After 14 beats have elapsed from the time of coronary artery ligation, measurements of myocardial segment length demonstrate significant abbreviation of the duration of systole in the schemic area, and after approximately 60 beats the intraventricular systolic pressure overcomes the

* Supported by Research Grants FR-5367, HE-12349 and HE-11734 from the USPHS; G5-G-61 from the American Heart Association, and N68-41 from the Chicago and Illinois Heart Associations.
† New evidence concerning this question has recently come to light. See references 164 and 165.

contractile tension developed by the ischemic myocardium.[5] At this time the ischemic myocardium (Fig. 1) lengthens, rather than shortens, so that it ceases to participate in ventricular contraction, but instead bulges outwards during systole.[5-7] Although contractility of the ischemic myocardium has been drastically impaired at this time, the ability to

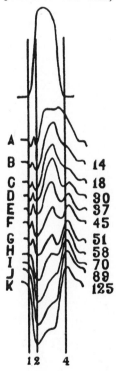

FIG. 1. Left ventricular myograms from a continuous record showing sequential changes following ligation of the left anterior descending coronary artery. The upper curve is the left ventricular pressure curve. Curves A through K were recorded after coronary ligation. The time (in seconds) at which the myographic record was made is indicated at the right of the diagram. In the myographic tracings, an upward deflection represents shortening and a downward deflection represents lengthening. Reproduced from Tennant and Wiggers, Am. J. Physiol., *112*:351, 1935.

shorten is not totally lost, for if the ischemic myocardium is excised and placed in saline, it will contract in response to electrical stimulation.[7] In the hypoxic heart which, unlike the ischemic heart, is not subject to the detrimental effects of extracellular K^+ accumulation, myocardial contractility also falls rapidly after the onset of anoxia.[8-11] However, a weak contractile response can be demonstrated after long periods of anoxia (see below) so that the rapid functional deterioration in both ischemic and hypoxic myocardium is attributable to severely impaired contractility, rather than failure to propagate an action potential or to respond with a contraction to excitation of the cell surface membrane.

Direct recordings of the electrical and mechanical responses of the hypoxic or ischemic myocardium confirm the view that rapid loss of contractility is not due to the absence of a propagated action potential. Electrical threshold has been found to be normal in the ischemic myocardium[5-7] and electrical activity persists in the hypoxic or ischemic myocardium at a time when contractility has fallen drastically.[9,11-14] Membrane potentials do, however, show abnormalities under these conditions. The most striking change in the hypoxic myocardium is an abbreviation of the action potential, which results primarily from shortening of the plateau,[9,11, 14-15] with relatively little change in the resting potential or the height of the action potential (Fig. 2). Similar changes have been found in the action potentials of the ischemic mammalian heart.[16] While impaired contractility has been suggested to result from the marked shortening of the action potential, apparently normal action potentials unaccompanied by a contractile response have been recorded from the hypoxic guinea pig ventricle.[14] Thus, the abbreviation of the action potential may be partly responsible for the impaired contractility of the ischemic or hypoxic heart, but other abnormalities in the mechanism linking excitation at the cell surface to the mechanical response generated by the heart's contractile proteins probably occur.

THE HEART'S CONTRACTILE PROTEINS

At this time, there is no definite evidence that

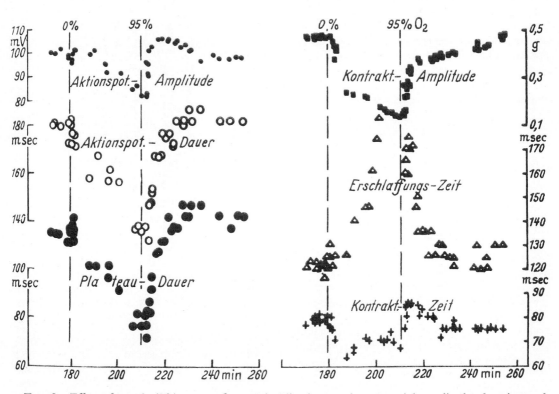

FIG. 2.   Effect of anoxia (0% oxygen, first vertical lines) on action potential amplitude, duration and plateau duration (left-hand graphs), and on contractile amplitude, relaxation time and contraction time (right-hand graphs). Reproduced from Trautwein and Dudel, Pflügers Arch. ges. Physiol. *263*:23, 1956.

ischemia or hypoxia causes irreversible changes in the contractile proteins of the heart. The shortening of actomyosin bands prepared from human hearts freshly obtained postmortem is similar to that of actomyosin bands prepared from hearts obtained up to 6 hours after death,[17] and changes in cardiac myofibrillar adenosine triphosphatase (ATPase) activity have not been noted over a 4–6 hour period postmortem.[18–19] It has been reported that as little as 30 minutes of anoxia causes permanent damage to the myosin molecule, manifested as impaired ATPase activity,[20] but active cardiac myosin can be prepared from rabbit hearts kept several days on ice.[21] The sulfhydryl reactivity of cardiac actin, which provides a sensitive index of the conformation of the actin molecule, is not affected by allowing the heart to remain at body temperature without coronary flow for up to an hour prior to extraction of the protein.[22]

These findings do not exclude the possibility that ischemia causes the contractile proteins to undergo conformational changes in situ, and which are reversed during the isolation and purification of the proteins. It is possible, for example, that the fall in intracellular pH which accompanies hypoxia (see below) may cause changes in the reactive groups or in the overall conformations of these proteins. Such a change in the Ca^{++}-receptor protein of the contractile apparatus may play a major role in decreasing myocardial contractility in the ischemic heart (see below).

CARDIAC EXCITATION-CONTRACTION COUPLING

In view of the potential importance of abnormal cardiac excitation-contraction coupling in the genesis of myocardial failure in the hypoxic or ischemic heart, our current views on the mechanism of this process as it normally occurs in cardiac and skeletal muscle will be described at this point.

Calcium ion appears to play a key role in the excitation-contraction coupling of skeletal muscle. Both the contractile response and adenosine triphosphatase (ATPase) activity of skeletal actomyosin and myofibrils are activated by Ca^{++},[23,24] and injection or application of small amounts of Ca^{++} causes skeletal muscle fibers to contract.[25,26] In the natural process of excitation-contraction coupling, in which contraction is initiated by an action potential, depolarization at the cell surface appears to trigger the release of calcium by structures deep within the skeletal muscle cell.[27] The possibility that excitation is effected by diffusion of Ca^{++} from the extracellular space to the interior of the skeletal

muscle fiber during excitation can be excluded because the interval between excitation and contraction is too brief to permit adequate amounts of Ca^{++} to enter the cell by passive diffusion.[28,29] It now appears that the intracellular release of free Ca^{++} is effected by the sarcoplasmic reticulum, a system of vesicles which is intimately associated with the contractile apparatus.[30] A central role for the sarcoplasmic reticulum in skeletal muscle excitation-contraction coupling is indicated by several lines of evidence. Sufficient Ca^{++} can be taken up by the sarcoplasmic reticulum in situ to effect relaxation,[31] and fragments of this system, recovered in the microsomal fraction of skeletal muscle, actively take up Ca^{++} against a concentration gradient.[32–34] Such Ca^{++} trapping is postulated to effect relaxation by inhibiting the interaction between actin and myosin.[22,23,24] Skeletal muscle contraction thus appears to be initiated when Ca^{++} is released by the sarcoplasmic reticulum, and relaxation occurs when this ion is reaccumulated within the sarcoplasmic reticulum.

Eighty-five years ago, Ringer[35] found calcium to be essential for cardiac contraction. Subsequently, a parallel relationship has been found between external Ca^{++} concentration and the force of cardiac contraction.[36–41] The effect of extracellular Ca^{++} to enhance myocardial contractility appears to reflect a competition between Na^+ and Ca^{++} for a membrane binding site, located at a portion of the myocardial fiber in contact with the extracellular fluid, which determines the force of the heart's contraction.[39,40,42] This view is based on the finding that myocardial contractility is directly proportional to the ratio $\frac{[Ca^{++}]_0}{[Na^+]_0^2}$.[39,40] An increase in this ratio appears to cause an increase in the amount of Ca^{++} available to the heart's contractile proteins during cardiac excitation-contraction coupling, thereby enhancing contractility. It is likely that changes in this ratio, like changes in external Ca^{++} bring about parallel changes in the much lower level of free Ca^{++} within the myocardial fiber during systole. This intracellular free Ca^{++} will further enhance the ATPase activity of the heart's actomyosin which, like that of skeletal actomyosin, is markedly stimulated when free Ca^{++} concentration is raised from 10^{-7} M to approximately 10^{-5} M.[43–46] When free Ca^{++} concentration is low, cardiac actomyosin is dissociated to myosin and actin, whereas additon of Ca^{++} causes reassociation of these proteins with activation of myosin ATPase by actin.[45] Thus, dissociation of the contractile proteins in solutions low in Ca^{++} can be considered to represent the state of the contractile proteins during diastole in the intact heart, where there is little or no interaction between the thick (myosin) and thin (actin) filaments. Increasing the concentration of free Ca^{++} causes an interaction to develop between the contractile proteins which resembles cardiac systole. Here, the thick and thin filaments interact in a manner that permits conversion of the chemical energy obtained from ATP hydrolysis into mechanical work. It is proposed that the degree of association between actin and myosin, and thus the extent of myocardial contractility, is determined by the amount of Ca^{++} made available to the contractile proteins during systole.[45,165]

Both fiber diameter and speed of contraction are less in mammalian cardiac muscle than in frog skeletal muscle, so that entry of Ca^{++} from the extracellular space could, in the heart, provide the link between excitation and contraction.[27,41,47] Such a view is supported by recent evidence that a significant Ca^{++} influx may be partly responsible for the inward current of the action potential.[48,49] On the other hand, a sarcoplasmic reticulum analogous to that found in skeletal muscle can be seen in the myocardial cell,[30,50,51] and cardiac microsomes, like those of skeletal muscle, inhibit the interaction between actin and myosin by removing Ca^{++} from solution.[43,52-59] Thus, two possible mechanisms for cardiac excitation-contraction coupling can be considered: that the Ca^{++} required to activate the cardiac contractile proteins is derived from the extracellular space; or that this Ca^{++} is derived from stores within the heart's sarcoplasmic reticulum. These mechanisms are not mutually exclusive, so that both intracellular and extracellular sources may provide Ca^{++} to the heart's contractile proteins following the excitatory event. In examining the quantitative relationships between enhanced myocardial contractility and the actions on actomyosin ATPase of the calcium-uptake that accompanies a positive rate staircase, we have suggested that the Ca^{++} taken up by the myocardium during an increase in contractility could, if added to a quantum of Ca^{++} released during systole by the sarcoplasmic reticulum, increase the extent of interaction between actin and myosin.[60] However, the exact mechanisms whereby such changes in Ca^{++} movement could be brought about remain to be determined.

Evidence has been obtained to indicate that the rapid decline in the contractility of the ischemic heart does not result from damage to the sarcoplasmic reticulum. The finding that calcium uptake by a cardiac microsomal preparation made from a heart subjected to 15 minutes of ischemia is unimpaired, indicates that the sarcoplasmic reticulum is not irreversibly damaged at a time when contractility is severely depressed.[61] However, the possibility that

transient impairment of this system, which might have occurred *in vivo,* was reversed during preparation of the microsomal fraction cannot be excluded.

Like hypoxia and ischemia, Ca^{++} depletion is rapidly followed by mechanical arrest in the face of continued electrical activity.[37,62-66] In skeletal muscle, as well, dissociation of electromechanical coupling can be brought about both by calcium removal or by metabolic inhibitors (see Reference 27 for a review of findings in skeletal muscle). Unfortunately, the mechanism responsible for this interruption in the coupling between excitation and contraction is not known for either skeletal or cardiac muscle. It has been suggested that a Ca^{++} mediated process links excitation of the cell surface membrane to activation of the sarcoplasmic reticulum, which in turn releases Ca^{++} into the region of the contractile proteins.[67] Such a hypothetical link, which could be the site of the Na^+- Ca^{++} competition described above, could be inactivated by Ca^{++}-depletion. Hypoxia or ischemia, by inhibiting the sodium pump, could lead to Na^+ accumulation at this site, thereby impairing the release of Ca^{++} to the contractile proteins (see reference 68 for a discussion of this hypothesis). Definitive experimental evidence for such a mechanism, and for these possible effects of hypoxia and ischemia, remains to be obtained.

One possible mechanism by which ischemia and hypoxia could depress myocardial contractility is based on the pH sensitivity of the calcium receptor site of cardiac actomyosin. Schädler[46] has shown that the sensitivity of the cardiac contractile proteins to Ca^{++} is greatly reduced at acid pH, so that greater amounts of calcium must be added to obtain full activation of both the ATPase activity and tension development by the cardiac contractile proteins. If this explanation is correct, the intracellular acidosis caused by anaerobic lactic acid production could depress the contractile response to the quantum of calcium delivered during excitation-contraction coupling and thereby cause the rapid fall in the mechanical performance of the ischemic and hypoxic heart.[164]

OXIDATIVE ENERGY PRODUCTION

Before discussing the altered pathways of energy production in the ischemic and hypoxic myocardium, it is useful to consider briefly the physiologic demands which are placed upon working cardiac muscle. Unlike a skeletal muscle, which contracts intermittently, the heart contracts without rest for the lifetime of the animal. Thus, the pathways of energy production must provide the heart's contractile system with a continuing supply of high-energy phosphate.[69] The high level of energy production is achieved primarily by the efficient pathways of oxidative metabolism which permit the heart to oxidize a wide variety of substrates derived from both coronary blood perfusing the myocardium and from intracellular stores.[70-73] Most important of these substrates is fat, which is taken from the bloodstream in the form of free (nonesterified) fatty acids.[74] Such dependence upon aerobic metabolism carries with it the requirement for a continuing delivery of oxygen by the coronary circulation, and interruption of the heart's supply of oxygen causes intramyocardial oxygen tension to fall to 10 per cent of its control value within 30 seconds[12] (Fig. 3). The large myocardial content of myoglobin, which is primarily responsible for the red color of cardiac muscle, has little functional importance as a site for storage of oxygen, but instead serves to facilitate diffusion of oxygen into the interior of the cell. [75-77] The heart's reliance upon the efficient pathways of oxidative energy production is therefore achieved at the price of dependence upon continuous oxygen delivery through the coronary arteries. Failure of this coronary arterial blood supply will bring the major energy-yielding reactions of myocardial metab-

olism to a halt (Table 1).

The major effect of myocardial ischemia upon aerobic energy production stems directly from oxygen lack, which deprives the mitochondrial transport system of its chief electron-acceptor. Evidence has been presented that intermediate metabolites of fatty acid synthesis may serve as electron-acceptors.[75-80] Though these latter reactions cannot maintain a functionally significant level of ATP

TABLE 1
Effects of Hypoxia or Ischemia on Intermediary Metabolism

Enzyme or Enzyme System	Enzyme Function	Effect of Brief Hypoxia or Ischemia
Oxidative phosphorylation	Aerobic ATP production	Inhibited
Phosphofructokinase	Anaerobic glycolysis	Activated
Phosphorylase a	Glycogenolysis	Increased
Phosphorylase b	Glycogenolysis	Activated
Glucose transport	Entry of glucose into cell	Activated
Hexokinase	Glucose phosphorylation	Activated
Glycogen synthetase	Glycogen synthesis	Inhibited

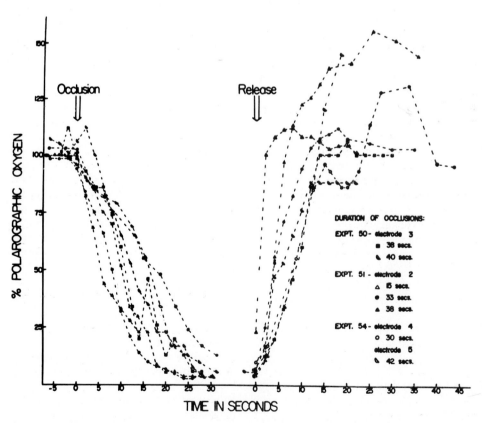

Fɪɢ. 3. Effect of coronary occlusion on myocardial oxygen tension. Reproduced from Sayen et al., Circulation Research, *6:*779, 1958 by permission of the American Heart Association.

production after coronary occlusion, they appear to be responsible for deposition of fat in the ischemic myocardium.[78-80] Electron microscopic studies have shown fat to appear near mitochondria 1–2 hours after infarction.[81-82] Active conversion of fatty acids to tissue lipids in the ischemic myocardium[78] is suggested by the finding that fat deposition is greatest at the periphery of the infarct and that the extent of fatty degeneration after infarction is much greater in areas of the myocardium to which arterial circulation was previously impaired.[83]

Relatively short periods of ischemia or anoxia cause irreversible damage to the enzymes of aerobic energy production.[84-95] As little as 5 minutes of anoxia is followed by impaired respiration when oxygen is resupplied. This impairment of oxidative metabolism probably reflects the rapid appearance of mitochondrial abnormalities, which can be detected anatomically after 15–20 minutes of ischemia.[96,97] The initial morphologic change is mitochondrial swelling,[97] which comes to be associated with considerable disorganization of mitochondrial structure after 30–40 minutes of ischemia.[74] The impaired oxidative metabolism of the ischemic heart is probably associated with breakage of mitochondrial membranes and unfolding of the cristae, changes which have been found to accompany the swelling of isolated mitochondria.[98]

Many details of mechanisms responsible for the swelling of mitochondria in the ischemic heart remain unclear, but it now appears that mitochondrial volume changes are due to osmotic changes rather than active contraction and relaxation.[99] Isolated mitochondria incubated under conditions favorable to oxidative phosphorylation, or in the presence of ATP actively maintain a low water content.[100] Inorganic phosphate, which accumulates in the ischemic myocardium, causes mitochondrial swelling *in vitro*,[101,102] and permeant anions such as phosphate appear to be required for certain types of mitochondrial swelling.[103] However, because many other factors are known to modify the volume of isolated mitochondria, further experimental work will be required to identify the precise cause of mitochondrial swelling in the hypoxic or ischemic heart.

ACTIVATION OF ANAEROBIC METABOLISM

Lactate, which is normally consumed by the myocardium[70,104,105] is released into the blood stream by the hypoxic or ischemic myocardium.[79,93,106-119] The heart's glycogen store, which provides the major source for this lactate, is rapidly utilized during prolonged hypoxia and ischemia.[106,108,110, 112,119-121] Loss of intramyocardial glycogen can be demonstrated histologically after as little as 5 minutes of myocardial ischemia.[96] An oxygen debt is incurred during brief periods of myocardial ischemia which is rapidly repaid during the period of reactive hyperemia that follows release of the coronary occlusion.[122] At the time of this reactive hyperemia, a transient rise in coronary venous lactate concentration is seen,[123] but the ability of the mammalian heart to go into oxygen debt is much less than that of skeletal muscle.[124]

The shift from aerobic to anaerobic ATP production during periods of ischemia or hypoxia reflects activation of the glycolytic pathway at steps mediated by phosphofructokinase and the phosphorylase system, and by stimulation of glucose uptake (Table 1).

The rate-limiting step in the normal glycolytic pathway, which is controlled by the enzyme phosphofructokinase,[125-130] can be modified by alterations in the intracellular concentrations of several metabolites. Phosphofructokinase activity is stimulated by elevated levels of inorganic phosphate and adenosine 5-monophosphate (AMP),[131] both of which accumulate in the anoxic heart.[128,132] The high ATP concentration present in the normal heart inhibits phosphofructokinase,[127,129] but this control mechanism is probably of little importance in stimulating glycolysis during the early stages of myocardial ischemia because ATP concentration falls significantly only after prolonged hypoxia (see below). A rise in intracellular pH may also contribute to the initial activation of phosphofructokinase.[129] Such an alkalosis could be brought about by phosphocreatine hydrolysis, which occurs when ATP production is impaired, because the pH of phosphocreatine is 4.58, whereas that of its hydrolysis products, creatine and inorganic phosphate, is 7.21.[129] Although the initial glycolytic response to hypoxia could be due partly to a rise in intracellular pH, the rapid accumulation of lactate would, within a short time, cause intracellular acidosis, and suppress glycolysis by direct inhibition of phosphofructokinase activity.[133-135]

The rate of myocardial glycogen breakdown is also enhanced by hypoxia and ischemia. This increased rate of glycogenolysis is due primarily to activation of the phosphorylase system,[136] which appears to be effected by two mechanisms: an increase in the proportion of phosphorylase in the active *a* form, and stimulation of the activity of the less active phosphorylase *b*. The increased proportion of phosphorylase *a* may result directly from myocardial hypoxia,[137,138] or it could be due to release of catecholamines from sympathetic nerve endings in the heart. It has been suggested that the rise in pH brought about by phosphocreatine breakdown (see above), may act to increase the proportion of phosphorylase in the *a* form,[129] but sustained glycolysis in the hypoxic heart, which rapidly becomes acidotic, must be achieved by other mechanisms. Phosphorylase *b* activity, like that of phosphofructokinase, is enhanced by elevated inorganic phosphate and AMP concentrations,[128,132] thereby supplementing the effects of the increased proportion of phosphorylase *a* to accelerate glycogenolysis.[137,138] Reductions in the concentrations of ATP and glucose-6-phosphate in the hypoxic or ischemic heart also enhance the activity of phosphorylase *b*.[138] In the turtle, myocardial glycogenolysis is increased primarily by activation of phosphorylase *b*, and the conversion of phosphorylase *b* to phosphorylase *a* assumes little or no functional importance.[139] In the ischemic or hypoxic mammalian heart, however, glycogenolysis is probably accelerated both by the increased proportion of phosphorylase *a* and by activation of phosphorylase *b*.

Hypoxia also increases the myocardial uptake of glucose,[136,140,141] thereby providing additional substrate for anaerobic glycolysis. The enhanced glucose uptake presents additional substrate for hexokinase, the enzyme which phosphorylates the free sugar prior to its entry into the glycolytic pathway. As hexokinase activity is inhibited by the relatively high intracellular level of glucose-6-phosphate in the normal myocardium, hypoxia or ischemia, by activating phosphofructokinase and thereby reducing glucose-6-phosphate concentration, will increase the activity of hexokinase,[128] thereby accelerating glycolysis.

Glycogen synthesis in the hypoxic or ischemic heart also may be impaired. Both ATP and ADP (and to a lesser extent inorganic phosphate) inhibit glycogen synthetase, the rate-limiting enzyme in glycogen synthesis.[142,143] This inhibition of glycogen synthesis by physiologic levels of these nucleotides is greatly increased at increasingly acid pH,[143] thus the accelerated lactic acid production in the anaerobic myocardium would inhibit glycogen synthesis. The inhibition of glycogen synthetase by ATP and ADP is partially reversed by glucose-6-phosphate[143] so that activation of phosphofructokinase could further inhibit glycogen synthesis by reducing glucose-6-phosphate concentration.

It is apparent that the heart is provided with a number of mechanisms which act to increase the rate of anaerobic ATP production during periods of hypoxia or ischemia. Such anaerobic energy production appears to provide for the low level of contractility which can be demonstrated to persist in the ischemic or anoxic myocardium,[9,10] but is clearly inadequate for the generation of useful cardiac work by the mammalian heart *in situ*. In the turtle heart, where contractility is well maintained under anoxic conditions, anaerobic glycolysis is more significant.[144] In other animals, the role of glycolytic pathways in maintaining the low level of contractility seen in the hypoxic or ischemic myocardium has been demonstrated by examination of the effects of iodoacetic acid (IAA), an inhibitor of glycolysis. IAA, which has no effect on the aerobically contracting frog heart, causes an abrupt loss of power under anaerobic conditions[145] in the mammalian myocardium. Both IAA and 2-deoxyglucose, another inhibitor of glycolysis, abolish the weak contractile activity seen in the absence of oxygen.[10] Although the accelerated rate of anaerobic ATP generation does not permit significant preservation of contractile function in the mammalian haert, anaerobic glycolysis does appear to play an important role in preserving myocardial integrity during transient hypoxia and ischemia.[146]

METABOLIC CAUSE OF MYOCARDIAL FAILURE

The ultimate cause of the impaired contractility of the hypoxic mammalian heart is undoubtedly the decreased rate of high-energy phosphate production. In the ischemic heart, as has already been mentioned, local increases in extracellular potassium may serve to prevent excitation of the cell surface membrane. In hypoxia, however, it appears that the deficit in energy production acts to deplete a key reaction, in the mechanism coupling excitation and contraction, of the chemical energy needed for this process.*

It is reasonable to predict that the reduced rate of energy production would cause a significant decrease in the concentrations of high-energy phosphate compounds. Both ATP and phosphocreatine concentrations have been found to be reduced after prolonged hypoxia.[8,89,107,108,113,128,132,147–159] Studies of the myocardium after brief periods of ischemia or hypoxia have generally shown a greater decline in the concentration of phosphocreatine than in that of ATP,[89,113,132,147,148,153,159] as have studies of the substrate-depleted heart.[160] The finding that ATP concentrations are nearly normal when myocardial function declined during [153,159] or after hypoxia[155] has been interpreted to indicate that a mechanism other than an imbalance

* For a more recent point of view, see reference 164.

between energy production and energy utilization causes the failure of the ischemic myocardium, because ATP now appears to be the immediate energy-source for muscular contraction. [161,162] However, such a conclusion appears to be incorrect because the total concentration of ATP in a myocardial biopsy specimen does not necessarily provide a valid index of the heart's ability to deliver ATP to all sites at which the ATP is rapidly hydrolyzed. For example, it has been found that the accelerated rate of energy utilization that accompanies increased cardiac work, like impaired energy production, causes a marked decline in phosphocreatine concentration with little or no decrease in overall ATP concentration.[155,163] Conversely, a reduction in cardiac work is accompanied by a rise in phosphocreatine content, but not a marked increase in ATP concentration. It is apparent, therefore, that phosphocreatine concentration, rather than ATP concentration, is the better measure of the steady state between energy production and energy utilization. In this way the heart resembles a storage battery in which the energy reserve (measured as specific gravity) of the battery acid, like phosphocreatine content, provides the best index of the ability to deliver energy; whereas resting voltage, like the average ATP concentration of a myocardial biopsy sample, can be virtually normal in a battery that is almost dead.

SUMMARY AND CONCLUSIONS

The rapid failure of the ischemic or hypoxic heart appears to result from a decline in myocardial contractility (the ability of the heart's contractil elements to develop tension and do work), rather than from failure of the cell surface membrane to propagate an action potential. This rapid deterioration of contractility may result from an abnormality in the mechanisms linking excitation of the cell membrane to the activation of the cardiac contractile proteins. For example, the Ca^{++} sensitivity of the heart's contractile proteins is depressed by a fall in pH. Thus, the intracellular acidosis caused by the lactic acid produced during anaerobic glycolysis in the ischemic or hypoxic heart, would decrease the mechanical response of the contractile proteins to a given quantum of calcium released during excitation-contraction coupling.

By depriving the heart of oxygen, the major acceptor for the electrons produced during oxidative phosphorylation, hypoxia or ischemia halts the efficient pathways of myocardial aerobic energy production. As a result, the myocardium is forced to obtain energy from the less well developed and less efficient anaerobic pathways of energy production. Although glycogenolysis, glucose transport and glycolysis all are accelerated in the ischemic myocardium, the rate of anaerobic energy production is insufficient to maintain significant myocardial function. On the other hand, anaerobic energy production probably serves to protect the myocardium from irreversible damage during short periods of hypoxia or ischemia.

At the time when failure becomes manifest in the ischemic myocardium, phosphocreatine concentration has fallen significantly. However, the concentration of ATP, which probably provides the immediate source of chemical energy for cardiac contraction, remains at or near its normal level. This finding, along with other evidence, indicates that phosphocreatine concentration provides a better index of the balance between energy production and energy utilization than does the average myocardial concentration of ATP.

REFERENCES

1. Wegria, R., Frank, C. W., Misrahy, G. A., Wang, H. H., Miller, R., and Case, R. B.: Immediate hemodynamic effects of acute coronary artery occlusion, Am. J. Physiol. *177*: 123, 1954.
2. Bing, R. J. Castellanos, A., Gradel, E., Lupton, C., and Siegel, A.: Experimental myocardial infarction: Circulatory, biochemical and pathological changes, Am. J. M. Sc. 232: 533, 1956.
3. Blumgart, H. L., Gilligan, D. R., and Schlesinger, M. J. Experimental studies of the effect of temporary occlusion of coronary arteries. II. The production of myocardial infarction, Am. Heart J. *22*:374, 1941.
4. Wiggers, C. J.: The functional consequences of coronary occlusion, Ann. Int. Med. 23:158, 1945.
5. Tennant, R., and Wiggers, C. J.: The effect of coronary occlusion on myocardial contraction, Am. J. Physiol. *112*:351, 1935.
6. Bronson, L. H.: Anatomical and chemical changes in the myocardium following short-term coronary artery occlusion in dogs, Yale J. Biol. & Med. *10*:405, 1938.
7. Prinzmetal, M., Schwartz, L. L., Corday, E., Spritzler, R., Bergman, H. C., and Kruger, H. E.: Studies on the coronary circulation. VI. Loss of myocardial contractility after coronary artery occlusion, Ann. Int. Med. *31*: 429, 1949.
8. Chang, I.: Asphyxial arrest of the isolated rabbit's auricle, Quart, J. Exper. Physiol. 27: 113, 1937.
9. Webb, J. L., and Hollander, P. B.: Metabolic aspects of the relationship between the contractility and membrane potentials of the rat atrium, Circulation Res. 4:618, 1956.
10. Yang, W. C.: Anaerobic functional activity of isolated rabbit atria, Am. J. Physiol. 205:781, 1963.
11. Trautwein, W., and Dudel, J.: Aktionspotential und Kontraktion des Herzmuskels in Sauerstoffmangel, Pflüger's Arch. ges. Physiol. 263:23, 1956.
12. Sayen, J. J., Sheldon, W. F., Pierce G., and Kuo, P. T.: Polarographic oxygen, the epicardial electro-

cardiogram and muscle contraction in experimental acute regional ischemia of the left ventricle, Circulation Res. *6*:779, 1958.

13. Redo, S. F., and Porter, B. Y.: The role of the lack of oxygen in irreversible cardiac arrest, Surg. Gynec. & Obstet. *109*:431, 1959.

14. Coraboeuf, E., Gargouil, Y. M., Lapland, J., and Desplaces, A.: Action de l'anoxie sur les potentiels électriques des cellules cardiaques de Mammiféres actives et inertes. (Tissu ventriculaire isolé de Cobaye), Compt. Rend. Acad. Sci, Paris *246*:3100, 1958.

15. Trautwein, W., Gottstein, W., and Dudel, J.: Der Actionsstrom der Myocardfaser in Sauerstoffmangel, Pflüger's Arch ges. Physiol. *260*:40, 1954.

16. Kardesch, M., Hogancamp, C. E., and Bing, R. J.: The effect of complete ischemia on the intracellular electrical activity of the whole mammalian heart, Circulation Res. *6*:715, 1958.

17. Kako, K., and Bing, R. J.: Contractility of actomyosin bands prepared from normal and failing human hearts, J.Clin, Invest. *37*:465, 1958.

18. Brown, A., Aras, A., and Hass, G. M.: Method for isolation of large quantities of human and canine cardiac myofibrils, J. Biol. Chem. *234*: 438, 1959.

19. Alpert, N. R., and Gordon, M. S.: Myofibrillar adenosine triphosphatase activity in congestive heart failure, Am. J. Physiol. *202*:940, 1962.

20. Luchi, R. J., and Kritcher, E. M.: Impaired cardiac myosin enzyme activity in acute anoxia, Circulation Suppl. II to vol. *36*: 175, 1967.

21. Bárány, M., Gaetjens, E., Bárány, K., and Karp, E.: Comparative studies of rabbit cardiac and skeletal myosins, Arch. Biochem. Biophys. *106*:280, 1964.

22. Katz, A. M., and Maxwell, J. B.: Actin from heart muscle: Sulfhydryl groups. Circulation Res. *14*: 345, 1964.

23. Weber, A., and Winicur, S.: The role of calcium in the superprecipitation of actomyosin, J. Biol. Chem. *236*:3198, 1961.

24. _____and Herz, R.: The binding of calcium to actomyosin systems in relation to their biological activity, J. Biol. Chem. *238*:599, 1963.

25. Heilbrunn, L. V., and Wiercinski, F. J.: The action of various cations on muscle protoplasm, J. Cell. & Comp. Physiol. *29*: 15, 1947.

26. Podolsky, R. J., and Costantin, L. L.: Regulation by calcium of the contraction and relaxation of muscle fibers, Fed. Proc. *23*: 933, 1964.

27. Sandow, A.: Excitation-contraction coupling in skeletal muscle, Pharmacol. Rev. *17*:265, 1965.

28. Hill, A. V.: On the time required for diffusion and its relation to processes in muscle, Proc. Roy. Soc. (Biol.) *135*:446, 1948.

29. _____The abrupt transition from rest to activity in muscle, Proc. Roy. Soc. (Biol.) *136*:399, 1949.

30. Porter, K. R., and Palade, G. E.: Studies on the endoplasmic reticulum: III. Its form and distribution in striated muscle cells, J. Biophys. & Biochem. Cytol. *3*:269, 1957.

31. Hasselbach, W.: Relaxation and the sarcotubular calcium pump, Fed. Proc. *23*:909, 1964.

32. Ebashi, S.: Calcium binding activity of vesicular relaxing factor, J. Biochem. (Tokyo) *50*:236, 1961.

33. Hasselbach, W., and Makinose, M.: Die Calciumpumpe der "Erchlaffungsgrana" des muskels und ihre Abhangigkeit von der ATP-spaltung, Biochem.

Zeitschr. *333*:518, 1961.

34. Weber, A., Herz, R., and Reiss, I.: Study of the kinetics of calcium transport by isolated fragmented sarcoplasmic reticulum. Biochem. Zeitschr. *345*:329, 1966.

35. Ringer, S.: A further contribution regarding the influence of the different constituents of the blood on the contraction of the heart, J. Physiol. (London) *4*:29, 1883.

36. Loewi, O.: Über den Zusammenhang Zwischen Digitalis-und Kalziumwirkung, Arch. exp. Path. U. Pharmakol. *82*:131, 1918.

37. Daly, I. de B., and Clark, A. J.: The action of ions upon the frog's heart, J. Physiol. (London) *54*:367, 1921.

38. McLean, F. C., and Hastings, A. B.: A biological method for the estimation of calcium ion concentration, J. Biol. Chem. *107*:337, 1934.

39. Willbrandt, W., and Koller, H.: Die calciumwirkung am Froschherzen als Funktion des lonengleichgewichts Zwischen Zellmembran und Umgebung, Helv. physiol. acta. *6*:208, 1948.

40. Lüttgau, H. C., and Niedergerke, R.: The antagonism between Ca and Na ions on the frog's heart, J. Physiol. (London) *143*:486, 1958.

41. Winegrad, S., and Shanes, A.: Calcium flux and contractility in guinea pig atria, J. Gen. Physiol. *45*:371, 1962.

42. Langer, G. A.: The ionic basis for control of myocardial contractility, Progr. Cardiov. Dis. *9*:194, 1966.

43. Fanburg, B., Finkel, R. M., and Martonosi, A.: The role of calcium in the mechanism of relaxation of cardiac muscle, J. Biol. Chem. *239*:2298, 1964.

44. Fanburg, B.: Calcium in the regulation of heart muscle contraction and relaxation, Fed. Proc. *23*:922, 1961.

45. Katz, A. M., Repke, D. I., and Cohen, B. R.: Control of the activity of highly purified cardiac actomyosin by Ca^{2+}, Na^+ and K^+, Circulation Res. *19*:1062, 1966.

46. Schädler, M. Proportional aktivierung von ATPase-aktivitat und durch Calciumionen in Isolierten contractilen Strukturen Verschiedener muskelarten. Pflüger's Arch. ges. Physiol. *296*:70, 1967.

47. Niedergerke, R.: Movements of Ca in beating ventricles of the frog heart, J. Physiol. (London) *167*:551, 1963.

48. Nakajima, S.: Differences in Na and Ca spikes as examined by application of tetrodotoxin, procaine, and manganese ions, J. Gen. Physiol. *49*:793, 1966.

49. Reuter, H. The dependence of slow inward current in Purkinje fibers on the extracellular calcium concentration, J. Physiol. (London) *192:* 479, 1967.

50. Fawcett, D. W.: The sarcoplasmic reticulum of skeletal and cardiac muscle, Circulation *24*:336, 1961.

51. Simpson, F. O., and Oertelis, S. J.: The fine structure of sheep myocardial cells; sarcolemmal invaginations and the transverse tubular system, J. Cell Biol. *12*:91, 1962.

52. Hasselbach, W.: Kontraktile Strukturen des Herzmuskels und Kontraktionszyklus, Verhandl. deutsch. Gesellsch. fur Kreislauf, *27*:114, 1961.

53. Fanburg, B., and Gergely, J.: Studies on adenosine triphosphate supported calcium accumulation by cardiac subcellular particles, J. Biol. Chem. *240:* 2721, 1965.

54. Katz, A. M., and Repke, D. I.: Quantitative aspects of dog microsomal calcium-binding and calcium-uptake, Circulation Res. *21*:767, 1967.

55. Inesi, A., Ebashi, S., and Watanabe, S.: Preparation of vesicular relaxing factor from bovine heart tissue, Am. J. Physiol. *207*:1339, 1964.

56. Carsten, M. E.: The cardiac calcium pump, Proc. Nat. Acad. Sc. (U. S.) *52*:1456, 1964.

57. Lee, K. S.: Present status of the cardiac relaxing factor, Fed. Proc. *24*:1432, 1965.

58. Briggs, F. N., Gertz, E. W., and Hess, M. L.: Calcium uptake by cardiac vesicles: Inhibition by amytal and reversal by ouabain, Biochem. Ztschr. *345*:122, 1966.

59. Weber, A., Herz, R., and Reiss, I.: The nature of the cardiac relaxing factor, Biochim. et biophys. acta. *131*:188, 1967.

60. Katz, A. M.: Regulation of cardiac muscle contractility, J. Gen. Physiol. *50* (No. 6, Pt. 2): 185, 1967.

61. Lee, K. S., Ladinsky, H., and Stuckey, J. H.: Decreased Ca^{2+} uptake by sarcoplasmic reticulum after coronary artery occlusion for 60 and 90 minutes, Circulation Res. *21*:439, 1967.

62. Locke, F. S., and Rosenheim, O.: Contributions to the physiology of the isolated heart. The consumption of dextrose by mammalian cardiac muscle, J. Physiol. (London) *36*:205, 1907.

63. Mines, G. R.: On functional analysis by the action of electrolytes, J. Physiol. (London) *46*:188, 1913.

64. Trautwein, W., and Zink, K.: Über Membran-und Aktionspotentiale einzelner Myokardfasern des Kalt and Warmblüterherzens, Pflüger's Arch ges. Physiol. *256*:68, 1952.

65. Nayler, W. G., and Emery, P. F.: Contractions of ventricular muscle in absence of certain cations, Am. J. Physiol. *206*:909, 1964.

66. Abe, Y., and Goto, M.: Effects of external ions on the excitation-contraction coupling of cardiac muscle of the rabbit, Jap. J. Physiol. *14*:123, 1964.

67. Bianchi, C. P., and Bolton, 'T. C.: Action of local anesthetis on coupling systems in muscle, J. Pharmacol. & Exper. Therap. *157*:388, 1967.

68. Shelburne, J. C., Serena, S. D., and Langer, G. A.: Rate tension staircase in rabbit ventricular muscle: relation to ionic exchange, Am. J. Physiol. *213*:1115, 1967.

69. Katz, A. M.: Patterns of energy production and energy utilization in cardiac and skeletal muscle, in Tanz, R. D., Kavaler, F., and Roberts, J. (eds.): Factors Influencing Myocardial Contractility. New York, Academic Press, 1967, p. 401.

70. Bing, R. J., Siegel, A., Vitale, A., Balboni, F., Sparks, E., Taeschler, M., Klapper, M., and Edwards, S.: Metabolic studies on the human heart in vivo. I. Carbohydrate metabolism of the human heart, Am. J. Med. *15*:284, 1953.

71. Bing, R. J., Siegel, A., Ungar, I., and Gilbert, M.: Metabolism of the human heart. II. Studies on fat, ketone, and amino acid metabolism, Am. J. Med. *16*:504, 1054.

72. Green, D. E., and Goldberger, R. F.: Pathways of metabolism in heart muscle, Am. J. Med. *30*:666, 1961.

73. Scheuer,. J: Myocardial metabolism in cardiac hypoxia, Am. J. Cardial. *19*:385, 1967.

74. Gordon, R. S., Jr., and Cherkes, A.: Unesterified fatty acids in human blood plasma, J. Clin. Invest. *35*:206, 1956.

75. Wittenberg, J. B.: Myoglobin-facilitated diffusion of oxygen, J. Gen. Physiol. *49* (No. 1, Pt. 2): 57, 1965.

76. Scholander, P. F.: Oxygen transport through hemoglobin solutions, Science *131*:585, 1960.

77. Lentini, E. A.: Myocardial developed tension and oxygen supply, Am. J. Physiol. *207*:341, 1964.

78. Evans, J. R.: Importance of fatty acid in myocardial metabolism, Circulation Res. *15* (Suppl. II) 96, 1964.

79. Scheuer, J., and Brachfeld, N.: Coronary Insufficiency: relations between hemodynamic, electrical, and biochemical parameters, Circulation Res. *18*: 178, 1966.

80. Gudbjarnason, S., Braasch, W., and Bing, R. J.: Mechanism of fatty degeneration in infarcted heart muscle, Circulation *36* (Suppl: II) 127, 1967.

81. Bryant, R. E., Thomas, W. A., and O'Neal, R. M.: An electron-microscopic study of myocardial ischemia in the rat, Circulation Res. *6*:699, 1958.

82. Wartman, W. B., Jennings, R. B., Yokoyama, H. G., and Clabaugh, G. F.: Fatty change of the myocardium in early experimental infarction, Arch. Path. *62*:318, 1956.

83. Mallory, G. K., White, P. D., Salcedo-Salger, J.: The speed of healing of myocardial infarction: A study of the pathologic anatomy in seventy-two cases, Am. Heart J. *18*:647, 1939.

84. Ruhl, A.: Über die bedeutung der milchsaure fur den herzstoffwechsel. Klin. Wchnschr. *13*:1529, 1934.

85. Bernheim, F., and Bernheim, M. L. C.: The effect of various conditions on the respiration of the rat heart muscle in vitro, Am. J. Physiol. *142*:195, 1944.

86. Govier, W. M.: The destruction of coenzyme I and cocarboxylase in skeletal and cardiac muscle after death, Science *99*:475, 1944.

87. Govier, W. M.: The effect of experimental coronary artery ligation on the coenzyme I and cocarboxylase content of the myocardium of the dog., Am. Heart J. *29*:384, 1945.

88. Christensen, W. R., and Pearson, O. H.: The effect of cytochrome *c* upon the respiration of tissue slices, J. Clin. Invest. *26*:1046, 1947.

89. Furchgott, R. F., and Shorr, E.: The effect of succinate on respiration and certain metabolic processes of mammalian tissues at low oxygen tensions in vitro, J. Biol. Chem. *175*:201, 1948.

90. Webb, J. L., Saunders, P. R., and Thienes, C. H.: The metabolism of the heart in relation to drug action. I. The endogenous aerobic metabolism of rat heart slices, Arch. Biochem. *22*:444, 1949.

91. Fuhrman, G. J., Fuhrman, F. A., and Field, J., II: Metabolism of rat heart slices, with special reference to effects of temperature and anoxia, Am. J. Physiol. *163*:642, 1950.

92. Lemley, J. M., and Meneely, G. R.: Effects of anoxia on metabolism of myocardial tissue, Am. J. Physiol. *169*:66, 1952.

93. Michal, G., Beuren, A., Hogancamp, C. E., and Bing R. J.: Effect of interruption of coronary circulation on metabolism of the arrested heart, Am. J. Physiol. *195*:417, 1958.

94. Kaltenbach, J. P., and Jennings R. B.: Metabolism of ischemic cardiac muscle, Circulation Res. *8*:207, 1960.

95. Calva, E., Mújica, A., Núñez, R., Aoki, K., Bisteni, A., and Sodi-Pallares, D. Mitochondrial biochemical changes and glucose-KCl-insulin solution in cardiac

infarction, Am. J. Physiol. *211*:71, 1966.

96. Caulfield, J., and Klionsky, B.: Myocardial ischemia and early infarction: An electron-microscope study, Am. J. Path. *35*:489, 1959.

97. Jennings, R. B., Baum, J. H., and Herdson, P. B.: Fine structural changes in myocardial ischemic injury, A. M. A. Arch. Path. *79*:135, 1965.

98. Wlodawer, P., Parsons, D. F., Williams, G. R., and Wojtczak, L.: Morphological changes in isolated rat-liver mitochondria during swelling and contraction, Biochim. et biophys. acta *128*:34, 1966.

99. Ogata, E., and Rasmussen, H.: Valinomycin and mitochondrial ion transport. Biochem. *5*:57, 1966.

100. Disabato, G., and Fonnesu, A.: Metabolic mechanisms involved in the swelling of isolated mitochondria and its prevention. Biochim. et Biophys. Acta. *35*:358, 1959.

101. Lehninger, A. L.: Water uptake and extrusion by mitochondria in relation to oxidative phosphorylation, Physiol. Rev. *42*:467, 1962.

102. Lehninger, A. L.: The Mitochondrion. Molecular Basis of Structure and Function, New York, W. A. Benjamin, 1964.

103. Rossi, C., Scarpe, A., and Azzone, G. F.: Ion transport in liver mitochondria. V. The effect of anions on the mechanism of aerobic K^+ uptake, Biochem. *6*:3902, 1967.

104. Evans, C. L.: The metabolism of cardiac muscle, *in* Newton, W. H. (ed.): Recent Advances in Physiology (6th ed.), Philadelphia, Blakiston's, 1939, p. 157.

105. Bing, R. J.: Cardiac metabolism, Physiol. Rev. *45*:171, 1965.

106. Clark, A. J., Gaddie, R., and Stewart, C. P.: The anaerobic activity of the isolated frog's heart, J. Physiol. (London) *75*:321, 1932.

107. Weicker, B.: Über den chemismus des tätigen Herzmuskels. Arch. exp. Path. U. Pharmakol. *174*:383, 1934.

108. Evans, C. L.: The metabolism of cardiac muscle, *in* Newton, W. H. (ed.): Recent Advances in Physiology (5th ed.), Philadelphia, Blakiston's, 1936, p. 33.

109. Hackel, D. B., Goodale, W. T., and Kleinerman, J.: Effects of hypoxia on the myocardial metabolism of intact dogs, Circulation Res. *2*:160, 1954.

110. Conn, H. L., Jr., Wood, J. C., and Morales, G. S.: Rate of change in myocardial glycogen and lactic acid following arrest of coronary circulation, Circulation Res. *7*:721, 1959.

111. DeHaan, R. L., and Field, J.: Mechanism of cardiac damage in anoxia, Am. J. Physiol. *197*:449, 1959.

112. Danforth, W. H., Naegle, S., and Bing, R. J.: Effect of ischemia and reoxygenation on glycolytic reactions and adenosinetriphosphate in heart muscle, Circulation Res. *8*:965, 1960.

113. Thorn, W.: Metabolitkonzentrationen im Herzmuskel unter normaler, hypoxischen, und anoxischen Bedingungen, Verhandl. deutsch. Gesellsch. fur Kreislauf *27*:76, 1961.

114. Ballinger, W. F., II, and Vollenweider, H.: Anaerobic metabolism of heart, Circulation Res. *11*:681, 1962.

115. Shea, T. M., Watson, R. M., Piotrowski, S. F., Dermksian, G., and Case, R. B.: Anaerobic myocardial metabolism, Am. J. Physiol. *203*:463, 1962.

116. Neill, W. A., Krasnow, N., Levine, H. J., and Gorlin, R.: Myocardial anaerobic metabolism in intact dogs, Am. J. Physiol. *204*:427, 1963.

117. Griggs, D. M., Jr., Nagano, S., Lipana, J. G., and Novack, P.: Myocardial lactate oxidation *in situ* and the effect thereon of reduced coronary flow, Am. J. Physiol. *211*:335, 1966.

118. Ruhl, A., and Thadden, S.: Anoxie und Milchsaurstoffwechsel von Herz und Lunge, Arch. exper. Path. U. Pharmakol. *191*:452, 1939.

119. Himwich, H. E., Goldfarb, W., and Nahum, L. H.: Changes of the carbohydrate metabolism of the heart following coronary occlusion, Am. J. Physiol. *109*:403, 1934.

120. Brachfeld, N., and Scheuer, J.: Metabolism of glucose by the ischemic dog heart, Am. J. Physiol. *212*:603, 1967.

121. Merrick, A. W., and Meyer, D. K.: Glycogen fractions of cardiac muscle in the normal and anoxic heart, Am. J. Physiol. *177*:441, 1954.

122. Coffman, J. D., and Gregg, D. E.: Reactive hyperemia characteristics of the myocardium, Am. J. Physiol. *199*:1143, 1960.

123. Coffman, J. D., and Gregg, D. E.: Oxygen metabolism and oxygen debt repayment after myocardial ischemia, Am. J. Physiol. *201*:881, 1961.

124. Katz, L. N., and Long, C. N. H.: Lactic acid in mammalian cardiac muscle. Part I. The stimulation mechanism, Proc. Roy. Soc. (Biol.) *99*:8, 1925.

125. Newsholme, E. A., and Randle, P. J.: Regulation of glucose uptake by muscle. V. Effects of anoxia, insulin, adrenaline and prolonged starving on concentrations of hexose phosphates in isolated rat diaphragm and perfused isolated rat heart, Biochem. J. *80*:655, 1961.

126. Karpatkin, S., Helmreich, E., and Cori, C. F.: Regulation of glycolysis in muscle. II. Effect of stimulation and epinephrine in isolated frog sartorius muscle, J. Biol. Chem. *239*:3139, 1964.

127. Passonneau, J. V., and Lowry, O. H.: The role of phosphofructokinase in metabolic regulation. Advan. Enzyme Regulat. *2*:265, 1964.

128. Regen, D. M., Davis, W. W., Morgan, H. E., and Park, C. R.: The regulation of hexokinase and phosphofructokinase activity in heart muscle. Effects of alloxan diabetes, growth hormone, cortisol and anoxia, J. Biol. Chem. *239*:43, 1964.

129. Danforth, W. H.: Activation of glycolytic pathway in muscle, *in* Control of Energy Metabolism, New York, Academic Press, 1965, p. 287.

130. Gevers, W., and Krebs, H. A.: The effects of adenine nucleotides on carbohydrate metabolism in pigeon-liver homogenates, Biochem. J. *98*:720, 1966.

131. Passonneau, J. V., and Lowry, O. H.: Phosphofructokinase and the Pasteur effect, Biochem. Biophys. Res. Comm. *7*:10, 1962.

132. Williamson, J. R.: Glycolytic control mechanisms. II. Kinetics of intermediate changes during the aerobic-anoxic transition in perfused rat heart, J. Biol. Chem. *241*:5026, 1966.

133. Delcher, H. K., and Shipp, J. C.: Effects of pH, pCO_2 and bicarbonate on metabolism of glucose by perfused rat heart, Biochim. et Biophys. Acta *121*:250, 1966.

134. Scheuer, J., and Berry, M. N.: Effect of alkalosis on glycolysis in the isolated rat heart, Am. J. Physiol. *213*:1143, 1967.

135. Halperin, M. L., Karnovsky, M. L., and Relman, A. S.: On the mechanism by which glycolysis responds

to pH: Implications for Acid-Base Homeostasis, Clin. Res. *15*:359, 1967.

136. Morgan, H. E., Cadenas, E., Regen, D. M., and Park, C. R.: Regulation of glucose uptake in muscle. II. Rate-limiting steps and effects of insulin and anoxia in heart muscle from diabetic rats, J. Biol. Chem. *236*:262, 1961.

137. Cornblath, M., Randle, P. J., Parmeggiani, A., and Morgan, H. E.: Regulation of glycogenolysis in muscle. Effects of glucagon and anoxia on lactate production, glycogen content, and phosphorylase activity of the perfused isolated rat heart, J. Biol. Chem. *238*:1592, 1963.

138. Morgan, H. E., and Parmeggiani, A.: Regulation of glycogenolysis in muscle. III. Control of muscle glycogen phosphorylase activity, J. Biol. Chem. *239*:2440, 1964.

139. Reeves, R. B.: Phosphorylase activity and glycogenolysis in the working turtle heart, Am. J. Physiol. *206*:898, 1964.

140. Morgan, H. E., Randle, P. J., and Regen, D. M.: Regulation of glucose uptake by muscle. III. The effects of insulin, anoxia, salicylate, and 2:4-dinitrophenol on membrane transport and intracellular phosphorylation of glucose in the isolated rat heart, Biochem. J. *73*:573, 1959.

141. Williamson, J. R.: Effects of insulin and diet on the metabolism of L(+)-lactate and glucose by the perfused rat heart, Biochem. J. *83*:377, 1962.

142. Rothman, L. B., and Cabib, E.: Allosteric properties of yeast glycogen synthetase. II. The effect of pH on inhibition and its physiological implications, Biochem. *6*:2107, 1967.

143. Piras, R., Rothman, L. B., and Cabib, E.: Regulation of muscle glycogen synthetase by metabolites. Differential effects on the I and D forms, Biochem. *7*:56, 1968.

144. Reeves, R. B.: Energy cost of work in aerobic and anaerobic turtle heart muscle, Am. J. Physiol. *205*:17, 1963.

145. Clark, J., Eggleton, M. G., and Eggleton, P.: Phosphagen in the perfused heart of the frog, J. Physiol. *75*:332, 1932.

146. Weissler, A. M., Kruger, F. A., Baba, N., Scarpelli, D. G., Leighton, R. F., and Gallimon, J. K.: Role of anaerobic metabolism in the preservation of functional capacity and structure of the anoxic myocardium, J. Clin. Invest. *47*:403, 1968.

147. Clark, A. J., and Eggleton, M. G.: Phosphagen changes in the iodoacetate poisoned frog's ventricle, Quart. J. Exper. Physiol. *26*:119, 1936.

148. Burns, W., and Cruickshank, E.W.H.: Changes in creatine, phosphagen, and adenylpyrophosphate in relation to the gaseous metabolism of the heart, J. Physiol. (London) *91*:314, 1937.

149. Chang, I.: Effect of asphyxia on the adenosinetriphosphate content of the rabbit's heart, Quart. J. Exper. Physiol. *28*:3, 1938.

150. Proger, S., Decaneas, D., and Schmidt, G.: The effects of anoxia and of injected cytochrome c on the content of easily hydrolyzable phosphorus in rat organs, J. Biol. Chem. *160*:233, 1945.

151. Miller, W. N., Anderson, P., and Dorfman, A.: Effect of anoxia and cytochrome c on readily hydrolyzable phosphate of rat tissues, Science *107*:421, 1948.

152. Khairallah, P. A., and Mommaerts, W.F.H.M.: Nucleotide metabolism in cardiac activity. I. Methods and initial observations, Circulation Res. *1*:8, 1953.

153. Fawaz, G., Hawa, E. S., and Tutunji, B.: The effect of dinitrophenol, hypoxaemia and ischaemia on the phosphorus compounds of the dog heart, Brit. J. Pharmacol. *12*:270, 1957.

154. Furchgott, R. F., and de Gubareff, T.: High energy phosphate content of cardiac muscle under various experimental conditions which alter contractile strength, J. Pharmacol. *124*:203, 1958.

155. Thorn, W., Heimann, J., Muldener, B., Isselhard, W., and Gercken, G.: Herzstoffwechsel in Abhängigkeit von Versuchsanordnung, Gewebsgewinnung und anoxischer Belastung, Pflüger's Arch. ges. Physiol. *269*:214, 1959.

156. Michal, G., Naegle, S., Danforth, W. H., Ballard, F. B., and Bing, R. J.: Metabolic changes in heart muscle during anoxia, Am. J. Physiol. *197*:1147, 1959.

157. Furchgott, R. F., and Lee, K. S.: High energy phosphates and the force of contraction of cardiac muscle, Circulation *24*:416, 1961.

158. Feinstein, M. D.: Effects of experimental congestive heart failure, ouabain and asphyxia on the high-energy phosphate and creatine content of the guinea pig heart, Circulation Res. *10*:333, 1962.

159. Pool, P. E., Covell, J. W., Chidsey, C. A., and Braunwald, E.: Myocardial high energy phosphate stores in acutely induced hypoxic heart failure, Circulation Res. *19*:221, 1966.

160. Thorn, W., Gerchen, G., and Hurter, P.: Function, substrate supply, and metabolite content of rabbit heart perfused in situ, Am. J. Physiol. *214*:139, 1968.

161. Infante, A. A., and Davies, R. E.: Effects of 2, 4-dinitrofluorobenzene on the activity of striated muscle, J. Biol. Chem. *240*:3996, 1965.

162. Mommaerts, W.F.H.M., and Wallner, A.: The breakdown of adenosine triphosphate in the contraction cycle of the frog sartorius muscle, J. Physiol. (London) *193*:343, 1967.

163. Hochrein, H., and Döring, H. J.: Die energiereichen phosphate des myokards bei variation der Belastungbedingunger, Pflüger's Arch. ges. Physiol. *271*:548, 1960.

164. Katz, A. M., and Hecht,H.H.: Editorial, The early "pump" failure of the ischemic heart, Am. J. Med. *47*:497, 1969.

165. Katz, A. M.: Contractile proteins of the heart, Physiol. Rev. *50*:63, 1970.

Pathogenesis of Coronary Artery Disease and Its Clinical Implications

Chairman

William Likoff, M.D.

The Diet and Plasma Lipids in the Etiology of Coronary Heart Disease

Ancel Keys, Ph. D.

The Possible Role of Behavior Patterns in Proneness and Immunity to Coronary Heart Disease

Ray H. Rosenman, M.D.

Meyer Friedman, M.D.

The Complex Pathogenesis of So-Called "Coronary" Heart Disease

Wilhelm Raab, M.D.

Relative Importance of Factors of Risk in the Pathogenesis of Coronary Heart Disease: The Framingham Study

William B. Kannel, M.D.

William P. Casteli, M.D.

Joel Verter

Patricia M. McNamara

The Diet and Plasma Lipids in the Etiology of Coronary Heart Disease[*]

Ancel Keys

For years, mention of the diet and coronary heart disease at a medical meeting was the signal for heated argument, largely because of the persistence of the one disease–one cause delusion. The protagonist was apt to ignore other factors in his enthusiasm about the importance of the diet; the antagonist countered by denying a role to the diet because it did not explain everything. The controversy continues today, but has been relatively muted because over the years the dialogue exposed the faults of oversimplification and over-emphasis. Also, the advance of factual knowledge has removed many questions from debate.

At present, there is general agreement on several points. The diet unquestionably affects the concentration of lipids, especially cholesterol, in the blood serum of man. Those lipids are certainly involved in atherogenesis, though there is argument about details and the sequence of events. It is also agreed that atherosclerosis is basic to coronary heart disease. Stated this way, it might seem that there is no longer room for debate on this issue and, in fact, it would be difficult not to conclude that the diet must play some role in the etiology of coronary heart disease. But the important question is the magnitude of that role and the extent to which dietary management might contribute to the control of coronary heart disease.

EXPERIMENTAL EFFECTS OF DIETARY LIPIDS ON SERUM CHOLESTEROL

Many years of controlled experiments on man

[*]Aided by grants in aid from the U.S. Public Health Service (HE 04697, HE 04997), the American Heart Association, New York, the California State Olive Advisory Board, San Francisco, and local sources in Finland, Yugoslavia and Greece. Some data cited here were obtained in work to be published in detail with collaborating investigators as co-authors: C. Aravanis (Athens), H. Blackburn (Minneapolis), R. Buzina (Zagreb), M. J. Karvonen (Helsinki), A. Menotti (Rome), H. L. Taylor (Minneapolis).

have provided empirical answers about the effects of the diet on the serum cholesterol concentration. The average cholesterol responses to given changes in dietary lipids are predictable.[1-3] If S and P represent, respectively, the percentage of total calories provided by saturated and polyunsaturated fatty acids in the diet and the subscripts 1 and 2 indicate two diets comparable except in respect to S and P, the average serum cholesterol response, mg. per deciliter of serum, resulting from the change from diet 1 to diet 2 is approximately:

$$1: \triangle \text{Cholesterol} \quad 2.7 \, (S_2 - S_1) - 1.3 \, (P_2 - P_1)$$

Alternatively, the simpler expression fits as well:

$$1\text{a}: \triangle \text{Cholesterol} = 1.35 \, (2\triangle S - \triangle P)$$

The above equation is an over-simplification, because all saturated fatty acids do not have identical effects. Saturated fatty acids with fewer than 12 or as many as 18 carbon atoms in the chain have little or no effect on serum cholesterol when they are isocalorically exchanged with starch in the diet.[4,5] Lauric, myristic and palmitic acids are similar in cholesterol-promoting power, but palmitic acid, being by far the most abundant of these fatty acids in ordinary diets, is the chief contributor to the "cholesterol problem." Stearic acid in the diet has little or no cholesterol effect,[4,5] a fact that brings comfort to cholesterol watchers because it means that chocolate is no longer on the dieter's blacklist.

Dietary cholesterol does not affect the blood of man to the degree it does the blood of rabbits and birds, but an effect can be shown when cholesterol is added to a cholesterol-free diet. The effect on serum cholesterol is proportional to the square root of the concentration of cholesterol in the diet.[6,7] If Z is the square root of the concentration of cholesterol in the diet, measured as mg. per 1000 calories, the average effect on the serum cholesterol, in mg./dl., of a change from Z_1 to Z_2 in the diet is:

$$2: \text{Chol}_2 - \text{Chol}_1 \quad 1.5 \, (Z_2 - Z_1)$$

Currently, the usual American diet contains something like 250 mg. of cholesterol per 1,000 calories. On such a diet, the average serum cholesterol level of middle-aged men is about 230 mg. dl. From controlled experiments it can be estimated that if all the cholesterol could be removed but the diet were otherwise unaltered, the average serum level of such men would be about 206 mg. dl. A decrease of almost 10 per cent in the serum level might have a significant effect on atherogenesis but a zero-cholesterol diet is beyond the bounds of practical possibilities. A reduction of 50 per cent in the cholesterol intake requires strict attention to the diet but is not too difficult. Unfortunately, change from 250 to 125 mg. of cholesterol per 1,000 calories of diet, with no other change in the diet, causes an average serum fall of only about 3 per cent. Egg yolk is the most concentrated source of cholesterol in most diets, but the addition of one egg yolk to the daily diet only increases the serum level by an average of about 2 to 3 per cent.

Differences Between Individuals

Even on exactly the same diet, individuals differ in serum cholesterol concentration. Among healthy, middle-aged white men in the United States, the inter-individual standard deviation is about 30 to 40 mg./dl., or some 15 per cent of the group mean. When groups of such men are maintained on the same fixed diet, the inter-individual standard deviation in cholesterol level is reduced very little. In other words, individuals differ intrinsically, the "cholesterolstat" has different settings in different people. Patients with familial hypercholesterolemia are extreme examples at one and of the scale.

In spite of such individual differences, in the great majority of people the serum concentration responds qualitatively in the same way to a given change in the diet. Change to a specific diet low in saturated fatty acids causes the level to drop in almost all persons, but they still tend to maintain their same rank order in cholesterol concentration. Quantitatively, however, the serum response to dietary change tends to reflect the intrinsic characteristic of the individual.[8,9] Men with intrinsically high levels tend to be correspondingly more responsive than men whose "cholesterolstats" are set at intrinsically lower levels. For example, 36 men in a metabolic unit were changed from one diet to another with an average effect of a serum change of 43.5 mg./dl. When the men were grouped into the upper and lower halves of the cholesterol distribution on the control diet and the data was re-analyzed, the average change for the 16 "high" men was 53.6, mg./dl. while for the 16 "low" men it was only 33.5. In the National Diet-Heart Study, men with

base period serum values of 242 mg./dl. or more (with an average of 269) had an average fall of 42 mg./dl. on the C diet, while men with control values less than 210 (with an average of 189) had a fall of only 23 mg./dl. on that diet.[10] Only a part of such differential responses can be ascribed to the so-called law of regression towards the mean. People with high serum cholesterol levels are generally unusually responsive to dietary changes and the average relationship between response and intrinsic characteristics has been formulated mathematically.[8,9]

Tests of the Predictability of Cholesterol Response

Figure 1 shows that the average serum cholesterol response to given changes in the lipid composition of the diet can be reasonably well predicated by equations 1 and 2, above. Each point in Figure 1 is the average response in a controlled experiment on a group of 6 to 24 men, prisoners studied by a team at Harvard[11] and mental patients studied in Minnesota.[2,3] Only 16 per cent of the variance of the group averages remains unaccounted for. Similar successes in predicting serum cholesterol responses

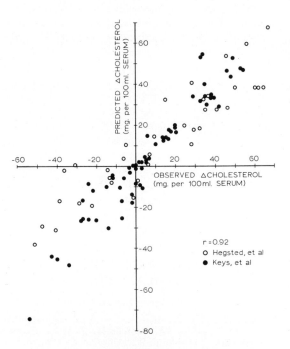

FIG. 1. Correlation between observed and predicted serum cholesterol response to known changes in lipid composition in the diet. Open circles are data from reference 11, closed circles are data from reference 2. Each point is the average response of a group of men.

to dietary changes from these equations have been reported in other studies. For example, in dietary trials in two mental hospitals in Finland, the predicted average responses were -26 and -13 mg./dl. and the observed values were -28 and -12, respectively.[12]

Such agreement between observed and expected averages should not be interpreted to mean that results of dietary changes by individuals can be equally well predicted. Unexplained intra-individual variability in serum cholesterol concentration is by no means negligible, even when the diet is constant and the comparison is made between cholesterol values from blood samples drawn only a few days apart. For middle-aged men, free-living but ostensibly on an unchanging diet, the average intra-individual standard deviation from the individual mean is about 20-24 mg./dl.[3,13] This means that, on the average, about one-third of repeated samples will be at least 20-24 mg./dl. away from (above or below) the true mean value of the individual. When comparison is made between single samples before and after dietary change, the apparent difference may be grossly unrepresentative of the true before and after averages of the individual.

Non-Lipid Items in the Diet

Severe dietary deficiencies of some nutrients may affect the lipids in the blood, but practical questions about the action of those nutrients are limited to less extreme conditions. Over the range of variation of ordinary diets in the United States and Europe, the serum cholesterol level is not affected significantly by differences in the intake of proteins,[14,15] vitamins or minerals. A recent conclusion about different cholesterol effects from different proteins[16] is not supported by a critical analysis of the data.[17] Carbohydrates are more interesting in this respect.

In spite of reiterated claims, it is not true that serum cholesterol falls when starch is isocalorically substituted for sugar in the diet.[3,16,18] it is also not true that dietary fiber lowers the serum cholesterol level or that the high fiber content of the diet accounts for the low cholesterol level characteristic of the Bantu people of South Africa.[19] However, some other complex carbohydrates do have an effect. Ten to 15 grams of pectin in the daily diet produces a modest fall of serum cholesterol in man.[19] The action of pectin and various mucilaginous gums that have a similar effect probably involves interference with intestinal absorption of cholesterol.

It is interesting that, when pectin is added to a high cholesterol diet fed to rabbits, the serum cholesterol falls and the result is a lesser degree of atherosclerosis.[20] Still, the experimental conditions required to produce this result are so extreme, both in the serum levels involved and in the amounts of pectin in the diet, that useful practical application to the human condition may be questionable.

More relevant, perhaps, is the fact that leguminous seeds—beans, peas, lentils, etc.—in the human diet have a cholesterol-lowering effect apparently due to complex carbohydrates in the seeds.[21] The high use of legumes in the diet of some populations, notably in India, Brazil, Greece and the Caribbean Islands, undoubtedly contributes to the maintenance of low serum cholesterol values, not only because the legumes are substituted for meats, with a resulting change in fatty acid intake, but also because of a specific property of the legumes. It seems likely that complex carbohydrates in the diet account for at least part of the fact that, as will be shown later, comparisons between populations often reveal larger average serum cholesterol differences than would be expected solely from differences in the lipid contents of the diets concerned.

THE DIET AND SERUM TRIGLYCERIDES

Effects of the diet on serum triglycerides have been studied much less, and only limited generalizations are possible at present. Compared with cholesterol, the measurement of triglycerides in the serum poses greater problems and involves much greater intra-individual variability. A good deal of propaganda has originated from the fact that abrupt change from a high-fat diet to a low-fat diet (meaning high carbohydrate diet) produces a prompt rise in serum triglycerides, especially in patients who already are hyperlipidemic. However, the fact is that metabolic adaptation to large changes in the fat-carbohydrate character of the diet takes time. In prolonged experiments in a prison, change to a very low-fat diet provoked the prompt rise in serum triglycerides noted in short-period experiments elsewhere, but continuation of the low-fat diet resulted after some months, in a return of the triglycerides to levels as low as, or lower than, those prior to the dietary change.[23]

In the National Diet-Heart Study, change from the usual 40 per cent fat calories of the United States diet to an average of slightly under 30 per cent fat calories (B diet), with corresponding increase in the carbohydrate proportion, produced no triglyceride rise but some tendency in the opposite direction.[10] However, the best evidence that low-fat diets do not promote lasting hyperlipidemia is seen in population surveys. Lifelong subsistence on extremely low-fat diets is not associated with elevated triglyceride values.[24]

Most studies on the effects of the diet on serum triglycerides have been made on patients with severe lipemia and obvious defects in fat metabolism.[25,26] Many such lipemic patients are best managed with restriction of carbohydrates, especially sugar, in the diet while others respond well to a low-fat diet.[27,28] Though the different types of patients may be recognized by their serum lipid patterns in paper electrophoresis,[26] there are no data on the frequency of the several metabolic types in the general population. Observations on patients with bizarre metabolic characteristics provide no reasonable basis for recommendations about diets for the general population.

THE DIET AND SERUM CHOLESTEROL LEVELS IN POPULATIONS

Population surveys in many parts of the world have repeatedly shown at least something like the relationships between the diet and the serum cholesterol concentration found in controlled experiments and expressed in equations 1 and 2, above. From time to time, exceptions to the rule are claimed and immediately receive wide publicity while the eventual disproof attracts far less attention. Unnecessary confusion has been caused by ill-founded claims that follow the "happy Hunza" tradition—stories about Eskimos, Navajo Indians and the like, that purport to show the virtue of the simple life. The latest claim of this type concerns the primitive Masai nomads in eastern Africa, who are said to refute the theory that saturated fatty acids in the diet promote coronary heart disease.[29] Actually, the data available is inadequate to allow *any* conclusions about the incidence of coronary heart disease among the Masai, so the question is only why the serum cholesterol level is low in the Masai—who get such a high proportion of dietary calories from milk which is kept from complete spoilage by a layer of urine. But the milk is mostly sour and the extraordinary thinness of the Masai attests to a chronic calorie shortage; periods of semi-starvation are common. The Masai and his diet seem to have little relevance to diet and coronary heart disease in the civilized world.

Few dietary surveys provide the details of fatty acid intake needed to examine the relationship between the serum cholesterol level and the composition of the diet. The extensive surveys of the International Cooperative Study on the Epidemiology of Cardiovascular Diseases[30] are exceptional in this regard, as well as in the attention paid to the sampling of subjects and the repetition of the surveys in different seasons of the year. Table 1 summarizes some results from these surveys. The data do not allow for differences in the diets in exogenous cholesterol or in complex carbohydrates but, even so, a definite relationship is indicated between the serum cholesterol level and the percentage of total calories provided by saturated fatty acids. It is also clear that in this regard differences in polyunsaturated fatty acid intake are unimportant and that the saturated fatty acid intake is not reliably indicated by the total fat in the diet.

When the serum cholesterol values are plotted against the percentages of calories from saturated fatty acids in the diet, as in Figure 2, the correlation

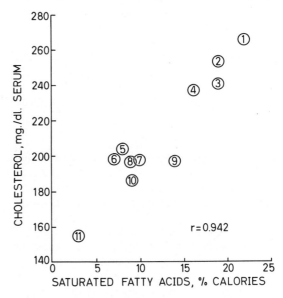

FIG. 2. Median concentration of cholesterol in the blood serum and percentage of calories from saturated fatty acids in the diet. Numbers in the circles identify the samples of men: 1—East Finland, 2—West Finland, 3—Zutphen, 4—U.S. railroad men, 5—Crete, 6—Corfu, 7—Crevalcore, 8—Montegiorgio, 9—Slavonia, 10—Dalmatia, 11—Kyushu, Japan.

is striking (r=0.94). In order to allow for the polyunsaturated fatty acids as in Equation 1, it would be better, theoretically, to compare the serum cholesterol values with the values of the expression 2 S-P as in Equation 1 a. However, as Figure 3 shows, this allowance makes very little difference. This emphasizes the point that, in natural diets, polyunsaturated fatty acids never make a large contribution to the blood lipid picture.

TABLE 1
Average Composition of Chemically Analyzed 7-Day Diets and Median Serum Cholesterol Concentration of Men Aged 40-59 in Different Populations.[30-36]

Area	Fats	% of Total Calories From: Saturated Fatty Acids	Poly-Unsat Fatty Acids	Cholesterol mg./dl. Serum
East Finland	39	22	3	265
West Finland	35	19	3	253
Zutphen, Netherlands*	40	19	5	240
U. S. Railroads**	40	17	5	237
Crete, Greece	40	8	3	204
Corfu, Greece	33	7	4	198
Crevalcore, Italy	27	10	3	198
Montegiorgio, Italy	25	9	3	197
Slavonia, Yugoslavia	33	14	3	197
Dalmatia, Yugoslavia	32	9	7	186
Kyushu, Japan	9	3	3	155

* Serum cholesterol value is the average of the men in the dietary survey sub-sample.
** Nutrients estimated from dietary questionnaires (no chemical analyses of the diets).

Therefore, the general levels of serum cholesterol in population samples correspond, at least qualitatively, to the expectations from the relationship shown in controlled experiments; it is interesting to ask how close the quantitative agreement is. The

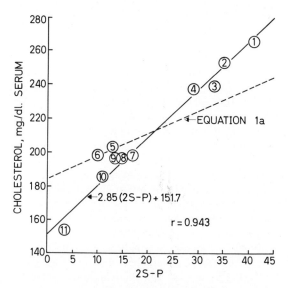

FIG. 3. Median serum cholesterol and the value of the expression 2 S-P, where S and P are percentages of dietary calories from saturated and polyunsaturated fatty acids, respectively. Samples of men identified by the numbers are the same as in Figure 2.

data in Figure 3 correspond to a linear relationship between serum cholesterol and 2 S-P, but the slope does not correspond to Equation 1 or 1 a. In Figure 3, the broken line corresponds to Equation 1 a, i. e., $\triangle$Chol.$=1.35$ $(2\triangle S-\triangle P)$; the solid line corresponds to a similar equation with twice the

slope; the actual least-squares solution for the data in Table 1, using the expression 2 S-P, is:

3: Chol.$=2.85$ $(2S-P)+152$

In other words, the equation for the difference in serum cholesterol value associated with a difference in dietary fats, corresponding to Equation 1 a from the controlled experiments, is:

1 b: $\triangle$Chol.$=2.85$ $(2\triangle S-\triangle P)$

It is interesting that, in population surveys, differences in the fat composition of the habitual diet are associated with considerably greater differences in serum cholesterol concentration than are found in controlled dietary experiments. Several possibilities come to mind. First, in natural populations, dietary items that tend to reduce the cholesterol level, such as pectin and leguminous seeds, may vary inversely with the saturated fatty acids in the diet. It is notable that legumes are eaten much more abundantly in Japan, Greece and Dalmatia than in the United States and especially in Finland. Second, there is a strong tendency for exogenous cholesterol and saturated fatty acids to be directly correlated in natural diets; both are provided by fatty meats and butterfat. Finally, it may be that lifelong subsistence on a diet produces greater effects on the blood than are revealed in relatively brief experiments on man.

Individuals Within the Population

It seems clear enough that when populations are compared there is at least a fair correspondence between the average serum cholesterol levels and the national diets. So clear a relationship does not appear when individuals within population samples are compared. When the population is culturally homogeneous, serum cholesterol differences among individuals often appear to be largely independent of dietary differences.[31,32,37-39] It is not difficult to understand why this should be the case. Besides the fact that variables other than the diet have large influences on the serum cholesterol level of the individual, it must be realized that even the most careful dietary surveys are subject to many errors in estimating the true habitual diet of the individual.[40] Repeated survey on the same individuals show that the intra-individual variance in critical nutrients often exceeds the inter-individual variance, so that in fact, within culturally homogeneous populations, it may not be possible to distinguish individuals reliably in regard to their habitual individual diets.

SERUM CHOLESTEROL AND LATER CORONARY HEART DISEASE

So much attention to the effect of the diet on the cholesterol concentration in the serum is justified by the well-established fact that the incidence of coronary heart disease is related to the cholesterol level. Figure 4 summarizes data from follow-up studies on men in Framingham, Massachusetts, in Albany, New York, and in Minneapolis-St. Paul, Minnesota.[41] On the average, men with serum cholesterol values of 260 or more proved to be 4.3 times more susceptible to coronary heart disease than men of the same age in the same community who had cholesterol values under 200. Follow-up studies in Chicago[39] and Los Angeles,[42] and in the Western Collaborative Group Study in California,[43] are in substantial agreement, the findings on busmen

in London[44] also concur.

The absence of any trace of a critical level or break to suggest a division between "normal" and "abnormal" serum cholesterol levels is notable in Figure 4 and in similar data from other investigators. In regard to the likelihood of future development of coronary heart disease, the higher the cholesterol the worse the outlook. Moreover, the risk does not rise merely in linear proportion to the cholesterol value; the relationship is more like risk being proportional to the third power of the serum cholesterol level.[41] The data on which Figure 4 is based were used to provide Figure 5, in which the observed relative incidence rates for the five cholesterol classes are plotted against the relative rates predicted from the third power of the mean cholesterol level for each class. These data suggest, in fact, that even the third power of the cholesterol concentration underestimates the importance of the influence of serum cholesterol on subsequent development of the disease.

Figure 4 probably underestimates the importance of the serum cholesterol concentration. In the first place, the men were classified in respect to cholesterol on the basis of single blood samples. Since, as noted earlier, intra-individual variability in this measure is substantial, it follows that many of the men must have been misclassified. The true relationship between coronary risk and serum cholesterol values of individuals is diluted by random errors when single values are used as estimates of the unavailable true averages.

In the second place, "coronary incidence" in the data used for Figure 5 includes the incidence of all manifestations of the disease—sudden coronary death, myocardial infarction and angina pectoris. But the relationship of serum cholesterol to these manifestations seems to be less for angina pectoris than for the more objective criteria of infarction and death.[39]

Finally, it should be noted that the data used for Figure 4 include a large number of cases of incidence after age 60. But the relationship of serum cholesterol level to incidence is very dependent on age, being most striking at the youngest ages and then diminishing until, in the sixties, the relationship is small and may not be statistically significant unless large numbers of persons are studied.[45,46] If it is agreed that the incidence of the disease is more important early in life than later, Figure 4 underemphasizes the picture.

In Figure 4, relative incidence rates are shown for men classified according to arbitrary fixed cutting points of serum cholesterol concentration. There are different numbers of men at risk in the several cholesterol classes. Furthermore, the material covers

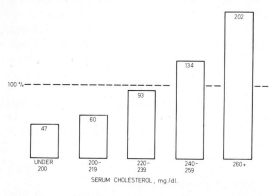

FIG. 4. Relative incidence rate of coronary heart disease among men classified according to entry level of serum cholesterol and followed thereafter for 31,197 man years during which 251 cases developed. Average of data from the Framingham Study (courtesy of Dr. T. R. Dawber), from the Albany Study (courtesy of Dr. J. T. Doyle), and from Minneapolis-St. Paul (Keys et al.[19]).

an extended range of age, and serum cholesterol as already seen, tends to be age-related, though not as much as blood pressure is. Therefore in analyses of rate of incidence as related to such variables as serum cholesterol, it is useful to classify the subjects at risk according to their place in regard to the variable, in the distribution of subjects of the same age examined at the same time in the same study population. The subsequent analysis is made in terms of relative incidence rates in specified proportions of the population at risk and is little affected by varying methods of measurement from sample to sample or from time to time. This avoids possible confounding with age and allows for pooling of data.

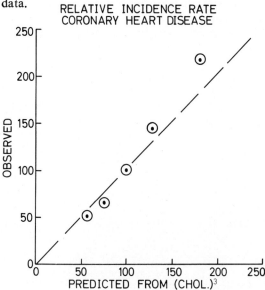

FIG. 5. Relationship between incidence rate of coronary heart disease and the cube of the serum cholesterol concentration. Same data as in Figure 4.

Figure 6 shows the distribution of 5-year coronary heart disease deaths among men, aged 40 to 59 at the outset, who were classified into deciles of the distributions of serum cholesterol and of systolic blood pressure values of men in the same quinquennium of age in the same population sample in the same examination period. These are preliminary and incomplete but unbiased data from the 5-year follow-up material of the International Cooperative Study on Cardiovascular Epidemiology[30] which will be reported in full with the collaborating investigators as co-authors. Both blood pressure and serum cholesterol are obviously important predictions of risk. Men in the top 20 per cent of the distribution of systolic blood pressure

had 2.7 times the coronary death rate of men in the bottom 20 per cent; the corresponding figure for the ratio of the rates for the top and bottom quintiles of serum cholesterol is 7.2 times. Note also that the death rate appears to be a linear function of place distribution, in the cholesterol distribution but that the relationship to blood pressure seems to be quite different; in the lower 60 per cent of the blood pressure distribution the blood pressure seems to be unimportant.

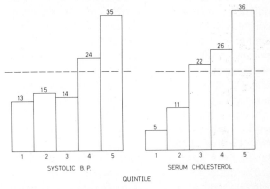

FIG. 6. Numbers of deaths in five years from coronary heart disease among men classified into age and sample specific quintiles of systolic blood pressure and of serum cholesterol concentration. European and American cohorts combined.

The data in Figure 6 include the results in both Europe and the United States, but the relationship is similar when the populations are analyzed separately. Figure 7 shows the relationship of coronary death rate to serum cholesterol for the men in Europe alone. The men in the top quintile had a death rate

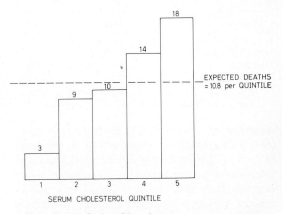

FIG. 7. Relationship between entry serum cholesterol concentration and coronary death rate in the next five years among rural and small-town men in Europe.

six times that of the men in the bottom quintile. It seems that the serum cholesterol level has much the same prognostic significance for farmers in Europe as for railroad employees in the United States.

CORONARY HEART DISEASE IN DIFFERENT POPULATIONS

In the International Cooperative Study,[30] large differences between populations in prevalence of coronary heart disease were seen at the entry examination. Table 2 shows examples. United States railroad employees and men in rural Finland were some ten times more apt than men in rural Greece and Dalmatia to be classified as having coronary heart disease. The discrepancy was similar whatever criterion was used—rigorously defined electrocardiographic evidence of definite old infarction, [47,48] classical angina pectoris and specified combinations of medical history and ECG peculiarities.

The difference between Finland, on the one hand, and Greece and Dalmatia, is on the other, particularly

from coronary heart disease and deaths from all causes. In regard to the coronary heart disease death rate, there is no statistically significant difference between the United states and the Finnish men or between the Dalmatians and the Greeks, so it is useful to compare the two pooled sets of cohorts in order to narrow the confidence limits. When this is done, the age-adjusted coronary death rate among the United States and Finnish men proves to be 16 times greater than among the Greeks and Dalmatians. To put it another way, among the Greeks and Dalmatians the coronary death rate was only 6 per cent of that among the Finns and American railroad men. This contrast is so great that it raises the question of whether some coronary deaths were attributed to other causes in Dalmatia and Greece. This suggestion is answered by the total all-causes death rates. The total all-causes death rate among the Greeks and Dalmatians was only 40 percent that among the Finns and Americans. If coronary deaths were being missed in Greece and Dalmatia they would show up in the deaths from other causes. But the deaths from other causes in Greece and

TABLE 2
*Prevalence of Coronary Heart Disease Among Men Aged 40-59 in Statistically Defined Samples**

Sample	N	Age-Standardized Cases/1000		
		Infarct	Angina	All CHD
U. S. Railroad men	2575	34.3	9.4	43.7
Rural Finland	1677	22.0	14.1	36.1
Rural Dalmatia	672	1.3	0	1.3
Rural Greece	1204	4.0	1.9	5.9

*Over 96 per cent of all men of this age in the defined rural areas were examined by the international teams. "Infarct" corresponds to Minnesota Code categories 1.1, or 1.2+5.1, or 1.2+5.2, or clinical judgment of definite heart disease and etiology specified as myocardial infarct plus any of code numbers 1.2, 1.3, 5.1, 5.2, 6.1, 7.1, 7.2, 7.4, or 8.3. See references 47 and 48.

TABLE 3
*Deaths in 5 Years Among Men Aged 40–59 at the Outset.**

Cohort	CHD Deaths			Deaths, All Causes		
	Observed	Expected	O/E	Observed	Expected	O/E
U.S. Railroad men	66	59.7	1.11	125	152.5	0.82
East Finland	17	17.7	0.96	64	45.5	1.41
Dalmatia	0	18.0	0.00	22	43.1	0.51
Crete and Corfu	3	27.7	0.11	21	70.0	0.30

*"Expected" deaths are the numbers corresponding to the death rates of white men matched by quinquennium of age in the United States in 1962. CHD=coronary heart disease.

impressive when we note that the subjects in those cohorts comprised over 96 per cent of all men aged 40 to 59 in geographically defined rural areas and that occupations and physical activity characteristics were similarly distributed in those cohorts. In contrast with most prevalence studies, self-selection could not play a significant role; these differences in prevalence, therefore, cannot be attributed to sampling bias.

Table 3 summarizes the 5-year data on deaths

Dalmatia are only about 60 per cent of the expectations calculated from deaths among United States white men of the same age.

Only one conclusion is possible: coronary heart disease is far less common among middle-aged men in these areas of Greece and Yugoslavia than in East Finland and the United States. Also, the dearth of coronary heart disease is not accompanied by any compensating rise in other causes of death; in fact, the reverse is indicated. These findings are

TABLE 4
Death Rates per 100,000 Men Aged 40–59 in 1962.*

Country	All Causes	CHD (=B 26)	Other Heart† (=B 26+B 27+B 28)
U. S. (White)	1647	654	69
Finland	1931	706	65
Greece	1014	104	71

*Data from World Health Statistics Annual for 1962 (published in 1965), for 5-year age groups, age-standardized by equal weight for each 5-year class rate.
†Not including rheumatic heart disease.

TABLE 5
Characteristics of Men Aged 40–59 at Start of the 5-Year Follow-up.

Item	U.S. Ry. Men	East Finns	Dalmatians	Greeks
Median Relative Weight, %	104	93	91	91
Median Sum of Skinfolds, mm.	32	14	14	14
% Non-smokers	42	32	41	39
% Heavy Smokers	22	31	23	27
% With Little Activity	52	11	8	17
% With Heavy Activity	5*	71	80	49
Median Serum Cholesterol, mg./dl.	236	265	186	201
% With Diast. B. P. 100 or more	14	21	8	6

*Rough estimate.

in remarkable agreement with such national vital statistics as are available. The latter are summarized in Table 4. No comparable data for Dalmatia are available.

Many factors have been examined in the search for explanations for these remarkable population differences in prevalence of coronary heart disease and the even more striking differences in death rates. The most important of these factors are summarized in Table 5. In this study differences in smoking habits are not involved; perhaps smoking cigarettes promotes coronary heart disease in general but, as Table 5 shows, there were no important differences among these cohorts in smoking habits. The east Finns tended to smoke somewhat more cigarettes than the men in the other cohorts but the actual amount of tobacco used was no greater; many of the east Finns smoke the Russian type of cigarette which contains less tobacco than the usual type. The United States men differed from the Finns, Greeks and Dalmatians in being, on the average, more overweight and much less active physically. Table 5 shows these differences as well as the fact that in these variables there was little difference among the Finnish, Greek and Dalmatian cohorts.

Blood pressure and serum cholesterol are the most interesting variables to consider in this material. Because the American men tended to differ so much in obesity and in physical activity from the men in the other cohorts, it is difficult to consider the possible role of serum cholesterol and blood pressure in accounting for differences in the incidence of coronary heart disease. On the other hand, comparison of the Finns with the Greeks and Dalmatians does not involve such possible confounding; those cohorts are similar at least in physical activity, relative weight, body fatness, occupation and smoking habits, but they do differ in serum cholesterol and in the prevalence of hypertension.

In prospective studies in the United States on men of the ages concerned here, the incidence of coronary heart disease, other things being equal, is increased two to three times by the presence of hypertension. In the present material, 21 per cent of the east Finns were hypertensive while only an average of 7 per cent of the Dalmatians and Greeks were hypertensive by the same definition. It is possible, therefore, to calculate the relative incidence rates expected in those contrasting cohorts if other things were equal and hypertension had a force something like that in the United States— giving the maximum estimated importance to hypertension, this would mean a three-fold rise in heart attacks and coronary deaths. If, in the absence of hypertension, the relative incidence rate is taken as 1.0, then the expected over-all incidence rate among the east Finns including their hypertensive men would be:

$$3 \times 0.21 + 1 \times 0.79 = 1.42.$$

The same kind of calculation applied to the Greeks and Dalmatians gives:

$$3 \times 0.07 + 1 \times 0.93 = 1.14.$$

Accordingly, other things being equal, the difference in prevalence of hypertension would lead to the expectation that the incidence of coronary heart disease among the east Finns would be 1.42/1.14= 1.25 times that among the Greeks and Dalmatians.

Though that would be an appreciable difference, it is obvious that the prevalence of hypertension could account for no more than a small fraction of the observed difference in coronary mortality.

Serum cholesterol can be examined in a similar way. Studies in the United States indicate that the incidence of coronary heart disease in middle-aged men followed for some years is roughly proportional to the third power of the serum cholesterol concentration. In the present material, the general average serum cholesterol level of the east Finns was 2.65 grams per liter while that for the Greeks and Dalmatians was about 1.95 grams per liter. The cubes of these values are 18.61 and 7.41, respectively, so, other things being equal, it might be predicted that the incidence of coronary heart disease among the east Finns would be 18.61/7.41 = 2.51 times that among the Greeks and Dalmatians.

Such considerations lead to several suggestions. First, in accounting for the great differences observed in the incidence rate, serum cholesterol is potentially much more important than blood pressure. Second, if the effects of the two variables are independent, we might predict that the east Finns would have 1.25 × 2.51 = 3.14 times greater incidence than the Greeks and Dalmatians. But that difference, great as it is, is much less than the observed difference in coronary mortality. The conclusion must be, then, that either some other powerful but unnoticed differentiating factor was at work, or the effects of blood pressure and serum cholesterol are much more than simply additive.

DIETARY TRIALS FOR SECONDARY PREVENTION

The first noteworthy trial of the use of diet for the prevention and control of coronary heart disease started more than twenty years ago in Los Angeles with a series of 100 survivors of myocardial infarction, half of whom received no dietary advice (controls) while the other half, said to be matched in clinical condition and relative characteristics, were put on a very strict diet which caused and maintained a large decrease in serum cholesterol concentration.[49]

That study on secondary prevention lasted 12 years, by which time all of the controls were dead but 19 out of 50 of the patients on the diet were still alive. The result would seem to show remarkable success of a diet very low in fats (15 per cent of calories) and severely restricted in exogenous cholesterol, but critics have been unsatisfied with the meager details reported and the absence of proof that the controls and diet patients were really com-

parable at the start and had identical medical management except in the matter of diet. Moreover, the investigator, a prominent internist but not a member of the "academic club," was judged from time to time to be imprudently over-enthusiastic. Accordingly, in "proper" medical circles, the Los Angeles story is virtually ignored.

Other favorable reports on dietary management in secondary prevention in California,[50] in Seattle[52] and in Hungary[52] have also been ignored because of one or another fault in the design of the trial or in the reporting. Far more impressive is the 5-year trial in Oslo, Norway, with 412 men under age 65 who had survived myocardial infarction.[53] The men were randomly assigned to control and diet treatment groups which proved to be well-matched at the start. The diet, sharply restricted in saturated fatty acids and enriched in polyunsaturates, promptly produced an average fall of about 18 per cent in serum cholesterol and the concentration changed little thereafter over the five years. At the end of five years, the clinical score was 37 coronary deaths in the diet group of 206 men and 50 among the 206 controls; 31 per cent of the diet group and 44 per cent of the controls had suffered relapses.

In the Oslo study, the younger men appeared to benefit from the diet more than the older men. This is not surprising and seems to be borne out by a dietary trial with 200 infarct survivors aged 20 to 50 in New Jersey.[54] Among the 100 patients on a fat-restricted diet, the rates of new heart attacks and of coronary death were only 62 and 43 per cent, respectively, of the rates among 100 control patients matched "with respect to age, age at the time of infarction, number of infarctions, prevalence of hypertension, degree of angina, height and weight, and serum cholesterol level."[54] But critics note the fact that the diet-treated patients and their controls were not randomly assigned from a master roster, as was done in Oslo.

In contrast with the results reported from the two studies in California and one each in Seattle, Oslo, Budapest and New Jersey, dietary trials aimed at secondary prevention in London have yielded negative results. One trial with corn oil and olive oil[55] can be dismissed from consideration because the number of patients was too small and the duration too short to allow any conclusions. A much larger trial with a dietary prescription aimed to produce a low-fat diet produced negative results,[56] but the comparison really was between two groups of men whose serum cholesterol values differed only trivially during the period of the trial. The patients on the diet showed a cholesterol fall of 15 per cent while the controls showed a fall of 10 per cent, so a significant difference in relapse rate could hardly be expected. The third negative report from London[57] cannot be so easily explained. The serum cholesterol response to the diet, a fall of around 20 per cent, was comparable to that in the Oslo study and agreed with the result predicted from equations 1 and 2, above. Also, the number of man-years was almost as great as in the Oslo study. In London, there seemed to be some tendency for the dieted group to do better, but a statistically significant benefit in terms of serious relapses and deaths could not be demonstrated. No explanation for this discrepancy from studies in other countries is forthcoming.

DIETARY TRIALS FOR PRIMARY PREVENTION

Except in London, experience with dietary management after myocardial infarction has been favorable but not spectacularly successful. Even enthusiasts for prevention by dietary control admit that there must be severe limitations as to how much can be accomplished after severe atherosclerosis has developed and been made manifest by a heart attack. It would be reasonable to have much more hope for primary prevention. But serious efforts at primary prevention have been few, small in scope and of relatively short duration. The first to start (1957) and the largest in terms of man-years is the "Anti-Coronary Club" program of the New York City Department of Health.[58,59]

The beginning program of the Anti-Coronary Club involved dietary prescription to middle-aged men who were judged to be at high risk for coronary heart disease because of high serum cholesterol concentration or obesity. The controls were men of the same age who were seen at one of the New York City Cancer Detection Centers and were not found to be at special risk; they had no dietary advice. The latest report on the findings covers up to the end of November, 1967, by which time 17 "confirmed new events" had occurred during 3954 man-years for the "active" club members, as compared with 32 such events in 3122 man-years of experience in the control group.[60] The difference in incidence rates, 2.4 times higher in the control than in the active club members, is indeed impressive besides being statistically significant.

Critics of the Anti-Coronary Club program object that, in selecting the treated and control cohorts, there was no random sampling or similar device to assure comparability of the two groups. This implies that if the diet-treated men had fewer heart attacks than the controls, several explanations are conceivable. Perhaps the treated men happened to be less susceptible for reasons other than the diet treatment. Or perhaps the control men, for some unknown reason, happened to be a high-risk group. These hypothetical explanations seem to fly in the face of two facts. Prior to going on the diet, the treated men certainly had a poorer outlook than ordinary men or than the controls, because of the high prevalence of recognized risk factors among the men in the "Club." Equally significant is the fact that, in comparison with the experience of other untreated groups of men of the same age, such as those in the Framingham Study, the Anti-Coronary controls had, if anything, an unusually *low* incidence rate in the follow-up.

A similar prevention program is operated by the Chicago Health Department in an effort to help men similarly judged to be coronary-prone. It is too early to arrive at final conclusions, but so far the results, according to the director, Dr. Jeremiah Stamler, resemble those in New York: the men selected as being high risks at the entry seem to be experiencing fewer heart attacks than would have been expected for ordinary men (that is, men not at high risk) in Chicago. But the same question about "control" subjects will be raised by statistical purists who believe that the only road to knowledge is one that follows a particular statistical design.

A somewhat similar objection may be raised about the favorable results reported from Finland from a trial of a fat-controlled diet at N Hospital, one of the two big mental hospitals in Helsinki. The other hospital, K Hospital, was the control.[12] Serum cholesterol decreased as predicted after the dietary change and, during the succeeding six years, the incidence rate of signs of coronary heart disease and of death was lower at N Hospital than at K Hospital. Electrocardiographic signs (Q, S-T and T) developed at only half the rate in N Hospital as compared with the rate in K Hospital, and the coronary death rate was similarly disparate. But were the mental patients at the two hospitals truly comparable at the outset? At the start of the study the prevalence of ECG abnormalities in N Hospital was somewhat greater than at K Hospital. On the other hand, before the dietary change, the average serum cholesterol level was lower at N Hospital than at K Hospital.

In an effort to rule out the possibility of bias between hospitals in basic patient susceptibility, after six years the Finnish investigators reversed the diets so that patients in N Hospital were changed to the control diet while the patients in K Hospital changed to the fat-modified diet. Serum[61] cholesterol levels promptly responded to the dietary switch-over as expected. More interesting is the fact that the morbidity pattern seems to be following suit, as shown in Table 6. After only two years of cross-over, it is too soon for final conclusions from the second phase, but the total picture from eight years is impressive.

One other study on attempted primary prevention by dietary means has been reported recently.[62] An 8-year study, double-blind, concerned 846 men aged 55 and over (mean: 66 years) randomly assigned to diet or control in a Veterans Administration domi-

TABLE 6
Incidence Rate, per 1000, of Appearance of Electrocardiographic Signs of Coronary Heart Disease Among Patients in Two Mental Hospitals in Finland With and Without a Modified-Fat Diet[61]

Diet	Hospital N	Hospital K
Modified fat	10*	20**
Control	25**	29*

*   1959–1965
** 1965–1967

ciliary unit. The men on the fat-modified diet "had a significantly lower incidence of major atherosclerotic events during the study than did the control group. Furthermore, fatal atherosclerotic events were less numerous in the experimental group than in the control group. Preliminary data suggest that most of this difference occurred in the younger subjects, aged 55–65 at the start of the study."[62]

So far, all experimental trials to evaluate the possible preventive value of dietary adjustment have begun with men of middle age or older, or who have already developed clinical coronary heart disease, or who have both characteristics. The concentration of effort on men who may be presumed, in most cases, to have advanced atherosclerosis is understandable; it guarantees a high rate of new coronary "events" in the control subjects and, therefore, offers the prospect of some conclusions in a few years from relatively small numbers of men. At the same time, however, the choice of such subjects assures that the preventive efforts are applied to persons least likely to benefit, persons whose atherosclerosis is so advanced and of such long-standing as to offer the least hope for reversal or prevention of clinical complications.

Accordingly, it is not surprising that, though the balance of evidence is strongly in favor of some preventive action of a suitable diet, it has not been easy to show a large measure of prophylaxis. Even in the primary prevention trials, where the apparent benefit of reducing saturated fatty acids and cholesterol in the diet is much more indicated than in secondary prevention, the differences in incidence rate between dieted and control groups do not approach those observed when natural populations are compared. Not all incidence differences, such as

between the Finns and the Greeks, may be attributed simply to the diet, but other variations between the populations do not begin to explain the 10-fold difference in age-standardized coronary mortality.

Consideration of the natural history of atherosclerosis and coronary heart disease leads one to believe that the magnitude of any dietary effect on the incidence of coronary heart disease must be inversely related to the age at which subsistence on the diet began and directly related to the duration of the subsistence on the diet. It may be confidently expected, then, that whatever prevention the diet can offer, the greatest benefit will be achieved in those persons whose diet control is started at the youngest age.

Sugar in the Diet

The idea that a high intake of sugar (sucrose) in the diet promotes coronary heart disease has been persistently argued by one English nutritionist.[63,64] This notion has been given considerable publicity at least partly because of two reasons that have nothing to do with the merit of the case. First, nutritionists have long been unhappy about diets loaded with the "empty calories" of sugar and are delighted to find arguments against sugar. Second, after years of so much talk about fats, many people find it refreshing to be told that there is another villain in the diet-atherosclerosis picture.

The case against sucrose is based on three points. First, the death rate attributed to coronary heart disease in Great Britain and in some other countries has risen greatly over the past half century and so has the per capita consumption of sugar. Great changes in diagnostic recognition and custom are ignored in the emphasis on some apparent parallelism in these trends. Second, for some selected countries, the national coronary death rates are correlated with the per capita sugar use in those countries. The statistics cited omit such countries as Cuba, Venezuela and Colombia, where sugar intake is very high but coronary heart disease is relatively infrequent, nor do the figures take into account that for the countries cited there is a high correlation between sucrose and saturated fats in the diet. If importance were to be attached to superficial appearances in national statistics, the sucrose theory would be destroyed by considering that Finland shows half the per capita sugar intake but twice the coronary death rate of next-door Sweden.

The third point used to bolster the sucrose theory is based on questionnaires about sugar put to 20 survivors of myocardial infarction, 25 patients with peripheral vascular disease and 25 persons not showing evidence of atherosclerosis. The latter "control" persons were estimated to consume much less sugar than the men in the other two groups. The reported difference in sugar intake was accounted for by differences in the number of cups of tea drunk—so tea could equally well be "blamed." A similar questionnaire-based comparison of coronary patients and controls in Canada found *no* difference in sugar intake.[65] Paul and others[66] have pointed out that how people use sugar, coffee and tea after developing a chronic disease is not necessarily an indication of their pre-disease custom; they have reported on sucrose intake of men in a prospective study in Chicago.[66] A positive association was found between high use of sugar and high use of both coffee and cigarettes. An analysis taking into account these interrelationships found no significant correlation between the intake of sucrose and the subsequent incidence of coronary heart disease.[66]

Meal Frequency—Nibbling

In experiments on animals, concentration of feeding into infrequent meals can increase the serum cholesterol level and degree of atherosclerosis as compared with nibbling the same diet.[67-69] Surveys of eating habits in Czechoslovakia showed that persons who took three or fewer meals a day tended more often to be overweight and to have high serum cholesterol values than persons who ate five or more meals a day.[70] More recently, the frequency in Prague of electrocardiographic indications of coronary heart disease was studied in men aged 60 to 64 who had been queried about their meal habits.[71] Among men eating 3 or fewer meals daily, the prevalence of ECG signs of probable or possible coronary heart disease was 50 per cent greater than among men eating 5 or more meals daily, with men eating 3 to 4 meals daily being intermediate.

While there is no proof that these findings in regard to meal frequency are relevant to etiology or the problem of prevention, it is easy to conceive of theoretical reasons why meal frequency should be important. Breaking up the day's food into more frequent but smaller meals would certainly mean smaller oscillations in the load of glucose and fats in the blood. And no physiologic or biochemical endorsement can be given to the current frequent American custom in which 50 to 70 per cent of the day's calories are concentrated in the evening meal.

Authoritative Opinion

In 1961, the American Heart Assocation issued a report calling for the reduction or control of fat in the diet, with reasonable substitution of poly-unsaturated for saturated fats. That report was directed to physicans and indicated that such dietary adjustment should be done under medical supervision, but in June, 1964, the Board of Directors of the American Heart Association extended these recommendations to the general public. The increasingly strong position of the American Heart Association on this matter was spelled out in a report approved by the Board of Directors in June, 1965, in which the public was advised:

1. To eat less animal (saturated) fat;
2. To increase the intake of unsaturated vegetable oils and other polyunsaturated fats, substituting them for saturated fats wherever possible;
3. To eat less food rich in cholesterol;
4. If overweight, to reduce caloric intake so that desirable weight is achieved and maintained;
5. To apply these dietary recommendations early in life;
6. To maintain the principles of good nutrition which are important with any change in the diet. Professional nutritional advice may be necessary in order to assure that correct adherence to the diet will not result in any imbalance or deficiency;
7. To adhere consistently to the above dietary recommendations, so that a decrease in the concentration of blood fats may be both achieved and maintained;
8. To make sound food habits a "family affair," so that the benefits of proper nutritional practices—including the avoidance of high blood fat levels—may accrue to all members of the family.

The position of the American Heart Association on these questions was most recently affirmed in a report released in October, 1968, by the Central Committee for Medical and Community Program. The Council on Foods and Nutrition of the American Medical Association may soon issue a new statement but, at least through 1965, it has been less positive except in insisting that all dietary advice must be the prerogative of the personal physician.[72] But the Council did say "that physicians should counsel young men on the advisability of diet modifications, to prevent the rise of serum-cholesterol and other lipids that occurs with increasing age."[72]

The Food and Nutrition Board of the National Research Council also was impelled to make a statement. Concern about dietary fads was evident: "Results of recent studies, while valuable and thought-provoking, do not provide sufficient data for firm recommendations for radical dietary changes."[73] However, the Board report was not entirely negative: "The Board considers that for many Americans moderate reduction in total fat intake and some substitution of polyunsaturated for saturated fat may be indicated."[73] It would be interesting to have a more recent evaluation by the Board.

So the major American non-governmental organizations that should be concerned about this matter of the diet have gone on record, with the American Heart Association, with the body most directly knowledgeable about the coronary problem taking the most positive position. But the official governmental watchdog of the public health, the United States Public Health Service, has only subsidized research and remained silent. The official word from the federal government comes from the Food and Drug Administration. In 1959, the FDA published a statement in the Federal Register denying a relationship between the serum cholesterol concentration and the development of atherosclerosis and warned "that any claim, direct or implied, in the labelling of fats and oils or other fatty substances offered to the general public that they will prevent, mitigate or cure diseases of the heart or arteries is false or misleading"[74] and would be grounds for prosecution by the government. While there is need to curb unjustified claims in the promotion of materials offered for sale to the public, the statement of the FDA about the lack of a relation between cholesterol and atherosclerosis was in itself "false and misleading" and could not be justified even on the basis of the evidence available in 1959.

The position of the FDA has not changed, the preposterous denial of the importance of serum cholesterol in the 1959 statement has not been retracted and, in 1964, the FDA made a further venture into arrogant obstructionism. The food industry was advised that disclosure of the chemical composition of fatty foods on labels would constitute an implied claim in the sense of the regulation of 1959 and would be cause for seizure. In other words, manufacturers were forbidden to tell the public the true composition of their foodstuffs. While that ruling was gratifying to certain food industries and their political friends, it meant, of course, that accurate dietary adjustment to prescription in regard to fatty acids was made difficult. In spite of appeals by many nutritionists and cardiologists, that 1964 ruling still stands as of early 1969.

In contrast to governmental negativity in the United States is a recent development in the Scandinavian countries. After several years of deliber-

ations and committee work, the Medical Boards of Norway, Sweden and Finland issued a joint statement, "Medical Views on Diet in the Scandinavian Countries."[75,76] However, "for reasons of principle the Medical Board of Denmark cannot officially endorse the . . . recommendations but nevertheless intends to see that they are published."[76] The statement, addressed to the general public as well as to the health professions, noted the growing problem of atherosclerosis and its clinical complications in the Scandinavian countries, pointed to the connection with the diet and told the peoples of the Scandinavian countries that: "The total consumption of fat should be reduced from 40 per cent—the present figure—to between 25 per cent and 35 per cent of the total number of calories. The use of saturated fat should be reduced and the consumption of polyunsaturated fats increased simultaneously."

Practicalities of Dietary Efforts

While debate continues on the benefit of reducing the serum cholesterol level late in life or after coronary heart disease is already evident, a great many people are asking practical questions about cholesterol-reducing diets. The response to the call for volunteers of the National Diet-Heart Study indicates that literally millions of Americans are concerned enough to seek help for dietary control. But not many physicians have the time and the knowledge to supply such guidance in practical detail.

Fortunately, at least a modest degree of serum cholesterol reduction is easily and safely made by following some simple rules. Since the first need is a large reduction in saturated fatty acids, there must be a sharp reduction in the consumption of the foods that provide most of those fatty acids—ordinary meats and particularly fatty meats, whole milk, cream, ice cream, butter, lard and heavily hydrogenated shortenings and margarines. Happily, most vegetable oils, except coconut and palm oils, can be recommended for liberal use in cooking and in salads. Most prepared salad dressings and some brands of imitation mayonnaise are acceptable. Many brands of margarines low in saturated fatty acids are available, though the stupid obduracy of the Food and Drug Administration prevents the American buyer from knowing the chemical composition. Restriction of fatty beef, pork, lamb and sausages is no hardship when they may be replaced with poultry, fish and carefully selected lean meats. Except in the most rigidly restricted diets, the fact that shellfish contain cholesterol is no bar to their reasonable use; the effect on the serum cholesterol is trivial. Pastries are frowned on, unless made with suitable oil instead of "hard" fat, but throughout the year there is an abundance of fruit now available for dessert and between-meal snacks. And, as noted earlier, chocolate is not forbidden. Finally, for this writer at least, there is no need for and some argument against swigging down one or another vegetable oil or cooking everything in a safflower or corn oil bath.

We have attempted to explain the principles and practicalities in detail in a book replete with menus, recipes and tables.[77] The American Heart Association has made available pamphlets on fat-controlled diets for physicians[78] and for the general public.[79] The abundance of books on low-fat cookery[80-90] attests to the interest in this subject. While all of the books listed in references 80 to 90 are useful in one way or another, it should be noted that many of them are directed only to restriction of total fats and do not take advantage of the newer knowledge of the role of different fatty acids in regard to effect on serum cholesterol. The judicious addition of vegetable oils to many basically low-fat recipes can make the difference between dull and delightful eating and produce a more favorable serum cholesterol response. Moreover, as indicated earlier, fats are not the entire story in dietary control. We have attempted to make it easy to exploit the legumes more[91] but undoubtedly much more can be done on the matter of the complex carbohydrates.

Nutritionists properly condemn "fad" diets because they rarely accomplish what they claim to do and frequently concentrate so much on a few food items as to be grossly unbalanced or even deficient in one or another essential nutrient. The type of diet advocated by responsible experts for possible prevention of coronary heart disease is not a fad diet at all. The type of diet eaten by the general population in southern Italy, along the Dalmatian coast of Yugoslavia and in Greece is not far from the prescription. A diet eaten by whole populations for centuries can hardly be called a new fad.

REFERENCES

1. Keys, A., Anderson, J. T., and Grande, F.: Serum cholesterol responses to changes in the diet. Metabolism, *14:*747, 1965.
2. Keys, A., and Parlin, R. W.: Serum cholesterol response to changes in dietary lipids. Amer. J. Clin. Nutrition, *19:*175, 1966.
3. Keys, A.: Blood lipids in man—a brief review. J. Amer. Diet. Assoc., *51:*508, 1967.
4. Keys, A., Anderson, J. T., and Grande, F.: Serum cholesterol responses to changes in the diet; IV. Particular fatty acids in the diet. Metabolism, *14:*776, 1965.
5. Grande, F., Anderson, J. T., and Keys, A.: Comparison of effects of palmitic and stearic acids in the diet on serum cholesterol in man. Amer. J. Clin. Nutrition, in press, 1969.
6. Keys, A., Anderson, J. T., and Grande, F.: Serum cholesterol responses to changes in the diet; II. The effect of cholesterol in the diet. Metabolism, *14:*759, 1965.
7. Grande, F., Anderson, J. T., Chlouverakis, C., Proja, M., and Keys, A.: Effect of dietary cholesterol on man's serum lipids. J. Nutrition, *87:*52, 1965.
8. Keys, A., Anderson, J. T., and Grande, F.: Serum cholesterol in man: diet fat and intrinsic responsiveness. Circulation, *19:*201, 1959.
9. Keys, A., Anderson, J. T., and Grande, F.: Serum cholesterol responses to changes in the diet; III. Differences among individuals. Metabolism, *14:*766, 1965.
10. National Diet-Heart Study Research Group: The National Diet-Heart Study final report. Circulation, *37,* No. 3, Supplement No. 1, 1968 (Am. Heart Assoc. Monograph No. 18)
11. Hegsted, D. M., McGandy, R. B., Myers, M. L., and Stare, F. J.: Quantitative effects of dietary fat on serum cholesterol in man. Amer. J. Clin. Nutrition, *17:*281, 1965.
12. Turpeinen, O., Roine, P., Pekkarinen, M., Karvonen, M. J., Ratanen, Y., Runeberg, J., and Alivirta, P.: Effect on serum-cholesterol level of replacement of dietary milk fat by soybean oil. Lancet, *1:*196, 1960.
13. Keys, A., Anderson, J. T, and Grande, F.: Prediction of serum-cholesterol responses of man to changes in fats in the diet. Lancet, *11:*959, 1965.
14. Keys, A., and Anderson, J. T.: Dietary protein and the serum cholesterol level in man. Amer. J. Clin. Nutrition, *5:*29, 1957.
15. Campbell, A. M., Swendseid, M. E., Griffith, W. H., and Tuttle, S. G.: Serum lipids of men fed diets differing in protein quality and linoleic acid content. Am. J. Clin. Nutrition, *17:*83, 1965.
16. Hodges, R. E., Krehl, W. A., Stone, D. B., and Lopez, A.: Dietary carbohydrates and low cholesterol diets: effects on serum lipids of man. Amer. J. Clin. Nutrition, *20:*198, 1967.
17. Keys, A.: Effects on serum lipids of different dietary proteins and carbohydrates. Letter to the editor, Amer. J. Clin. Nutrition, *29:*1249, 1967.
18. Porte, D., Jr., Bierman, E. L., and Bagdade, J. D.: Substitution of dietary starch for dextrose in hyperlipemic subjects. Proc. Soc. Exp. Biol. Med., *123:* 814, 1966.
19. Keys, A., Grande, F., and Anderson, J. T.: Fiber and pectin in the diet and serum cholesterol concentration in man. Proc. Soc. Exp. Biol. Med., *106:*555, 1961.
20. Fisher, H., Griminger, P., and Siller, W. G.: Effect of pectin on atherosclerosis in the cholesterol-fed rabbit. J. Atheroscl. Res., *7:*381, 1967.
21. Grande, F., Anderson, J. T., and Keys, A.: Effect of carbohydrates of leguminous seeds, wheat and potatoes on serum cholesterol concentration in man. J. Nutrition, *86:*313, 1965.
22. Hollister, L. E., Beckman, W. G., and Baker, M.: Comparative variability of serum cholesterol and serum triglycerides. Amer. J. Med. Sci., *248:*329, 1964.
23. Antonis, A., and Bersohn, I.: The influence of diet

on serum triglyceride levels in South African white and Bantu prisoners. Lancet, *1*:3, 1961.

24. Scott, R. F., Lee, K. T., Kim, D. M., Morrison, E. S., and Goodale, F.: Fatty acids of serum and adipose tissue in six groups eating natural diets containing 7 to 40 per cent fat. Amer. J. Clin. Nutrition, *14*:280, 1964.

25. Kuo, P. T., and Bassett, D. R.: Primary hyperlipidemias and their management. Ann. Internal Med., *59*:495, 1963.

26. Lees, R. S., and Fredrickson, D. S.: The differentiation of exogenous and endogenous hyperlipemia by paper electrophoresis. J. Clin. Invest., *44*:1968, 1965.

27. Kuo, P. T.: Hyperglyceridemia in coronary artery disease and its management. J. Am. Med. Assoc., *201*:87, 1967.

28. Reissell, P. K.: Mandella, P. A., Poon-King, T. M. W., and Hatch, F. T.: Treatment of hypertriglyceridemia. I, Total caloric restriction followed by refeeding a low carbohydrate, high fat diet in the carbohydrate-induced type (eight cases). II, Low fat diet plus medium-chain triglycerides in the fat-induced type (two cases). Amer. J. Clin. Nutrition., *19*:84, 1966.

29. Mann, G. V., Shaffer, R. D., Anderson, R. S., and Sandstead, H. H.: Cardiovascular disease in the Masai. J. Atheroscl. Res., *4*:289, 1964.

30. Keys, A., Aravanis, C., Blackburn, H., van Buchem, F. S. P., Buzina, R., Djordjevic, B.S., Dontas, A. S., Fidanza, F, Karvonen, M. J., and Kimura, N.: Epidemiological studies related to coronary heart disease: characteristics of men aged 40-59 in 7 countries. Acta Med. Scand. Suppl. No. 460, 1967, 392 pp.

31. den Hartog, C., van Schaik, Th. F. S. M., Dalderup, L. M., Drion, E. F., and Mulder, T.: The diet of volunteers participating in a long-term epidemiological field survey on coronary heart disease at Zutphen, the Netherlands. Voeding, *26*:184, 1965.

32. Fidanza, F., Fidanza Alberti, A., Ferro-Luzzi, G., and Proja, M.: Dietary surveys in connection with the epidemiology of heart disease: results in Italy. Voeding, *25*:502, 1964.

33. Roine, P., Pekkarinen, M., and Karvonen, M. J.: Dietary studies in connection with epidemiology of heart diseases: results in Finland. Voeding, *25*:384, 1964.

34. Buzina, R., Keys, A., Brodarec, A., Anderson, J. T., and Fidanza, F.: Dietary surveys in rural Yugoslavia. II. Chemical analyses of diets in Dalmatia and Slavonia. Voeding, *27*:31, 1966.

35. Keys, A., Aravanis, C., and Sdrin, H.: The diets of middle-aged men in two rural areas of Greece. Voeding, *27*:575, 1966.

36. Keys, A., and Kimura, N.: Diets of middle-aged farmers in Japan. Amer. J. Clin. Nutrition, in press, 1969.

37. Rosenman, R. H., Friedman, M., and Boasberg, S.: Lack of correlation of serum cholesterol and habitual diet of male and female adults. Circulation, *24*:Part 2, 1024, 1961.

38. Morris, J. N., Marr, J. W., Heady, J. A., Mills, G. L., and Pikingen, T. R. E.: Diet and plasma cholesterol in 99 bank men. Brit. Med. J., *1*:571, 1963.

39. Paul, O., Lepper, M. H., Phelan, W. H., Dupertuis, G. W., McKean, A., and Park, H.: A longitudinal

study of heart disease. Circulation, *28*:20, 1963.

40. Keys, A.: Dietary survey methods in studies on cardiovascular epidemiology. Voeding, *26*:463, 1965.

41. Keys, A., Taylor, H. L., Blackburn, H., Brozek, J., Anderson, J. T., and Simonson, E.: Coronary heart disease among Minnestoa business and professional men followed fifteen years. Circulation, *28*:381, 1963.

42. Chapman, J. M., and Massey, F. J., Jr.: The interrelationships of serum cholesterol, hypertension, body weight, and risk of coronary disease. Results of the first ten years' follow-up in the Los Angeles Heart Study. J. Chronic Dis., *17*:933, 1964.

43 Rosenman, R. H., Friedman, M., Straus, R., Wurm, M., Jenkins, C. D., and Messinger, H. B.: Coronary heart disease in the Western Collaborative Group Study: a follow-up experience of two years. J. Amer. Med. Assoc, *195*:130, 1966.

44. Morris, J. N., Kagan, A., Pattison, D. C., Gardner, M. J. and Baffle, P. A. B.: Incidence and prediction of ischaemic heart-disease in London busmen. Lancet *11*:553, 1966.

45. Kannel, W. B., Kagan, A., Dawber, T. R., and Revotskie, N.: Epidemiology of coronary heart disease. Implications for the practicing physician. Geriatrics *17*:675, 1962.

46. Gofman, J. W., Young, W., and Tandy, R.: Ischemic heart disease, atherosclerosis and longevity. Circulation *34*:679.

47. Blackburn, H., Keys, A., Simonson, E., Rautaharju, P. and Punsar, S.; The electrocardiogram in population studies: classification system. Circulation, *21*:1160, 1960.

48. Rose, G. A., and Blackburn, H.: Cardiovascular survey methods. World Health Organization Monograph Ser. No. 56, 1968.

49. Morrison, L. M.: Diet in coronary atherosclerosis. J. Amer. Med. Assoc., *173*:884, 1964.

50. Lyon, T. P., Yankely, A., Gofman, J. W., and Strisower, B.: Lipoproteins and diet in coronary heart disease. Calif. Med., *84*:325, 1956.

51. Nelson, A. M.: Phospholipids and coronary mortality. Use of ratio between phospholipid and cholesterol levels to determine successful treatment. Northwest Med., *61*:47, 1962.

52. Koranyi, A.: Prophylaxis and treatment of the coronary syndrome. (In Hungarian) Therap. Hung, *11*:17, 1963.

53. Leren, P.: The effect of plasma cholesterol lowering diet in male survivors of myocardial infarction. Acta Med. Scand. Suppl. No. 466, 1966.

54. Bierenbaum, M. L., Green, D. P., Florin, A., Fleischman, A .I. and Caldwell, A. B.: Modified-fat diet management of the young male with coronary disease. J. Amer. Med. Assoc., *202*:1119, 1967.

55. Rose, G. A., Thomson, W. B., and Williams, R. T.: Corn oil in treatment of ischaemic disease. Brit. Med. J., *1*:1531, 1965.

56. London Hospitals Research Committee: Low fat diet in myocardial infarction. A controlled clinical trial. Lancet, *11*:501, 1965.

57. Research Committee: Controlled trial of soyabean oil in myocardial infarction. Lancet, *11*:693, 1968.

58. Christakis, G., Rinzler, S. H., Archer, M., Winslow, G., Jampel, S., Stephenson, J., Friedman, G., Fein, Kraus, A., and James, G.: The anti-coronary club.

H., A dietary approach to the prevention of coronary heart disease—a seven-year report. Amer. J. Pub. Health, *56:*299, 1966.

59. Christakis, G., Rinzler, S. H., Archer, M., and Kraus, A.: Effect of the anti-coronary club program on coronary risk status. J. Amer. Med. Ass., *198:* 597, 1966.

60. Rinzler, S. H.: Primary prevention of coronary heart disease by diet. Bull. New York Acad. Med., *44:*936, 1968.

61. Turpeinen, O., Mitettinen, M., Karvonen, M. J., Roine, P., Pekkarinen, M., Lehtosuo, E. J., and Alivirta, P.: A controlled study on the effects of diet modification on blood lipids and primary coronary events. Minnesota Symposium on Prevention in Cardiology, Rochester, Minnesota. Minnesota Med., in press, 1969.

62. Dayton, S.: A controlled clinical trial of a diet high in unsaturated fat. Minnesota Symposium on Prevention in Cardiology, Rochester, Minnesota, Minnesota Med., in press, 1969.

63. Yudkin, J.: Diet and coronary thrombosis. Lancet, *11:*155, 1957.

64. Yudkin, J., and Roddy, J.: Levels of dietary sucrose in patients with occlusive arteriosclerotic disease. Lancet, *11:*6, 1964.

65. Papp, O. A., Padilla, L., and Johnson, A. L.: Dietary intake in patients with and without myocardial infarction. Lancet, *11:*259, 1965.

66. Paul, O., MacMillan, A., McKean, H., and Park, H.: Sucrose intake and coronary heart disease. Lancet, *11:*1049, 1968.

67. Cohn, C., Pick, R., and Katz, L. N.: Effect of meal eating compared to nibbling upon atherosclerosis in chickens. Circulation Res. *9:*139, 1961.

68. Gopalan, C., Srikantia, S. G., Jagannathan, S. N., and Ramathan, K. S.: Effect of mode of feeding of fats on serum cholesterol levels and plasma fibrinolytic activity of monkeys. Amer. J. Clin. Nutr. *10:*332, 1962.

69. Wells, M. M., Quan-Ma, R., Cook, C. R., and Anderson, S. C.: Lactose diets and cholesterol metabolism. II. Effect of dietary cholesterol, succinylsulfathiazole and mode of feeding on atherogenesis in rabbits. J. Nutrition, *76:*41, 1962.

70. Fábry, P., Fodor, J., Hejl, Z., Braun T., and Zvolánková, K.: The Frequency of meals. Its relation to overweight, hypercholesterolemia and decreased glucose-tolerance. Lancet, *11:*614, 1964.

71. Fábry, P., Fodor, J., Hejl, Z., Geizerová, H., Balcarová, O., and Zvolánková, K.: Meal frequency and ischaemic heart-disease. Lancet, *11:*190, 1968.

72. Council on Foods and Nutrition. Diet and possible prevention of coronary atheroma. J. Amer. Med. Assoc., *194:*1148. 1965.

73. Food and Nutrition Board. Dietary fat and human health. Nat. Acad. Sci.-Nat. Res. Council Pub. No. 1147, 1966:

74. Food and Drug Administration. Status of articles offered to the general public for the control or reduction of blood cholesterol levels and for the prevention or treatment of heart and artery disease under the Federal Food, Drug and Cosmetic Act. Fed. Register, Dec. 10, 1959.

75. Keys, A.: Prevention of coronary heart disease. Official recommendations from Scandinavia. Circulation, *38:*227, 1968.

76. Keys, A.: Official collective recommendation on diet in the Scandinavian countries. Nutrition Rev., *26:*259, 1968.

77. Keys, A., and Keys, M. H.: Eat well and stay well. Rev. ed. Garden City, New York, Doubleday, 1963.

78. American Heart Association: Planning fat-controlled meals for 1200-1800 calories. (EM 288). Planning fat-controlled meals for 2000-26000 calories (EM 288A).

79. American Heart Association: The way to a man's heart (EM 455). Recipes for fat-controlled, low cholesterol meals (EM 455A).

80. Stead, E. S., and Warren, G. K.: Low-fat cookery. Rev. ed. New York, McGraw-Hill, 1959.

81. Cavanna, E., and Welton, J.; Gourmet cookery for a low-fat diet. New York, Prentice Hall, 1956, 153 pp.

82. Hooper, A. R.: Fat-free cookery. London and New York, Oxford University Press, 1958.

83. Swank, R. L., and Grimsgaard, A., Low-fat diet. Reasons, rules and recipes. Eugene, Oregon, University of Oregon Books, 1959.

84. Payne, A. S., and Callahan, D.: The low sodium, fat-controlled cookbook Rev. ed. Boston, Little, Brown & Co., 1960.

85. Rosenthal, S.: Live high on low fat. Philadelphia, J. B. Lippincott, 1962.

86. Waldo, M.; Cooking for your heart and health. New York, Pocket Books, 1962.

87. Whyte, H. M., and Whyte, P., Eat to your heart's content. New York, Hawthorne, 1962.

88. Belinkie, H.; The low-fat cookbook for gourmets. New York, David McKay, 1964.

89. Zugibe, F. T.: Eat, drink and lower your cholesterol. New York, McGraw-Hill, 1964.

90. Lichty, J. A., Bickel, J. H., and Gray, J. C.: A low cholesterol diet manual. Iowa City, Iowa, University of Iowa, 1968.

91. Keys, M. H., and Keys, A.: The benevolent bean. Garden City, New York, Doubleday, 1967.

The Possible Role of Behavior Patterns in Proneness and Immunity to Coronary Heart Disease*

Ray H. Rosenman and Meyer Friedman

Although some degree of coronary atherosclerosis is likely to have occurred in all progenitor hominids and is known to have occurred in men of the early historical milleniums, it is nevertheless difficult to conceive of atherosclerosis as primarily an inherited disease process. The development of atherosclerosis may be structured in part by such genetically related, pertinent factors as the vascular anatomy, blood pressure and blood sugar, the body habitus, the serum lipids and possibly by some as yet unknown inherited factor concerned with intimal structure and permeability. However, the relatively recent and rapidly progressive increase in incidence of clinical coronary heart disease (CHD) in selective populations would imply the occurrence of some strange and all too rapid genetic alteration. Thus, although coronary atherosclerosis probably has always occurred in man, its severe expression with occlusive CHD was rather rare until recent decades.[1]

Clinicians of earlier centuries clearly recognized angina pectoris, but even Osler[2], at the beginning of this century, considered angina to be rare and either did not observe or recognize acute myocardial infarction. Syndromes such as gout and migraine have been recognized since antiquity and it is difficult to believe that the superb clinical observers of nineteenth century England and America, such as Osler, would fail to note the even more dramatic syndrome of acute myocardial infarction, had they observed its occurrence.[3] We must conclude that angina pectoris was quite rare and myocardial infarction also infrequent until the past four or five decades.[3] Since coronary incidence has increased even in the most recent decades, particularly in middle-aged males, it cannot be ascribed simply to improved diagnostic technics or to a larger population base of older individuals.[1] Again we must conclude that there has been a true increase in the frequency and severity of basic coronary atherosclerosis, and occurring increasingly in younger individuals.[1,4] However, the recent increase in coronary morbidity may be ascribable, in part, to a disproportionately greater increase in the incidence of coronary thrombosis, above and beyond any altered frequency of severe basic atherosclerosis.[5,6]

Coronary incidence has been essentially restricted to populations with higher socioeconomic standards. Primitive groups today still exhibit only minimal basic coronary atherosclerosis and still enjoy almost total freedom from symptomatic CHD.[1] Since occlusive CHD is thus an accompaniment of civilization, its recent increase must be largely attributable to the environmental changes associated with the processes of civilization. Coronary atherosclerosis doubtlessly results from the complex interaction of multiple factors, and any influence that enhances the rate of intimal damage and hyperplastic repair or the intimal deposition of lipid and thrombotic material may accordingly accelerate atherogenesis and the advent of clinical CHD.[7]

Epidemiologic studies have shown that the rate of CHD is substantially higher in populations characterized by a plethoric diet and relative physical indolence than in more primitive groups whose diet is lower in calories and fats and who are more physically active.[1] However, the decades witnessing the rising CHD rate in the more privileged societies have not been characterized by any parallel changes of diet, which has altered surprisingly little in fat intake during the past century or more.[8] There is no linear relationship between national dietary fat intakes and coronary morbidity rates; on the contrary, coronary morbidity rates have increased almost fourfold while at the same levels of fat intake.[9] Moreover, there are several groups, such as the African Samburu, which exhibit almost total freedom from CHD despite habitual ingestion of a high-saturated fat diet.[10] It is also unclear why

*The studies described in this paper were supported by United States Public Health Service Research Grant No. HE-03429 from the National Heart Institute and the Irwin Strasburger Memorial Medical Foundation of New York.

coronary morbidity was so astonishingly low in earlier decades of this century and in the 19th century, for example, among the host of older individuals in Britain and America who ingested an habitually plethoric diet abundantly enriched with animal fat.[3] Finally, despite the undoubted pathogenetic role of the diet, prospective studies, including our own, have not shown differences of diet between subsequently victimized individuals and those who remained free of CHD.[11] In this regard, although the low serum lipids of primitive groups and the higher serum lipids of more privileged groups are correlated with major differences of dietary fat intakes,[12] there are important exceptions, such as the African Samburu[10] and American prison inmates,[13,14] both of which groups exhibit low serum lipids despite habitual high dietary fat intakes. Finally, among members of any group ingesting an habitual, high fat diet, the serum cholesterol shows extreme variability, and there is no correlation between the individual serum cholesterol and the dietary intake of saturated fat, nor for that matter with the intake of any diet fraction.[15,16]

In general, the same experience prevails with respect to exercise habits. Thus, primitive groups with very low coronary morbidity are also usually characterized by high levels of physical activity when compared to more privileged societies where relative physical indolence prevails and coronary rates are high; but a causal relationship has not been established.[1] Although the level of physical activity may influence the age of onset and the type of initial manifestation of CHD and mortality rates[1,17] by influencing the development of collateral circulation,[1] there is as yet little evidence that it is significantly related to basic coronary atherosclerosis per se.[18] In this regard, it is again important to point out that CHD was rare in large 19th century British and American populations that also did not indulge in significant physical activity.[3] Finally, prospective studies of CHD have not shown significant differences in levels of physical activity between the victimized and the healthy subjects.[19,22] It must be concluded that, despite the undoubted role of the diet in the pathogenesis of coronary artery disease and the possible influencing role of physical activity, the recent advent and progressive increase of coronary morbidity in the more privileged societies cannot be ascribed *per se* either to dietary excess or physical indolence, alone or together.

Epidemiologic studies in this country have shown that the incidence of CHD is significantly increased in individuals who prospectively exhibit certain characteristics or risk factors, alone or in combination.[1] Our own prospective study, the Western Collaborative Group Study, was initiated in 1960 with 3,500 men, aged 39 to 59 years at intake and employed in 10 participating California companies.[20-22] Clinical CHD had been observed in 195 of 3,182 initially well men at risk during the first mean $61\frac{1}{2}$-year period of follow-up. Since the findings in the two intake age decades are generally similar,[21,22] the subjects have been combined for the present purpose in order to simplify presentation of the data. The findings are similar to other prospective studies[1] in that (Table 1) a significantly increased

TABLE   1
$6\frac{1}{2}$-Year Incidence of CHD in Subjects
with Various Characteristics

Risk Factor	No. at Risk	No. of CHD Cases	Annual Incidence of CHD*
All subjects	3182	195	9.4
Cigarettes:			
0	1651	72	6.7
16 and over per day	1183	108	14.0
Parental CHD:			
History no	2536	142	8.6
History yes	623	53	13.1
Diastolic Blood Pressure:			
94 or less	2866	161	8.6
95 and over	293	34	17.9
Cholesterol:			
224 or less	1619	53	5.0
260 and over	642	77	18.5
Triglycerides:			
99 or less	851	28	5.1
177 and over	706	63	13.7
Beta/Alpha LP ratio:			
2.03 or less	1815	81	6.9
2.36 and over	989	88	13.7

*No. of CHD cases/1,000 men/year at risk.

TABLE 2
Prevalence of Various Characteristics

	Subjects at Risk		CHD Cases ($6\frac{1}{2}$ Years)	
	No.	% of Total	No.	% of Total
All Subjects	3182	100.0	195	100.0
Cigarettes 16+/day	1183	37.4	108	55.4
B/A LP Ratio 2.36+	989	31.4	88	45.4
Triglycerides 177+	706	23.5	63	34.8
Cholesterol 260+	642	20.4	77	39.4
Parental CHD+History	623	19.5	53	27.2
*Chol. 225+, Tglyc. 148+, B/A 2.04+	467	15.6	55	30.4
Tglyc. 177+, B/A 2.36	381	12.7	43	23.8
Chol. 260+, B/A 2.36+	370	11.8	49	25.2
Diast. Blood Pressure (DBP) 95+	293	9.3	34	17.4
Chol. 260+, Cigs. 16+	289	9.2	43	22.1
Chol. 260+, Tglyc. 177+	253	8.4	32	17.6
Chol. 260+, Tglyc. 177+, B/A 2.36+	168	5.6	25	13.8
Chol. 260+, Diast, BP 95+	77	2.4	15	7.7
Chol. 260+, Cigs. 16+, DBP 95+	33	1.0	7	3.6

*Mean lipid levels for total population.

incidence of CHD was observed in men who prospectively exhibited elevated blood pressure, elevated serum levels of cholesterol, triglycerides or beta/alpha lipoprotein ratios, heavy cigarette smoking, or a parental history of CHD, compared to men who were more favorably endowed. An increased incidence also occurred in subjects with glucose intolerance.[21,22]

The prevalence of the various adverse prospective characteristics, alone and in various representative combinations, in the total population and in the men who later suffered the advent of clinical CHD is shown in Table 2. It can be seen that although the coronary incidence was significantly increased in men who exhibited such attributes, the risk factors were present in only a minority of both the total and the later coronary population. It should also be noted that the vast majority of men at risk with such unfavorable characteristics still remain free of clinical disease over the passage of time.

It is clear, then, that epidemiologic studies have identified various characteristics that enhance coronary-proneness, but the findings are pertinent only to *groups* of men and lack *individual* predictive specificity, since the group of men living with any of the high risk factors exceeds the later morbidity by at least tenfold. An even more important corollary can be derived from the above findings, namely that a considerable incidence of CHD occurs in men who do not prospectively exhibit these classical risk factors, and even in subjects with relatively low serum lipid and lipoprotein concentrations.[23]

Consideration of the above and other pertinent findings[24,25] led our group, to conclude more than a decade ago, that neither the diet, the serum lipids nor any of the classic culprits provided a satisfactory basis to explain the recent selective, rapid rise of coronary morbidity in groups enjoying higher socioeconomic standards. It was clear that most epidemiologic and allied studies had failed to consider the possible role of socioeconomic stresses and various individual personality and behavioral factors.[24,25] This was surprising to us in view of; (1) the findings of Bronte-Stewart and associates[26] in their Cape Town population studies that if "job responsiblilty" were employed as an indicator of stress, as good a correlation could be found between its variations and the varying incidence of clinical coronary disease as that which they believed existed between the dietary fat intake and clinical coronary disease; (2) the fact that population groups exhibiting freedom from CHD, although not invariably ingesting a low fat diet, also were not exposed to the socioeconomic stresses characterizing the high coronary areas;[24,25] (3) Osler's, writings[27], more than 70 years ago, which pointed out that: "in the worry and strain of modern life, arterial degeneration is not only very common but develops at a relatively early age. For this, I believe that the high pressure at which men live, and the habit of working the machine to its maximum capacity, are responsible, rather than excesses in eating and drinking," and some years later Osler's observation[2] that "it is not the delicate, neurotic person who is prone to angina but the robust, the keen and ambitious man, the indicator of whose engine is always at 'full speed' ahead"; and (4) the more recent studies of young patients with CHD in which Gertler and White[28] found that, in their series of patients, "those in managerial and executive positions" did exhibit a relatively high frequency of appearance. Thus, the impression was gained throughout the interviews "that these patients wanted to succeed in anything they attempted and, furthermore, that they were able to do so," and that, more often than the controls, those afflicted were significantly "hard-driving and goal-directed."

There thus appeared to be valid reason to wonder if the rising coronary incidence might stem from some emotional interplay associated with newer socioeconomic stresses, acting in pathogenetic conjunction with our high fat diets, relatively high serum lipids, physical indolence and other classic factors. This suspicion appeared possible in spite of the fact that stress of various types has always been integral to all civilizations, even primitive ones today. However, societies with rising socioeconomic standards were fraught with new stresses unique to industrialization and not prevalent in earlier or more primitive groups. Possibly the most unique aspect of these newer stresses is the fast "pace," recognized by our most famous historian, Toynbee,[29] when he wrote that "at the earliest moment at which we catch our first glimpse of man on earth, we find him not only on the move but already moving at an accelerating pace. This crescendo of acceleration is continuing today. In our generation, it is perhaps the most difficult and dangerous of all the current problems of the human race."

Our suspicions about the effects of socioeconomic stresses were strengthened when we examined a group of younger coronary patients and found that the substantial majority of them exhibited a particular personality structure and behavior pattern that we later termed *pattern type A*.[30]

Behavior pattern type A is characterized primarily by aggressiveness, ambition, drive, competitiveness and a profound sense of time urgency. Some or most of these traits are present in various degrees in most men, but the man with pattern type A has them to an excessive and often inordinate degree. Certain typical muscular or motor phenomena are often associated with these emotional traits. Speech[31] is usually forceful, rather rapid, often explosively uneven and emphatic, and accompanied by sudden gestures such as fist clenching and taut facial grimaces. Locomotion and mannerisms are rapid, reflecting enhanced drive, competitive striving, chronic restlessness, impatience and a sense of time urgency. The man with pattern type A appears to be excessively driven to achieve and willingly committed to getting things done, while struggling against the inflexible factor of time itself and the competing and obstructing influences of other persons and things. Thus, he habitually lives under time pressure.

Pattern type A, then, is an interplay of certain personality (endogenous) and environmental (exogenous) factors. It exists particularly in the milieu that characterizes our modern urban civilization.

Because it so commonly accompanies the new socioeconomic stresses unique to our industrialized, mechanized, fast-moving society, it is probably increasingly prevalent in western populations. The pattern type A man, immersed in these new stresses, often seems to be content with his multiple vocational and avocational commitments despite their propensity to produce deadlines enhancing his sense of time urgency. This behavior pattern should not be confused with such emotional responses as simple nervous anxiety and the garden variety of neuroses, as indicated earlier by Osler.[27]

Although we have designated the absence of the type A emotional interplay as the converse pattern type B, it would be erroneous to think of this cleavage as being sharply defined. The man with pattern type A simply exhibits an excessive degree of certain specific emotional traits that may be variously present to a much lesser degree in a man with pattern type B. Thus, the facets of type A can be likened to an elevated body temperature or blood pressure, both of which are normally present in lesser degree in all men. Although no electronic device can quantitate the interplay of such behavioral traits, we have found that a specially devised interview[20] can usually identify the presence of pattern type A. This method has allowed a high degree of rater agreement and has shown that the behavior pattern is stable over a period of time.[32]

In our earlier studies we found that the substantial majority of younger and middle-aged coronary patients exhibited behavior pattern type A, and in prevalence studies found that both male[30] and female[33] groups of type A individuals exhibited significantly higher rates of CHD than did their counterparts with type B. The Western Collaborative Group Study[20-22] already referred to, was undertaken in 1960 as a comprehensive prospective study of the role of behavior pattern and of all factors having possible relevance to the future incidence of CHD. The behavior pattern of these 3,500 participants was determined by means of the structured psychological interview described elsewhere in detail.[20] Clinical CHD has been observed in 195 of 3,182 initially healthy men during the first mean $6^1/_2$ years of follow-up, an annual incidence of 9.4 per 1,000 subjects at risk. CHD occurred in 139 of 1,584 men classified at intake as exhibiting behavior pattern type A, compared to 56 of 1,598 men initially classified as exhibiting pattern type B. The annual incidence of CHD thus was 13.5/1,000 type A men compared to 5.4/1,000 type B men, the differences in morbidity rates being highly significant statistically in the total subjects as well as in two age decades.

TABLE 3

Incidence of CHD in Type A and Type B Subjects

Risk Factor	No. at Risk			No. of CHD (6½ Yr.)			Annual Incidence of CHD (No./1,000 Men at Risk)			
	Total	Type A	Type B	Total	Type A	Type B	Total	Type A	Type B	Significance†
All subjects	3182	1584	1598	195	139	56	9.4	13.5	5.4	.001
Cigarettes:										
0	1651	781	870	72	53	19	6.7	10.4	3.4	.01
16+	1183	643	540	108	78	30	14.0	18.7	8.5	.01
Parental CHD:										
History no	2536	1248	1288	142	104	38	8.6	12.8	4.5	.01
History yes	623	338	285	53	35	18	13.1	15.8	9.7	NS
Diastolic Blood Pressure:										
94—	2866	1415	1451	161	110	51	8.6	12.0	5.4	.01
95+	293	171	122	34	29	5	17.9	26.1	6.3	.01
Cholesterol:										
*224+	1619	778	841	53	37	16	5.0	7.3	2.9	.01
260+	642	354	288	77	54	23	18.5	23.5	12.3	.01
Triglycerides:										
99—	851	403	448	28	20	8	5.1	7.6	2.7	.01
177+	706	358	348	63	45	18	13.7	19.3	8.0	.01
Beta/Alpha LP Ratio:										
*2.03—	1815	892	923	81	62	19	6.9	10.7	3.2	.01
2.36+	989	526	463	88	61	27	13.7	17.8	9.0	.01

*Mean lipid levels for total population.

†P values are based on chi square test with correction for continuity (Yates).

If the relationship of pattern type A to the coronary incidence is merely result of its association with some other risk factor, then stratifying by values of that factor should reduce the relationship to negligible levels. The results of such an exercise are shown in Table 3, where it can be seen that the significantly higher incidence of CHD in type A men was found to prevail even when the behavior pattern was stratified by high or low levels of the classic risk factors. Indeed, in most instances it can further be noted that the coronary incidence in type A men with a *low* level of some other risk factor approximated the incidence in type B men with a *high* level of the respective other characteristic. The CHD incidence in type A and type B men exhibiting various combinations of risk factors at high and low levels is shown in Table 4, with similar results. It is worthy of emphasis that, among subjects with low levels of these multiple risk factors, a significant incidence of CHD was still observed in type A men, but was very low in men with pattern type B, as previously noted.[23]

The results of our own studies would appear to indicate clearly that the personality and behavior pattern of an individual is significantly and independently related to his prospective candidacy for CHD. These results also indicate that clinical assessment of an individual's behavior pattern not only helps to define coronary-proneness but also considerably enhances the individual predictive specificity of other more widely-used risk attributes.

Psychological factors, as they relate to the occurrence of CHD, have undergone considerable clinical and experimental research, but much of this earlier work has resulted in equivocal or even ambiguous findings.[34] Some of the more recent studies have indicated that the incidence of CHD may be increased in individuals who have experienced increased sociocultural mobility and other marked change within their cultural settings,[35] as well as in individuals with enhanced occupational stress.[36] The extensive literature in this regard cannot be reviewed here, particularly since only empirical investigation rather than opinion biased pro or con, can answer the question of whether social and psychological factors are involved in the pathogenesis of CHD.

One study should be described, however, since it is the first independent assessment of the role of pattern type A in the incidence of CHD. Quinlan, Barrow and their associates utilized our psychological interview[20] in an extensive survey of Benedictine and Trappist monks in North America. Their investigating psychologist, Dr. Bernard Caffrey,[34] visited our laboratory to gain precise knowledge of our interview methods in order to accomplish this survey. Their preliminary results lend considerable confirmation to the role of the behavior pattern in the pathogenesis of CHD. Thus they found that the prevalence of angina pectoris was more than twice as frequent and that of myocardial infarction more than four times as frequent in monks who had been assessed as exhibiting the type A behavior pattern, compared to otherwise comparable monks with pattern type B behavior.[37]

It is also pertinent that Brozek, Keys and Blackburn[38] employed psychological investigations in the course of their prospective study and found that their potential candidates for CHD, compared to men who remained clinically normal during 14 years of follow-up, had exhibited a higher activity drive, were more "masculine" in their interests, were more likely to be "on the go" and to "speak, walk, write, drive, work and eat fast", even when they did not have to do so—a quite accurate description of the type A individual. The differences between the potential coronary candidates and the control group were statistically significant.

Epidemiological correlations do not establish a cause-and-effect relationship per se. Accordingly, if pattern type A bears a causal relationship to clinical CHD, it should be possible to ascertain the pathogenetic relationships. One possible association, of course, would merely be that pattern type A enhances proneness to the thrombotic complications of an already diseased coronary artery. However, a more significant relationship is indicated by the fact that men with pattern type A not only exhibit higher coronary morbidity and mortality rates but also significantly more severe basic coronary atherosclerosis than do men with the converse pattern type B.[39] Moreover, we have found that men with fully developed type A also exhibit various congeners related to the pathogenesis of CHD. Thus, type A individuals exhibit more rapid blood coagulation,[25,30] higher blood levels of cholesterol, triglycerides and beta lipoproteins,[30,33,41] augmented postprandial hypertriglyceridemia and capillary sludging with delay in clearance of an ingested test fat meal,[42] and augmented excretion of norepinephrine during their challenging daytime occupational milieu.[43]

Additional possible neurohumoral pathways are under current investigation. The considerable number of studies of serum lipids and lipoproteins in correlation with different personality and behavioral traits has recently been reviewed.[41] The results leave little doubt that an individual's serum lipid levels are significantly related to his personality, higher levels being variously observed in men who are more competitive, ambitious, aggressive, restlessly impatient, active and over-conscientious.

Taken in their entirety, the present results indicate that a certain emotional interplay plays an important causal role in the pathogenesis of coronary heart disease. Although much remains to be learned about this relationship, the data indicate that at this juncture both the researcher and the clinician must include an evaluation of such factors in their respective approaches if progress is to be made in the prevention of this major affliction.

REFERENCES

1. Epstein, F.: The epidemiology of coronary heart disease: A review. J. Chronic Dis., *18:*735, 1965.
2. Osler, W.: The Lumleian lectures on angina pectoris. Lancet, *1:*839, 1910.
3. Michaels, L.: Aetiology of coronary artery disease: An historical approach. Brit. Heart Jr., *28:*258-264, Mar. 1966.
4. Spain, D. M.: Problems in the study of coronary atherosclerosis in population groups. Ann. N. Y. Acad. Sci. *84:*816, 1960.
5. Morris, J. N.: Recent history of coronary disease.

TABLE 4

Prospective High and Low Risk Factors and Incidence of CHD in Type A and B Subjects

Risk Factors	Type A Subjects		Type B Subjects		Annual Incidence of CHD (No./1,000 Men at Risk)			
	No. at Risk	No. CHD	No. at Risk	No. CHD	All Subjects	Type A	Type B	Significance†
All Subjects	1584	139	1598	56	9.4	13.5	5.4	.001
Subjects with High Risk Factors								
Tglyc. 177+, B/A 2.36+	201	30	180	13	17.4	23.0	11.1	.05
Chol. 260+, Cigs. 16+	167	30	122	13	22.9	27.6	16.4	—
Chol. 260+, Tglyc. 177+	137	24	116	8	19.5	26.9	10.6	.05
Chol. 260+, Tglyc. 177+, B/A 2.36+	99	19	69	6	22.9	29.5	13.4	—
Chol. 260+, Diast. BP 95+	49	14	25	1	31.2	44.0	6.2	.05
Chol. 260+, Cigs. 16+, DBP 95+	22	7	11	0	32.6	48.9	0.0	—
Subjects with Low Risk Factors								
Chol. 259−, DBP 94−	1110	70	1188	29	6.6	9.7	3.8	.01
Chol. 259−, Cigs. 0, DBP 94−	554	27	669	10	4.7	7.5	2.3	.01
Chol. 259−,Tglyc.176−,B/A 2.35−	750	44	807	17	6.0	9.0	3.2	.01
*Chol. 224−,Tglyc.147−,B/A 2.03−	446	20	471	6	4.4	6.9	2.0	.01
*Chol. 224−, Cigs. 0	411	15	517	7	3.7	5.6	2.1	.05

* Mean lipid levels for total population.

† P values are based on chi square test with correction for continuity (Yates).

Lancet, *1:*1-7, Jan. 6, 1951.

6. Saphir, O., Ohringer, L. and Silverstone, H.: Coronary arteriosclerotic heart disease in younger age groups: Its greater frequency in this group among increasingly older necropsy population. Amer. J. Med. Sci., *231:*494-501, May 1956.

7. Friedman, M. and Rosenman, R. H.: Etiology and pathogenesis of coronary heart disease. In Cardiovascular Disorders. Philadelphia, F. A. Davis, 1968.

8. Trulson, M. F.: The American diet: Past and present. Amer. J. Clin. Nutr., *7:*91-97, 1959.

9. Yudkin, J.: Diet and coronary thrombosis; hypothesis and fact. Lancet, *2:*155-162, July 27, 1957.

10. Shaper, A. G.: Cardiovascular studies in the Samburu tribe of northern Kenya. Amer. Heart J., *63:*437, 1962.

11. Paul, O., Lepper, M. H., Phelan, W. F., Dupertuis, G. W., MacMillan, A., McKean, H. and Park, H.: A longitudinal study of coronary heart disease. Circulation, *28:*20, 1963.

12. Keys, A. and Blackburn, H.: Background of the patient with coronary heart disease. Progr. Cardiovasc. Dis., *6:*14, 1963.

13. Gofman, J. W., Hanig, M., Jones, H. B., Lauffer, M. A., Lowry, E. Y., Lewis, L. A., Mann, G. V., Moore, F. E., Olmstead, F., Yeager, J. F., Andrus, E. C., Barach, J. H., Beams, J. W., Fertig, J. W., Page. I. H., Shannon, J. A., Stare, F. J. and White, P. D.: Evaluation of serum lipoprotein and cholesterol measurements as predictors of clinical complications of atherosclerosis. Report of a cooperative study of lipoproteins and atherosclerosis. Circulation, *14:*691, 1956.

14. Hatch, F. T., Reisell, P. K., Poon-King, T. M. W., Canellas, G. P., Lees, R. S. and Hagopian, L. M.: A study of coronary heart disease in young men: Characteristics and metabolic studies of patients and comparison with age-matched healthy men. Circulation, *33:*679, 1966.

15. Rosenman, R. H., Friedman, M. and Boasberg, S.: Lack of correlation of serum cholesterol and habitual diet. Circulation, *24:*1024, 1961.

16. Morris, J. N., Marr, J. W., Heady, J. A., Mills, G. L. and Pilkington, T. R. E.: Diet and plasma cholesterol in 99 bank men. Brit. Med. J., *1:*571, 1963.

17. Morris, J. N., Heady, J. A., Raffle, P. A. B., Roberts, C. G. and Parks, J. W.: Coronary heart disease and physical activity of work. Lancet, *2:*1053, 1111, 1953.

18. Morris, J. N. and Crawford, M. D.: Coronary heart disease and physical activity of work. Brit. Med. J., *2:*1485, 1958.

19. Rosenman, R. H.: The influence of different exercise patterns on the incidence of coronary heart disease in the Western Collaborative Group Study. Medicine and Sport, Vol. 4, Physical Activity and Aging. Basel/New York, Karger, 1969.

20. Rosenman, R. H., Friedman, M., Straus, R., Wurm, M., Kositchek, R., Hahn, W. and Werthessen, N. T.: A predictive study of coronary heart disease: The Western Collaborative Group Study. J.A.M.A., *189:*15-26, July 6, 1964.

21. Rosenman, R. H., Friedman, M., Straus, R., Wurm, M., Jenkins, C. D., Messinger, H. B., Kositchek, R., Hahn, W. and Werthessen, N. T.: Coronary heart disease in the Western Collaborative Group Study: A follow-up experience of two years. J.A.M.A., *195:*86-92, Jan. 10, 1966.

22. Rosenman, R. H., Friedman, M., Straus, R., Jenkins, C. D., Zyzanski, S. J., Wurm, M. and Kositchek, R.: Coronary heart disease in the Western Collaborative Group Study. A follow-up experience of 4½ years. Submitted for publication.

23. Rosenman, R. H., Friedman, M., Jenkins, C. D., Straus, R., Wurm, M. and Kositchek, R.: The prediction of immunity to coronary heart disease. JAMA, *198:*1159-1162, 1966.

24. Friedman, M. and Rosenman, R. H.: Comparison of fat intake of American and men women; possible relationship to incidence of clinical coronary artery disease. Circulation, *16:*339-347, Sept. 1957.

25. Friedman, M., Rosenman, R. H. and Carroll, V.: Changes in the serum cholesterol and blood clotting time in men subjected to cyclic variation of occupational stress. Circulation, *17:*852-861, May 1958.

26. Bronte-Stewart, B., Keys, A. and Brock, J. F.: Serum cholesterol, diet and coronary heart disease: An inter-racial survey in the Cape Peninsula. Lancet, *2:*1103, 1955.

27. Osler, W.: Lectures on angina pectoris and allied states. New York, D. Appleton & Co., 1897.

28. Gertler, M. and White, P. D.: Coronary disease in young adults: A multidisciplinary study. Cambridge, Harvard Univ., 1954.

29. Toynbee, A.: A study of history. Vol. 12. London, Oxford University Press, 1961, p. 603.

30. Friedman, M. and Rosenman, R. H.: Association of specific overt behavior pattern with blood and cardiovascular findings; blood cholesterol level, blood clotting time, incidence of arcus senilis, and clinical coronary artery disease. JAMA, *169:*1286-1296, Mar. 21, 1959.

31. Friedman, M., Brown, A. E. and Rosenman, R. H.: Voice analysis test for detection of behavior pattern. J. Am. Med. Assoc., *208:*828-836, 1969.

32. Jenkins, C. D., Rosenman, R. H. and Friedman, M.: Replicability of ratings the coronary-prone behavior pattern. Brit. J. Prev. & Social Med., *22:*16-22, 1968.

33. Rosenman, R. H. and Friedman, M.: Association of specific behavior pattern in women with blood and cardiovascular findings. Circulation, *24:*1173-1184, Nov. 1961.

34. Caffrey, B.: Interpersonal and psychological characteristics in cardiovascular disease: A review of empirical findings. Milbank Memorial Fund Quarterly, Part 2, *45:*119-139, 1967.

35. Syme, S. L. and Reeder, L. G. (eds.): Social stress and cardiovascular disease. Milbank Memorial Fund Quarterly, Part 2, *45:*9-192, 1967.

36. Russek, H. I.: Stress, tobacco, and coronary disease in North American professional groups. J. Amer. Med. Assoc., *192:*189-194, Apr. 19, 1965.

37. Quinlan, C. B., Barrow, J. G., Hayes, C. G., Moinuddin, M. and Goodloe, M. H.: The association of risk factors and coronary heart disease in Trappist and Benedictine Monks. Proceedings of Conference on Epidemiology, American Heart Assoc., New Orleans, March 3, 1969.

38. Brozek, J., Keys, A. and Blackburn, H.: Personality difference between potential coronary and non-coronary subjects. Ann. N. Y. Acad. Sci., *134:*

1057-1064, 1966.

39. Friedman, M., Rosenman, R. H., Straus, R., Wurm, M. and Kositchek, R.: The relationship of behavior pattern A to the state of the coronary vasculature. Am. J. Med., *44:*525-537, 1967.

40. Jenkins, C. D., Hames, C. G., Zyzanski, S. J., Rosenman, R. H. and Friedman, M.: Psychological traits and serum lipids. I. Findings from the California Psychological Inventory. Psychosomatic Med. Vol. XXXI, No. 2, Mar.-Apr. 1969.

41. Rosenman, R. H. and Friedman, M.: Behavior patterns, blood lipids, and coronary heart disease.

J.A.M.A., *184:*934-938, June 22, 1963.

42. Friedman, M., Rosenman, R. H. and Byers, S. O.: Serum lipids and conjunctival circulation after fat ingestion in men exhibiting Type-A behavior pattern. Circulation, *29:*874–886, June 1964.

43. Friedman, M., St. George, S., Byers, S. O. and Rosenman, R. H.: Excretion of catecholamines, 17-ketosteroids, 17-hydroxycorticoids and 5-hydroxy-indole in men exhibiting a particular behavior pattern (A) associated with high incidence of clinical coronary artery disease. J. Clin. Invest., *39:*758-764, May 1960.

The Complex Pathogenesis of So-Called "Coronary" Heart Disease

Wilhelm Raab

Scientific concepts in biology and medicine are not much less subject to change than political, ethical and esthetic views, and dissensions between defenders of older and proponents of newer thoughts constitute natural ingredients of progress. There have been times when miasmas and ptomaines were accepted causes of disease, but the terms have disappeared with the development of keener insight based on more precise facts.

In the problem area of pathogenesis of degenerative heart disease, changes of interpretation have not occurred with dramatic speed, but it is being increasingly realized that we have imperceptibly entered a new era. After a half-century of nearly complete preoccupation with the heart muscle's vascular "plumbing," the myocardium itself and its highly vulnerable metabolic equilibrium are gradually becoming recognized as the most immediately concerned victims of coronary vascular, as well as of usually coincident nonvascular, potentially fatal, pathogenic mechanisms.

Significant advances in formerly technically inaccessible realms of information concerning myocardial oxygen economy and electrolyte balance, and their regulation by powerful neuroendocrine and hormonal interferences, have made it clear that the traditional, one-sidedly vascular approach to basic problems of cardiac pathophysiology has become inadequate, and that it is in need of drastic modifications and amplifications.

A wider and faster acceptance of emerging modern concepts would probably be possible were it not for a deeply ingrained, but outdated and chaotic, clinical nomenclature which has for decades revolved around the conveniently intelligible and acoustically appealing, but often misplaced word "coronary." It exemplifies J. W. Hurst's recent statement[1] that "words can prevent learning."

In order not to antagonize the still numerous,

This work was, in part, supported by research grants from the National Heart Institute (HE-02169 and HE-09184), and from the Vermont Heart Association (AG-48).

staunch adherents of the popular cliché, "CHD" (Coronary Heart Disease), and to employ it instead as a subtle disguise for the gradual dissemination of up-to-date concepts, it is suggested that its use be continued by alerted contemporaries for the time being, with the tacit understanding that it should stand for the more realistic (even though cumbersome) "Cardiac Hypoxic Dysionism." Reasons for this subversive proposal will be give in the following discussion.

In the first place, it must be pointed out that, apart from the no longer tenable view concerning an exclusive primacy of "atherosclerosis" in myocardial degenerative pathology, the legitimacy of the term "infarction," with reference to commonly designated instances of major necrotic myocardial tissue destruction, has likewise come under serious doubt.

No evidence of vascular occlusion was found in more than 50 per cent of meticulously examined freshly "infarcted" human hearts,[2-5] and where thrombi actually did exist, their estimated age and their location suggested in many cases that they had developed later than the clinically observed "heart attack," and in no regular topical relation to the areas of necrosis.[3,5,6] On the other hand, severely stenosing, or even occluding coronary arterial lesions remain not infrequently unassociated with significant structural lesions of the heart muscle.[3,7]

Thus, a vascular obstructive origin, i.e., the logical prerequisite for correct use of the term "infarction," has become questionable for a not clearly determined but probably overwhelming majority of more or less extensive myocardial necroses.

An increasing number of pathologists[8-11] are leaning toward the view that the *formation of composite "infarcts" is to be explained by a confluence of pre-existing or fresh, separate, multifocal, non-thrombotic micronecroses* in areas of poor collateral development and under the impact of acutely triggering circumstances, such as an increase in mechanical workload or an emotionally or physically stressful situation.

METABOLIC PHYSIOPATHOLOGICAL ELEMENTS

From this point of view, the primary pathogenesis of previously overlooked microfocal myocardial lesions steps into the foreground of pathogenic considerations, and it becomes mandatory that more attention be given to a vast body of available but widely disregarded experimental observations concerning the origin of focal necroses.

Since Josué's discovery[12] that *injection of large doses of epinephrine is followed by the appearance of scattered necrotic foci in the myocardium,* this phenomenon has been confirmed in numerous subsequent studies over the following 60 years, but its clinical pathological implications remained largely ignored, until causal relations between the syndrome of angina pectoris and the sympathoadrenal system were recognized.[13]

Identical necrotic lesions can be produced by the exogenous administration of the catecholamines, epinephrine and norepinephrine, and by intensive stimulation of the central and peripheral neurones of the sympathetic nervous system.[7,14]

The *hypoxic nature of catecholamine-induced cardiac lesions* is suggested by the analogous morphologic appearance and local distribution, as well as by the histochemical characteristics (e.g., loss of glycogen and potassium) of changes, induced by oxygen deprivation and by toxic catecholamine action.[23]

The specific location of most of the catecholamine-induced necrotic foci in the subendocardial layers of the left ventricle[14,15] and in the papillary muscles seems to be due to the microcirculatory disadvantages of intraventricular, hydrostatic, vascular compression[16] and of falling intramural perfusion pressure gradients[17] in those areas of the heart muscle.

The peculiar confinement of hypoxic changes to scattered, spotty cell groups may be explained by microcirculatory mechanisms ("breadline" hypothesis[7,15] which jeopardize the oxygen supply, particularly of cells which are located at the end of long capillaries (Fig. 1).

Under normal circumstances, the inevitable *augmentation of myocardial oxygen consumption under increased adrenosympathetic catecholamine action* (physical effort, emotional excitement, nicotine, etc.) does not induce hypoxia in the myocardial tissue because of the simultaneous compensatory dilatation of the coronary system and the resulting increase in blood supply.[18,19]

However, if amounts of catecholamines are ex-

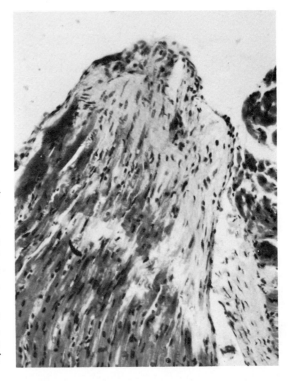

Fig. 1.   Necroses at the end of long capillaries in tip of papillary muscle of the rat, induced by stress plus cortisol plus sodium sulphate. (After J. Văsků et al.[20])

cessive (e.g., due to pheochromocytomas or overdosage), or if compensatory coronary dilatability is impaired by atherosclerosis or experimental restriction, sympathetic stimulation results promptly in hypoxia of the myocardial areas involved.[21]

This long opposed but now generally accepted concept applies to situations known to cause anginal pain.[22] The anginal syndrome is associated with usually marked elevations of the catecholamine level in the blood.[7,22,23] In recent years it has been studied in detail by Gorlin,[24] employing a method whereby an excess production of lactate in hypoxic regions of the left ventricle could be located by means of catheterization of the coronary venous system.[25]

In assessing the quantitative relationship between the amounts of oxygen consumed by the heart muscle and simultaneously performed external mechanical work, it should be kept in mind that *under catecholamine action, oxidative energetic "efficiency" is considerably reduced* in an uneconomic fashion, presumably due to the typical, adrenergic acceleration of intrinsic velocity of ventricular contraction.[26] Thus, the pain-producing, sympathogenic augmentation of myocardial oxygen consumption cannot be attributed simply to an increase of ventricular "work" but rather to the specifically adrenergic, "oxygenwasting" mechanism which causes it.

A cardiometabolic factor of the utmost importance for anomalies of myocardial structure as well as of contractile function and rhythmicity are the *electrolyte derangements which are inseparably connected with any significant lack of oxygen within the myocardial cells.*

The normally functioning so-called "ionic pump" guarantees the transmembranous re-entry of systolically extruded potassium and magnesium against

toxic catecholamine action causes marked focal, potassium displacements in the myocardium within minutes (Fig. 2).

The need of adequate potassium and magnesium stores, as such, for maintenance of myocardial cell structural integrity is evident from the fact that mere dietary withholding of these ions causes severe, massive, subendocardial necrosis[27] in the absence of any hypoxia-producing, vascular or other noxious factors, and that these necroses can be prevented by timely administration of potassium and magnesium

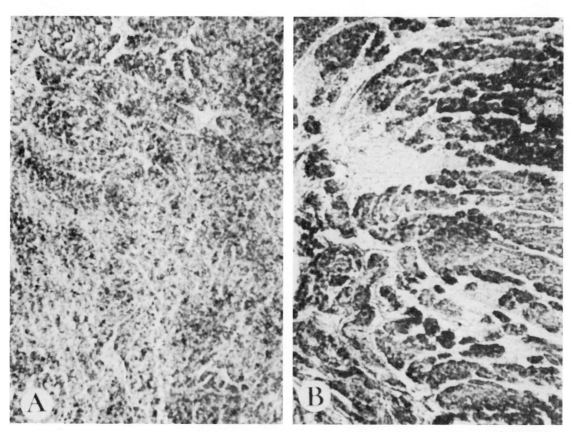

FIG. 2. Potassium distribution in the rat's left ventricular subendocardium. (A) Control. Homogenous distribution of potassium ions. (B) 35 minutes after s.c. injection of *epinephrine* (4.5 μg/g): Spotty depletion and adjacent accumulation of potassium. (After E. Bajusz: Electrolytes and Cardiovascular Diseases, Baltimore, Williams and Wilkins, 1966, vol. I, p. 303).

their respective gradients into the cellular space during the diastolic phase of "restitution," and it expels sodium ions which had replaced intracellular potassium during systole.

If this mechanism, which depends primarily on oxidative energy production, fails, the cells lose potassium and gain extra sodium to the detriment of their structure, contractility, and electrical equilibrium.[27] Histochemical studies have shown that

salts.

Myocardial contractility likewise depends to a large extent on the availability of sufficient intracellular potassium. This was domonstrated by the fact that totally anoxic, adynamic hearts can be, at least temporarily, restored to full contractile power by perfusion with "polarizing" potassium solutions without added oxygen.[28] Relations between potassium, sodium and calcium ions in the mechanism of

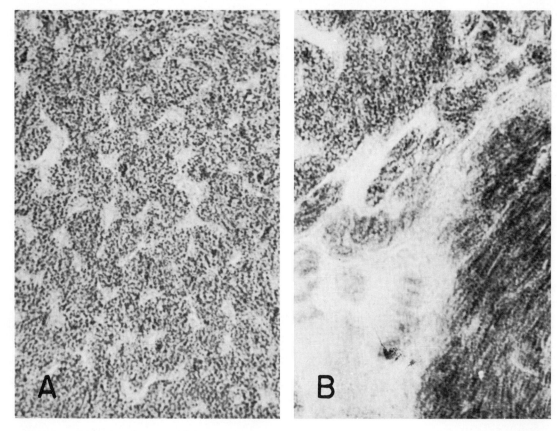

FIG. 3.   Corollary to Fig. 2. (A) Control. Small gray spots are artifacts caused by freezing. (B) Similar potassium displacements as in Fig. 2, produced in isolation-stressed, corticoid-sensitized rat by injection of only 1/18th of epinephrine dose, used in experiment of Fig. 2 (30 minutes after injection). (After W. Raab, E. Bajusz, H. Kimura and H. C. Herrlich: Proc. Soc. Exper. Med. & Biol., *127*:142, 1968.)

myocardial contractility are still incompletely understood.[27]

The crucial role of an adequate electrolyte balance in the heart muscle's physiology and pathophysiology seems to constitute the basis for the cardiac complications arising from adrenergically or otherwise induced states of myocardial, potassium-depleting, cell hypoxia.

Beyond the neurohormonal aspects of pathogenic myocardial electrolyte derangements, the important phenomenon of *adrenal corticoid-induced, marked potentiation of catecholamine cardiotoxicity*[29-34] (Fig. 3) seems to be attributable to an additional, equidirectional interference of glucocorticoids (notably cortisol), and, to a lesser degree, of mineralocorticoids (aldosterone) in myocardial electrolyte balance[27] (Fig. 4).

So far, the apparent pathogenic role of adrenal cortical overactivity in human myocardial pathology has, unfortunately, not been studied in depth, and Selye's extensive experimental investigations concerning that fundamental problem[29,30] have not yet

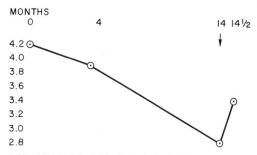

REDUCTION OF K/Na RATIO DURING PROLONGED ISOLATION AND RISE AFTER RETURN INTO COMMUNITY

FIG. 4.   Electrolyte imbalance (reduction of K/Na) in the rat's myocardium, caused by the environmental-emotional stress of prolonged isolation, which is associated with an increased production of corticoids and a marked augmentation of catecholamine cardiotoxicity; return toward normal after termination of stress (Conf. Figs. 2 and 3) (After W. Raab, E. Bajusz, H. Kimura and H. C. Herrlich: Proc. Soc. Exper. Biol. & Med. *127*:142, 1968.)

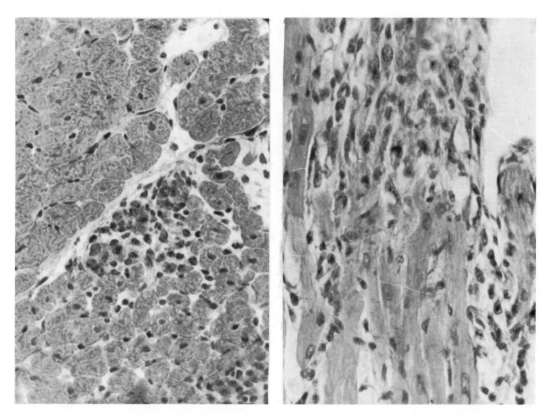

FIG. 5. Subendocardial necroses, produced in wild rats (69% of series) by one-week exposure to anxiety stress (tape-recorded noise of cat-rat fight; alternating 15 minute periods of noise and of quiet). (After W. Raab, J. P. Chaplin and E. Bajusz, Proc. Soc. Exper. Biol. & Med., *116:*665, 1964.)

been widely incorporated into clinical reasoning.

However, clues concerning an outstanding involvement of adrenocortical overfunction in the origin of degenerative heart disease are available in the well-known facts that (a) Cushing's syndrome (hyperadrenocorticism) is frequently complicated by myocardial necrotic lesions and failure,[14,35-37] but only relatively rarely by coronary atherosclerosis[36] (b) that such features are practically nonexistent in Addison's disease; (c) that in certain cases of congestive heart failure adrenalectomy has been found therapeutically effective; and (d) that substitutive overtreatment of hypoadrenocorticism with corticoids is prone to provoke severe cardiac complications.[14]

The highly cardiotoxic, necrotizing effect of an experimental combination of per se subthreshold doses of injected or secreted catecholamines and glucocorticoids[29-34] (Fig. 4) suggests that both components may contribute jointly to clinical heart disease under notoriously catecholamine-plus corticoid-liberating conditions; i.e. environmental emotional stresses[38,39] (Fig. 5) and tobacco smoking.[40]

The apparently dual, neurogenic plus hormonal pathogenic background of degenerative, so-called "coronary" heart disease is conspicuously reflected in an increased incidence of hyperglycemia and diabetes in such cases,[41,42] since both catecholamine and glucocorticoid overactivity are known to elicit corresponding disturbances in carbohydrate metabolism.[23]

CLINICAL IMPLICATIONS OF MYOCARDIAL METABOLIC PATHOPHYSIOLOGY

The longest known causal connection between cardiac neurogenic adrenergic mechanisms and pathologic clinical manifestations exists in the one syndrome in which the primacy of coronary vascular pathology is also most convincingly established,[24,44] namely, *angina pectoris.* Here, a major degree of usually atherosclerotic vascular narrowing can be held responsible for the vast majority of instances.

Apart from the known elevations of the plasma catecholamine level during anginal attacks,[7,43] indirect evidence of the latters' adrenergic nature is provided by the therapeutic effectiveness of various antiadrenergic measures (thoracic sympathectomy, beta receptor blockade, vagal stimulation, hyper-catecholemia-reducing roentgen irradiation of the adrenal glands, catecholamine-inactivating thyrostatic procedures, etc.)[22,14]

We do not know exactly what is going on behind the scenes in the heart muscle's microstructure during and after the brief episodes of intensive myocardial hypoxia which constitute the essence of the anginal attacks, but the opinion has frequently been expressed that many, if not all of them, leave their marks in the form of necrotic foci, the apparent forerunners and "building stones" of later developing "infarctions."

This concept, if true to facts, would assign to the *catecholamine-liberating adrenosympathetic system* and to its well-known civilization-induced overactivity (sedentary living; automobile-driving[45,46] environmental-emotional and other stresses; nicotine[7,27] an initiating role in the *pathogenic antecedents of the "infarction" process*. However, the difference in appearence between the typically catecholamine-induced, focal distribution of small tissue necroses, and the full-fledged, massive "infarct" would require the assumption of an additional factor or factors for explanation. In view of the ability to produce experimentally widespread "infarctoid,"[29,31] myocardial necroses by catecholamine action (injected or stress-induced) in corticoid-pretreated animals, one might suspect a significant contribution of *exaggerated glucocorticoid action* to be involved in expansive tissue destructions also in man.

Glucocorticoids (especially cortisol) are liberated in excess together with catecholamines under a great variety of physical, emotional, and sensory stresses and everyday annoyances[27,38,39] (Fig. 6) (with exception of the "pseudo-stress" of moderate physical exercise,[27] as well as during and after automobile-driving[45] and tobacco smoking.[40,47] Their prolonged metabolic action in the heart muscle is not limited to certain vascularly handicapped areas like the focally circumscribed, cardiotoxic, hypoxia-producing effects of adrenergic neurohormones. This may account for the wider dimensions and more diffuse character of jointly coronary vascular, neurogenic-adrenergic, and adrenocortical myocardial tissue destructions of the "infarction" type.

It is a matter of common knowledge that *myocardial "infarction" involves severe derangements of the affected heart muscle's electrolyte balance.* The necrotic center of an "infarcted" area is depleted of potassium and magnesium, and contains a high concentration of sodium. Fresh "infarcts" are tem-

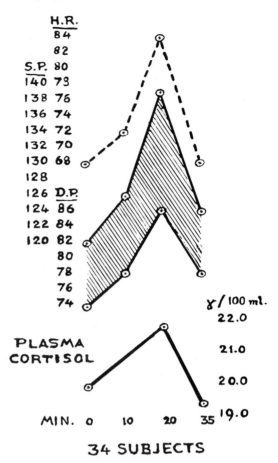

FIG. 6. Simultaneous adrenergic cardiovascular (heart rate, blood pressure) and adrenocortical (plasma cortisol) response to 20 minutes of sensory plus mental annoyances (mental arithmetic, telephone bell-ringing, flicker light), followed by 15 minutes of recovery. (After W. Raab.[39])

porarily surrounded by "walls" of extruded potassium.[27] Similarly, extruded potassium accumulates near catecholamine-induced hypoxic microfoci (Figs. 2, 3). Both types of abnormal potassium gradients (intra-extracellular and topical) seem to be essentially responsible for the post-"infarction" changes of T and S-T in the electrocardiogram.

Aside from electrolyte shifts in and around the "infarct" itself, it was found in autopsied hearts that after recent "infarction" all other ventricular areas display similar electrolyte derangements (low potassium and magnesium, high sodium) of a major degree[27] (Fig. 7).

It is not yet possible to decide whether and to what extent these marked distortions of the general electrolyte equilibrium of both ventricles had preceded the "infarction" as a result of pre-existing,

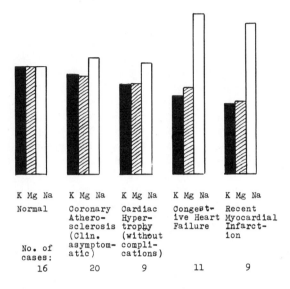

K Mg Na	K Mg Na	K Mg Na	K Mg Na	K Mg Na
Normal	Coronary Athero- sclerosis (Clin. asymptom- atic)	Cardiac Hyper- trophy (without compli- cations)	Congest- ive Heart Failure	Recent Myocardial Infarct- ion

No. of cases:

| 16 | 20 | 9 | 11 | 9 |

FIG. 7. Electrolytes in 5 pooled sections each from the left ventricles of autopsied human hearts; represented as percentile deviations from "normal" averages. (After W. Raab.[27]) (This study is still in progress.)

vascularly induced hypoxia (Fig. 7) and the presence of microfocal lesions, or originated during the postinfarction stress period, when both catecholamines and cortisol circulate within the blood in abnormally large amounts.[27]

Presumably, all of these vascular and nonvascular factors participate in creating a metabolic situation which is functionally highly critical and which is also characterized by a ubiqitous loss of high energy phosphates.[48] It can be assumed to account for the hazards of the first postinfarction days with regard to both rhythmicity and contractility of the heart.

Myocardial electrolyte derangements are of fundamental importance for *abnormalities in electrical stimulus formation and conduction.*[49-51] Localized "trigger zones"[49] exist in myocardial areas, affected by vascular and/or catecholamine-induced, cardiotoxic hypoxia and electrolyte imbalance. Specific features of catecholamine action which promote the occurrence of atrial and ventricular arrhythmias, ranging from isolated premature contractions to fatal ventricular fibrillation, are: an augmentation of pacemaker activity, shortening of the action potential and of the refractory period, and an increased asynchrony of recovery and excitability.[52,55] These changes contribute to a lowering of the threshold for the emergence of ectopic beats in response to accessory electrical, mechanical and other stimuli.

Such stimuli arise frequently under emotionally and physically stressful conditions. *Sudden, unexpected cardiac death* occurs in cases of pheochromocytoma and in seemingly healthy individuals during "sympathetic storms." Excessively high catecholamine concentrations have been found post mortem in the blood[56] and heart muscle[57-59] in such instances, and abnormally low myocardial K:Na ratios seem to be characteristic of sudden deaths which had occurred from apparently cardiac causes.[60]

Vagal cholinergic overactivity, if colliding with sympathetic stimulation, seems to be involved in the origin of atrial fibrillation[61] and, by itself, in the mechanism of potentially fatal cardiac standstill due to atrioventricular conduction block.[62,63]

Contractile failure of the ventricles develops basically as a result of metabolic derangements which derive largely from cellular hypoxia and from its detrimental effects on myocardial phosphate metabolism, energy utilization, and electrolyte balance.[28,64]

Apart from predisposing structural alterations of the heart muscle (necroses, fibrosis), congestive heart failure is commonly elicited by acute or chronic, hypoxia-producing, adrenergic overaction in the presence of coronary, flow-limiting, vascular changes, and/or by mechanical overstrain of the heart muscle which induces similar metabolic reactions.[28,64] The levels of potassium and magnesium in the myocardium of patients who had died from congestive heart failure are always found to be deeply depressed, whereas sodium is markedly increased[27] (Fig. 7) in accordance with the typical hypoxia-and/or corticoid-induced pattern of electrolyte imbalance.[27]

Acute congestive heart failure of the left ventricle (pulmonary edema) occurs in cases of pheochromocytoma or after intensive stimulation of the adrenosympathetic system, especially in predamaged hearts.

The myocardial contractile protein fraction, myosin, was found diminished in hypoxia[65] and under the influence of cardiac protein-catabolic glucocorticoid overaction[66,67] which is usually present in chronic congestive heart failure,[23] possibly as a secondary, stress-induced phenomenon.

A complicating overproduction of aldosterone[68] probably mediated by angiotensin,[69] often contributes to the retention of sodium and water, thus constituting an additional aggravating factor in established congestive heart failure.

The epinephrine content of failing human hearts is not infrequently augmented, especially in an acute episode culminating in death.[59] By contrast, myocardial neurogenic norepinephrine has been found considerably decreased in congestive heart failure, [59,70] as well as in other types of myocardial damage without overt cardiac decompensation (myocardial hypertrophy, fibrosis, infarction, uremia, etc.)[59] in man and in animals.[71,72] This phenomenon does not seem to play a major causal role in the initiating mechanisms of contractile failure, also in view of the fact that cardiac catecholamine-depleting sympathectomy and drugs do not usually elicit contractile insufficiency.

Plasma catecholamine levels are frequently elevated in cases of congestive heart failure, especially during exercise[73,74] and during acute episodes of left ventricular failure.[13,75]

A certain degree of participation of *extracardiac adrenergic mechanisms* in the perpetuation of chronic congestive left ventricular failure is suggested both by the above mentioned indications of increased catecholamine production and by functional and metabolic criteria, such as a usually accelerated heart rate, a reduced efficiency of myocardial oxidative energy production,[76,77] and the occasional therapeutic effectiveness of essentially antiadrenergic measures, such as ganglionic blockade, sympathectomy, and catecholamine-desensitizing thyrostatic therapy.[14]

Elimination of corticoid overproduction by subtotal or total adrenalectomy has been found therapeutically useful in cases of intractable cardiac failure with severe hypertension[14] and antiadrenocortical drugs (spironolactone, aldactone) have proved effective in the control of cardiac edema.[78,79]

Thus, the principle of combined catecholamine and corticoid cardiotoxicity appears to be involved not only in the development of preinsufficiency myocardial, metabolic and structural alterations but also in that of final contractile failure itself.

PREVENTIVE ASPECTS

Rational preventive action against any disease depends largely, if not entirely, on an up-to-date insight into its fundamental causes. Pluricausal degenerative, so-called "coronary" or "ischemic" heart disease is no exception to this axiom.

Clinical observations and epidemiology have contributed much toward a tentative correlation of some superficially conspicuous, functional and morphologic, cardiovascular phenomena from the point of view of their possible cardiopathogenic significance. However, like the bulk of the proverbial iceberg, the originally obscure fundamental principles of myocardial metabolism under interacting vascular, autonomic nervous, and hormonal influences were hidden

for a long time beneath the surface in the semi-darkness of basic animal and laboratory experimentation. Thus the, as it were, underwater information explosion of recent years remained widely unnoticed by clinicians and policy-making health agencies. Consequently, certain fundamental points were and still are being missed in the current interpretation of the results of otherwise valuable, statistical mass studies, which had been tailored from the beginning to fit customary, but too narrowly limited, concepts of pathogenesis.

In the foregoing pages, a clearer semantic and cogitative discrimination between the pathology of the coronary arteries on the one hand, and that of the heart muscle on the other, has been postulated. The need for categorical clarity applies likewise to the definitions of preventive angiology (referring chiefly to vascular atherogenesis) and preventive cardiology (referring to the pathophysiology and vulnerability of the myocardium as such).

This writer initiated nearly 40 years ago a preliminary worldwide epidemiologic inquiry concerning the role of dietary factors (animal fats and cholesterol) in atherogenesis,[80] and was gratified by the later vindication[82-86] of his early prophylactic dietary recommendations.[81] However, he has also for many years emphasized that the traditional, solely vascular approach to the problem of degenerative myocardial disease needs broadening to include the entire discernible spectrum of fundamentally contributing, pathogenic mechanisms (Figs. 8, 9, 10).

At the present time, principles generally considered for practical preventive application are the following: dietary restriction of saturated fats and cholesterol[15,86] and essentially antiadrenergic adjustments of living habits; namely, abstinence from smoking[87,88] regular physical activity,[89-98] and avoidance of emotional-environmental stresses.[99,100]

In nearly all lay educational, and in many professional publications these measures are represented as preventing or retarding the development of coronary atherosclerosis. With the exception of dietary rules, these claims are largely, if not entirely, unfounded and misleading.[23]

For communication with the lay public, the continued use of no longer adequately descriptive but popular terms, such as "coronary" heart disease, coronary "occlusion," and myocardial "infarction," may remain temporarily justifiable as a psychologically expedient compromise. However, within the domains of organized research and of scientific planning for future, more sophisticated and more deliberately individualized, preventive devices, there would appear to be desirable a realistic adaptation of thought and terminology to contemporary

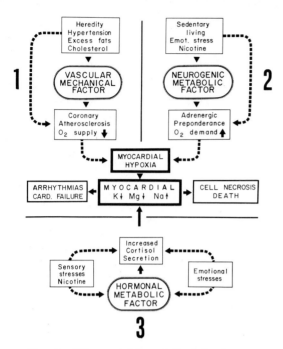

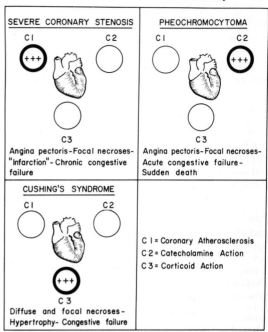

FIG. 8. "Structural formula" of the three categories of interrelated pathogenic factors, contributing to degenerative, so-called "coronary" heart disease by ultimately deranging myocardial electrolyte balance: (*1*) Vascular limitation of O_2 supply; (*2*) Neurogenic-adrenergic increase of myocardial O_2 consumption, both combined cause hypoxic loss of K and Mg, accompanied by gain in Na; (*3*) Adrenocortical overactivity aggravates adrenergic catecholamine cardiotoxicity, apparently by additional interference in myocardial electrolyte balance. (All details of this schema are documented by clinical and/or experimental observations.) (After W. Raab.[27])

FIG. 9. Three basic elements contributing to pluricausal, so-called "coronary" degenerative disease of the myocardium.

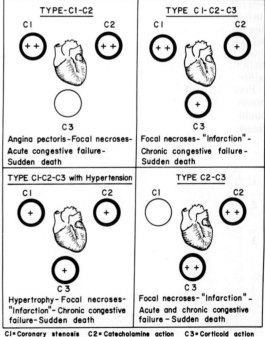

FIG. 10. Examples of common pathogenic patterns of pluricausal, so-called "coronary" disease of the myocardium.

knowledge and concepts with regard to basic pathogenic principles.

In view of the crucial, health-preserving importance of the myocardial electrolyte equilibrium, the maintenance of which is actually being served by the above-mentioned primitive preventive measures, particular attention should be focused on this, so far only rudimentarily explored, complex and challenging problem. Both the transfer of potassium from the contracting skeletal muscles into the myocardium during exercise, and the exogenous administration of "polarizing" potassium and magnesium salts,[27] appear to be possibilities for metabolic cardioprotection. The latter approach is at present being investigated in a cooperative long-range testing program in some of the several thousand preventive Heart Reconditioning Centers[101] abroad.

SUMMARY

Modern developments in basic cardiology have

provided a deeper insight into the complex and interdependent pathogenic mechanisms of pluricausal, degenerative, so-called "coronary" heart disease.

Coronary vascular atherogenesis constitutes an important predisposing and contributory element but can no longer be regarded as solely or necessarily dominant in myocardial degenerative pathogenesis.

Metabolic vulnerability, the ultimately decisive feature of degenerative myocardial disease, depends essentially on the heart muscle's oxygen economy and electrolyte balance. Both of these are critically deranged by jointly hypoxia-producing discrepancies between coronary vascular oxygen supply and adrenergic catecholamine-induced, uneconomical, oxygen consumption. Cell hypoxia, in turn, causes a potentially fatal, myocardial ionic imbalance which is further aggravated by largely civilization-induced states of catecholamine, cardiotoxicity-enhancing, adrenal cortical overactivity.

A "structural formula," integrating the basic causal elements of CHD (Cardiac Hypoxic Dysionism) has been presented.

Certain traditional, but no longer adequately descriptive, unduly generalizing and confusing terms, such as "coronary" heart disease, coronary "artery" disease (if referring to plurifactorial lesions of the myocardium), coronary "occlusion" and "infarction," need more precise specification, or replacement by a less prejudicial and more realistic nomenclature.

Preventive angiology (concerning arteries) and preventive cardiology (concerning the myocardium) ought to proceed on intimately correlated but clearly distinguished lines.

REFERENCES*

1. Hurst, J. W.: Notes on teaching: How some words prevent learning, J. A. M. A. 74:858, 1967.
2. Baroldi, G.: Acute coronary occlusion as a cause of myocardial infarct and sudden coronary heart death, Am. J. Cardiol. 16:859, 1965.
3. Baroldi, G., and Scomazzoni, G.: Coronary Circulation in the Normal and the Pathologic Heart, Office of the Surgeon General, Dept. of the Army, U.S. Govt. Printing Office, Washington, D.C., 1967.
4. Ehrlich, J. C., and Shinohara, Y.: Low incidence of recent thrombotic coronary occlusion in hearts with acute myocardial infarction studied by serial block technique, Circulation 26:710, 1962.
5. Spain, D. M., and Bradess, V. A.: The relationship of coronary thrombosis to coronary atherosclerosis and ischemic heart disease, Am. J. M. Sc. 240:701, 1960.
6. Branwood, A. W., and Montgomery, G. L.: Observations on morbid anatomy of coronary artery disease. Scottish. M. J. 1:367, 1956.

*More extensive bibliographies can be found in reference numbers 7, 14, and 23.

7. Raab, W.: The non-vascular metabolic myocardial vulnerability factor in "coronary heart disease," Am. Heart J. 66:685, 1963.
8. Fulton, W. F.: The Coronary Arteries, Springfield, Ill., Charles C Thomas, 1965.
9. Hort, W.: Mikroskopische Beobachtungen an menschlichen Infarktherzen, Virchows Arch. path. Anat. (Abt. A) 345:45, 1968.
10. Myasnikov, A. L.: Myocardial necroses of coronary and noncoronary genesis, Am. J. Cardiol. 13:435, 1964.
11. Snow, P. J. D., Morgan Jones, A., and Duber, K. S.: Coronary disease, Brit. Heart J. 17:503, 1955.
12. Josué, O.: Hypertrophie cardiaque causée par l'adrénaline et la toxine typhique, Compt. rend. soc. biol. de Paris 63:285, 1907.
13. Raab, W.: The pathogenic significance of adrenalin and related substances in the heart muscle, Exp. Med. & Surg. 1:188, 1943.
14. Raab, W.: Hormonal and Neurogenic Cardiovascular Disorders, Baltimore, Williams & Wilkins, 1953.
15. Raab, W.: The adrenergic-cholinergic control of cardiac metabolism and function, Advances Cardiol. 1:65, 1956. (Basel/New York, S. Karger).
16. Salisbury, P. F., Cross, C. E., and Riebens, P. A.: Acute ischemia of inner layers of ventricular wall, Am. Heart J. 66:650, 1963.
17. Honig, C. R., Kirk, E. S., and Myers, W. W.: Transmural distributions of blood flow, oxygen tension and metabolism in myocardium: mechanism and adaptations, International Symposium on Coronary Circulation and Energetics of the Myocardium, Milan, 1966, Basel/New York, S. Karger, 1967, p. 31.
18. Gregg, D. E.: The coronary circulation in the unanesthetized dog. International Symposium on Coronary Circulation and Energetics of the Myocardium, Milan, 1966, Basel/New York, S. Karger, 1967, p. 45.
19. Gorlin, R.: Physiologic studies in coronary atherosclerosis, Fed. Proc. 21:93, 1962 (suppl. no. 11).
20. Vašků, J., Urbánek, E., and Nevrtal, M.: The influence of K-Mg aspartate upon the incidence and development of nonspecific cardiac necroses in the young albino rat, Exp. Med. & Surg. 24:210, 1966.
21. Raab, W., van Lith, P., Lepeschkin, E., and Herrlich, H. C.: Catecholamine-induced myocardial hypoxia in the presence of impaired coronary dilatability, independent of external cardiac work, Am. J. Cardiol. 9:455, 1962.
22. Raab, W.: The sympathetic biochemical trigger mechanism of angina pectoris, Am. J. Cardiol. 9:576, 1962.
23. Raab, W.: Fundamentals and Targets of Preventive Cardiology, Springfield, Ill., Charles C Thomas, (in press).
24. Gorlin, R., and Elliott, W. C.: The coronary circulation, myocardial ischemia and angina pectoris, Mod. Concepts Cardiovas. Dis. 35:111, 1966 (I, II).
25. Herman, N. V., Elliott, W. C., and Gorlin, R.: An electrocardiographic, anatomic and metabolic study of zonal myocardial ischemia in coronary heart disease, Circulation 35:834, 1967.
26. Sonnenblick, E. H., Ross, J., Jr., Covell, J. W., and Braunwald, E.; The effects of catecholamines on the mechanics and energetics of the heart, in International Symposium on Coronary Circulation and Energetics of the Myocardium, Basel/New York, S.

Karger, 1967, p. 143.

27. Raab, W.: Myocardial Electrolyte Derangement-Crucial Feature of Pluricausal, so-called "Coronary" Heart Disease (Dysionic Cardiopathy), Monograph, Ann. New York Acad. Sc. (in press).

28. Hochrein, H.: Electrolytes in heart failure and myocardial hypoxia, Vascular Dis. *3*:196, 1966.

29. Selye, H.: The Chemical Prevention of Cardiac Necroses, New York, The Ronald Press Company, 1958.

30. Selye, H.: The Pluricausal Cardiopathies, Springfield, Ill., Charles C Thomas, 1961.

31. Raab, W., Stark, E., Macmillan, W. H., and Gigee, W.: Sympathogenic origin and antiadrenergic prevention of stress-induced myocardial lesions, Am. J. Cardiol. *8*:203, 1961.

32. Rona, G., Kahn, D. S., and Chappel, C. J.: The effect of electrolytes on experimental infarct-like myocardial necrosis, *in* Bajusz, E. (ed.): Electrolytes and Cardiovascular Diseases, Baltimore, Williams & Wilkins, vol. I, 1966, p. 181.

33. Nahas, G. G., Brunson, J. G., King, W. M., and Cavert H. M.: Functional and morphological changes in heart-lung preparations following administration of adrenal hormones, Am. J. Path. *34*:717, 1958.

34. Fizel', A., and Fizel'ova, A.: Studium einiger metabolischer Prozesse des versagenden Herzens im Experiment, XI. Adrenokortikale Mechanismen, Ztschr. Kreislaufforsch. *55*:804, 1966.

35. Kalinin, A. P., and Kilinsky, E. L.: Characteristics of myocardial alterations in Itsenko-Cushing's disease before and after adrenalectomy, Kardiologiya *6*:85, 1966. (Russian)

36. Zairatyants, V. B., and Kilinsky, E. L.: Changes of the cardiac muscle in Itsenko-Cushing disease, Kardiologiya *7*:126, 1967. (Russian)

37. Plotz, C. M., Knowlton, A. J., and Ragan, C.: The natural history of Cushing's syndrome, Am. J. Med. *13*:597, 1952.

38. Raab, W.: Emotional and sensory stress factors in myocardial pathology, Am. Heart J. *72*:538, 1966.

39. Raab, W.: Correlated cardiovascular adrenergic and adrenocortical responses to sensory and mental annoyances in man, Psychosom. Med. (in press.)

40. Kershbaum, A., Pappajohn, D. J., Bellet, S., Hirabayashi, M., and Shafiiha, N.: Effect of smoking and nicotine on adrenocortical secretion, J. A. M. A. *203*:275, 1968.

41. Epstein, F. L.: Hyperglycemia: a risk factor in coronary heart disease, Circulation *36*:609, 1967.

42. Datey, K. K., and Nanda, N. C.: Hyperglycemia after acute myocardial infarction, N. England J. Med. *276*:258, 1967.

43. DiBiase, G. and Labriola, E.: Contributo allo studio della catecholaminemia nell' insufficienza coronarica, Cardiol. prat. *15*:511, 1964.

44. Proudfit, W. L., Shirey, E. K., and Sones, F. M.: Selective cinecoronary arteriography. Correlation with clinical findings in 1000 patients, Circulation *33*:901, 1966.

45. Bellet, S., Roman, L., and Kostis, J.: Effect of auto driving on urinary catecholamine and cortisol excretion, Circulation *38* (suppl. VI): 40, 1968.

46. Simonson, E., Baker, C., Burns, N., Keiper, C., Schmitt, O. N., and Stackhouse, S.: Cardiovascular stress (ECG changes) induced by automobile driving, Am. Heart J. *75*:125, 1968.

47. Hökfelt, B.: The effect of smoking on the production of adrenocortical hormones, Acta med. scandinav. *170*: (suppl. 369): 123, 1961.

48. Gudbjarnason, S., Braasch, W., Cowan, C., and Bing, R. J.: Metabolism in infarcted heart muscle during tissue repair, Am. J. Cardiol. *22*:360, 1968.

49. Harris, A. S., Russell, R. A., Bocage, A. J., and Toth, L. A.: Arrhythmias that follow experimental coronary occlusion. Proc. Internat. Union Phys. Sciences VII. XXIVth Internat. Congr., Washington, D.C. 1968, p. 181, no. 542.

50. Hoffman, B. F., and Cranefield, P.: Electrophysiology of the Heart, New York, McGraw-Hill Book Company Inc., 1960.

51. Pick, A.: Arrhythmias and potassium in man, Am. Heart J. *72*:295, 1966.

52. Papp, J. Gy., and Szekeres, L.: Analysis of the mechanism of adrenergic actions on ventricular vulnerability, Europ. J. Pharmacol. *3*:15, 1968.

53. Hoffman, B. F., Siebens, A. A., Cranefield, P. F., and Brooks, C.McC.: The effect of epinephrine and norepinephrine on ventricular vulnerability, Circulation Res. *3*:140, 1955.

54. Scherf, D., and Schott, A.: Extrasystoles and Allied Arrhythmias, Melbourne, London, Toronto, Capetown, William Heinemann Ltd., 1953.

55. Bellet, S.: Clinical Disorders of the Heart Beat, 2nd ed. Philadelphia, Lea & Febiger, 1963.

56. Lund, A.: Adrenaline and noradrenaline in postmortem blood. Med. Sc. & Law, July 1964, p. 194.

57. Raab, W.: Sudden death of a young athlete with an excessive concentration of epinephrine-like substances in the heart muscle, Arch. Path. *36*:388, 1943.

58. Raab, W.: Sudden death with an excessive myocardial concentration of epinephrine-like substances in a case of obesity and cystic thyroid disease, Arch. Path. *38*:110, 1944.

59. Raab, W., and Gigee, W.: Norepinephrine and epinephrine content of normal and diseased human hearts, Circulation *11*:593, 1955.

60. Zugibe, F. T., Bell P., Conley, T., and Standish, M.L.: Determination of myocardial alterations at autopsy in the absence of gross and microscopic changes, Arch. Path. *81*:409, 1966.

61. Rothberger, C. J., and Winterberg, H.: Ueber die Bezichungen der Herznerven zur automatischen Reizerzeugung und zum plötzlichen Herztode, pflüger's Arch. ges. Physiol. *141*:343, 1911.

62. Wolf, S.: Sudden death and the oxygen-conserving reflex, Am. Heart J. *71*:840, 1966.

63. Hellerstein, H. K., and Turell, D. J.: The mode of death in coronary artery disease, an electrocardiographic and clinicopathological correlation, *in* B. Surawicz and E.D. Pellegrino (ed.), Sudden Cardiac Death. New York, Grune & Stratton, 1964, p. 17.

64. Wollenberger, A.: Relation between work and labile phosphate content in the isolated dog heart, Circulation Res. *5*: 175, 1957.

65. Bondaryenko, M. F., and Rajskina, N. E.: Influence of Pavlovi's augmenting nerve upon myocardial proteins, Bull. Eksperim. Biol. y Meditsinyi *8*: 39, 1956. (Russian)

66. Sobel, H., Myers, S. M., and Cohen, F.: Proteins of heart and kidney of the rat following starvation and cortisone administration, Exper. Med. & Surg. *17*:

119, 1959.

67. DeGrandpré, R., and Raab, W.: Interrelated hormonal factors in cardiac hypertrophy, Circulation Res. *1*:345, 1953.

68. Lenzi, F.: Sulla patogenesi dello scompenso congestizio, Minerva Medica *49*:677, 1958.

69. Urquarth, J., and Davis, J. O.: Role of the kidney and the adrenal cortex in congestive heart failure, Mod. Concepts Cardiovas. Dis. *32*:781, 1963.

70. Chidsey, C. A., Braunwald, E., Morrow, A. G., and Mason, D. T.: Myocardial norepinephrine concentration in man. Effects of reserpine and congestive failure, New England J. Med. *269*:653, 1963.

71. Ito, Y.: The tissue catecholamine concentration of the rabbit in experimental cardiac failure, Jap. Circul. J. *32*:761, 1968.

72. Meerson, F. Z., and Karlyev, K. M.: The role of neuro-endocrine factors in the mechanism of development of cardiac hypertrophy and insufficiency, Kardiologiya 7:78, 1967. (Russian)

73. Chidsey, C. A., Harrison, C., and Braunwald, E.: Augmentation of plasma norepinephrine response to exercise in patients with congestive heart failure, New England. J. Med. *267*:650, 1962.

74. Tomomatsu, T., Ueba, Y., Kondo, Y., Oda, M, Ijiri, Y., Kogame, H., Itto, Y., and Yao, T.: Catecholamine in congestive heart failure, Jap. Heart J. *8*: 242, 1967.

75. Labriola, E., DiBiase, G., and Scola, R.: La catecolaminemia nello scompenso sinistro, Boll. Soc. Ital. di Cardiol. *9*:76, 1964.

76. Jokl, E., and Wells, J. B.: Exercise training and cardiac stroke force, *in* Raab, W. (ed.): Prevention of Ischemic Heart Disease, Springfield, Ill. Charles C Thomas, 1966, p. 135

77. Levine, H. J., and Wagman, R. J.: Energetics of the human heart, Am. J. Cardiol. *9*:372, 1962.

78. Selye, H.: Stress and Cardiovascular Disease, World-Wide Abstracts of General Med. *4*:8, 1961.

79. Antalóczy, Z., and Ludvigh, G.: Sekundärer Aldosteronismus als Zweitkrankheit in intraktabler kardialer Dekompensation, Ztschr. f. ärztl. Fortbildung *59*:757, 1965.

80. Raab, W.: Alimentäre Faktoren in der Entstehung von Arteriosklerose und Hypertonie, Med. Klinik No 14/15: *521*, 1932.

81. Raab, W.: Möglichkeiten der Arterioskleroseverhutung München. med. Wchnschr. *18*:689, 1939.

82. Keys, A., and Keys, M.: Eat Well and Stay Well, New York, Doubleday & Company, Inc. 1963.

83. American Heart Association: Dietary fat and its relation to heart attacks and strokes, Circulation *23*, Jan. 1961.

84. American Medical Association: Dietary fat and its relation to heart attacks and strokes, J.A.M.A. *175*, 389, 1961.

85. Stamler, J.: Lectures on Preventive Cardiology, New York/London, Grune & Stratton, 1967.

86. Rinzler, S. H.: The role of diet in the prevention of coronary heart disease, *in* Raab, W. (ed.): Prevention of Ischemic Heart Disease, Springfield, Ill., Charles C Thomas, 1966, p. 278.

87. U.S. Department of Health, Education and Welfare. Office of the Surgeon General: Smoking and Health, U.S. Gov't Printing Office, Washington, D.C., 1964.

88. Doyle, J. T.: Tobacco and cardiovascular disease, *in* Raab W. (ed.): Prevention of Ischemic Heart Disease, Springfield, Ill., Charles C Thomas, 1966, p. 186.

89. Fox, S. M. III, and Skinner, J. S.: Physical activity and cardiovascular health, Am. J. Cardiol. *14*:731, 1964.

90. Kraus, H., and Raab, W.: Hypokinetic Disease, Charles C Thomas, 1961.

91. Mellerowicz, H.; The effect of training on heart and circulation and its importance in preventive cardiology, *in* Raab, W. (ed.): Prevention of Ischemic Heart Disease, Springfield, Ill., Charles C Thomas, 1966, p. 309.

92. Hollmann, W.: Der Arbeits-und Trainingseinfluss uud Kreislauf und Atmung, Dr. D. Steinkopff, Darmstadt, 1959.

93. Roskamm. H., Reindell, H., und König: Körperliche Aktivität und Herz-und Kreislauferkrankungen, München, Johann Ambrosins Barth, 1966.

94. Hellerstein, H. K.: A primary and secondary coronary prevention program-in-progress report, *in* Raab, W. (ed.): Prevention of Ischemic Heart Disease, Springfield, Ill., Charles C Thomas, 1966, p. 331.

95. Cureton, T. K.: The relative value of various exercise programs to protect adult human subjects from degenerative heart disease, Ibid, p. 321.

96. Gottheiner, V.: Long-range strenuous sports training for cardiac reconditioning and rehabilitation, Am. J. Cardiol. *22*:426, 1968.

97. Brunner, D.: The influence of physical activity on incidence and prognosis of ischemic heart disease, *in* Raab, W. (ed.): Prevention of Ischemic Heart Disease, Springfield, Ill., Charles C Thomas, 1966, p. 236.

98. Cooper, K. H.: Aerobics, New York, M. Evans & Co. and J. B. Lippincott Co., 1968.

99. Russek, H.I.: Emotional stress, tobacco smoking and ischemic heart disease, *in* Raab, W. (ed.), Prevention of Ischemic Heart Disease, Springfield, Ill., Charles C Thomas, 1966, p. 190.

100. Rosenman, R. H.: The role of a specific overt behavior pattern in the genesis of coronary heart disease, Ibid, p. 201.

101. Rabb, W.: Preventive medical reconditioning abroad–why not in U.S.A.? Ann. Int. Med. *54*: 1191, 1961.

Relative Importance of Factors of Risk in the Pathogenesis of Coronary Heart Disease: The Framingham Study

William B. Kannel*, William P. Castelli*, Joel Verter†, and Patricia M. McNamara*

The natural history of coronary heart disease (CHD) may be discerned with a minimum of distortion from an investigation of the way in which it evolves and terminates fatally in a general population sample. Because asymptomatic as well as symptomatic cases, cases not hospitalized as well as those reaching medical care and cases dying too suddenly to reach the hospital are included, a more comprehensive picture of its entire spectrum is realized.

Such a study has been conducted in Framingham, Massachusetts, where 5,127 men and women, constituting a reasonably representative sample of the adult population of the town, have been followed biennially for the development of initial attacks of CHD since 1949. Details of the sampling procedure, composition of the study group, clinical and laboratory methods employed and diagnostic criteria have been reported previously.[1-4] After 14 years of biennial cardiovascular surveillance, follow-up has been reasonably complete. Of those who took the initial examination and survived the 14 years of follow-up about 80 per cent took all seven biennial examinations and over 97 per cent took more than one examination. By means of examination in the clinic, daily surveillance of admissions to the only general hospital in town, information from spouses and physicians and evaluation of death certificates and medical examiners' reports, very few infarctions and deaths due to CHD have escaped detection. Less than 2 per cent of the original population sample have been entirely lost to follow-up.

CRITERIA FOR CHD

The criteria employed for the diagnosis of CHD

*From the Heart Disease Epidemiology Study, Framingham, Massachusetts and the National Heart Institute, National Institutes of Health, Public Health Service, U. S. Department of Health, Education and Welfare, Washington, D. C. 20201.
†Biometrics Research Section, National Heart Institute, National Institutes of Health, Bethesda, Maryland 20014.

have been described in detail in previous reports.[1-2] A diagnosis of angina pectoris was made from the minimal criteria of substernal discomfort of brief duration clearly related to exertion or excitement and could be relieved by rest or nitroglycerin. The symptoms had to be absent at rest and sufficiently clear so that two independent medical observers could agree. Myocardial infarction was diagnosed only in the presence of either serial ECG changes of myocardial infarction or transient diagnostic elevations of serum enzymes (SGOT, LDH) in an appropriate clinical setting. Comparison was made by study personnel between antecedent premorbid ECG's and those obtained during and subsequent to hospitalization. The development of an unequivocal ECG pattern of myocardial infarction since the previous tracing, in the absence of a suggestive history of chest discomfort, was regarded as evidence of an unrecognized myocardial infarction. A syndrome of "coronary insufficiency" was recognized when clinical findings suggesting a myocardial infarction were present, accompanied by documented transient ECG evidence of myocardial ischemia or injury, but without evidence of myocardial necrosis. When sudden unexpected death was documented to have occurred in less than one hour in persons not suffering from some potentially lethal disease and with medical histories suggesting no other cause, it was attributed to CHD.

NEED FOR PREVENTION

Knowledge of the natural history gained from this study of the epidemiology of CHD makes it clear that a substantial proportion of "heart attack" victims cannot be protected by modern medical management, no matter how sophisticated it may become. If a substantial reduction in CHD mortality is to be achieved, management must be directed against its precursors and not delayed until the clinical onset of symptomatic disease. All too often, in CHD, the very first symptom is also the terminal event, and a substantial proportion of attacks are either silent or so atypical that they go unrecognized. In this community, where even suspected heart attacks are routinely hospitalized, about 40 per cent of those with documented attacks did not reach the hospital. Sudden death and silent or unrecognized myocardial infarctions were responsible for 75 per cent of those cases not hospitalized (Table 1). One in every six initial "heart attacks" involved sudden death. Of all deaths occurring during such an attack, 65 per cent were sudden and unexpected (Fig. 1).

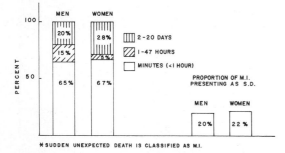

FIG. 1. Immediate mortality of initial myocardial infarction (sudden unexpected death is classified as myocardial infarction) in men and women, ages 30 to 62 at entry. (Framingham Heart Study, 14-year follow-up)

Most attacks occurred unheralded; only one in five were preceded by angina pectoris (Table 2). A sizeable proportion of ECG-documented myocardial

TABLE 1

Proportion of Initial "Heart Attacks" Hospitalized;
Men and Women 30–79: Framingham Heart Study

	Hospitalized		Not Hospitalized	
	No.	%	No.	%
Men	161	63	95	37
Women	42	54	36	46

	Not Hospitalized: Clinical Categories							
	Sudden Death		Other Death		Unrecognized M.I.		Other	
	No.	%	No.	%	No.	%	No.	%
Men	42	44	8	8	33	35	12	13
Women	12	33	4	11	11	31	9	25

infarctions were subclinical and about one in four were either silent or went unrecognized, thereby escaping proper medical attention (Table 3). Among those hospitalized, the case fatality rate before the acquisition of a coronary care unit by the hospital was about 17 per cent—virtually identical, excluding the sudden deaths, to that in those not hospitalized. Even if the mortality during the acute stage of a myocardial infarction in those who survive long enough to reach the hospital is substantially reduced as a result of modern innovations in management, it is clear that mortality from attacks will not be greatly reduced. A substantial proportion of persons sustaining "heart attacks" cannot be protected by modern medical management in coronary care units because their attacks occur undetected or because they die suddenly before medical resources can be mobilized in their behalf.

Clearly, a preventive approach aimed at cor-

TABLE 2

Proportion of "Heart Attacks" Preceded by Angina Pectoris; Men and Women 30–62 at Entry: Framingham Heart Study

Clinical Manifestation of Attack	Men			Women			Both Sexes		
	Total No.	No. with A. P.	% with A. P.	Total No.	No. with A. P.	% with A. P.	Total No.	No. with A. P.	% with A. P.
Myocardial Infarction	172	35	20	42	9	21	214	44	21
Coronary Insufficiency	26	6	23	19	7	37	45	13	29
CHD Death Not Sudden	16	6	38	5	0	—	21	6	29
Sudden Death	42	7	17	12	3	25	54	10	19
Total	256	54	21	78	19	24	334	73	22

TABLE 3

Proportion of ECG-Documented Myocardial Infarctions Unrecognized;
Men and Women 30–79

Age at time of infarction	Men			Women			Both Sexes		
	Total No.	Proportion Unrecognized No.	%	Total No.	Proportion Unrecognized No.	%	Total No.	Proportion Unrecognized No.	%
Under 50	34	7	21	5	2	40	39	9	23
50 and over	117	26	22	32	9	28	149	35	23
All ages	151	33	22	37	11	30	188	44	23

recting predisposing factors, identified years in advance of the first symptoms, is required if substantial inroads against this leading cause of death are to be made. Prevention requires a knowledge of the pathogenetic factors which predispose to the underlying atherosclerotic process, precipitate attacks in those so predisposed and affect survival once an attack occurs. Precursors of CHD can be identified from an examination of the epidemiology of the clinically overt disease. While most myocardial infarctions occurred without premonitory symptoms and a surprising proportion were subclinical, such patients were seldom free of stigmata characteristic of the coronary candidate—most could have been identified as particularly vulnerable or already afflicted with asymptomatic coronary heart disease. Only a small proportion (less than 25 per cent) were free of one or more of a limited number of personal characteristics known to be associated with increased vulnerability to CHD.

These hallmarks of unusual susceptibility have been ascertained from an exploration of the incidence of CHD in relation to antecedent personal traits and living habits suspected of being associated with the development of CHD in prospective epidemiologic studies.[5-10]

The purpose of this report is to review the factors contributing to risk of CHD, using data both from Framingham and elsewhere. The magnitude of the risk associated with these factors according to age in each sex will be determined. Then, based on data from Framingham, an attempt will be made to assess the net effect of a number of the major predisposing factors in a vulnerable subgroup of the male population.

HOST FACTORS INFLUENCING SUSCEPTIBILITY

A review of the medical literature, including reports from a variety of epidemiologic and other sources as well as from Framingham, reveals a number of host factors which are well established as precursors of CHD and other factors which, while reasonable, are more speculative.

Coronary artery atherosclerosis is an insidious process that may properly be considered a pediatric disease since there is evidence that it has its inception shortly after birth.[11] It then pursues a relentless course, progressing so that by age 20 extensive involvement of the coronary vessels with atherosclerosis is commonplace.[11-17] However, since a drastic encroachment on the lumen is required to produce impairment of flow and since thrombus formation is often required to produce a clinical

attack, the occurrence of clinically overt CHD is rare before age 40.[5]

It is well documented that the risk of clinical attacks is proportional, among other things, to the extent of coronary artery involvement with atherosclerosis.[18-21] No acceptable method currently exists for *directly* assessing the condition of the coronary vessels without hazard or discomfort to asymptomatic persons. Certain physiologic and biochemical concomitants of atherosclerosis do exist, however, which are sufficiently correlated with the rate of coronary atherogenesis so as to allow an assessment of the probability of extensive asymptomatic coronary artery involvement. Such an assessment requires only simple, inexpensive, atraumatic and safe office procedures and some readily available laboratory tests. Thus, aside from age and sex, risk has been shown to be proportional to serum lipid concentration, blood pressure, impaired carbohydrate tolerance and adiposity.[5-10,22-24] The more abnormal these characteristics are, the greater the risk of clinically overt coronary attacks and fatal outcomes.

Age and Sex

Because of the study of necropsy material, it has long been recognized that the severity of coronary atherosclerosis increases with age.[11] Clinical manifestations of CHD are also highly related to sex, predominantly afflicting the male. Age and male sex constitute the most powerful of the atherogenic host factors thus far identified. Age may well be atherogenic per se, but it very likely also reflects the duration of exposure to adverse living habits, biochemical abnormalities and physiologic disturbances which predispose to coronary disease. Age also reflects the greater chance of acquiring one or more of these abnormalities over a longer period of time. Sex may well play a biologic role, since the relative immunity of the pre-menopausal female is apparently lost after the menopause. However, such differences in relevant biochemical and physiologic parameters and living habits as have been noted in women as compared to men cannot explain entirely the relative resistance of women to this disease. The immunity of women to CHD is only relative to men, since even in women it is a distressingly common disease and a leading cause of death.[25]

It is clear that coronary atherosclerosis is not simply an inevitable consequence of biologic or genetic make-up since at any age in either sex some persons proved distinctly more vulnerable than others, based on a number of identified characteristics.[5-10,25] While genetic factors undoubtedly play a role and most of the rare instances of extremely precocious disease are clearly a consequence of inborn errors of metabolism, faulty living habits and acquired disorders appear to contribute the most prominently in the usual case of CHD encountered in the general population.

Serum Lipids

Based on autopsy studies, epidemiologic investigations of populations, animal experiments, clinical investigation of cases of CHD in comparison to controls, and metabolic studies in humans, a variety of lipids and their lipoprotein vehicles have been implicated in atherogenesis.[5-10,22,25-39] Uncertainty exists over which lipid or lipoprotein is most basic to the atherosclerotic process and whether the problem is primarily one of faulty transport, uncontrolled biosynthesis, dietary overloading of normal metabolic pathways, or faulty lipolytic enzymes.[29-40] Despite incomplete information on the details of atherogenesis and the nature of the metabolic defect responsible and without consideration of other related factors, there is little doubt that each of the major lipids and lipoproteins encountered in the blood is related to the incidence of CHD.[25,35]

While risk of CHD can be shown to increase in proportion to the number of lipid "abnormalities" noted in an individual's blood, it is not at all clear whether each particular lipid is, in fact, contributing to the risk. The net contribution of each of the lipids and lipoproteins to risk of CHD is uncertain since, in the general population, the various lipids and lipoproteins are highly correlated. Those with multiple lipid abnormalities are also likely to have the highest level of any particular lipid component.[25] Gradients of risk observed in prospective study in relation to percentile of serum lipid concentration are reasonably similar, with no particular lipid standing out clearly to a degree that would suggest it as most atherogenic.[41] Thus, it is not easy to state what the net effect of each of the major lipids and lipoproteins incriminated is, nor which is most atherogenic as judged by propensity to subsequent clinical CHD. Because of the generally high levels of lipid and lipoprotein present in this population, everyone appears to have enough lipid to manufacture atheromata—the rate and extent of its development being proportional to the lipid content of the blood. No particular concentration of any of the lipids that have been investigated has been demonstrated to be critical in propensity to CHD; the risk is simply proportional to the concentration of lipid from the lowest to the highest levels recorded for each lipid.[25,41]

Hypercholesterolemic persons appear to have a high risk regardless of the associated lipoprotein pattern, the risk being roughly proportional to the total cholesterol concentration in the blood. Knowledge of the lipoprotein pattern, however, appears to be important in understanding the reason for the hypercholesterolemia and in selecting the measures likely to be most effective in correcting the lipid abnormality.[29,32,42-45]

A number of factors have been observed to exert a marked influence on the risk associated with any particular lipid concentration. The most important of these is the coexisting blood pressure.[25,48] It seems clear that correction of lipid abnormalities is most urgent in hypertensive persons. The excessive risk associated with elevated serum cholesterol levels cannot be attributed to overt metabolic defects, such as diabetes, gout, obesity and hypertension, known to be associated with both CHD and lipid abnormalities. Risk of CHD appears to be proportional to the serum lipid content of the blood, even in the absence of overt evidence of these metabolic defects.

Blood Pressure

At any level of lipid in the blood, hypertension appears to accelerate atherogenesis as reflected by the incidence of clinical CHD events. To a greater extent than the associated lipoprotein pattern, the concomitant level of the blood pressure appears to determine the magnitude of the risk associated with an elevated serum cholesterol concentration.[25] Epidemiologic data demonstrate prospectively that coexisting hypertension in humans further augments the risk associated with an elevated serum lipid level.[25] This is entirely consistent with animal experiments which have demonstrated that lipid-induced atherogenesis can be further accelerated by also inducing hypertension.

As is the case for lipids, no "safe" level of blood pressure has been demonstrated—the risk of clinical CHD in prospective studies is simply proportional to the blood pressure level from the lowest to the highest recorded.[5-10,48] Apparently all grades and types of "hypertension" are potent contributors to CHD at all ages in both sexes. The commonly accepted notions that the cardiovascular consequences of hypertension are due principally to the diastolic component and that isolated systolic elevation is an innocuous accompaniment of advancing age appear to have little foundation. Nor is there much evidence that hypertension is innocuous in women.

High blood pressure is not only a potent contributor to risk, but is commonly encountered in the general population as well. Elevated blood pressure and hyperlipemia are entirely asymptomatic conditions for decades, while they silently promote accelerated atherogenesis. They are detected early only by periodic medical surveillance of well persons. In assessing risk of CHD by the simple clinical observation of blood pressure, it is important to take cognizance of the fact that elevated systolic pressure may be as important as diastolic pressure, particularly in older persons, and that casual elevations, as well as those which persist under basal conditions, may be clinically significant.

Impaired Glucose Tolerance and Gouty Diathesis

A large body of evidence has accumulated indicating that diabetics have an unusual propensity to precocious atherosclerosis and to its clinical consequences. There is also evidence that they are particularly liable to silent myocardial infarctions and to a fatal outcome once an attack occurs.[47-52] A gouty diathesis has been shown to be associated with lipid abnormalities,[53,54,58,60,61] with obesity[57] and with hypertension.[59] On this account alone, such persons can reasonably be expected to have an increased susceptibility to CHD.[55,56,60]

INDICATORS OF OCCULT CHD

Just as advanced coronary artery atherosclerosis may exist for long periods without provoking symptoms, so myocardial involvement due to CHD can be silently present. It is not unreasonable to assume that a silent, asymptomatic phase of myocardial involvement is also part of the clinical spectrum of CHD. At present, the only practicable means for the detection of occult CHD is routine periodic ECG examination.

The earliest evidence of compromised coronary circulation is provided by the postexercise ECG. Asymptomatic persons with ischemic S-T segment depression provoked by a standard exercise stimulus have been convincingly shown by others to have a substantial increase in risk of attacks of clinically overt CHD.[62-64] Certain abnormalities in the ECG at rest also undoubtedly reflect myocardial involvement due to advanced coronary artery atherosclerosis.

Finding ECG evidence of a myocardial infarction provides unequivocal evidence, in almost every instance, of myocardial damage as a result of a severely compromised coronary circulation. Silent or atypical actual myocardial infarctions are far from rare, occurring at almost one-third the rate of symptomatic attacks. This virtually pathognomonic evidence of coronary myocardial damage can be detected readily by periodic ECG examination of all persons beyond age 45 or, more profitably, of those demonstrated to be highly vulnerable to accelerated atherogenesis.

More speculative but highly suggestive evidence of myocardial involvement with coronary artery disease is the finding of left ventricular hypertrophy, or possibly intraventricular block.[25,65] Persons with such symptoms have a risk of an overt manifestation of CHD comparable to the likelihood of another CHD event in persons with angina pectoris, although not quite as close to the likelihood of those with a prior myocardial infarction.[66]

Persons with these possible occult evidences of myocardial involvement, presumed due to a compromised coronary circulation, deserve the same careful management as that afforded survivors of a symptomatic myocardial infarction, since survival and recurrence rates are quite comparable.

LIVING HABITS

Diet

Over the past century, agricultural technology and the food industry have wrought profound changes in the composition of the American diet, to a degree unequaled in the history of mankind. The resulting diet, rich in saturated fat, cholesterol, refined carbohydrates and calories, has reduced nutritional deficiency diseases almost to the vanishing point. With a concomitant reduction in demand for physical work as a result of advances in industrial technology, the problem of over-nutrition has now replaced that of undernutrition in Western civilization. There is a considerable amount of indirect evidence that this overnutrition is exacting a toll in cardiovascular disease and that altered dietary habits have played a prominent role in determining the generally high level of cholesterol and other blood lipids encountered in affluent Western civilizations.[67,70]

There is also direct evidence from experiments in animals and from metabolic studies in humans that specific alterations in the nutrient content of the diet can produce predictable changes in the serum lipid content and pattern.[34,71-77] Also, there is much to suggest that the composition of the diet with respect to refined carbohydrate, cholesterol and saturated fat has a greater impact in persons with positive energy balance than in those whose energy requirements equal or exceed their calorie intake.[78-80]

Despite this body of evidence incriminating diet

in atherogenesis, there is little direct prospective evidence demonstrating that persons under observation actually develop clinical CHD in relation to their habitual dietary intake. Most prospective studies attempting to evaluate the relation of diet to subsequent CHD incidence have failed to demonstrate a relationship between what people eat and either their serum lipids or their propensity to clinical CHD.[81-82] This apparent paradox may stem from the difficulties in obtaining valid estimates of long-term nutrient intake, from the relative homogeneity of dietary habits in free-living affluent population subgroups, or from the lack of a biologically important range of nutrient intakes in Western population samples. Most population samples studied have, in general, been partaking of a uniformly high calorie, cholesterol, refined carbohydrate and saturated fat intake, with an insignificant proportion of the population on intakes within the range noted in populations reporting a low CHD prevalence or at a level required to alter significantly serum lipid levels in metabolic studies.

High cholesterol levels in the blood may be associated primarily with elevated Sf 0-20 beta lipoprotein and with sensitivity to the saturated fat and cholesterol content of the diet.[43] Less commonly. "hypercholesterolemia" may be associated with an increase only in the Sf20–400 "pre-beta" lipoprotein content and may show particular sensitivity to the carbohydrate content of the diet.[43] More commonly, it is associated with an elevation of both lipoprotein fractions, requiring modification of both the fat and carbohydrate content of the diet.

For therapeutic purposes and prevention, these distinctions can be quite important. However, whatever the type of hypercholesterolemia or lipoprotein pattern with which it is associated, a high blood cholesterol concentration appears to be associated with an increased risk of CHD, proportional to its level. No lipid has been demonstrated in prospective studies to be distinctly superior to the total serum cholesterol for the purpose of assessing risk of CHD.

Emotional Factors

Conditions favorable for the development of an increasing incidence of CHD have evidently resulted to some degree from a modern technology that has substantially altered living habits. It has been alleged that "emotional stress" is one consequence of modern living and that this has exacted a toll by enhancing the occurrence of CHD.[83-88] The hypothesis that "emotional" (i. e., social and psychological) stress plays a role in the pathogenesis of CHD

has appeared in medical and social science literature for decades. A number of investigators have reported that certain "personality types" are coronary-prone, presumably as a consequence of inability to cope with their environment.[89-93] Epidemiologists have reported that social mobility, with its emotional implications, is associated with an increased rate of development of CHD. Serum lipids, blood clotting and urinary catecholamine output have been reported to be influenced acutely by various "stressful situations" such as examinations, preparing tax returns and appearing before congressional committees.[94-101]

Reasonable pathogenetic mechanisms have been suggested by animal experiments in which emotional stress, by affecting the autonomic nervous system, produced changes in circulatory dynamics, lipid metabolism and blood coagulation that could result in accelerated atherothrombosis.[102-105]

While the evidence presented to support the "stress hypothesis" is intriguing and provocative, it is still a good way from being conclusive. Investigation of a possible relation between "emotional stress" and CHD has been severely hampered by methodologic problems. The principal handicaps have been the lack of agreement on a uniform acceptable definition of the phenomenon and a failure to develop reliable and valid methods for measuring the intensity of the stress. Clearly these problems should receive the bulk of the attention of investigators. In spite of these basic difficulties, the concept of emotional stress as a potent force of morbidity and mortality in cardiovascular disease has gained increasing prominence and acceptance.

Although reasonable pathogenetic mechanisms may be hypothesized to explain any demonstrated relationship of emotional stress to CHD, evidence to support the contention of a major contributory role of emotional stress in the development of CHD is meager indeed. While acute changes in cardiovascular physiology, clotting and certain metabolic alterations are known to occur as a consequence of catecholamine release in response to stress, apprehension and anxiety, it is not clear that these transient effects produce lasting pathology. It is also not clear whether emotional stress is atherogenic or is merely a mechanism precipitating attacks in those already predisposed by atherogenic traits. In any event, it is somewhat discouraging to contemplate the preventive implications of a demonstrated relationship of emotional stress to CHD; behavioral and psychological difficulties have been, thus far, quite resistant to preventive and corrective efforts.

Obesity

Adiposity may result from sloth, gluttony, metabolic aberration or some combination of these. It is often accompanied by atherogenic traits including hypertension[106] abnormal blood lipids,[107] and impaired glucose tolerance.[108,109] As a consequence, the obese could be expected to exhibit an excess risk of CHD. A prospective examination of the incidence of CHD in the obese in contrast to their more lean cohorts has indeed revealed an association of adiposity with an increased propensity to CHD, but apparently for other reasons. While adiposity may well enhance atherogenesis, its principal contribution to CHD morbidity and mortality may well derive from the increased cardiac workload imposed by the adipose condition.[110] Prospective epidemiologic and physiologic investigation strongly suggests that obesity acts primarily as a precipitating factor in those already having a compromised coronary circulation and not as an accelerating factor in the atherosclerotic process common to all manifestations of CHD. While a relationship of obesity to development of angina pectoris and sudden death has been demonstrated, an association with increased risk of myocardial infarction has not.[24]

Physical Activity

Sedentary living appears to predispose to a fatal outcome in attacks.[111-113] In persons with a compromised coronary circulation, exercise under medical guidance may afford some measure of protection against a fatal outcome when an attack occurs. At any rate, it may be unwise rather than prudent to advise severe restriction of physical activity in persons who have recovered from a myocardial infarction without symptoms of congestive failure, who have evidence of occult CHD or who are prime coronary candidates.

The Cigarette Habit

In persons with one or more atherogenic traits or with occult CHD, the cigarette habit appears to be distinctly hazardous.[114-115] The effect of the cigarette habit appears to be noncumulative, transient and reversible. The risk is related to the daily consumption of cigarettes, but appears unrelated to the habit.[114] This is difficult to evaluate since people begin smoking at about the same ages and the effect of the duration of the habit is most difficult to disentangle from age. Much appears to be gained in giving up the habit, the ex-smoker having a

considerably lower risk than those who never stop smoking.[114-115] Abstinence would seem most imperative for those having one or more atherogenic traits. It would appear likely that those with angina pectoris or survivors of a myocardial infarction who continue to smoke are placing their life in jeopardy. For those who cannot give up the tobacco habit, substitution of non-inhaling tobacco practices would seem reasonable, since pipe and cigar smokers have a substantially lower risk of CHD than do those who use cigarettes.

NEED FOR SECONDARY PREVENTION

In addition to primary prevention, a need for secondary prevention is also quite evident. Immediate mortality in those under medical care with recognized myocardial infarction is still high. An examination of those dying within the same examination interval as their infarction, excluding the attack presenting as sudden death, reveals a case fatality rate ranging from three to 35 per cent, rising with age (Table 4). Now that coronary care units are available, this may be expected to improve. Selection of patients for limited coronary care unit

TABLE 4
Short Term Mortality After a
Recognized Myocardial Infarction;
Men 30–62 at Entry

Age at Examination Preceding the Event	Number M. I.'s	Number Dying in Same Examination Interval as M. I.	Case Fatality Rate (%)
Under 50	39	1	2.6
50–59	56	7	12.5
60 and over	49	17	34.7
Total	144	25	17.4

facilities is difficult, since sudden demise is all too frequent even in those without alarming findings at the time of hospital admission. There is a need to identify those who based on antecedent personal characteristics and medical findings, are particularly prone to a fatal outcome.

Even those fortunate enough to survive their initial attack, while they can expect surprisingly little disability on the whole, do not by any means have a bright future. The prospects for a long life free of recurrent attacks are quite dim. Within five years, one in every three attacks will recur—and half of these recurrences will be fatal. Risk of a stroke is increased almost threefold. Risk of death in survivors of an initial myocardial infarction was almost triple that of their cohorts, and following onset of angina, the risk was double (Table 5).

The probability of a second episode of coronary heart disease was, of course, quite high. Over an eight year period, depending on length of follow-up, from 23 to 59 per cent of infarctions recurred. After onset of angina, from 7 to 44 per cent developed a myocardial infarction or fatal episode. This represents a relative risk from five to 10 times that of the general population in those who have had myocardial infarctions, and three to six times the risk in angina patients. The relative risk tended to decrease with age (Table 6).

results to date are quite consistent with most but not all of the findings reviewed and serve to illustrate the epidemiologic features of CHD.

In 14 years of biennial observation, 323 men and 169 women developed some clinical manifestation of CHD for the first time out of a population at risk of 2,282 men and 2,845 women aged 30 to 62 years and found free of CHD at entry. The average annual incidence was observed to increase from about 2.5 per 1000 in the 30's to a peak of 22 per 1000 in the early 60's, after which it remained either constant or declined slightly. In general, the in-

TABLE 5
Risk of Death Following a Myocardial Infarction and Angina Pectoris*
Men and Women 30–62

Age at Entry	Death Following Myocardial Infarction Observed	Expected	Mortality Ratio	Death Following Angina Pectoris Observed	Expected	Mortality Ratio
Men						
30–44	7	1.3	5.4	2	0.9	—
45–54	17	6.6	2.6	13	6.7	1.9
55–62	16	8.0	2.0	19	8.7	2.2
Total	40	15.9	2.5	34	16.3	2.1
Women						
30–44	—	0.1	—	—	0.3	—
45–54	2	1.0	—	7	2.8	2.5
55–62	7	1.3	5.4	10	5.1	2.0
Total	9	2.4	3.8	17	8.2	2.1

*The expected number of deaths for any age-sex group are computed as follows: Let p_i be the proportion surviving from exam i to $i+1$ ($i=1,2,\ldots,$ 7) and $P_i=p_i$, $pi+1\ldots.p7$, and n_i. be the number of persons first appearing with the characteristic (myocardial infarction or angina pectoris) at Exam i, then $\sum_i n_i (1-P_i)$ is the expected number of deaths.

TABLE 6
Probability of a Second CHD Episode After Onset of Angina or Myocardial Infarction
Men 30–62

No. of Years After Onset	Probability of Second Episode After Myoc. Inf. 30–44	45–54	55–62	After Angina 30–44	45–54	55–62	Relative Risk* of Second Episode After Myoc. Inf. 30–44	45–54	55–62	After Angina 30–44	45–54	55–62
	No. %	No. %	No. %	No. %	No. %	No. %						
2	†(38) 16	(45) 29	(38) 24	(24) 8	(48) 8	(33) 6	9.9	8.0	6.8	5.9	2.7	1.3
4	(21) 36	(21) 42	(23) 40	(18) 24	(40) 22	(26) 24	11.2	5.8	5.5	8.1	3.5	2.7
6	(11) 53	(12) 47	(18) 47	(12) 30	(27) 25	(19) 40	11.4	4.3	4.4	6.5	2.6	3.1
8	(7) 67	(8) 74	(14) 47	(12) 30	(19) 49	(14) 49	10.1	5.1	3.4	4.8	3.7	3.2

*Risk of myocardial infarction, coronary insufficiency, or fatal coronary heart disease event relative to the population as a whole in the same age cohort coming at risk in the same examination as the first appearance of angina or myocardial infarction.

†( )=Number of cases at beginning of specified interval.

SOME RESULTS OF 14 YEARS OF FOLLOW-UP AT FRAMINGHAM

Now that 14 years of follow-up experience are available for analysis at Framingham and 492 cases of CHD have accumulated, it is possible to examine prospectively and in detail some of the foregoing findings reported from a variety of sources. The

cidence in women lagged about 10 years behind that in men. The male predominance was most pronounced for sudden death and for myocardial infarction, with the incidence in women becoming comparable to that in men some 20 years later in life (Fig. 2). While angina pectoris as a presenting complaint was in general more common in men than women, angina uncomplicated by a myocardial infarction was seen as frequently in women as in

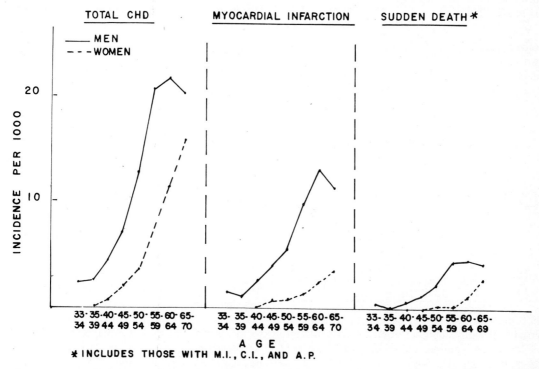

FIG. 2. Smoothed average annual incidence of manifestations of coronary heart disease in men and women, ages 33 to 70. (Framingham Heart Study)

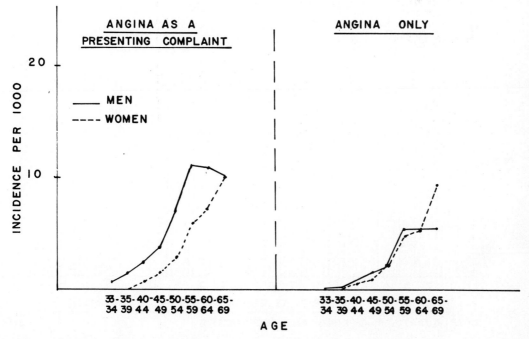

FIG. 3. Smoothed average annual incidence of angina pectoris in men and women, ages 33 to 70. (Framingham Heart Study)

men, the male predominance being evident only up to age 60 (Fig. 3).

Put another way, the probability of developing some manifestation of CHD was quite high. Within two years of entry, it rose from about 1.4 per cent in men 30 to 44 to 4.6 per cent at age 55 to 62. The probability of CHD rose within 14 years from

TABLE 7
Probability of Developing CHD According to Length of Follow-Up and Age at Entry Men and Women 30–62

Years of Follow-Up	Men 30–44	Men 45–54	Men 55–62	Women 30–44	Women 45–54	Women 55–62
		Probability (%) of Coronary Heart Disease				
2	1.4	3.1	4.6	0.2	1.4	2.6
4	2.9	6.3	8.9	0.4	2.7	5.3
6	4.6	9.5	12.8	0.7	4.1	8.2
8	6.3	13.1	15.4	0.9	5.6	10.8
10	8.0	16.8	18.4	1.3	7.3	13.1
12	9.6	19.8	21.8	1.5	8.9	16.0
14	11.8	22.9	24.8	1.7	10.5	19.6

11.8 per cent to 24.8 per cent in these same age groups. The probability in women was one-seventh of this in the younger age group and 80 per cent as great in the older age group (Table 7).

In each sex at any age, some persons identifiable by certain traits proved distinctly more susceptible to the development of overt evidence of the disease. An understanding of the pathogenesis and relative importance of the factors, along with a knowledge of the chain of events leading to overt disease, to recurrences and to mortality, is essential if effective prophylactic measures are to be developed and implemented. Thus far, no essential etiologic factor has been identified in clinical CHD. Multiple interrelated factors which appear to contribute to the underlying precocious atherosclerosis, to precipitate attacks in those so predisposed, to reflect asymptomatic myocardial involvement and to affect immediate and long-term survival have been identified.

ATHEROGENIC FACTORS

Serum Lipids

The concentration in the blood of the lipid cholesterol, phospholipid, and of the lipoprotein vehicles was determined at the time of the initial examination. Each was distinctly and impressively related to the subsequent rate of development of CHD.[41] As illustrated in younger men whose lipids were measured between the ages of 35 and 54, the risk

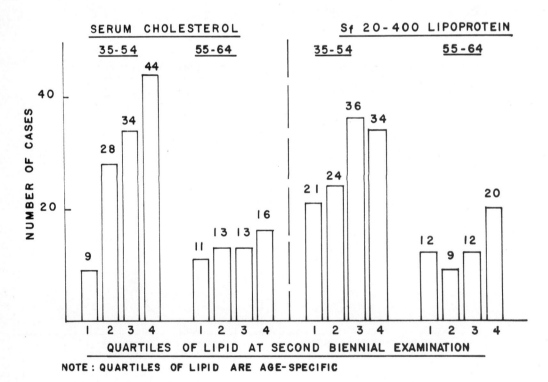

FIG. 4.   Risk of coronary heart disease in men, ages 35 to 64, according to serum lipid content. (Framingham Heart Study, 14 years)

of CHD is proportional to the concentration of each of the major lipids in the blood, including cholesterol and endogenous triglyceride (as reflected by the concentration of Sf20–400 "pre-beta" lipoprotein). This is evidenced by a distinct clustering of cases in the higher quartiles of the distribution of lipids. No safe or critical level of any of these lipids could be identified, the risk increasing in proportion to the concentration of each lipid from the lowest to the highest recorded in this population sample, with the high lipid levels characteristic of an affluent society. Risk gradients beyond age 55 were less steep (Fig. 4).

Blood Pressure

The coexisting blood pressure had a pronounced effect on the magnitude of the risk associated with any particular concentration of any of the major lipids. Elevated lipid concentrations were distinctly more ominous in hypertensive than in normotensive persons.[25,46] Risk of every major clinical manifestation of CHD was impressively related to antecedent blood pressure in both sexes at all ages. As illustrated here for men, risk was proportional to the blood pressure level (Table 8).

DETECTION OF OCCULT CHD

In persons with atherogenic traits and a high probability of developing a coronary circulation compromised by precocious atherosclerosis, the appearance of certain electrocardiographic abnormalities may herald the onset of myocardial involvement with coronary heart disease. Electrocardiographic evidence of myocardial infarction in asymptomatic persons is neither rare nor innocuous. Such silent or clinically–unrecognized myocardial infarctions were noted to occur in the general population at a rate almost one-third that of clinically-overt infarctions (Table 3).

In addition to this unequivocal ECG evidence of myocardial involvement due to coronary artery disease, the occurrence of ECG-left ventricular hypertrophy may also indicate occult CHD. Persons with definite ECG-LVH—including S-T and T wave abnormality along with increased QRS voltage—had a pronounced increase in risk of overt CHD. When hypertensive individuals developed this ECG abnormality, they further increased, by as much as threefold, their risk of a symptomatic manifestation of CHD. That the excess risk is not simply a reflection of hypertension common to both

TABLE 8
Risk of Manifestations of CHD (14 Yrs.) According to Blood Pressure Status: Men 30–62

Population at Risk			
	At Entry		
Blood Pressure Status	30–39	40–49	50–62
Normotensive	424	323	252
Borderline	311	310	251
Hypertensive	93	137	181

Risk of CHD Events									
Clinical Manifestation of CHD	Normotensive			Borderline			High Blood Pressure		
	Obs.	Exp.	M. R.	Obs.	Exp.	M. R.	Obs.	Exp.	M. R.
Total CHD									
30–49	51	73.4	69	76	65.1	117	38	26.4	144
50–62	41	58.0	71	64	58.2	110	53	41.8	127
Fatal CHD (C. D. and N. S. D.)									
30–49	6	12.7	47	12	11.5	105	11	4.8	227
50–62	4	10.6		11	10.6	103	14	7.7	181
Myoc. Inf.									
30–49	32	40.2	80	43	35.0	123	14	13.9	101
50–62	18	30.4	59	37	30.7	121	28	21.9	128
Angina Pectoris									
30–49	9	12.4	73	12	11.7	103	8	4.9	162
50–62	17	14.1	121	12	13.9	86	9	10.1	90
Coronary Insuff.									
30–49	4	8.2		9	7.0	128	5	2.8	180
50–62	2	2.9		4	3.0		2	2.1	

Normotensive= <140/90
High blood pressure=> 160/95
Borderline high blood pressure=the rest.

left ventricular hypertrophy and coronary heart disease is indicated by the demonstration of a distinct residual risk after adjustment for the associated blood pressure level. Electrocardiographic left ventricular hypertrophy unaccompanied by S-T and T wave abnormality does not have this implication, since the increased risk associated with its appearance is virtually obliterated when adjustment is made for coexisting hypertension (Table 9).

TABLE 9
*Factor of Increased Risk (14 Years) According to
ECG-LVH Status at Comparable Blood Pressure Levels
Men and Women 30–62*

Men	Possible ECG-LVH			Definite ECG-LVH		
	Obs.	Exp.	M. R.*	Obs.	Exp.	M. R.
45–54	6	7.2	83	13	4.8	271
55–62	6	4.0	150	19	5.3	358
Total	12	11.2	107	32	10.1	317
Women						
45–54	7	3.4	206	10	1.5	667
55–62	6	4.4	136	6	3.5	171
Total	13	7.8	167	16	5.0	320
Men and Women						
45–54	13	10.6	123	23	6.3	365**
55–62	12	8.4	143	25	8.8	284**
Total	25	19.0	132	48	15.1	318**

*Ratio of obs./exp. x 100.
**M. R. significantly greater than standard at P= <.05 level.
Note: Incidence at ages 29–44 was too low to be evaluated and was omitted from this table.

RELATIVE CONTRIBUTION OF HOST FACTORS

A variety of interrelated factors appear to play a role in the occurrence of CHD. While no one is immune, some are more susceptible than others and the more unfavorable characteristics they have, the greater their probability of acquiring the disease. Because of the correlation among the factors contributing to risk, the net effect of each is difficult to assess. The impact of the major host factors also appears to be related to and influenced by certain living habits such as cigarette smoking and lack of physical activity.

A detailed examination of a vulnerable segment of the population, men 38 to 61, was carried out in an effort to assess the net contribution to risk of the most important host factors in CHD. The factors included in the analysis were two of the major lipid entities incriminated (cholesterol and Sf20-400 "pre-beta" lipoprotein), systolic and diastolic pressure, casual blood sugar and relative weight. Also, since persons predisposed by these atherogenic traits have been shown to exhibit a further enhancement of risk of lethal coronary attacks if they smoke, analysis was done separately for cigarette smokers and for non-smokers. Among the smokers, the number of cigarettes smoked each day was taken into account. In an effort to measure the joint contribution of these factors to the incidence of CHD, the data were submitted to discriminant analysis. The procedure employed was to examine those persons free of CHD at the end of the second, fourth and sixth biennial examinations for the variables enumerated above. When a measurement was missing in a particular examination but present at an earlier examination, the policy adopted was to refer back to the earlier measurement.

The discriminant function analysis revealed a somewhat different effect of relative weight in cigarette smokers than in non-smokers. Among non-smokers, relative weight seemed to contribute to CHD incidence while in cigarette smokers, relative weight appeared to have little if any effect. However, among both cigarette smokers and non-smokers, serum cholesterol and blood pressure were important factors contributing to risk. In general, the contribution of other factors to CHD incidence is more difficult to discern (Table 10).

Comparing those in the lowest against those in the highest decile of risk, as judged by the constellation of the specified risk attributes, it is clear that an excess number of cases clusters in the highest

TABLE 10
*Average Standardized Discriminant Weights for CHD Specified Variables: Smokers Versus Non-Smokers
Men 38–61*

Characteristic	Cigarette Smokers		Non-Smokers
	Age: 38–61 years	46–61 years	46–61 years
Sf20–400 lipoprotein	.008	.007	.190
Cholesterol	.475**	.436**	.278*
Systolic blood pressure	.251*	.360**	.703**
Diastolic blood pressure	.017	−.078	−.512
Relative weight	.130	.145	.379**
Glucose	.152*	.221*	−.055
Number of cigarettes	.217**	.280**	—

*Significantly positive at 5% level.
**Significantly positive at 1% level.

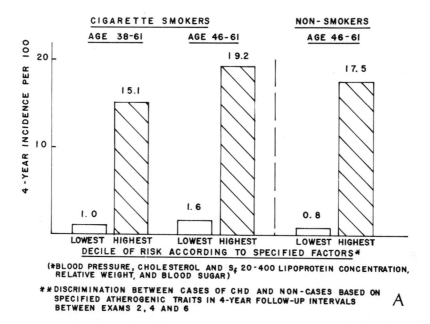

FIG. 5 A. Risk of coronary heart disease in men, ages 38 to 61, according to specified factors and cigarette habit. Discrimination between cases of coronary heart disease and other disorders was based on the observation of specified atherogenic traits in the 4 year follow-up intervals between the second, fourth and sixth examination. (Framingham Heart Study)

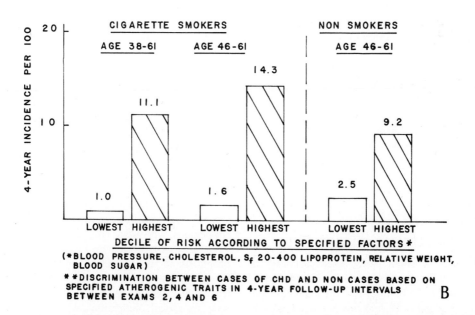

FIG. 5 B. Risk of death from myocardial infarction or coronary heart disease in men, ages 38 to 61, according to specified factors and the cigarette habit. Discrimination between death from coronary heart disease and those from other disorders was based on the observation of specified atherogenic traits in the 4 year follow-up intervals between the second, fourth and sixth examination. (Framingham Heart Study)

decile and that a deficiency of cases is present in the lowest decile. About a fifteenfold difference exists between these polar deciles of risk characteristics. In both smokers and non-smokers, risk is proportional to the intensity of the specified atherogenic traits (Fig. 5 A, B).

Smokers have a higher incidence of CHD, particularly of myocardial infarction and CHD death, than do non-smokers (Fig. 6). At a very low level

presents, for the first time, as sudden, unexpected death.

While CHD is a multifactorial disease for which, at the present time, no essential etiologic factor can be specified, a profile of the likely coronary candidate can be constructed and the degree of vulnerability can be estimated. From a preventive standpoint, the importance of the various factors contributing to risk depends not only on the strength of the

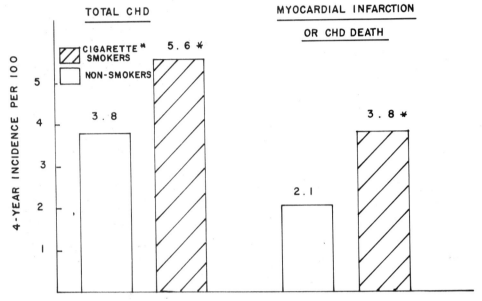

Fig. 6.   Four year incidence of coronary heart disease in men, ages 38–61, smokers vs. non-smokers. Adjusted to age distribution of non-smoker. (Framingham Heart Study)

of the other factors, there is relatively little excess incidence of myocardial infarction or coronary mortality associated with cigarette smoking (Fig. 5 B). This suggests that predisposing factors may well be a necessary prerequisite for the harmful cardiovascular effects of cigarettes. This is quite consistent with the hypothesis that the cigarette habit triggers lethal consequences in persons predisposed and presumed to have an already compromised coronary circulation.

PREVENTIVE IMPLICATIONS

A considerable latent period exists between the time of occurrence of a pathological degree of coronary artery narrowing and the appearance of symptomatic disease. It is in this latent period that preventive measures must be implemented in an effort to delay the onset of myocardial damage—damage which is often asymptomatic, frequently occurs without warning and distressingly often

contribution they make, but on the ease with which they can be detected and measured, their prevalence in the general population and their amenability to correction or control without undue hazard or cost.

In the general population the key factors which appear to determine the development rate of the clinical consequences of coronary atherosclerosis are the serum lipid content and the blood pressure. Persons identified as prone to precocious coronary atherosclerosis because they have hypertension or serum lipid abnormalities deserve special attention. In persons who also have occult myocardial involvement as indicated by ECG abnormalities, the prognosis as to recurrences and premature death is so serious as to warrant the vigorous use of every reasonable means—including hygienic measures such as weight reduction, dietary manipulation, exercise and, should these fail, pharmacologic agents—to lower blood pressure, alter serum lipids and correct impaired glucose tolerance. Prohibition of cigarettes in such individuals seems prudent.

A good case can be made not only for instituting prophylactic measures in those identified as highly vulnerable or afflicted with CHD, but for altering the living habits of the general population as well, since susceptibility is almost universal. It seems clear that health education alone is less than adequate, since the human condition is such that persons can seldom be successfully motivated to give up that which they enjoy in order to achieve some future benefit. Thus, it can be advocated that physical activity be engineered back into daily work and leisure, that substitutes for refined carbohydrate and saturated fat be used more widely in prepared foods, that more lean animal products be bred and marketed and that denicotinized cigarettes be promoted and smoking advertising be designed to suggest non-inhaling cigar and pipe substitutes. Corrective measures that deserve emphasis are those which are directed against common as well as potent contributors to risk of CHD. The cigarette habit, hypertension and elevated blood lipids all qualify in this regard. Those prophylactic measures which are safe as well as effective, such as weight reduction, antihypertensive, antilipemic and hypoglycemic pharmacologic agents correctly and prudently employed, should be seriously considered for young persons with multiple coronary precursors.

Field trials and clinical trials are urgently needed to demonstrate the efficacy of the preventive measures which seem rational. While the efficacy of such prophylactic use of the indicated hygienic measures and pharmacologic agents in delaying attacks and prolonging life remains to be demonstrated, the problem is so grave that further temporizing is difficult to defend. The measures advocated are usually indicated for other reasons as well. There is already preliminary evidence to suggest that in those already afflicted with CHD such measures may be helpful. Unless unforseen hazards related to their long-term use appear, it is reasonable to assume that such measures employed early in the disease process will be even more effective. More studies of the efficacy of such procedures in asymptomatic individuals with one or more high risk attributes are urgently needed.

REFERENCES

1. Kannel, W. B., Dawber, T. R., Kagan, A., Revotskie, N., and Stokes, J., III.: Factors of risk in the development of coronary heart disease-six year follow-up experience. The Framingham Study. Ann. Intern. Med., *55:*33, 1961.
2. Dawber, T. R., Kannel, W. B., and Lyell, L. P.: An approach to longitudinal studies in a community: The Framingham Study. Ann. N. Y. Acad. Sci., *107:*539, 1963.
3. Dawber, T. R., Meadors, G. F., and Moore, F. E., Jr.: Epidemiological approaches to heart disease: The Framingham Study. Amer. J. Public Health, *41:*279, 1951.
4. Gordon, T., Moore, F. E., Shurtleff, D., and Dawber, T. R.: Some methodologic problems in the long-term study of cardiovascular disease: Observations on the Framingham Study. J. Chronic. Dis., *10:*186, 1959.
5. Kannel, W. B., Dawber, T. R., and McNamara, P. M.: Detection of the coronary-prone adult: The Framingham Study. J. Iowa Med. Soc., *52:*26, 1966.
6. Doyle, J. T., Heslin, A. S., Hilleboe, H. E., Formel, P. F., and Korns, R. F.: Measuring the risk of coronary heart disease in adult population groups: III. Prospective study of degenerative cardiovascular disease in Albany: Report of three years' experience. I. Ischemic heart disease. Amer. J. Public Health 47 (suppl., Apr 1957), *25:* 1957.
7. Chapman, J. M., Goerke, L. S., Dixon, W., Loveland, D. B., and Phillips, E.: Measuring the risk of coronary heart disease in adult population groups: IV. The clinical status of a population group in Los Angeles under observation for two to three years. Amer. J. Public Health, *47:*33, Suppl., Apr. 1957.
8. Stamler, J., Lindberg, H. A., Berkson, D. M., Shaffer, A., Miller, W., and Poindexter, A.: Prevalence and incidence of coronary heart disease in strata of the labor force of a Chicago industrial corporation. J. Chronic Dis., *11:*405, 1960.
9. Keys, A., Taylor, H. L., Blackburn, H., Brozek, J., Anderson, J. T., and Simonson, E.: Coronary heart disease among Minnesota business and professional men followed fifteen years. Circulation, *28:*381, 1963.
10. Paul, O., Lepper, M. H., Phelan, W. H., Duopertuis, G. W., MacMillan, A., McKean, H., and Park, H.: A longitudinal study of coronary heart disease. Circulation, *28:*20, 1963.
11. Strong, J. P., and McGill, H. C., Jr.: The history of coronary atherosclerosis. Amer. J. Path., *40:*37, 1962.
12. Von den Velden, R.: Feldarztliche Hertzfragen. Zentralblatt für Herzund Gefässkrankheiten, *7:*1, 1915.
13. French, A. J., and Dock, W.: Fatal coronary arteriosclerosis in young soldiers. JAMA, *124:*1233, 1944.
14. Yater, W. M., Traum, A. H., Brown, W. G., Fitzgerald, R. P., Geisler, M. A., and Wilcox, B. B.: Coronary artery disease in men 18 to 39 years of age; report of 866 cases, 450 with necropsy examinations. Amer. Heart J., *36:*334, 481, 683, 1948.
15. Enos, W. F., Holmes, R. H. and Beyer, J.: Coronary disease among United States soldiers killed in action in Korea; preliminary report. J.A.M.A., *152:*1090, 1953.
16. Mason, J. K.: Asymptomatic disease of coronary arteries in young men. Brit. Med. J., *2:*1234, 1963.
17. Rigal, R. D., Lovell, F. W., and Townsend, F. M.: Pathologic findings in the cardiovascular systems of military flying personnel. Amer. J. Cardiol., *6:*19, 1960.
18. Blumgart, H. L., Schlesinger, M. J., and Davis, D.: Studies on the relation of the clinical manifestations

of angina pectoris, coronary thrombosis, and myocardial infarction to the pathologic findings, with particular reference to the significance of the collateral circulation Amer. Heart J., *19:*1, 1940.

19. Horn, H., and Finkelstein, L. E.: Arteriosclerosis of the coronary arteries and the mechanism of their occlusion. Amer. Heart J., *19:*655, 1940.

20. Saphir, O., Priest, W. S., Hamburger, W. W., and Katz, L. N.: Coronary arteriosclerosis, coronary thrombosis, and the resulting myocardial changes; an evaluation of their respective clinical pictures including the electrocardiographic records, based on the anatomical findings. Amer. Heart J., *10:*567, 762, 1935.

21. Roberts, J. C., Jr., Wilkins, R. H., and Moses, C.: Autopsy studies in atherosclerosis. II. Distribution and severity of atherosclerosis in patients dying with morphologic evidence of atherosclerotic catastrophe. Circulation, *20:*520, 1959.

22. Hatch, F. T., Reissell, P. K., and Poon-King, T. M. W., Canellos, G. P., Less, R. S., and Hagopian, L. M.: A study of coronary heart disease in young men. Characteristics and metabolic studies of the patients and comparison with age-matched healthy men. Circulation, *33:*679, 1966.

23. Ostrander, L. D., Jr., Francis T., Jr., Hayner, N. S., Kjelsberg, M. O., and Epstein, F. H.: The relationship of cardiovascular disease to hyperglycemia. Ann. Intern. Med., *62:*1188, 1965.

24. Kannel, W. B., LeBauer, E. J., Dawber, T. R., and McNamara, P. M.: Relation of body weight to development of coronary heart disease. The Framingham Study. Circulation, *35:*734, 1967.

25. Kannel, W. B., Castelli, W. P., and McNamara, P. M.: The coronary profile: 12-year follow-up in the Framingham Study. J. Occup. Med, *9:*611, 1967.

26. Buck, R. C., and Rossiter, R. J.: Lipids of normal and atherosclerotic aortas; chemical studies. Arch. Path. *51:*224, 1951.

27. Katz, L. N., and Stamler, J.: Experimental Atherosclerosis. Springfield, Ill., Charles C. Thomas, 1953.

28. Roberts, J. C., Jr., and Straus, R. (eds.): Comparative Atherosclerosis. New York, Harper and Row, 1965.

29. Fredrickson, D. S., Levy, R. I., and Less, R. S.: Fat transport in lipoproteins—an integrated approach to mechanisms and disorders. New Eng. J. Med., *276:*34, 94, 148, 215, 273, 1967.

30. Siperstein, M. D., Chaikoff, I. L., and Chernick, S. S.: Significance of endogenous cholesterol in arteriosclerosis: synthesis in arterial tissue. Science, *113:*747, 1951.

31. Zilversmit, D. B., McCandless, E. L., Jordan, P. H., Henly, W. S., and Ackerman, R. F.: The synthesis of phospholipids in human atheromatous lesions. Circulation, *23:*370, 1961.

32. Kuo, P. T.: Current metabolic-genetic interrelationship in human atherosclerosis. With therapeutic considerations. Ann. Intern. Med., *68:*449, 1968.

33. Keys, A.: Diet and the epidemiology of coronary heart disease J.A.M.A., *164:*1912, 1957.

34. McGandy, R. B., Hegsted, D. M., and Stare, F. J.: Dietary fats, carbohydrates and atherosclerotic vascular disease. New Eng. J. Med., *277:*186, 242, 1967.

35. Gofman, J. W., Young, W., and Tandy, R.: Ischemic heart disease, atherosclerosis, and longevity.

Circulation, *34:*679, 1966.

36. Albrink, M. J., Meigs, J. W., and Man, E. B.: Serum lipids, hypertension and coronary artery disease. Amer. J. Med., *31:*4, 1961.

37. Antonis, A., and Bersohn, I.: Serum-triglyceride levels in South African Europeans and Bantu and in ischemic heart disease. Lancet, *1:*998, 1960.

38. Gertler, M. M., Garn, S. M., and Lerman, J.: The interrelationships of serum cholesterol, cholesterol esters and phospholipids in health and in coronary artery disease. Circulation, *2:*205, 1950.

39. Nothman, M. M., and Proger, S.: Cephalins in the blood. Patients with coronary heart disease and patients with hyperlipemia. J.A.M.A., *179:*40, 1962.

40. Engelberg, H., Kuhn, R., and Steinman, M.: A controlled study of the effect of intermittent heparin therapy on the course of human coronary atherosclerosis. Circulation, *13:*489, 1956.

41. Kannel, W. B., Dawber, T. R., Friedman, G. D., Glennon, W. E., and McNamara, P. M.: Risk factors in coronary heart disease. An evaluation of several serum lipids as predictors of coronary heart disease. The Framingham Study. Ann. Intern. Med., *61:*888,1964.

42. Hatch, F. T., Abell, L. L., and Kendall, F. E.: Effects of restriction of dietary fat and cholesterol upon serum lipids and lipoproteins in patients with hypertension. Amer. J. Med., *19:*48, 1955.

43. Nichols, A. V., Dobbin, V., and Gofman, J. W.: Influence of dietary factors upon human serum lipoprotein concentrations. Geriatrics, *12:*7, 1957.

44. Ahrens, E. H., Jr., Hirsch, J., Oette, K., Farquhar, J. W., and Stein, Y.: Carbohydrate-induced and fat-induced lipemia. Trans. Ass. Amer. Physicians, *74:*134, 1961.

45. Kritchevsky, D., Tepper, S. A., Alaupovic, P., and Furman, R. H.: Cholesterol content of human serum lipoproteins obtained by dextran sulfate precipitation and by preparative ultracentrifugation. Proc. Soc. Exp. Biol. Med., *112:*259, 1963.

46. Cornfield. J.: Joint dependence of risk of coronary heart disease on serum cholesterol and systolic blood pressure: a discriminant function analysis. Fed. Proc. 21. (4) Pt. 2:58, 1962.

47. Root, H. F., and Bradley, R. F.: Cardiovascular-renal disease *in* The Treatment of Diabetes Mellitus, 10th ed. Joslin, E. P., Root, H. F., White, P., and Marble, A., (eds.) Philadelphia, Lea Febiger, 1969, p. 407.

48. Bradley, R. F., and Schonfeld, A.: Diminished pain in diabetic patients with acute myocardial infarction. Geriatrics, *17:*322, 1962.

49. Marble, A.: Coronary artery disease in the diabetic. Diabetes, *4:*290, 1955.

50. Aarseth, S.: Cardiovascular-renal disease in diabetes mellitus; clinical study. Acta Med. Scand. (Suppl. 281), *146:*1, 1953.

51. Rubin, H. B., and Weiss, M. J.: Diabetic patients with myocardial infarction; the diagnostic accuracy of the electrocardiogram. Calif. Med., *86:*254, 1957.

52. Agar, J. M.: Silent myocardial infarction in diabetes mellitus. Med. J. Aust., *49* (2):284, 1962.

53. Schoenfeld, M. R., and Goldberger, E.: Serum cholesterol-uric acid correlations. Metabolism, *12:*714, 1963.

54. Kuzell, W. C., Glover, R. P., Gibbs, J. O., and Blau, R. A.: Effect of sulfinpyrazone on total serum

cholesterol in gout: a long-term study. Amer. J. Med. Sci., *248:*164, 1964.

55. Kohn, P. M., and Prozan, G. B.: Hyperuricemia-relationship to hypercholesterolemia and acute myocardial infarction. J.A.M.A., *170:*1909, 1959.

56. Gertler, M. M., Garn, S. M., and Levine, S. A.: Serum uric acid in relation to age and physique in health and in coronary heart disease. Ann. Intern. Med., *34:*1421, 1951.

57. Hall, A. P., Barry, P. E., Dawber, T. R., and McNamara, P. M.: Epidemiology of gout and hyperuricemia. A long-term population study. Amer. J. Med., *42:*27, 1967.

58. Harris-Jones, J. N.: Hyperuricemia and essential hypercholesterolemia. Lancet, *1:*857, 1957.

59. Kinsey, D., Walther, R., Sise, H. S., Whitelaw, G., and Smithwick, R.: Incidence of hyperuricemia in 400 hypertensive patients. (Abstract) Circulation, *24:*972, 1961.

60. Benedek, T. G.: Correlations of serum uric acid and lipid concentrations in normal, gouty, and atherosclerotic men. Ann. Intern. Med., *66:*851, 1967.

61. Feldman, E. B., and Wallace, S. L.: Hypertriglyceridemia in gout. Circulation, *29:Suppl.:*508, 1964.

62. Mattingly, T. W.: The postexercise electrocardiogram. Its value in the diagnosis and prognosis of coronary arterial disease. Amer. J. Cardiol., *9:*395, 1962.

63. Brody, A. J.: Master two-step exercise test in clinically unselected patients. J.A.M.A., *171:*1195, 1959.

64. Rumball, A., and Acheson, E. D.: Latent coronary heart disease detected by electrocardiogram before and after exercise. Brit. Med. J., *1:*423, 1963.

65. Grant, R. P.: Left axis deviation. An electrocardiographic-pathologic correlation study. Circulation, *14:*233, 1956.

66. Kannel, W. B., Gordon, T., and Castelli, W. P.: Electrocardiographic left ventricular hypertrophy and risk of coronary heart disease: The Framingham Study. In preparation.

67. Keys, A., Kimura, N., Kusukawa, A., Bronte-Stewart, B., Larson, N., and Keys, M. H.: Lessons from serum cholesterol studies in Japan, Hawaii and Los Angeles. Ann. Intern. Med., *48:*83, 1958.

68. Bronte-Stewart, B., Keys, A., and Brock, J. F.: Serum-cholesterol, diet, and coronary heart disease; an inter-racial survey in the Cape Peninsula. Lancet, *2:*1103, 1955.

69. Lee, K. T., Nam, S. C., Kwon, O. H., Kim, S. B., and Goodale, F.: Geographic pathology of arteriosclerosis: a study of the "critical level" of dietary fat as related to myocardial infarction in Koreans. Exper. Molec. Path., *2:*1, 1963.

70. Katz, L. N., Stamler, J., and Peck, R.: Nutrition and Atherosclerosis. Philadelphia, Lea and Febiger, 1958.

71. Hartroft, W. S., and Thomas W. A.: Induction of experimental atherosclerosis in various animals. *In* Atherosclerosis and Its Origin. edited by M. Sandler and G. H. Bourne. 570 pp. New York, Academic Press, 1963, pp. 439–457.

72. Keys, A., Anderson, J. T., and Grande, F.: Prediction of serum cholesterol responses of man to changes in fats in the diet. Lancet, *2:*959, 1957.

73. Brown, H. B., and Page, I. H.: Lowering blood lipid levels by changing food patterns. J.A.M.A., *168:*1989, 1958.

74. Connor, W. E., Hodges, R. E., and Bleiler, R. E.: Effect of dietary cholesterol upon serum lipids in man. J. Lab. Clin. Med., *57:*331, 1961.

75. Ahrens, E. H., Jr., Insull, W. Jr., Blomstrand, R., Hirsch, J., Tsaltas, T. T., and Peterson, M. L.: The influence of dietary fats on serum lipid levels in man. Lancet, *1:*943, 1957.

76. Beveridge, J. M. R., Connell, W. F., Haust, H. L., and Mayer, G. A.: Dietary cholesterol and plasma cholesterol levels in man. Canad. J. Biochem. Physiol., *37:*4, 575, 1959.

77. Kuo, P. T.: Hyperglyceridemia in coronary artery disease and its management. J.A.M.A., *201:*87, 1967.

78. Gsell, D., and Mayer, J.: Low blood cholesterol associated with high calorie, high saturated fat intakes in a Swiss alpine village population. Amer. J. Clin. Nutr., *10:*471, 1962.

79. Morris, J. N., Heady, J. A., Raffle, P. A. B., Roberts, C. G., and Parks, J. W.: Coronary heart-disease and physical activity of work. Lancet, *2:*1053, 1953.

80. Karvonen, M. J., Pekkarinen, M., Metsala, P., and Rautanen, Y.: Diet and serum cholesterol of lumberjacks. Brit. J. Nutr., *15:*157, 1961.

81. Browe, J. H., Morlley, D. M., Logrillo, V. M., and Doyle, J. T.: Diet and heart disease in the cardiovascular health center. III. Dietary intake and physical activity of male civil service employees. J. Amer. Diet. Ass., *50:*376, 1967.

82. Dawber, T. R., Kannel, W. B., Pearson, G., and Shurtleff, D.: Assessment of diet in the Framingham Study. Methodology and preliminary observations. Health News, *38:*4, 1961.

83. Friedman, M., and Rosenman, R. H.: Association of specific overt behavior pattern with blood and cardiovascular findings. J.A.M.A., *169:*1286, 1959.

84. Minc, S., Sinclair, G., and Taft, R.: Some psychological factors in coronary heart disease. Psychosom. Med., *25:*133, 1963.

85. Jenkins, C. D., Rosenman, R. H., and Friedman, M.: Development of an objective psychological test for the determination of the coronary-prone behavior pattern in employed men. J. Chronic Dis. *20:*371, 1967.

86. Wardwell, W. I., Hyman, M., and Bahnson, C. B.: Stress and coronary heart disease in three field studies. J. Chronic. Dis., *17:*73, 1964.

87. Weiss, E.: Emotional factors in cardiovascular disease. Springfield, Ill., Charles C Thomas, 1951.

88. Russek, H. I., and Zohman, B. L.: Relative significance of heredity, diet and occupational stress in coronary heart disease of young adults. Amer. J. Med. Sci., *235:*266, 1958.

89. Bahnson, C. and Wardwell, W. I.: Personality factors predisposing to myocardial infarction. In Psychosomatic Medicine (Proceedings of the First International Congress of the Academy of Psychosomatic Medicine, Palma de Mallorca, Spain, September). New York, Excerpts Medical International Congress Series, No. 134, 1966.

90. Arlow, J. A.: Identification mechanisms in coronary occlusion. Psychosom. Med., *7:*195, 1945.

91. Keith, R. A., Lown, B., and Stare, F. J.: Coronary heart disease and behavior patterns. An examination of method. Psychosom. Med., *27:*424, 1965.

92. Miles, H. H., Waldfogel, S., Barrabee, E. L., and Cobb, S.: Psychosomatic study of 46 young men with coronary artery disease. Psychosom. Med., *16:*455, 1954.

93. Miller, C. K.: Psychological correlates of coronary artery disease. Psychosom. Med., *27*:257, 1965.

94. Syme, S. L., Hyman, M. M., and Enterline, P. E.: Some social and cultural factors associated with the occurrence of coronary heart disease. J. Chronic. Dis., *17*:277, 1964.

95. Syme, S. L., Hyman, M. M., and Enterline, P. E.: Cultural mobility and the occurrence of coronary heart disease. J. Health. Hum. Behav., *6*:178, 1965.

96. Syme, S. L.: Social stress and cardiovascular disease. Implications and future prospects. Milbank Mem. Fund Quart., *45:Suppl.*:175, 1967.

97. Friedman, M., Rosenman, R. H., and Carroll, V.: Changes in the serum cholesterol and blood clotting time in men subjected to cyclic variation of occupational stress. Circulation, *17*:852, 1958.

98. Wold, S.: Emotional stress *in* coronary heart disease. New York J. Med., *15*:826, 1959.

99. Groover, M. E.: quoted *in* Fat and stress, medicine. Time, *69*:79, (Jan. 28), 1957.

100. Thomas, C. B., and Murphy, E. P.: Further studies on cholesterol levels in the Johns Hopkins Medical students: The effect of stress at examination. J. Chronic. Dis., *8*:661, 1958.

101. Levi, L.: The urinary output of adrenalin and noradrenalin during experimentally induced emotional stress in clinically different groups. A preliminary report. Acta Psychother., *11*:218, 1963.

102. Cannon, W. B., and Mendenhall, W. L.: Factors affecting the coagulation time of blood. I. The graphic method of recording coagulation used in these experiments. Amer. J. Physiol., *34*:225, 1914.

103. Uhley, H. N., and Friedman, M.: Blood lipids, clotting and coronary atherosclerosis in rats exposed to a particular form of stress. Amer. J. Physiol., *197*:396, 1959.

104. Myasnikov, A. L., Kipschidze, N. N., and Tchazov, E. I.: The experimental induction of myocardial infarction. Amer. Heart J., *61*:76, 1961.

105. Schneider, R. A.: The relation of stress to clotting time, relative viscosity and certain other biophysical alterations of blood in normotensive and hypertensive subjects. A. Res. Nerv. & Ment. Dis. Proc.

(1949), *29*:818, 1950.

106. Kannel, W. B., Brand, N., Skinner, J. J., Jr., Dawber, T. R., and McNamara, P. M.: The relation of adiposity to blood pressure and development of hypertension. The Framingham Study. Ann. Intern. Med., *67*:48, 1967.

107. Kannel, W. B., Dawber, T. R., Glennon, W. E., and Thorne, M. C.: Preliminary report: The determinants and clinical significance of serum cholesterol. Mass. J. Med. Tech., *4*:11, 1962.

108. Joslin, E. P., Dublin, L. I., and Marks, H. H.: Studies in diabetes mellitus; interpretation of variations in diabetes incidence. Amer. J. Med. Sci., *189*:163, 1935.

109. Albrink, M. J., and Meigs, J. W.: Interrelationship between skinfold thickness, serum lipids and blood sugar in normal men. Amer. J. Clin. Nutr., *15*:255, 1964.

110. Alexander, J. K., Dennis, E. W., Smith, W. G., Amad, K. H., Duncan, W. C., and Austin, R. C.: Blood volume, cardiac output, and distribution of systemic blood flow in extreme obesity. Cardiovasc. Res. Cent. Bull., *1*:39, 1962–1963.

111. Eckstein, R. W.: Effect of exercise and coronary artery narrowing on coronary collateral circulation. Circ. Res., *5*:230, 1957.

112. Spain, D. M., and Bradess, V. A.: Occupational physical activity and the degree of coronary atherosclerosis in "normal" men. A postmortem study. Circulation, *22*:239, 1960.

113. Morris, J. N., and Crawford, M. D.: Coronary heart disease and physical activity of work. Evidence of a national necropsy survey. Brit. Med. J., *2*:1485, 1958.

114. Kannel, W. B., Castelli, W. P., and McNamara, P. M.: Cigarette smoking and risk of coronary heart disease. Epidemiologic clues to pathogenesis: The Framingham Study. Nat. Cancer Inst. Monograph No. 28., pp. 19–20, 1968.

115. Doyle, J. T., Dawber, T. R., Kannel, W. B., Kinch, S. H., and Kahn, H. A.: The relationship of cigarette smoking to coronary heart disease. J.A.M.A., *190:* 886, 1964.

Pathophysiology and Pathogenesis

Chairman
Wilhelm Raab, M.D.

The Life History of an Atheromatous Plaque
Meyer Friedman, M.D.

**The Role of Vascular Dynamics (Mechanical Factors)
in the Development of Atherosclerosis**
Meyer Texon, M.D.

The Role of Arterial Hypertension in Coronary Atherosclerosis
John H. Moyer, M.D.
James Flynn, M.D.

Diseases Accelerating Atherosclerosis
William Likoff, M.D.

Metabolic Changes in Myocardial Infarction
Sigmundur Gudbjarnason, M.D.
Richard J. Bing, M.D.

Collateral Circulation and Myocardial Infarction
Donald E. Gregg, Ph.D., M.D.

The Natural History of Coronary Atherosclerosis
Henry I. Russek, M.D.
Burton L. Zohman, M.D.

Panel Discussion: Can We Prevent Ischemic Heart Disease?

Moderator: Eliot Corday, M.D.

Panelists: Meyer Friedman. M.D.

Ancel Keys, Ph.D.

Campbell Moses, M.D.

Wilhelm Raab, M.D.

The Life History of an Atheromatous Plaque*

Meyer Friedman

The life history of a coronary atheromatous plaque is actually a sequence of violences which condition its origin, its growth, its decay and only too often its final and tragic transformation into a lumen-occluding instrumentality. These violences are perpetrated both by hemodynamic and by biochemical processes and it may well be that the pitiful inadequacy of our attempts to forestall the consequences of these same processes may later be discovered to have been due to our almost willful insistence in preoccupying ourselves with only the biochemical violences that possibly attend the life history of an atheromatous plaque.

Certainly there can be little doubt after the painstaking and repeatedly confirmed studies of Moon and Rinehart[1] that the initial phenomenon signalling the origin of a coronary atheromatous plaque is a fracture and fragmentation of segments of the internal elastica of the coronary artery, a phenomenon of violence that may and frequently does take place within days or weeks after expulsion of the human subject from his intrauterine abode. Following, but never preceding this fracture of elastica, a tiny, mucopolysaccharide laden nubbin of hyperplastic intimal cells arises and the life history of a plaque may be said to have begun. At this early stage, there need be and usually is no trace of excess lipid or cholesterol; the perpetrating trauma is sheerly an hemodynamic one, namely the arterial trauma probably induced by a newly activated left ventricle that for the first time must itself contract vigorously enough to supply *all* the blood the infant needs and to do this, notwithstanding the suddenly elevated extrauterine systemic blood pressure against which it must expel its contents. In short, one of the first vascular penalties the human subject appears to pay for extrauterine living is a fragmentation and attempted cellular repair of portions of the elastica of his coronary vasculature. And it is precisely in these very same vascular areas that later in life, atheromatous plaques, if present at all, will be found.

*Aided by a grant from the National Institutes of Health, National Heart Institute, HE-00119.

It is quite probable, however, that this particular traumatic event alone, despite its relative ubiquity and constancy, is itself inadequate to promote the development or continued growth of a typical lipid/cholesterol-rich coronary plaque. Seemingly, the *continual* intrusion of cholesterol itself into the initial lesion is necessary for the evolution of the full fledged atheromatous plaque. Thus if besides the initial hemodynamic violence, a second or biochemical violence is presented to the lesion, the development of an atheromatous plaque appears to be assured. Thus the deposition of cholesterol once it enters the lesion in sufficient amount, serves, if we can extrapolate from experimental data,[2,3,4] as a "neoplastic" agent. Just how excess cholesterol serves to incite the continued proliferation of endothelial and smooth muscle cells remains to be determined. We only know that this substance appears to accumulate in any locus of the body which is undergoing cellular hyperplasia whether such hyperplasia has been incited by mechanical, chemical or bacterial injury.[4,5] Moreover, it is the cholesterol derived from chylomicronous sources that appears to be so tenaciously persistent in its residence in such hyperplastic tissue.[4] Even beta-lipoprotein cholesterol appears capable once it leaves the lumen of a blood vessel to return therein but not so chylomicronous cholesterol.

With these facts in mind, it is interesting to recall that whereas Enos and his associates[6] observed that the majority of their young American soldiers killed in the Korean War exhibited a *significant atheromatous* plaque in one or more of their coronary vessels, almost none of their control Japanese male subjects did likewise. However, and I believe that this was a very important observation, these Japanese subjects did exhibit the *same* number of coronary lesions as the American soldiers, except that their lesions were simple scars, not cellular masses teeming with excess lipid/cholesterol substances. Seemingly the Japanese subjects had experienced the same initial hemodynamic violence and the resultant damage to their coronary elastica as frequently as the Americans but their lesions had evolved into simple scars rather than into continually growing atheromatous processes. Again from experimental data,[7] the resolution of their initial lesions into scars appears to be due to the relative absence of cholesterol in their diet and, as a result, a failure of such dietary derived cholesterol to enter into and aggravate the healing process attendant to the initial elastica injury.

Unfortunately cholesterol itself also appears capable of damaging elastic tissue and its continued entrance into a plaque thus not only directly stimulates the continued proliferation of various species of arterial cells but also damages successively deeper layers of the artery. This latter damage evokes a proliferation of the smooth muscle cells of the tunica media and eventually, a proliferation of fibroblastic cells lying in the tunica adventitia. Stemming apparently from this latter proliferation, the plaque receives a dense collagenous covering or "cap." When this cap is laid down, further expansion of the plaque ceases for an indefinite period. This inhibition to further immediate growth is probably due to the fact that the cap resists the easy entrance of additional lipid/cholesterol substances. It is at this stage that the lesion takes on its "pearly plaque" appearance[8] and as a fibrolipid or pearly plaque, the total process may remain dormant for years, decades or forever.

Nevertheless, the atheromatous plaque in its fibrolipid or "pearly plaque" stage only too often still carries a great potential for further development. Thus the lipid/cholesterol substances which initially were deposited chiefly within the hyperplastic cells of the plaque eventually lead to the rupture of such cells, and gradually accumulate at the base of the plaque as an extracellular mass. Such a mass, undoubtedly aggrandized by the continual or intermittent escape of additional lipid/cholesterol substances from the small adventitia-derived blood vessels entering into the base of the plaque, always carries the potential of instigating two possible complications, namely, the frank necrosis and liquefaction of the area which it occupies or a partial calcification of this same area. Either event appears capable of eliciting the continued ingrowth of new adventitia-derived but poorly structured blood vessels, thus promoting an additional escape of excess lipid/cholesterol substances.

Although it has been and still is widely believed that intraplaque necrosis and liquefaction result chiefly from ischemia, our own studies[3] make it clear that necrosis and liquefaction in the depths of a plaque do not take place because of an inadequate blood supply but rather because of the interference offered by the excess lipid/cholesterol substances themselves to adequate cellular nutrition and maintenance.

Without question, if a pearly plaque never suffered from necrotic or calcific degeneration, the potential lethality of an atheromatous plaque would be almost nil. Thus such plaques in the experimental animals never occasion any sort of significant hemodynamic distress. But either of these "complications," ostensibly by encouraging the adventitia to continue to supply new cells and new lipid/cholesterol "leaking" vessels, lead to the aggrandizement and even more widespread internal necrosis of the once dormant plaque.

The lethality of the plaque is compounded when one of these areas of necrosis begins to extend from its original central basal area toward the lumen-bordering portions of the plaque. This extension, heralded as it is by a vanguard of lipid-engorged macrophages (originally surrounding the initial area of necrosis), erodes away the originally dense fibrous covering of the plaque until the latter ruptures, allowing contact between the blood coursing through the lumen of the coronary artery and the necrotic interior of a plaque. Such contact promotes the aggregation of platelets[9] and other coagulative elements of the blood, a process which is responsible for the overwhelming majority of all coronary thromboses.[9]

If this acute thrombotic process completely occludes a major branch of the coronary artery, an infarct of course usually occurs. If the patient survives this insult, the original thrombus becomes converted into a fibrous mass which supports a system of newly formed blood vessels. These latter provide an "intraluminal collateral vasculature"[10] whose importance heretofore has been almost completely overlooked. It is probable that the eventual well-being of many patients who have suffered from an acute thrombotic occlusion depends not only upon the extent of this "intraluminal collateral vasculature" but also upon its future integrity. Our own studies,[10] however have made it clear that these newly formed vessels are extraordinarily susceptible to rupture and such rupture appears to have been the cause of many fatal episodes of coronary heart disease.

The erosion of the wall of a plaque need not result in total luminal occlusion, in which case the mural thrombus resulting is eventually converted into tissue indistinguishable from that of a typical atherosclerotic plaque. This conversion of thrombus to plaque tissue, which was suggested by Duguid[11] as taking place, has been actually demonstrated to take place by us both in the experimental animal[12] and in man.[13]

Until quite recently, it was generally considered that many coronary thromboses were caused by an initial hemorrhage arising in an atherosclerotic plaque. It was theorized that such hemorrhages burrowed to the intimal surface and in so doing led to coronary thrombus formation. However, it now has been demonstrated[14] that significant intraplaque or intramural hemorrhages arise in the same manner that thrombi do; namely by rupture of a plaque wall which then fosters the entrance of luminal blood into the interior of a plaque.

SUMMARY

The life history of an atheromatous plaque has been briefly described. The initial lesion is occasioned by a traumatic fragmentation of segments of the internal elastica. This lesion in many members of Western society later accumulates excess lipid/cholesterol substances and it is the accumulation of these substances which appear to promote the evolution of a simple wound into a proliferating mass of endothelial, smooth muscle and fibroblastic cells, all engorged with lipid/cholesterol substances. With the acquisition of a fibrous cap, the plaque becomes dormant frequently for decades. Only too frequently, however, the extracellularly sequestered excess lipid/cholesterol substances promote internal necrosis and/or calcification. The advent of these two complications initiates a new cycle of cellular and new blood vessel invasion carrying additional excess lipid/cholesterol substances in their wake. If and when an area of necrosis extends to and erodes the fibrous wall of the plaque, fracture of the latter allows contact between the luminal blood and the internal structure of the plaque. Such contact results in coronary thrombosis or intramural hemorrhage or both. The thrombus resulting, if completely occluding the lumen, eventually (if the patient survives) becomes transformed into fibrous tissue, which in turn supports a system of newly formed blood vessels which frequently can and do serve as an important vehicle for collateral circulation.

Thrombi which do not completely occlude the lumen evolve in tissue which appears identical to that comprising a typical atherosclerotic plaque.

REFERENCES

1. Moon, H. D., and Rinehart, J. F.: Histogenesis of coronary arteriosclerosis, Circulation *6*:481,1952.
2. Friedman, M.: Pathogenesis of the spontaneous atherosclerotic plaque, Arch. Path. *76*:318,1963.
3. Friedman, M., and Byers, S. O.: Experimental thrombo-atherosclerosis. J. Clin. Invest. *40*:1139, 1961.
4. Friedman, M., and Byers, S. O.: The atherogenic potential of dietary derived cholesterol, Brit. J. Exper. Path , *46*:1-5, 1965.
5. Friedman, M., and Byers, S. O.: Excess lipid leakage: Property of very young vascular endothelium, Brit. J. Exper. Path., *43*:363, 1962.
6. Enos, W. F., Jr., Beyer, J. C., and Holmes, R. H.: Pathogenesis of coronary disease in American soldiers killed in Korea, J.A.M.A. *158*:912, 1955.
7. Friedman, M., and Byers, S. O.: Endothelial permeability in atherosclerosis, Arch. Path. *76*:99, 1963.
8. Holman, R. L., McGill, H. C., Jr., Strong, J. P., and Geer, J. C.: The natural history of atherosclerosis. The early aortic lesions as seen in New Orleans in the middle of the 20th Century, Am. J. Path. *34*:209, 1958.
9. Friedman, M., and Van den Bovenkamp, G. J.: The pathogenesis of a coronary thrombus, Am. J. Path. *48*:19, 1966.
10. Friedman, M.: The coronary canalized thrombus: Provenance, structure, function, and relationship to death due to coronary artery disease, Brit. J. Exper. Path. *48*:556, 1967.
11. Duguid, J. B.: Thrombosis as a factor in the pathogenesis of coronary atherosculerosis, J. Path. & Bact. *58*:207, 1946.
12. Friedman M., and Byers, S. O.: Induction of thrombi upon pre-existing arterial plaques, Am. J. Path. *46*:567, 1965.
13. Friedman, M., and Van den Bovenkamp, G. J.: Role of thrombus in plaque formation in the human diseased coronary artery, Brit. J. Exper. Path. *47*:550, 1966.
14. Friedman, M., and Van den Bovenkamp, G. J.: The pathogenesis of coronary intramural haemorrhages, Brit. J. Exper Path. *47*:347, 1966.

The Role of Vascular Dynamics (Mechanical Factors) in the Development of Atherosclerosis*†

Meyer Texon

INTRODUCTION

The hemodynamic concept of atherosclerosis considers the effects of the laws of fluid mechanics—vascular dynamics—as the primary causative factor in the development of atherosclerosis.[1,2] Vascular dynamics relate the effect of mechanical factors to the biologic response of blood vessels. The forces and principles involved are fully comparable to those which prevail in any hydraulic system, with due regard to local conditions of flow and hydraulic specifications. This report identifies the localization, inception and progressive pathology of atherosclerosis in relation to forces which derive from the effects of mechanical factors inherent in the circulatory system.

Application of the laws of fluid mechanics to the natural conditions in the circulatory system reveals a demonstrable basis for the localization of atherosclerotic lesions at specific areas of predilection in the arterial tree as well as for its absence in identical adjacent areas of intima. Atherosclerosis does not occur at random locations. The sites of predilection for atherosclerosis can be precisely defined, predicted and produced by applying the principles of fluid mechanics. The areas of predilection for atherosclerosis are found to be consistently the sites of diminished lateral or static pressure. Such areas are characterized by curvature, branching, bifurcation, tapering or external attachment. These anatomic patterns occur in various combinations and in many variations of geometry. Their common feature is the production of segmental zones of diminished lateral pressure.

Atherosclerotic lesions observed at autopsy[1] correlate uniformly with mechanical forces which determine their localization in the circulatory system.

Rigid and flexible model hydraulic systems built to simulate the specifications of human blood vessels with respect to pulsatile flow, volumetric flow, velocity of flow, and anatomic patterns confirm the localization of atherosclerosis at specific areas of predilection, namely, areas of diminished lateral pressure.

The experimental production of hemodynamically-induced atherosclerosis in dogs[3] by surgical alteration of vascular configurations under controlled conditions further supports the central role of mechanical factors in the development of atherosclerosis.

The variations in the severity of atherosclerosis found in individual patients are demonstrated in this report to be due principally to the composite effect of individual differences in their hydraulic specifications. The velocity of blood flow, the caliber of the lumen, and the anatomic pattern are of importance. Biologic factors must also be considered; namely, the local reparative reaction or physiopathologic response of the intima to the diminished lateral pressure (suction effect) generated by the flowing blood. It is here that the nature and degree of atherosclerotic change may be influenced by differences in tissue structure and differences in tissue response to injury arising from genetic and species characteristics.

*Portions of the this article have appeared in the *Archives of Internal Medicine;* in the *Bulletin of the New York Academy of Medicine;* in *Atherosclerosis and its Origin* edited by M. Sandler and G.H. Bourne, and *Atherosclerotic Vascular Disease* edited by A.N. Brest and J.H. Moyer.

†From the Department of Forensic Medicine, New York University Medical Center, and the Office of the Chief Medical Examiner, City of New York.

This study was supported in part by: U. S. Public Health Service (N.I.H.) Research Grant H-3590, Emanuel Frank Foundation, Harry Kurnitz Research Award, Swift Newton Foundation and the Fan Fox and Leslie R. Samuels Foundation.

FLUID MECHANICS; HYDRAULIC CONDITIONS

The flow of rivers and streams, the flight of the airplane, the bird and the insect, the movement of a ship on the water or a fish in its depths, and the circulation of blood in our arteries and veins are varied phenomena determined by the laws of fluid mechanics.

The motion of fluids may be streamline or turbulent. In a streamline or laminar flow, the fluid moves in definite layers or smooth paths. In turbulent motion the fluid moves in an eddying mass, and at a given point the velocity varies irregularly from instant to instant. At a low velocity the motion of fluid is usually laminar. As the velocity increases the laminar motion breaks down and becomes turbulent. Because blood flow is laminar or streamline in all the smaller blood vessels, their pressure-flow relations can be analyzed with considerable mathematical precision. In the large arteries, some turbulence exists, and some differences from laminar flow may be expected. However, the significant feature of low pressure areas occurs in both laminar and turbulent flow.

The distribution of pressure in any hydraulic system is determined by the composite effect of many factors. In the circulatory system the relevant parameters include the following:

A. Physical Characteristics of the Blood
1. Viscosity, μ=centipoise
2. Specific gravity=S, or density=ρ=Gm/cm³
3. Homogeneity
4. Particulate content and hematocrit
5. Temperature

B. Flow Characteristics
1. Velocity of Flow=V=cm/sec
2. Pressure=p=dynes/cm²
3. Volumetric rate of flow=Q=cm³/sec
4. Pulsation of flow
5. Pulse rate, rhythm and amplitude
6. Reynolds Number Re=VDρ/μ

C. Anatomic Pattern (Geometry)
1. Caliber of lumen=D=cm
2. Bifurcation
3. Tapering
4. Branching characteristics
5. Curvature
6. Total area of flow

D. Fabric or Local Mural Factors
1. External attachment
2. External pressure
3. Thickness
4. Elasticity
5. Porosity
6. Strength of bond between layers

When lines of flow converge there is a tendency toward stability or streamline flow. Flow in tubes with converging boundaries or narrowed lumens is characterized by an increase in velocity and a decrease in static or lateral pressure. The decrease in

lateral pressure is predictable in an inviscid fluid on the basis of Bernoulli's theorem, which states that the sum of the pressure and the square of the velocity times $\rho/2$ is constant for any two points of flow on the same streamline:

$$P_1+\tfrac{1}{2}\rho V_1{}^2=P_2+\tfrac{1}{2}\rho V_2{}^2 \qquad \text{(Equation 1)}$$

The effect of gravity has been neglected in Equation 1 since gravity is not expected to have any influence in the distribution of rebution in local pressure referred to in this presentation.

Regions of low pressure can readily be identified in a variety of local situations:

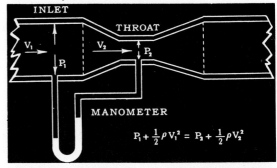

FIG. 1.   Venturi meter and Bernoulli's Equation.

1. Fluid in a Venturi meter (Fig. 1), as in a tube or vessel with converging boundaries, causes the lateral pressure to be reduced at the narrow portion where the velocity is increased.

2. In curvilinear motion (Fig. 2) the lateral pressure is increased along the outer wall and decreased along the inner wall by virtue of the effective centrifugal force.

3. The velocity of flow at a cross section of a

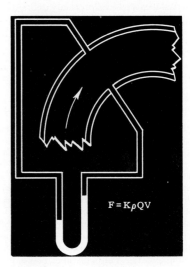

FIG. 2.   Elbow flow meter and equation for force developed at a given angle or curvature.

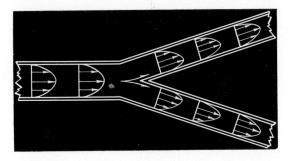

FIG. 3. Velocity distribution for streamline flow along a tube and at a bifurcation.

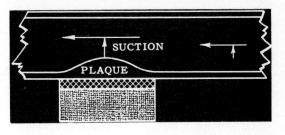

FIG. 4. Velocity and pressure (suction) changes associated with atherosclerotic plaque at zone of attachment.

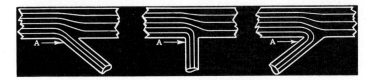

FIG. 5. Flow patterns at sites of branching. A indicates areas of low pressure.

tube (Fig. 3) increases from the wall toward the center. Division of the stream at a site of bifurcation results in a relative increase in velocity and a decrease in lateral pressure at the medial walls due to the local curvatures required of the streamlines.

4. At areas of external attachment (Fig. 4), a relative diminution in lateral pressure is developed by the fixation which resists any tendency of the flowing blood to move the wall of the vessel inward toward the axis of the stream.

5. At sites of branching, the flow patterns vary but tend to develop a low pressure region on the inner wall (Fig. 5, Points A), the tendency increasing as the angle of branching or deflection of the stream increases.

These anatomic patterns occur in various combinations and in many variations of geometry. In each instance low pressure or suction zones are produced as a common feature in accordance with the laws of fluid mechanics. The sites of predilection for atherosclerosis are uniformly found to be locations characterized by a relative reduction in lateral pressure.

HEMODYNAMIC MECHANISM FOR LOCALIZATION, INCEPTION AND PROGRESSIVE CHANGES

The pressure difference between the outside and the inside of the wall of a blood vessel is the net force per unit area exerted on the wall which tends to move the wall of the blood vessel. For a given geometry of curve, taper, bifurcation, branch or attachment, the maximum pressure difference is a function of the Reynolds number of the flow and is proportional to ρV^2 where ρ is the density and V is the velocity. A localized decrease in static pressure at points of predilection produces, in effect, a local suction action upon the wall. The intima is here subjected to the lifting or pulling effect of the flowing blood upon the endothelial layer and subjacent cells. This represents the initial stimulus. The initial response is a local biologic change, a reparative process of reactive thickening (Fig. 6) due to the proliferation of endothelial cells and fibroblasts from subjacent layers. There is no evidence of cellular reaction, vascularization or lipid change in the earliest stage of intimal thickening. The endothelial and internal elastic layers appear to remain intact and unchanged in the early lesion. With continuing

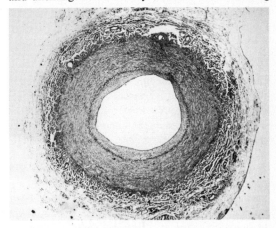

FIG. 6. Carotid artery of dog fed normal diet. Early concentric plaque in a "taper" lesion.

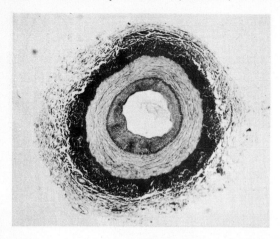

FIG. 7.   Carotid artery of dog fed normal diet. Moderately advanced concentric atherosclerosis in a "taper" lesion.

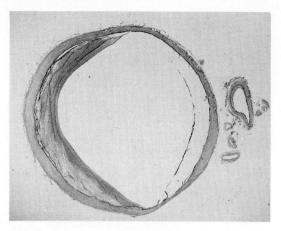

FIG. 8.   Female, age 65, internal carotid artery showing eccentric atherosclerosis in a "curvature" lesion. Orientation of layers of fibroblastic proliferation of intima reflect successive hydraulic forces.

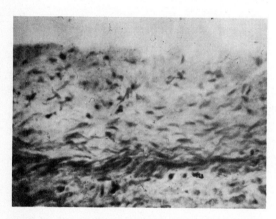

FIG. 9.   Lipid droplets in basement zone of intimal plaques. (*Above*) Aorta of a human female, age 56. (*Right*) Aorta of a dog fed normal diet.

blood flow, the thickening intima encroaches upon the lumen where an increased Venturi effect is produced. The lateral pressure becomes further reduced as the caliber of the lumen diminishes (Fig. 7). The plaque assumes characteristics of shape and degrees of further pathologic change which correspond to zones of varying diminution in lateral pressure. The orientation of cells to successive hydraulic forces is manifested by successive layers of fibroblastic proliferation (Fig. 8) which appears as the dominant pathologic change at all stages. Cellular elements and lipids are added to the intimal fibroblastic proliferation as part of the pathologic change in situ.

The earliest lipid change is noted as droplets within fibroblasts in the basement zone of the intimal plaque (Fig. 9). More advanced lesions reveal free lipid droplets which coalesce and extend toward the luminal surface subjacent to the plaque's fibrous cap. In some lesions the intimal proliferation extends across the lumen as tonguelike projections producing a multiluminal channel (Fig. 10). The growth and direction of such tonguelike lesions are influenced by the hydraulic forces present. Vascularization and hemorrhage (Fig. 11) within an intimal plaque has been observed. Advanced lesions may be partially or completely occlusive (Fig. 12) and consist of layered

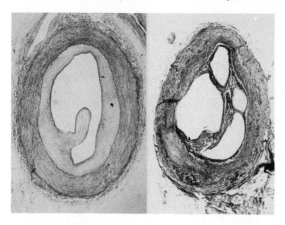

FIG. 10. (*Left*) Femoral artery of dogs showing concentric atherosclerosis with tonguelike intimal proliferation. (*Right*) Femoral artery of dog showing multiluminal channel and intimal proliferation.

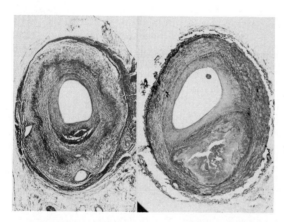

FIG. 11. Carotid artery of dog showing hemorrhage within eccentric atherosclerotic plaque.

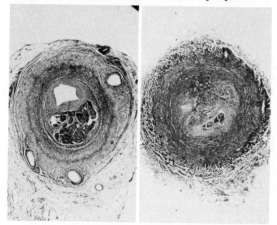

FIG. 12. Carotid artery of dog showing almost total obliteration (occlusion) of lumen by fibroblastic proliferation.

fibroblastic proliferation with occasional evidence of fatty change or cellular proliferation.

The atherosclerotic plaque, which begins as a minute reactive thickening due to proliferation of endotheliumand fibroblasts at sites of diminished lateral pressure in the circulatory system, evolves through progressive stages which vary in their rate of development as well as in the nature and severity of pathologic change. These are in situ pathologic processes which may include elastic tissue changes, collagen deposition, cellular infiltration, lipid changes, and occasional calcification. Vascularization of the intima may also occur by growth of capillaries from the adventitia or, more rarely, from the lumen.

The continuous operation of local hydraulic factors makes progressive pathologic changes inherently possible. The pathologic process may be relatively stationary for long periods, slowly progressive, or episodic in nature. A critical stage in the pathogenesis may arrive when a quick or dramatic change occurs (Fig. 13): 1. The superficial layers of an atherosclerotic plaque may become ruptured, lifted, or sheared off. The atheromatous content of the plaque is drawn into the blood stream and embolized distally. A raw or ulcerated surface is exposed to the flowing blood elements. These may become deposited or adherent to the plaque to form a thrombus. The thrombus may enlarge to a partially or totally occlusive degree by the accretion of additional blood elements. 2. An intramural or intimal hemorrhage may result from the same hydraulic forces which tend to draw the plaque toward the lumen. The intima is split or torn locally

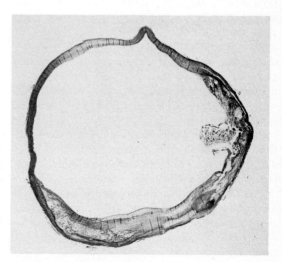

FIG. 13. Atherosclerosis of the thoracic aorta showing "attachment" lesion and mechanism for embolization (see text). Microscopic specimen.

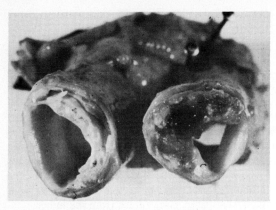

FIG. 14. Bifurcation of the aorta showing "crotch," "bifurcation," or "Y" lesions of the common iliac arteries. Note intramural hemorrhage.

to produce a microscopic hemorrhage in a manner comparable to a gross medial dissecting hematoma of the aorta. Intimal hemorrhages in association with or as part of the atherosclerotic plaque are frequent (Figs. 11, 14). They vary in size; although a small hemorrhage may not be sufficient to affect significantly the caliber of the lumen, a large hemorrhage may reduce an already narrowed lumen to the stage of total occlusion.

The pathologic process inherent in atherosclerosis produces occlusive changes of all degrees as the net result of the vascular response to local hemodynamic factors. Partial to complete occlusion may result locally from (1) progressive intimal thickening, (2) thrombosis superimposed upon the ulcerated luminal surface of an atherosclerotic plaque, and (3) intimal hemorrhage within or in association with an atherosclerotic plaque. While encroachment upon the lumen of a blood vessel may be due to any or any combination of these pathologic changes, the most commonly encountered completely occlusive lesion is that in which the lumen is obliterated by progressive thickening of the intima with incorporated old hemorrhage in various stages of transformation.

Partial to complete distal occlusion may result from embolization of the atherosclerotic contents of a plaque by rupture of the overlying fibrous cap as it is drawn by the axial stream.

The localization and progressive changes in naturally occurring lesions in humans are fully comparable to the lesions experimentally produced in dogs[3] by the surgical alteration of vascular configurations under controlled conditions. Atherosclerotic lesions, whether occurring naturally or induced by altering the hemodynamics, are consistently found at sites of diminished lateral pressure. These low

pressure areas are sites of predilection which derive from local hydraulic specifications.

BLOOD FLOW CHARACTERISTICS IN ARTERIES

Solution of the equations of fluid mechanics have been given for both steady and oscillatory flow in straight rigid tubes. Additional modifications of flow in the animal or human circulatory system are due to (1) the elasticity of the blood vessels, (2) the pulsatile character of the flow, (3) the viscous properties of the blood as a suspension of particles in a colloid solution, (4) the complex ejection pattern of blood flow in the aorta, and (5) the flow pattern determined by the intricate accommodations of structure or anatomic design which characterize the arterial and venous circulation. Some simplification of the analysis of blood flow in arteries is justified here because the major hydraulic conditions pertaining to the development of atherosclerosis occur in both steady and pulsatile flow.

Laminar Flow; Poiseuille's Law; Turbulence; Reynolds Number

Laminar or streamline flow in a circular tube is also called "Poiseuille flow" because Poiseuille, a physician, first studied the steady flow of liquids in cylindrical tubes. Poiseuille's law states that the pressure drop is directly proportional to the length of the tube, to the rate of flow, and to the viscosity, while it is inversely proportional to the fourth power of the radius. If the velocity of flow is increased to a critical point the laminar motion breaks down and becomes turbulent; Poiseuille's law no longer applies. The laws governing pressure-flow relations in turbulent flow are less easily subjected to precise analysis.

The transition from laminar to turbulent flow occurs at critical conditions which depend on the velocity of flow, the density and viscosity of the liquid, and the diameter of the tube. These factors are combined in the Reynolds number defined by:

$$Re = VD\rho/\mu \qquad \text{(Equation 2)}$$

A Reynolds number of 2000 is usually given as the critical value for transition from laminar to turbulent flow. However, this number may vary with other conditions of flow such as varying rates of flow and disturbances in the flow. The Reynolds number for blood flow in the circulatory system, except in the larger arteries, is generally found to be well below the critical level for turbulence. In the larger arteries, despite the existence of local areas of turbulence during a part of the cardiac cycle, essentially laminar flow may be assumed for calculation of average pressure-flow relations without the introduction of any significant error.

Pulsatile Flow; Viscosity; Movement of the Arterial Wall; Elasticity; Pressure-Flow Relations

Arterial blood flow is characterized by the recurring pulsation imparted by systolic contraction of the heart. Pulsations modify the instantaneous pressure-flow relations found in steady flow.[5,6] At all frequencies of oscillatory or pulsatile flow a variable lag is produced between the applied pressure and the ensuing movement of the fluid. The laminae nearest the wall have the lowest velocity due to the effect of viscosity. The flow near the wall has relatively less kinetic energy and reverses easily with each half-cycle. In the more central streamlines the velocity and kinetic energy are greatest. With reduction in pressure gradient and reversal of flow at the half-cycle, the axial streamline may be still flowing forward when reversal of the direction of flow may be occurring in the peripheral laminae. In such conditions the average velocity may approach zero. As the frequency of pulsation increases, the axial stream's velocity is reduced and the parabolic distribution of velocity across the tube flattens.

Blood Viscosity. A precise theoretical analysis of the flow of liquids generally assumes the fluid to be homogeneous, of uniform viscosity, and a "Newtonian" fluid. Blood is not a simple fluid; it has anomalous viscous properties. In the flowing blood the relatively cell-free zone of plasma which appears close to the wall of the blood vessel causes a local decrease in viscosity. This effect becomes important in the relatively slow rate of capillary blood flow and in vessels of less than 0.5 mm. in diameter. Under conditions of relatively high velocity as in the arteries which develop atherosclerosis, the variable viscosity of the blood does not alter appreciably the pressure-flow calculations. Blood may, in such instances, be considered to behave as a Newtonian fluid. Variation in viscosity, as a physical characteristic of blood, does not appear to influence significantly the role of hemodynamics in the development of atherosclerosis.

Movement of the Arterial Wall, Elasticity. Arteries vary in diameter and length during the cardiac cycle. The transient dilatation following systole is relatively small, and its effect on the stability of flow is negligible when compared with the effects of the average or peak velocity of flow. Likewise, the longitudinal movement of the arteries is usually slight because of their anatomic attachments. The behavior of the arterial wall as an elastic tube affects the propagation and damping of the pulse wave but has no appreciable effect on the average pressure-flow relationships which pertain to the development of atherosclerosis. In a larger artery, notably the arch of the aorta, vascular elasticity helps to produce streamline flow by reducing the pressure and velocity fluctuations throughout the cardiac cycle by its action as a surge chamber.

Pressure-Flow Relations. In a steady flow the rate of discharge through a tube is directly proportional to the pressure gradient in accordance with Poiseuille's law. The pressure gradient is the difference in pressure between two points in a continuous hydraulic system divided by the distance between the two points. This difference in pressure rather than the absolute values of pressure determines the velocity of flow. The chief determinants of the pressure gradient are the flow rate, the vessel diameter, and the viscosity of the fluid. A rise or fall in absolute pressure in a tube will not, per se, influence volumetric flow significantly. Similarly, the cyclic changes in absolute pressure levels of the arterial tree do not affect appreciably the flow volume. The variable pressure gradient inherent in pulsatile flow produces a variable velocity of flow. The peak velocity may be significantly greater than the average velocity with consequently greater effect on the development of atherosclerosis.

An equation relating volumetric flow to a varying pressure gradient may be derived by methods similar to the derivation of Poiseuille's equation. Although steady flow rate is dependent chiefly on the magnitude of the average pressure gradient, pulsatile flow rate is dependent on the frequency of oscillation of the pulse pressure as well as its amplitude.

The arterial tree branches progressively so that the cross-sectional area of the branches generally increases peripherally. However, the total wall area of the branches, hence the friction or resistance, also increases with the number of branches and causes an increased pressure gradient. The velocity of flow is related to the total cross-sectional area of a vascular bed rather than the caliber of a single vessel. The velocity of flow in the arterial system thus generally reduces with increasing distance from the heart.

The velocity of flow may also be influenced by external pressure or arteriolar constriction. Blood flow may then cease or be directed to alternate channels.

Cavitation; Boundary Layer; Separation

Cavitation. There is no evidence that the phenomenon of cavitation occurs in the circulatory system. Cavitation occurs as liquid flows, usually at high velocity, past a surface or through a passage when the pressure falls below vapor pressure at a particular temperature. The liquid vaporizes and a cavity or void forms. The alternate formation and collapse of the vapor bubbles is responsible for noise, reduced efficiency and the pitting of metal parts by the intermittent pressure of high intensity on small areas. These intermittent pressures can exceed the tensile strength of many metals. Particles of metal broken out by cavitation can progressively erode and weaken even metals of high strength.

Boundary Layer Theory. The boundary layer theory is based on the assumptions that (1) for high

enough Reynolds numbers, close to the wall of a blood vessel there exists a thin layer of fluid in which the velocity gradient is large enough to produce viscous stresses of a significant magnitude and (2) in the remaining portion of the fluid outside the boundary layer viscous forces may be neglected.

Separation of Boundary Layers. The boundary layer remains in contact with the entire surface of a body such as an airfoil (Fig. 15) or wall of a blood vessel provided the inclination of the surface to the direction of motion is not too great. When the angle of divergence is excessive, the boundary layer may detach itself and a surface of discontinuity forms. This surface of discontinuity usually rolls up into vortices and forms a wake.

Downstream of a point of separation of the boundary layer in a tube there is usually a region of increasing pressure. The pressure distribution on the surface of the body or on the wall of the channel is determined by the shape of the body or channel.

Separation of the flow from a boundary surface produces a change in velocity distribution within the boundary layer (Fig. 16). The point of separation is a point of stagnation on that streamline which divides the oncoming flow from the reverse flow of a region of discontinuity. The change in curvature of the velocity profile is due to the adverse pressure gradient; namely, the positive gradient. The point of separation is also determined by the stage of development already attained by the boundary layer in the upstream region. A laminar boundary layer will lead to separation at an earlier point than a turbulent layer; in both cases a region of appreciable deceleration will cause separation.

In a converging channel the flow is accelerated in the converging section and some pressure head is

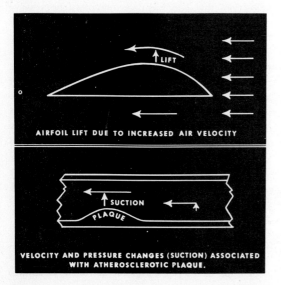

FIG. 15. Similarity of dynamic factors involving an airfoil and an atherosclerotic plaque.

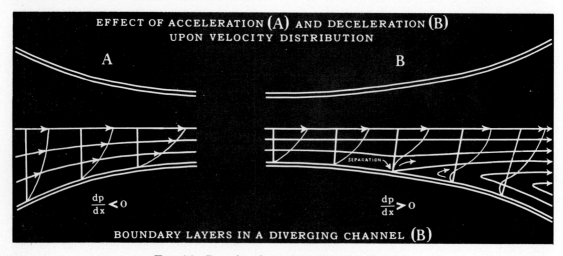

FIG. 16. Boundary layers in a diverging channel.

converted to velocity head. This is a stable and efficient process with only small losses of energy and no eddy formation.

In a diverging channel the flow may be unstable if the angle of divergence is considerable. Some velocity head is converted to pressure head. Some of the kinetic energy is converted to thermal energy because of the viscosity of the fluid. The fluid may not fill the channel and separation may take place, just as the stall of a lifting vane. Flow in a diverging channel is unstable, less efficient and may produce large energy losses and eddy formation.

If P is the static pressure and X is the distance along the channel, the derivative dp/dx is the pressure gradient, In a straight channel dp/dx would be zero if no friction were present. If friction were present, dp/dx would be negative; there would be a pressure drop. In a converging channel dp/dx would be negative. In a diverging channel dp/dx is positive; the pressure rises along the channel. This rise in pressure may account in part for the poststenotic dilatation frequently seen in atherosclerotic vessels.

In summary, when lateral pressure decreases with acceleration, the velocity distribution becomes more uniform and stable. On the other hand, when the pressure increases with deceleration, the velocities become unequal until one eventually reaches zero velocity. At this point, separation may occur and the main stream of the flow leaves the surface of the body or vessel wall. This results in a discontinuity of flow—but not in fluid, as in the case of cavitation—for the region of discontinuity is generally filled with fluid moving in the upstream direction along the wall.

THEORETICAL CALCULATIONS; FLOW PATTERNS

The forces generated by the flowing blood can be computed in certain idealized situations. The values calculated will be increasingly reliable as technologic instrumentation improves and as hydraulic specifications are more accurately defined.

Taper

Bernoulli's equation $(P_1 + \frac{1}{2}\rho V_1^2 = P_2 + \frac{1}{2}\rho V_2^2)$ provides a basis for computing the velocity and pressure relations in a tapering vessel. The computations must consider the effect of branch run-offs if present between the points under study. In some instances the effect of gravity may be important.

Curvature; Bends; Force Equation

The total force required to deflect a steady stream of fluid through a given angle (Figs. 2 and 17) is given by the equation:

$$F = K\rho QV \qquad \text{(Equation 3)}$$

where F=total force in dynes, K=coefficient (see Table 1), ρ=density in Gm./cm.^{3}, Q = flow rate in cm.^{3}, and V= velocity in cm./sec. The value of the coefficient K depends on the angle θ (Table 1). If ρ=1 Gm./cm.^{3}, A = 0.20 cm.^{2}, V =20 cm./sec., then Q =AV = 4 cm.^{3} /sec. and from the formula F = Kρ QV, at 45°, F =61 dynes, at 90°, F = 113 dynes; at 135°, F=148 dynes; and at 180°, F = 160 dynes.

It is clear that at a constant velocity and volumetric flow an increase in the angle θ increases the force required to divert the stream. By halving the diameter and maintaining the volumetric flow, the velocity must increase fourfold; thus, the force is increased by increasing the velocity. (See Table 1)

The computation of the forces described here, it should be noted, does not describe their distribution. However, it is reasonable to assume that the net

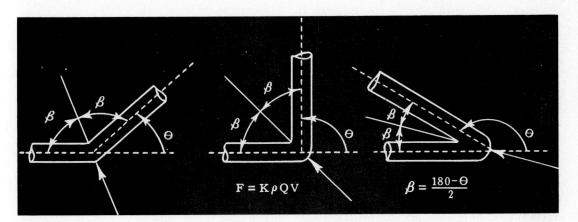

FIG. 17.   Diagrams and force equation at bends.

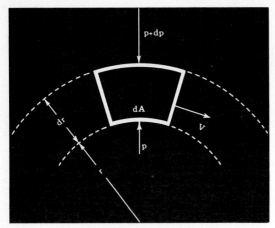

FIG. 18.   Flow in a curved path.

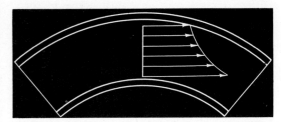

FIG. 19.   Velocity of flow in mainstream at bend.

effect must be an increased pressure on the outer curvature and a decreased pressure (net suction action) on the inner curvature. It is this suction effect which evokes the atherosclerotic response.

Relation Between Pressure and Radius of Curvature, Flow in a Curved Path. Flow in a curved path is so common in the circulatory system that special emphasis on this type of flow is appropriate.

Consider the flow of an infinitesimal element between two concentric stream lines an infinitesimal distance apart (Fig. 18). The radius of curvature of this path is r, and the tangential linear velocity is V. If the height of the element is dr and the area is dA then the mass of the element is ρdr dA (Mass = density × volume). The normal or radial acceleration is V^2/r. The effective centrifugal force acting on the element is the product of mass and acceleration or ρ dr dA (V^2/r). The pressure varies from p to p+dp as the radius varies from r to r+dr. The effective centrifugal force on the fluid element is balanced by the resultant forces over the surfaces. A force balance in the radial direction gives:

$$dpdA = \rho V^2/r\ dr\ dA \qquad \text{(Equation 4)}$$
$$\text{and}\quad dp = \rho V^2/r\ dr. \qquad \text{(Equation 5)}$$

TABLE 1
Value of Coefficient K with Angle θ

DEGREES	K	DEGREES	K
0	0	105	1.58
15	0.26	120	1.73
30	0.52	135	1.85
45	0.76	150.	1.93
60	1.00	165	1.97
75	1.22	180	2.00
90	1.41	$\beta=\dfrac{180-\theta}{2}$	

The pressure increases with radius in a curved flow. There is a fall in pressure per unit radial distance toward the center of curvature by the amount

$\rho V^2/r$; i.e., the pressure gradient $dp/dr=\rho V^2/r$.

While Bernoulli's equation usually applies to flow along a streamline, Equation 5 defines the fundamental relation $dp=\rho V^2/r\ dr$ which provides a method for studying conditions in a direction normal to the streamlines. If the streamline is straight, the pressure change normal to the streamline is zero because r is infinitely large. For streamlines of finite curvature, the pressure varies from p to p + dp in the distance dr. Since dp is positive if dr is positive, Equation 5 shows that pressure increases for successive points from the concave to the convex side of the stream. The exact variation in pressure depends upon the variation in velocity with radius and the local radius of curvature of the streamlines.

The velocity distribution for certain ideal curvilinear flows is known; the case of a free vortex is illustrated (Fig. 19). In this case the velocity increases as the radius decreases. In an actual flow around a bend, viscous effects, the pulsatility of the flow, and the elasticity of the wall will produce modifications of this idealized pattern. However, for any case of curved flow, the pressure will increase with the radius, and the order of magnitude can be approximated by assuming a free vortex velocity distribution. On a meteorologic scale, the low pressure found in the eye of tornadoes and hurricanes is explained on the same basis.

The pressure distribution in a free vortex can be determined by substituting the relation $V=K/r$ in the equation $dp=\rho V^2/r\ dr$ and integrating between limits. K is determined by the known velocity and radius at a particular point.

$$\int_1^2 dp= \rho \int_1^2 V^2/r\ dr \qquad \text{(Equation 6)}$$
$$P_2-P_1=\rho K^2 \int_1^2 dr/r^3=(1/r_1^2-1/r_2^2)\ \rho K^2/2$$

Since $V_1 r_1=V_2 r_2=K$, the equation may be written

$$P_1+\tfrac{1}{2}\ \rho V_1^2=P_2+\tfrac{1}{2}\rho V_2^2$$
$$P_1/w+V_1^2/2g=P_2/w+V_2^2/2g=\text{Constant}$$
$$\text{(Equation 7)}$$

Equation 7 shows that the total energy in each stream tube is the same as in each of the other stream tubes. No energy is added to the vortex by a torque and no energy is dissipated by friction. Such a free vortex may be found in the two-dimensional flow in the main body of a stream flowing around a bend.

Calculations. In a free vortex the difference in pressure per unit radial distance toward the center is $\rho V^2/r$. Thus, $dp = \rho V^2/r \ dr$. Q (volumetric flow) and A (cross sectional area) are determined by direct measurement and give V_1(velocity) because $Q = AV$. Knowing V_1 (velocity) and measuring the internal radius of curvature (r_1) and the internal diameter of the vessel (dr) the difference in pressure on the inner and outer walls of a bend can be calculated from the above equation.

Thus, at a velocity of 25 cm./sec. and an internal radius of curvature of 1 cm., in a vessel having a diameter of 0.3 cm. the difference in pressure is 173 dynes assuming $\rho = 1.06$ (the density of blood). The radius of curvature of the center line of the vessel is used as the average radius of curvature.

$V_1 = 25$ cm./sec.

$r_1 = 1.15$ cm. $dp = \rho V^2/r \ dr$

$dr = 0.3$

$dp = 173.0$ dynes/cm^2.

The difference in pressure (dp) will be lessened if the radius of curvature (r) is increased or the velocity (V) is decreased.

An increase in differential pressure at a bend may be produced by increasing the blood velocity, increasing the diameter (volumetric flow) of the blood vessel at a constant velocity or by decreasing the radius of curvature. It is known that the potential velocity distribution assumed here will not apply precisely in any actual viscous flow. In actual flow viscous effects cause a portion of the fluid in the region near the wall to be retarded. Outside the wall region the flow may be closer to a free vortex. However, any velocity distribution through the same bend having the same volumetric flow will give the same order of magnitude of pressure differential.

Secondary flow occurs in the flow around a bend in tubes, pipes and blood vessels. The secondary flow, consisting of two spirals, is superimposed upon the primary or main flow. In rivers and streams the secondary flow tends to pile up sand and gravel at the inner side of the bend and deepen the channel toward the outer side of the bend. No evidence of such deposition of blood elements has been noted in the pathologic studies of early lesions. Rather it is constantly noted that the diminished lateral pressure on the convex surface of bends stimulates the endothelium to proliferate with production of a progressively thickened intima which gradually encroaches upon the lumen as an atherosclerotic plaque. In brief, viscous effects and secondary flow

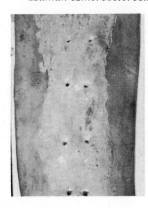

Fig. 20. Atherosclerosis of the thoracic aorta showing attachment lesion on dorsal surface. Gross specimen.

may modify flow in a curved path. These effects may modify the pressure distribution to some extent but cannot eliminate the basic effect of the production of low pressure areas on the convex surface of curved blood vessels which provides the initial stimulus for the development of atherosclerosis.

Attachment

A free elastic tube has no motion of its wall when the pressures on each side of the wall are equal. The flowing blood, whether steady or oscillating, produces varying pressures which move the wall toward the lesser pressure. Motion of an arterial wall is relatively unrestricted at most points compared to the limitation of motion imposed at zones of attachment (Fig. 20). It may be expected that mechanical stress at points of attachment stimulates intimal proliferation, the initial change in the development of atherosclerosis. There may be local diminished lateral pressure at tethered sites during some portion of each heart cycle.

Branching

Patterns of blood flow are determined by the anatomic pattern of a branch and the rate of flow through each branch. The ratios of branch to parent stem's diameter and angles of branching vary greatly. The flow patterns, therefore, necessarily vary and change in accordance with the local hydraulic conditions. In the flow pattern of each branch a zone of relatively low pressure is produced. If a sufficient suction effect due to the diminished lateral pressure is produced, an intimal response leading to atherosclerosis may appear. Low pressure areas are identified by points A in Figure 5 and correspond precisely to sites of atherosclerotic change.

Bifurcation

The velocity distribution and result of flow patterns at a bifurcation are illustrated in Figs. 3 and 14.

The sites of relative diminution in pressure or suction effect are determined in each instance by the velocities and curvatures of the flow at the wall of each branch, the angles of branching, the anatomical attachments and the ratio of trunk to branch diameter.

Other Considerations

In each of the above patterns of flow which relate to the anatomical design, an ideal geometry was described. Modifications of flow will be produced by the natural asymmetry or imperfections in the anatomic geometry of blood vessels. Further modifications will be produced progressively as the atherosclerotic process influences the velocity and volumetric flow by encroachment on the lumen.

It should be emphasized that several hydraulic conditions may be found concurrently. Thus, a tapering vessel may at the same time branch or have an attachment, etc. The composite effect of all the local hydraulic specifications—i.e., curvature, taper, branch, bifurcation, and attachment—will influence the velocity of flow and lateral pressure at a given site with respect to its predilection for atherosclerotic change.

HUMAN ATHEROSCLEROSIS

Vascular Embryology and Subsequent Development

The vascular system develops embryologically by means of endothelial sprouts from an early capillary network formed by the growth and coalescence of blood islands in the mesoderm. The vascular outgrowths are guided in their course by epithelial obstructions which determine the position of the capillary plexuses. Favorable channels enlarge and become main arteries and veins sending forth new branches. The hydraulic characteristics change both generally and locally while the anatomic design elaborates in response to the growth needs of the organism as a whole and the needs of individual organs. Hydraulic conditions conducive to atherosclerosis appear in utero as soon as blood begins to flow in definitive channels. The anatomic design of the vascular system and the natural laws of fluid mechanics provide hydraulic specifications which are prerequisite and conducive to atherosclerosis. The

earliest lesions, intimal thickening, are found at certain sites of predilection, namely, regions of relative decrease in lateral pressure such as are produced by curvature, tapering, bifurcation, branching, or external attachments. The continuous operation of local hydraulic forces throughout life makes further pathologic changes inherently possible. In fact, atherosclerosis, as a progressive occlusive arterial disease, or its pathologic complications, is a major cause of human disability and death.

Illustrative Examples

The human circulatory system is necessarily characterized by specific hydraulic-biologic conditions. The precise correlation of atherosclerotic lesions with their localization at sites of predilection,—namely, regions of diminished lateral pressure,—in accordance with the laws of fluid mechanics is demonstrated by the following examples, each of which is discussed under the appropriate heading: (1) The coronary arteries, (2) the aorta, (3) bifurcation of the aorta and common iliac arteries, (4) splenic artery, (5) pulmonary artery, and (6) veins.

1. The Coronary Circulation. The coronary circulation is unique with respect to its hydraulic characteristics. The flow of blood is intermittent as a result of systolic contraction of the heart. The blood stream is subject to abrupt, rapid and wide fluctuations in velocity, increased velocity and volumetric flow occurring during diastole and reduced velocity and volumetric flow occurring during systole. Retrograde or reversal of flow under certain conditions also occurs. The coronary arteries are unique in the body with respect to such wide phasic variations in blood flow. It is notable that the caliber of the extramural coronary arteries tapers rapidly. The anatomic curvatures inherent in the coronary circulation are also notable. The composite effect of these hydraulic factors,—namely, the rapid changes in velocity of flow, the nozzle effect of tapering, and the inherent anatomical curves—seem to be significant factors in the predisposition of the coronary arteries toward atherosclerotic changes. Pathologic examination of coronary arteries reveals uniformly that the atherosclerotic process develops at sites of predilection which are determined by the local hydraulic conditions. A free and straight vessel presents correspondingly more concentric atherosclerotic change. The forces generated by blood flow in a zone of curvature determine a greater degree of involvement of the inner (convex) wall compared with the outer wall (Fig. 21). The free epicardial aspect of a coronary artery may be less affected by atherosclerotic change than the tethered or attached

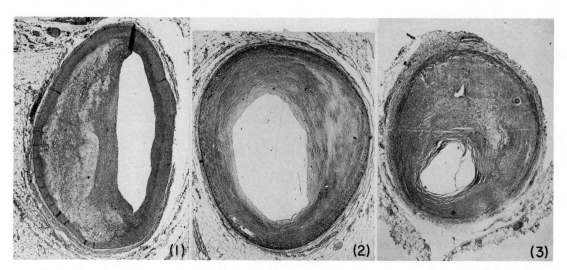

FIG. 21. Coronary atherosclerosis. Showing relatively advanced occlusive disease—eccentric "curvature" lesions.

surface. The reduced lumen at the site of atherosclerosis due to curvature or attachment will be, of necessity, eccentrically placed. A frequent finding is a segmental linear atherosclerotic plaque involving the left coronary artery beginning approximately 1 cm. from its origin at a zone where it curves and continues to form the left anterior descending branch. This is a "curvature" lesion aptly described as a "waterfall" lesion.

2. The Aorta. The predilection of the aortic arch for atherosclerotic changes and dissecting hematomas appears to be determined by the high velocity of blood flow and reduced static pressure or suction effect which characterize the hydraulic specifications in this region. A common finding is a large atherosclerotic plaque on the inner curvature of the aortic arch, a "sentinel patch." The sudden release of intra-abdominal pressure in the Valsalva maneuver causes a sudden increase in aortic blood velocity. The accompanying suction effect due to the sudden diminution in lateral pressure may tear the aortic wall by overcoming the bond between the layers to produce a dissecting hematoma. One of the earliest plaques to appear is located at the obliterated exit of the ductus arteriosus, an "attachment" lesion. The thoracic aorta typically and invariably presents atherosclerotic changes predominantly on the dorsal surface (Figs. 13 and 20). Tapering of the aorta and effects of gravity result in a relative increase in blood velocity in the abdominal portion of the aorta with consequently more severe atherosclerosis in this area. In advanced instances of atherosclerosis of the aorta, the involvement may be diffuse, affecting both dorsal and ventral walls.

3. Bifurcation of the Aorta and Common Iliac Arteries. The bifurcation of the aorta divides the more central stream lines. Under such hydraulic conditions a relative increase in velocity and decrease in lateral pressure are produced at the medial walls of the crotch zone compared with the lateral walls. These forces determine the medial walls of the crotch zone as sites of predilection for atherosclerotic changes (Fig. 14). It is notable that the proximal margins of the atherosclerotic plaques in the common iliac arteries may be about 1 cm. distal to the carina or the margin of bifurcation. This area, as a stagnation point, is free of atherosclerosis because of the local increase in pressure where impingement of the blood stream occurs. The high impingement pressure is less prone to produce atherosclerotic changes than the diminished lateral pressure at the immediately distal medial walls of the crotch zone.

It may be noted that the angles of bifurcation of the common iliac arteries vary among different individuals. When the angle of bifurcation is relatively acute the medial wall or "crotch" lesion develops. As the angle of bifurcation increases the lateral walls of the iliac arteries assume their anatomic importance as convex walls of curvatures in continuity with the aorta. Under such conditions, "curvature" lesions may appear on the lateral walls of the iliac arteries. The geometry or anatomic design of the aortic bifurcation will determine the hydraulic characteristics and sites of predilection for atherosclerosis in each individual.

4. Splenic Arteries. The splenic artery is remarka-

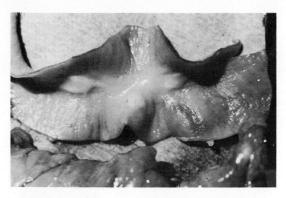

FIG. 22. Human splenic artery showing normal tortuosity. Note atherosclerotic plaque at convex surface of curvatures.

ble for its tortuosity and relatively large caliber. The large caliber serves to decrease the velocity of the blood flow. Atherosclerosis is therefore less frequent. Nevertheless, atherosclerosis will be found as a result of the local hydraulic characteristics in accordance with the laws of fluid mechanics. An atherosclerotic plaque is noted on the inner walls of the curvatures in the specimen illustrated (Fig. 22).

5. Pulmonary Artery. The pulmonary ring and pulmonary artery have a greater circumference than the aortic ring and ascending aorta. Since, normally, the same volume of blood per unit time must pass these sections, it is obvious that the velocity of flow is lower in the pulmonary artery compared with the ascending aorta. Therefore, atherosclerosis due to the suction effect of the blood stream is uncommon or minimized in the pulmonary artery.

6. Veins. Veins present gradually diverging lines of flow and have a larger caliber than corresponding arteries. The velocity of blood flow is relatively low and comparatively steady in veins (Fig. 23). The suction effect upon the walls of veins is therefore minimal, and occlusive sclerotic changes are comparatively rare.

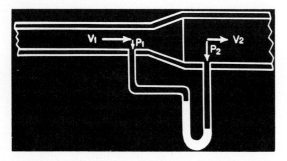

FIG. 23. Diagram of velocity changes in veins.

EXPERIMENTAL ATHEROSCLEROSIS IN DOGS

An approach to scientific proof that the effect of the laws of fluid mechanics is the primary factor in the causation, localization and progressive pathology of atherosclerosis may be achieved by altering hydraulic specifications under controlled conditions in order to observe arterial wall changes.

Vessels examined in 30 dogs at intervals up to three years following surgically produced s-shaped curvatures, attachments, and tapers consistently revealed atherosclerotic changes at all stages of development from the earliest intimal thickening to the most advanced occlusive fibroblastic proliferation (Figs. 6, 7, 10). The atherosclerotic plaque assumes characteristics of localization and shape corresponding to zones of varying diminution in lateral pressure. The pathologic changes evolve through progressive stages which vary in their rate of development as well as in their nature and severity. The in situ pathologic processes may include collagen deposition, elastic tissue changes, cellular infiltration, lipid changes, and occasional calcification. Vascularization of the intima, intimal hemorrhage, and subdivision of the channel by transluminal intimal proliferation have been noted. Fibroblastic proliferation appears to be the dominant pathologic change at all stages.

The localization and progressive changes in atherosclerotic lesions produced in dogs by the surgical alteration (Fig. 24) of vascular configuration under controlled conditions are fully comparable to the naturally occurring atherosclerotic lesions in humans. Atherosclerosis invariably develops at sites of predilection, namely, segmental zones of low pressure which derive from local hydraulic specifications.

DISCUSSION

The characteristics of pulsatile flow in arteries can be analyzed by applying the same basic equations of fluid mechanics which apply to flow in rigid tubes. Operation of the laws of fluid mechanics under the hydraulic conditions found in the human circulatory system is prerequisite and conducive to atherosclerosis.

Atherosclerosis begins as a change in the intima at sites of predilection characterized by tapering, curvature, bifurcation, branching or external attachment. Such locations are subject to a relative decrease in lateral pressure in accordance with the applicable laws of fluid mechanics. The initial change is a reparative response of the intima to the local

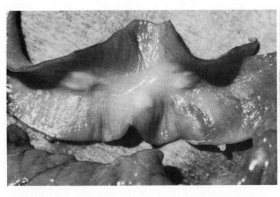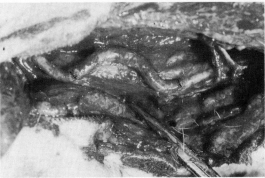

FIG. 24. Comparison of curvatures in human splenic artery with curvatures in dog formed by interposing a segment of femoral artery between ends of transected carotid artery.

suction effect of the flowing blood upon the vessel's wall. The biologic reaction is a thickening of the intima due to proliferation of the endothelial cells and fibroblasts from subjacent layers. Continuous operation of the local hydraulic factors causes further pathologic alterations. These may include cellular infiltration, lipid changes and further fibroblastic proliferation. The plaque thickens and gradually encroaches on the arterial lumen producing varying degrees of occlusion. The hemodynamic mechanism is also described for intimal ulceration, intimal hemorrhage and dissecting hematoma occurring as complications inherent in the pathogenesis of atherosclerosis.

The variations in the severity of atherosclerosis found in individual patients are shown to be due principally to the composite effect of variations in their hydraulic specifications. The velocity of blood flow, the caliber of lumen and anatomical pattern are of importance. Biologic factors must also be considered, namely, the physiopathologic response or local reparative reaction of the intima to the diminished lateral pressure (suction effect) generated by the flowing blood. It is here that the nature and degree of atherosclerotic change may be influenced by differences in tissue structure and differences in tissue response to injury arising from genetic and species characteristics.

The roles of other contributing atherogenic factors such as age, sex, race, diet, nutritional status, habitus, lipid metabolism, obesity, drugs, hormones, associated diseases, enzyme systems, hypertension, occupation, and emotional stress, require re-evaluation as secondary or modifying factors. Not one of these factors is always present, nor is any particular combination present as a common denominator (sine qua non) or as a primary factor responsible in a causative sense for atherosclerosis.

None of these factors can create atherosclerosis. Atherosclerosis is found in both men and women, in the relatively young as in the aged, in hypertensive persons as well as in normotensives and in lean as well as in obese individuals. Notwithstanding available studies of the statistical association of atherosclerosis with lipids, diet, sex, habitus, occupation, emotional stress, and ethnic groups, proof of the causal relation of these factors to atherosclerosis is not thereby demonstrated or proved. Statistical associations, per se, cannot be considered scientific proof of causal relation.

The experimental production of hemodynamically-induced arterial lesions in dogs by surgical alterations of vascular configurations under controlled conditions supports the central role of vascular dynamics in the development of atherosclerosis.

By identifying the role of hemodynamics as the specific primary factor in the development of atherosclerosis, a direction for further research is indicated. Atherosclerosis has been demonstrated to be due to a specific stimulus—namely the diminished lateral pressure—produced by local hemodynamic characteristics. Each hydraulic factor must be critically analyzed, and control of relevant hydraulic specifications must be sought in order to control directly the atherosclerotic process. It may be noted that the hydraulic factors which contribute to the development of atherosclerosis are not all of equal importance, nor are all the hydraulic factors amenable to change, manipulation, or control. Thus, anatomic patterns, such as angles of branching, curvature, attachment, and calibers of lumens are largely determined by heredity and development. Similarly, the biologic response of the intima to the stimulus of the hydraulic forces is probably determined by heredity as a racial or species characteristic.

An area of specific research suggested by the present approach lies in the study of the velocity of blood flow. Control of blood velocity provides a method of control of lateral pressure or suction effect which is proposed and identified in this report as the immediate stimulus for the inception and progressive pathology of atherosclerosis. An increased velocity, if other factors remain unchanged, must produce more severe atherosclerosis. Conversely, a decrease in blood velocity, if achieved without impairing the metabolic requirements of vital centers or organs, may be expected to minimize the atherosclerotic process and its progressive pathologic development. Research in this area is in progress. A pharmacologic agent or physiologic method may be found or developed to achieve this goal.

SUMMARY AND CONCLUSION

Correlated data[1,2,3,7,8,9] derived from autopsy findings, model hydraulic systems, and the experimental production of hemodynamically-induced arterial lesions in dogs support the concept that the effect of the laws of fluid mechanics are the primary causative factor in the localization and pathogenesis of atherosclerosis.

Atherosclerosis begins as a minute reactive thickening of the tunica intima due to proliferation of endothelium and fibroblasts from subjacent layers at sites of diminished lateral pressure in the circulatory system.

Progressive pathologic changes occur in situ as fibroblastic proliferation continues and encroaches upon or even occludes the vessel's lumen.

The biologic response of blood vessels and vascular dynamics (mechanical factors) are integrated by the hemodynamic concept of atherosclerosis which considers the role of fluid mechanics—vascular hemodynamics—as the primary factor in the causation, localization, and progressive pathology of atherosclerosis.

Study of factors which determine blood velocity may yield data useful in controlling vascular dynamics and the intimal response to hydraulic forces.

Further study of vascular dynamics and its control may be expected to provide the main key to the solution of the problem of atherosclerosis.

REFERENCES

1. Texon, M.: A hemodynamic concept of atherosclerosis with particular reference to coronary occlusion, Arch. Int. Med. *99*:418, 1957.
2. Texon, M.: The hemodynamic concept of atherosclerosis, Bull. New York Acad. Med. *36*:263, 1960.
3. Texon, M., Imparato, A. M., Lord, J. W., Jr., and Helpern, M.: Experimental production of arterial lesions, Arch. Int. Med. *110*:50, 1962.
4. Weinberg, S. B., and Helpern, M.: Circumstances related to sudden, unexpected death in coronary heart disease, *in* Work and the Heart, Rosenbaum, F., and Belknap, E. L., (eds.) New York, Harper & Row, 1959, pp. 288–92.
5. McDonald, D. A.: Blood Flow in Arteries, Baltimore, The Williams and Wilkins Co., 1960.
6. Womersley, J. R.: WADC–TR 56–614, 1957.
7. Texon, M.: The role of vascular dynamics in the development of atherosclerosis, *in* Atherosclerosis and its Origin, Sandler, M., and Bourne, G. H., (eds.) New York, Academic Press Inc. 1963, pp. 167–95.
8. Texon, M., Imparato, A. M., and Helpern, M.: The role of vascular dynamics in the development of atherosclerosis. J.A.M.A. *194*:1226, 1965.
9. Texon, M.: Mechanical factors in atherosclerosis, *in* Atherosclerotic Vascular Disease, Brest, A.N., and Moyer, J. H. (eds.) New York, Appleton-Century-Crofts, 1967, pp.23–42.

The author wishes gratefully to acknowledge the cooperation and encouragement of Dr. Milton Helpern, Chief Medical Examiner of the City of New York, Professor and Chairman of the Department of Forensic Medicine, New York University School of Medicine.

Dr. Richard Skalak, Professor of Civil Engineering and Engineering Mechanics at Columbia University reviewed the manuscript and offered helpful suggestions for which the author here records his deep appreciation and thanks.

The author also records his appreciation and gratefully acknowleges the cooperation in the surgical experiments of Dr. Anthony M. Imparato, Assistant Professor of Clinical Surgery, Department of Surgery, New York University School of Medicine.

The Role of Arterial Hypertension in Coronary Atherosclerosis

John H. Moyer and James Flynn

In the United States today, cardiovascular disease is the leading cause of death, and coronary atherosclerosis accounts for two thirds of the deaths from this cause. One third of all deaths of white men aged 45 to 74 and one fifth of the deaths among white men aged 35 to 44 are due to coronary heart disease.[1] Many of these men have concurrent essential hypertension. The significance of this disease complex is readily apparent, not only in the older age groups, but in the younger ones as well.

Although women are affected by coronary artery disease, as well as by essential hypertension alone, they are not as severely affected as men. A review of the medical literature reveals that the ratio of incidence of coronary artery atherosclerosis in men as compared to the incidence in women varies between 4.7:1 and 2:1, depending on age distribution and other variable factors in different groups studied.[2-6] In the past decade the Framingham study[7] has separated the male-to-female ratio on the basis of age groups. The authors found in the younger group, ages 30 to 44, a ratio of 13:1. In the older group, ages 45 to 62, the ratio decreased to 2:1. Gordon, Bland and White[8] reported the incidence at age 70 and over to be equal in both sexes.

The factors that predispose to coronary heart disease can be divided into two groups: disease processes occurring in the individual and factors associated with the environment. In the former group are included hypertension, hypercholesterolemia, hyperlipemia, obesity, diabetes mellitus, hyperuricemia, hypothyroidism, estrogen deficiency states, and left ventricular hypertrophy as demonstrated by either electrocardiograph or x-ray. [7,9-11] Environmental factors include diet, geographical area, emotional stress, smoking, and habits of physical activity or inactivity. [7,10-12]

As Murphy[13] suggests, hereditary and environmental factors may interact either to reinforce or to modify the influence that any one of them might exert. The extent to which these various factors contribute to the development of atherosclerosis, and in what proportion, is therefore difficult to evaluate. Nevertheless, of all those mentioned above, the two that appear to be most significant are hypertension and hypercholesterolemia. These factors are not independent of each other, but are closely interrelated in accelerating the atherosclerotic process. In this discussion, however, we are primarily concerned with the former.

EARLY STUDIES

For more than 60 years investigators have been aware of the close association of hypertension and atherosclerosis. In 1906 Carrel and Guthrie[14] published a paper concerning the accelerated development of atherosclerosis in patients with elevated blood pressure. During the next decade Anitschkow[15] associated cholesterol with atherosclerosis and suggested that constituents of the serum are filtered through the blood vessel walls. Bell and Clawson,[16] in 1928, published their classic monograph in which they analyzed post-mortem findings in 420 deceased patients with a history of hypertension. The authors stated, "Coronary sclerosis must have some causal relation to hypertension since the association is too frequent to be accidental." They further stated, ". . . when hypertension is associated, the increased strain accelerates and intensifies the arterial disease and makes it more prominent anatomically and clinically than in cases in which hypertension is not present." Eleven years later Clawson[17] analyzed 928 cases of coronary heart disease and concluded that hypertension was the most significant etiologic factor.

QUANTITATIVE RELATIONS BETWEEN DEGREE OF BLOOD PRESSURE ELEVATION AND ATHEROSCLEROSIS

The level of the blood pressure and the degree of atherosclerosis appear to be related in a linear fashion. In low pressure systems, such as the venous system and the pulmonary circulation, atherosclerosis is practically nonexistent under normal circumstances. In veins subjected to increased pressure, such as occurs in arteriovenous fistulas or in veins used for arterial bypass, atherosclerosis develops. This phenomenon is also seen in the portal and mesenteric vasculature of patients with portal hypertension. Pulmonary hypertension of any origin predisposes the pulmonary vasculature to the development of atherosclerotic lesions. The arterial system is more commonly subjected to the deleterious effects of increased pressure. In patients with coarctation of the aorta, the proximal area will show extensive atherosclerosis, whereas the distal area is usually free of this process.

Interesting observations have been made on the relation between blood pressure and atherosclerosis in persons who are normotensive—that is, whose systolic pressure is 140 mm. of mercury or less and whose diastolic pressure is 90 mm. of mercury or less. The lower the blood pressure, the less apt the person is to have atherosclerosis.[18–21] With progressively higher levels of pressure (either systolic or diastolic, or both), even within the normotensive range, the degree of atherosclerotic change appears to increase. Once the hypertensive range of pressure is reached, the atherosclerotic process is greatly accelerated and continues to increase as the pressure gets higher.

The dividing line between hypertension and normal blood pressure is only relative. Once the systolic pressure rises above 140 mm. of mercury or the diastolic pressure rises above 90 mm. of mercury, no abnormal physiologic processes are called into action. Rather, the biochemical and physiologic processes taking place in the normotensive range are merely accelerated. Master, Dack and Jaffe[5] summed up this problem concisely when they concluded: *"Hypertension accelerates the aging process."*

A rapid and sustained rise in pressure affects the arterioles (in contrast to the larger arteries), and the hypertensive process goes into a malignant phase. Persons with this acute form of hypertension die before the atherosclerotic process involves the larger arteries. The renal arterioles (glomeruli) are most severely involved, as indicated by deteriorating renal function (Fig. 1). In this phase, if the disease is untreated, death usually ensues within a year (Fig. 2).

Figure 2 summarizes graphically the mortality in untreated and treated patients with malignant hypertension. Of those who were not treated, 80 per cent had died after one year. Effective treatment of

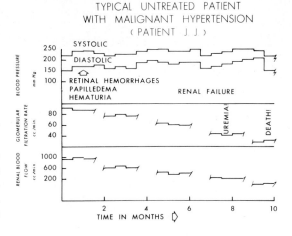

FIG. 1. Deterioration of renal function in a typical untreated individual with malignant hypertension. The graph shows a progressive reduction in glomerular filtration rate, leading to renal excretory failure. The reduction in glomerular filtration rate (inulin clearance) is a good index of renal damage. (Reprinted from Am. J. Med. *24*:177, 1958[39].)

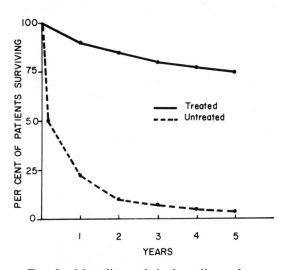

FIG. 2. Mortality statistics in malignant hypertension—treated vs. untreated. The mortality when the disease is untreated is 100 per cent within five years, but treatment reduces it to 25 per cent in that period of time. Patients who die early after treatment is begun still tend to die of progressive renal failure; but after two years of blood pressure control, when death occurs it is likely to result from atherosclerotic occlusive disease. (See also Table 1)

the hypertension in a comparable group of patients reduced the mortality to 25 per cent after five years. The malignant vascular process can be arrested by controlling the hypertension if treatment is begun early enough in this phase of the disease, before advanced excretory renal failure develops. It is of some interest that most of the untreated patients died of renal failure. Of the treated patients, those who died of renal failure did so within the first year or two. However, when the blood pressure was regulated, so that only intermittent hypertension might be expected, few patients died subsequently of renal failure. Deaths after this initial period were due to atherosclerosis. Apparently, these patients died of major vascular occlusions; i.e., the cause of death was similar to that found in mildly hypertensive patients, which is primarily coronary artery disease or cerebral atherosclerosis. These vascular accidents usually happen at a time when the blood pressure has escaped from control. Briefly then, if you keep them alive long enough, patients whose hypertension is controlled will eventually succumb to atherosclerotic complications rather than as a result of renal failure; however, this occurs only if the period of survival is adequate to permit the development of advanced atherosclerosis.

As Table 1 shows, in a group of 48 patients treated with antihypertensive drugs and followed up for a period of five years, 12 died. Of the three patients who died within the first year, two died of renal failure and only one from occlusion of a major vessel. However, during the second year only one of three deaths resulted from renal failure; the remaining two were due to vascular occlusion. Subsequent to the second year six patients died, all from a major arterial occlusion associated with atherosclerotic disease.

TABLE 1
Cause of Death in 12 of 48 Patients Treated for Malignant Hypertension

Year of Treatment	Cause of Death		
	Renal	*CVA*	*Coronary*
First	2	1	
Second	1	1	1
Third		2	
Fourth		1	2
Fifth			1
TOTAL	3	5	4

Mortality after 5 years due to hypertension: 25%. Unrelated cause of death: 3 patients.

NATURAL HISTORY OF HYPERTENSION

Perera[22] studied the natural history of hyper-

tension. He found the average life expectancy of an untreated person with essential hypertension to be approximately 20 years from the time the hypertension was detected (Fig. 3). The first three quarters of this period were relatively symptom-free, but in

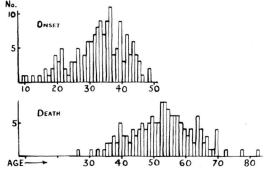

Fig. 3. Age at onset and age at death of the same 150 patients with hypertensive vascular disease. (Reprinted from Perera, G. A.: J. Chron. Dis. *1*:33, 1955[22].)

the last quarter the complications of hypertension began to appear. These included congestive heart failure, renal insufficiency, cerebrovascular accidents and myocardial infarction. The latter two are primarily the result of the accelerated atherosclerotic process generated by the hypertension.

The effect of blood pressure on the arterial system begins in utero or shortly after birth[23] and is characterized by elastic tissue changes in the intima of the vessels. These changes, which are continuous and progressive, appear to be degenerative in nature. In the young adult, lipid is deposited for the first time in the intima.[24] The lipid accumulations progress, and by the fifth and sixth decades the morbidity and mortality resulting from the atherosclerotic process become strikingly apparent.

We must now consider the pathophysiologic changes occurring in the blood vessels which lead to the formation of the atherosclerotic plaque.

PATHOPHYSIOLOGIC RELATION BETWEEN HYPERTENSION AND ATHEROSCLEROSIS

Two of the current theories that attempt to relate hypertension with atherosclerosis are the theory of vascularization [25,26] and the theory of lipid filtration.[15,27] The former theory postulates that following some undefined degenerative changes in the arterial intima, capillaries develop which communicate with the arterial lumen. Under the stress of elevated pressure, transient or persistent, such capillaries are prone to rupture. This leads to intimal

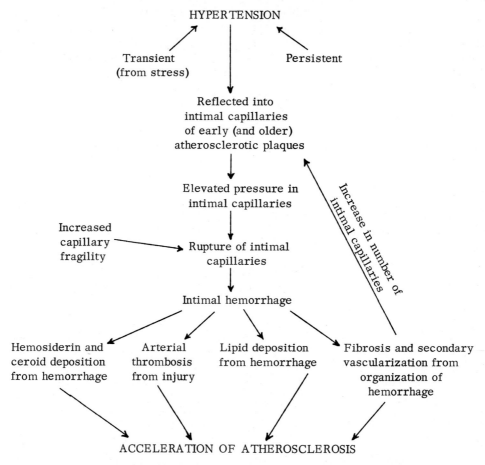

FIG. 4. Diagrammatic representation of how atherosclerosis develops, according to the "vascularization" theory. (Reprinted from Paterson, J. C. et al.: Canad. M. A. J. *82*:65, 1960 [26].)

hemorrhage, which lays the foundation of the atherosclerotic plaque, and the subsequent deposit of lipids and hemosiderin causes an increase in the size of the plaque. The lesions become organized to form the fibrous tissue seen in atherosclerosis. The process of organization also leads to the development of new capillaries, thereby initiating a vicious cycle (Fig. 4). The more capillaries, the more hemorrhage; and the more hemorrhage, the larger the plaque will be. The principal drawback to this theory is that it does not account for the increased atherosclerosis seen in nonhypertensive states such as diabetes mellitus, hypercholesterolemia and hyperlipemia. However, an amplification of this theory recently described by Paterson[26] in a personal communication to the authors may partly account for accelerated development of atherosclerosis even in the absence of sustained hypertension. He states: " . . . stress might produce other significant changes than simple elevation of blood pressure, e.g., the release of epinephrine during severe emotional or physical

stress also mobilizes the fat in the various depots, resulting in an elevation of serum cholesterol; and further, epinephrine is now known to favor the conglutination of platelets, thus enhancing the predilection for thrombosis."

The lipid filtration theory had its origin with Anitschkow[15] more than 50 years ago. Wilens[27] later demonstrated that serum could be filtered through blood vessel walls. The resulting filtrate was markedly different in appearance and chemical composition from the original serum. The fluid was much more watery in character and had lost most of its cholesterol and protein content. Wilens's investigation showed that some of the cholesterol had entered the arterial wall and had been deposited in it.

Watts[28] has refined the work of his predecessors and explained the filtration theory on a cellular and histochemical level. He suggests that plasma lipoproteins are filtered from the lumen of the vessel, passing through the intima and media to the adventitia, where the lymphatics pick them up. During passage through the cell wall, the beta-lipoproteins are taken up in the muscle cells by the process of pinocytosis. The lipids are then metabolized by enzymes contained in the mitochondria of these cells. If the process of lipid metabolism becomes ineffective for any reason, or if the lipid content increases beyond the capacity of the enzymes to metabolize it, the lipids accumulate in the mitochondria. As the mitochondria become overloaded they degenerate, fragment, and release their products (enzymes and lysozymes) as well as the lipid into the cytoplasm. The myocytes then become foam cells, which continue to absorb lipid but can no longer effectively metabolize it. As a result the cell eventually dies and disintegrates, thereby releasing its own substances and the lipid into the connective tissue of the vessel wall, where they remain to impede the filtration of plasma proteins and lipids through the wall.

The end stage of this process is, of course, the atherosclerotic plaque. In hypertensive patients, the amount of lipids filtered would be increased because the elevated pressure would drive more through the vessel wall. This theory also takes into account the diseases that result in hyperlipemic states and therefore increase the amount of lipid available for filtration.

Laboratory observations confirm an association between hypertension and atherosclerosis. Deming et al.[29] showed that in rats with hypercholesterolemia and hyperlipemia resulting from a high-cholesterol diet, experimentally induced hypertension greatly increased the severity and rapidity of development of the atherosclerotic process. Later, with other co-workers,[30] he demonstrated in a similar study that hypertensive rats whose blood pressures were subsequently controlled exhibited much less atherosclerosis than found in the rats with uncontrolled hypertension.

Heptinstall and Bronte-Stewart[31,32] found that in rabbits fed a diet high in cholesterol, a slight rise in blood pressure over a short period of time greatly accelerated the atherosclerotic process. Subsequently, Heptinstall and Porter[33] studied similarly fed rabbits divided into three groups according to whether or not the animals were hypertensive, and if so, whether for a short or long period of time. At post-mortem examination, those rabbits that were hypertensive the longest were found to have aortic atheroma of the severest grade. Moses[34] and Wakerlin et al.[35] found the onset of atherosclerosis to be accelerated and its severity increased in hypercholesterolemic dogs that had been made hyper-

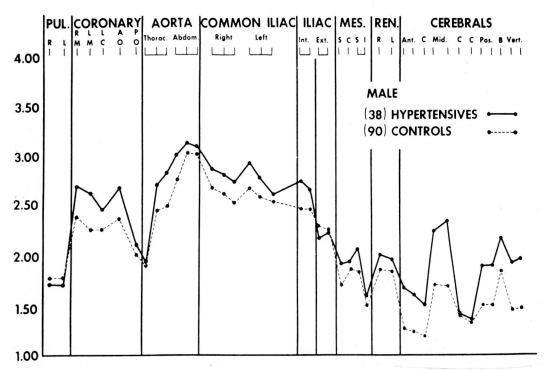

FIG. 5. Atherosclerosis profiles of hypertensive men compared with age-matched controls (normotensive). (Reprinted from Moses, C.: Atherosclerosis, Philadelphia, Lea and Febiger, 1963. [12])

tensive.

The objection may be raised that the conditions under which atherosclerosis was induced in these animals differ markedly from the conditions under

mortem examinations, Wilkens et al.[36] studied the degree of atherosclerosis in various parts of the body relative to predisposing diseases and other conditions. It appeared to be greater in the coronary

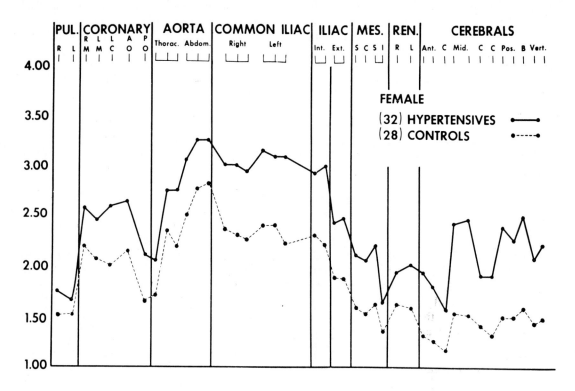

FIG. 6. Atherosclerosis profiles of hypertensive women and age-matched normotensive controls. (Reprinted from Moses, C.: Atherosclerosis, Lea and Febiger, 1963[12].)

which it occurs in man. The animals are fed an abnormal diet, and atherosclerosis develops during the first half of their life span. Despite this difference, we are unable to escape the conclusion that: Hypercholesterolemia+hypertension=atherosclerosis.

DISTRIBUTION OF ATHEROSCLEROSIS IN MAN

Although atherosclerosis affects all of the vascular beds in man, the two areas most consistently involved to the greatest extent are the heart and the brain. As previously mentioned, much of the morbidity and mortality resulting from essential hypertension is related to coronary heart disease and cerebral vascular disease, in which the underlying disease process is atherosclerosis. The distribution of the lesions in hypertensive persons appears to differ according to sex. In a large series of post-

and cerebral circulations of hypertensive men than in normotensive men (Fig. 5). In hypertensive women, all of the vascular beds examined were more atherosclerotic than corresponding sites in a similar group of normotensive women (Fig. 6). With the exception of those who were diabetic or obese, no significant differences were found between the distribution and extent of atherosclerosis in normotensive men and women.

It seems reasonable to assume that the extent to which atherosclerosis affects the vessels in different areas is reflected in the clinical manifestations of severe vascular disease in those areas. One of us has previously reported[37] that among patients with essential hypertension, the incidence of fatal myocardial infarction is four times greater in men than in women. Cerebral vascular disease, on the other hand, was found to be a more common cause of death in women. Renal failure (resulting largely from vascular damage) occurred with almost equal frequency in both men and women (Fig. 7) and was

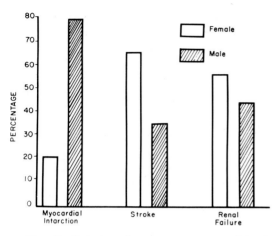

FIG. 7. Relation of sex to some causes of death in patients with nonaccelerated hypertension. Comparison of the incidence in men and women of some major vascular complications of hypertension. (Reprinted from Am. J. Cardiol. *17*:673, 1966.)

found to be related primarily to the severity of the blood pressure elevation. This indicates a greater preponderance of atherosclerotic involvement in the cerebral circulation of women than Wilkens found in his study, but is not necessarily inconsistent with his findings. Moses[12] suggests that differences in sex may influence the outcome of vascular disease as well as its distribution.

RESULTS OF THERAPY AND PROGNOSIS

During the past 15 years drug therapy has greatly altered the outlook for hypertensive patients, thus providing indirect evidence of the relation between elevated blood pressure and atherosclerotic vascular disease. Prior to this time, uremia and congestive heart failure were leading causes of death in the hypertensive population; but now that we are able to control blood pressure effectively, the malignant phase of essential hypertension is rarely seen. A decade ago one of us, working with a group, demonstrated the detrimental effect of elevated blood pressure on renal function.[38,39] The results of this early study proved that drug therapy could arrest the renal vascular deterioration and prolong the lives of patients with severe, premalignant hypertension. More recent studies have borne out the original observations (Fig. 2).

The effect of drug therapy on the longevity of patients with non-malignant essential hypertension has been more difficult to evaluate especially when atherosclerotic disease of the major arteries complicates the picture. The reasons for this are that the natural history of the disease runs a prolonged course, and it is not always possible to demonstrate early atherosclerotic changes in the living person. The era of effective drug therapy is only beginning to approach two decades, which is the average life expectancy of a person with untreated essential hypertension from the time of onset. Nevertheless, lowering of elevated blood pressure to the normal range appears to decrease the incidence of atherosclerotic complications, although it does not eliminate them entirely.

Indirect evidence of this is summarized in Table 2. A group of 32 patients who were retired because of intractable angina and hypertension were treated for the latter condition with drugs that depress the sympathetic nervous system. Their response was evaluated against that of placebo-treated controls. When the blood pressure was initially reduced, the angina improved so that 20 of the 32 patients experienced rather dramatic improvement and an additional 10 patients received partial relief of symptoms. This was apparently related to the decreased cardiac work load and the reduced need for blood delivered through the obstructed coronary arteries to the myocardium. However, after three years many of these patients, though still normotensive, experienced a return of severe anginal pain. Presumably the advancing atherosclerotic disease led to greater obstruction of the coronary circulation. During the three-year period of study, eight patients died, of whom six had experienced only partial relief of symptoms and two had experienced no relief with blood pressure control. We can thus conclude that blood pressure elevation is a complicating phenomenon here rather than a condition of primary significance.

TABLE 2
Intractable Angina with Hypertension:
Results of Therapy (32 Patients)

Results	First Two Months After Control of Blood Pressure	After 3 Years Normotensive
Complete relief	20	8
Partial relief	10	6
No change	2	10
Death	–	8

Probably one of the reasons hypertensive patients with controlled blood pressure have a greater incidence of coronary heart disease and cerebral vascular accidents is that they have not been treated from the onset of their disease. They are experiencing the untoward effects of hypertension already established during the several years before the elevated pressure was discovered and treated.

The degree to which hypertension contributes to the morbidity caused by atherosclerosis when both phenomena are present in the same patient may be difficult to determine. Nevertheless, some insight is provided by observing the results in such patients when their blood pressure has been controlled for an extended period of time, and then the control is

TABLE 3
Results in 17 Severely Hypertensive Patients with Remission Who Discontinued Therapy

Period off Drug* Before Recurrence	No. of Patients	No. of Deaths
6 months	8	4†
18 months	3	1†
3 years	2	1†
5 years	1	

*Two of 16 patients remained normotensive after drug therapy was discontinued, and one additional patient had a persistent labile hypertension but not complete relapse.
†3 cerebrovascular accidents and 3 myocardial infarctions.

suddenly withdrawn. Table 3 summarizes the results of such circumstances. As the blood pressure rises to pretreatment levels, vascular occlusion occurs within months in a large number of patients, thus demonstrating the prophylactic value of controlling the blood pressure. Undoubtedly, major vascular occlusions will eventually occur in most of these patients even if they are kept normotensive, but at a much later date.

We might conclude, then, that although the blood pressure of most hypertensive patients can be maintained at normal levels, the aging process of atherosclerosis continues, though more slowly (Table 4). The goal of blood pressure control in essential hy-

TABLE 4
Therapeutic Considerations: Hypertension vs. Atherosclerosis

Hypertension:——→(Retinal; Nephrons; Cerebral)= A direct therapeutic response to control of blood pressure has been proved.

Atherosclerosis: (Coronary; Renal Vascular; Cerebrovascular)= A dual therapeutic problem—i.e., atherosclerosis and hypertension. Hypertension is only a complicating factor, while the basic atherosclerosis is the fundamental abnormality of the disease complex. The effectiveness of therapy remains to be proved.

pertension complicated by atherosclerosis is to decrease the accelerated development of atherosclerosis that characterizes this group of patients and to prevent major arterial occlusions. If this is accomplished, the incidence of coronary heart disease and cerebral vascular disease may be reduced, though certainly not eradicated. For maximum effectiveness, treatment must be started to control the atherosclerosis in the early phase of the disease, and adequate therapy must also be provided to maintain the blood pressure within normal limits.

REFERENCES

1. Enterline, P.E., and Stewart, A. H.: Geographic patterns in death from coronary heart disease, Pub. Health Rep. 77:849, 1956.
2. White, P. D.: Heart Disease, New York, Macmillan Company 1931, p. 609.
3. Clawson, B. J.: Coronary sclerosis, Am. Heart J. 17:387, 1939.
4. Levy, H., and Boas, E. P.: Coronary artery disease in women, J.A.M.A. 107:97, 1936.
5. Master, A. M., Dack, S., and Jaffe, H. L.: Age, sex and hypertension in myocardial infarction due to coronary occlusion, Arch. Int. Med. 64:767, 1939.
6. Master, A. M.: Incidence of acute coronary artery occlusion. Am. Heart J. 33:135, 1947.
7. Kannel, W. B., Dawber, T. R., Kazan, A., Revatskie, W., and Stokes, J.: Factors of risk in the development of coronary heart disease—six-year follow-up experience, Ann. Int. Med. 55:33, 1961.
8. Gordon, W. H., Bland, E. F., and White, P. D.: Coronary artery disease analyzed post mortem, Am. Heart J. 11:10, 1939.
9. Brest, A. N.: Diseases predisposing to atherosclerosis, in Likoff, W., and Moyer, J. H.: Coronary Heart Disease, New York, Grune and Stratton, 1963, p. 120.
10. Dawber, T. R., and Kannel, W. B.: Susceptibility to coronary heart disease, Mod. Concepts Cardiovas. Dis. 30:671, 1961.
11. Ostrander, L. D.: Alterations of factors predisposing to coronary heart disease, Ann. Int. Med. 68: 1072, 1968.
12. Moses, Campbell: Atherosclerosis, Philadelphia, Lea and Febiger, 1963, p. 15.
13. Murphy, E. A.: Genetics and atherosclerosis, in Likoff, W., and Moyer, J. H.: Coronary Heart Disease, New York, Grune and Stratton, 1963, p. 89.
14. Carrel, A., and Guthrie, C. C.: Arteriosclerose par modification chirurgicale dela circulation, Compt. rend. Soc. de Biol. 60:730, 1906.
15. Anitschkow, N. N.: Über die Atherosklerose der Aorta beim Kaninchen und uber deren Entstehungsbedingungen, Beitr. path. Anat. 59:306, 1914.
16. Bell, E. T., and Clawson, B. J.: Primary (essential) hypertension—a study of four hundred and twenty cases, Arch. Path. 5:939, 1928.
17. Clawson, B. J.: Coronary sclerosis—an analysis of nine hundred twenty-eight cases, Am. Heart J. 17:387, 1939.

18. Hunter, A., cited by Gubner, R., and Ungerleider, H. E.: Arteriosclerosis: Statement of the problem, Am. J. Med. *6*:60, 1949.

19. Bender, S. R.: Clinical relationship of atherosclerosis and hypertension, *in* Brest, A. N., and Moyer, J. H.: Hypertension: Recent Advances—The Second Hahnemann Symposium on Hypertensive Disease, Philadelphia, Lea and Febiger, 1961, p. 164.

20. Young, W., Gofman, J. W., and Tandy, R.: The quantitation of atherosclerosis. II. Quantitative aspects of the relationship of blood pressure and atherosclerosis, Am. J. Cardiol. *6*:294, 1960.

21. Build and Blood Pressure Study, 1959. Society of Actuaries.

22. Perera, G.: Hypertensive vascular disease: Description and natural history, J. Chron, Dis. *1*:33, 1955.

23. Stehbens, W. E.: Focal intimal proliferation in the cerebral arteries, Am. J. Path. *36*:289, 1960.

24. Geer, J. C., and McGill, H. C.: The fine structure of coronary atheroma, *in* Likoff, W., and Moyer, J. H.: Coronary Heart Disease, New York, Grune and Stratton, 1963, p. 125.

25. Mills, J., Moffatt, T., and Paterson, J. C.: Incidence of intimal hemorrhage in the aorta in normotensive and hypertensive men. A preliminary report, Lab. Invest. *7*:606, 1959.

26. Paterson, J. C., Mills, J., and Lockwood, C. H.: The role of hypertension in the progression of atherosclerosis, Canad. M. A. J. *82*:65, 1960.

27. Wilens, S. L.: The experimental production of lipid deposition in excised arteries, Science *114*:389, 1951.

28. Watts, H. F.: The mechanism of arterial lipid accumulation in human coronary artery atherosclerosis, *in* Likoff, W., and Moyer, J. H.: Coronary Heart Disease, New York, Grune and Stratton, 1963, p. 98.

29. Deming, Q. B., Mosback, E. H., Bevans, M., Daly, M. M., Abell, L. L., Martin, E., Brun, L. M., Halpern, E., and Kaplan, R.: Blood pressure, cholesterol content of serum and tissues, and atherosclerosis in the rat, J. Exper. Med. *107*:581, 1958.

30. Deming, Q. B., Daly, M. M., Bloom, J., Brun, L., and Kaplan, R.: Effect of antihypertensive treatment in the rat on the potentiation of atherogenesis by experimental hypertension, J. Clin. Invest. *39*:980, 1960.

31. Heptinstall, R. H., and Bronte-Stewart, B.: Visceral and plasma changes in cholesterol-fed rabbits with raised blood pressure, J. Path. & Bact. *68*:202, 1954.

32. Bronte-Stewart, B., and Heptinstall, R. H.: The relationship between experimental hypertension and cholesterol-induced atheroma in rabbits, J. Path. & Bact. *68*:407, 1954.

33. Heptinstall, R. H., and Porter, K. A.: The effect of a brief period of high blood pressure on cholesterol-induced atheroma in rabbits, Brit. J. Exper. Path. *38*:55, 1957.

34. Moses, C.: Development of atherosclerosis in dogs with hypercholesterolemia and chronic hypertension, Circulation Res. *2*:243, 1954.

35. Wakerlin, G. E. Moss, M. G., and Kiley, J. P.: Effect of experimental renal hypertension on experimental thiouracil-cholesterol atherosclerosis in dogs, Circulation Res. *5*:426, 1957.

36. Wilkens, R. H., Roberts, J. C., and Moses, C.: Autopsy studies in atherosclerosis. III. Distribution and severity of atherosclerosis in the presence of obesity, hypertension, nephrosclerosis and rheumatic heart disease, Circulation *20*:521, 1959.

37. Moyer, J. H., and Brest, A. N.: The changing outlook for the patient with hypertension, Am. J. Cardiol. *17*:673, 1966.

38. Moyer, J. H., Heider, C., Pevey, K., and Ford, R. B.: The vascular status of a heterogeneous group of patients with hypertension, with particular emphasis on renal function, Am. J. Med. *24*:164, 1958.

39. Moyer, J. H., Heider, C., Pevey, K., and Ford, R. B.: The effect of treatment on the vascular deterioration associated with hypertension, with particular emphasis on renal function, Am. J. Med. *24*:177, 1958.

Diseases Accelerating Atherosclerosis

William Likoff

Regrettably, the cause of coronary atherosclerosis is not known. Numerous hypotheses attempt to explain how the granulomatous lesions develop in the arterial wall and encroach upon the vascular channel. Some contend the basic fault resides in the arterial wall.[1] Others indict the plasma and its contents.[2] Many acknowledge a multifactorial responsibility in both host and environment embracing such items as age, hepatic function, endocrine status, thrombogenesis, hemodynamics, diet, exercise and occupation.[3] The nature and magnitude of the differences included in these concepts become quite apparent when two prevailing postulates, platelet conglutination and abnormal lipid metabolism are compared.

The first of these concepts holds that atherogenesis is initiated with the deposition of platelets along the vascular endothelium. Presumably an intrinsic or acquired abnormality in the arterial wall, a biophysical or biochemical defect in the platelets, or an imbalance in the clotting-anti-clotting forces is responsible for this phenomenon. Additionally, it is influenced by the size of the artery, its configuration and the turbulence, velocity and force of blood flow.[4]

Repetitively, as platelets accumulate at specific points in the artery, they are said to pass into the intima by transendothelial imbibition. Here acting as foreign cells, they initiate an inflammatory reaction. With time an intramural abscess matures, ultimately undergoing hemorrhagic, lipid, fibrotic or calcific degeneration. Lipid infiltration is believed to take place because the capillaries which pervade the inflammatory mass are exceptionally permeable, particularly when plasma lipid concentrations are abnormally high.

As the atheromatous lesion enlarges it impinges upon and narrows the arterial channel. It may occlude the vessel completely. Occasionally, a thrombus forms in the slowly moving blood stream where the artery is narrowed and obstructs the lumen. At times the atheroma ruptures, discharging its contents into and occluding a smaller distal vessel.

In brief, the platelet conglutination theory holds a number of factors responsible for atherogenesis not the least of which reside in the platelets, the arterial wall or both. Lipids, however, are considered only secondary agents in the final development of the atheromatous lesion.

On the other hand, the lipid metabolic theory relates atherogenesis directly to circulating lipids although it does not define whether the process evolves because of the type of lipids, their levels in the plasma, or both. Support for this concept is impressive and is derived from the facts that: (1) Atherosclerotic lesions are composed largely of lipids, notably free cholesterol and cholesterol esters, in concentrations corresponding closely to those in plasma; (2) the only means by which atheroma can be produced in experimental animals is by producing an elevation of plasma lipids; (3) patients suffering from atherosclerosis have higher plasma-lipid levels than those not afflicted with the disease; and (4) patients with disturbed lipid metabolism have a high incidence of atherosclerosis.

However obscure the exact etiology, it is clear that atherogenesis is influenced by a great number of factors including age, sex and dietary habits. The current discussion concerns specific diseases which are believed to accelerate the development and progress of atherosclerosis.

First among these is essential hypertension. Experimentally, hypertension intensifies atherosclerosis in a number of laboratory animals.[5] Epidemiologic surveys suggest that in patients with blood pressure levels higher than 145/95 mm. Hg there is a 2-to 6-fold increase in the likelihood of coronary heart disease.[6] The incidence increases with the severity of the hypertension.

Theoretically, hypertension may exercise its effect by influencing the mechanical factors believed involved in atherogenesis; namely, intravascular pressure, and the turbulence, force and velocity of blood flow. Additionally, the neurohumoral factors which increase arterial resistance may have a profound effect upon the physicochemical structure of the arterial wall and its metabolic function.

Patients with overt and latent diabetes and those with a family history of the disorder have an increased incidence of clinical atherosclerosis. The frequency and precociousness of coronary heart disease in diabetics and the prevalence of abnormal glucose tolerance curves in "nondiabetics" with clinical coronary atherosclerosis suggest that both diseases share a common metabolic fault.[7] It is unlikely that this is influenced by diet since the incidence of atherosclerosis in diabetics has not changed even though dietary regulations have been materially altered over the years.

Clinical atherosclerosis is encountered commonly in patients with disturbed lipid metabolism.[8] Included in this group are the following phenotypes: (1) *Type 2.* This is known as familial hypercholesterolemia and may be encountered with or without xanthomatosis. It is characterized by increased beta lipoprotein and serum cholesterol concentration but normal triglycerides. (2) *Type 3.* This is also recognized as carbohydrate induced hyperglyceridemia (hyperlipemia) with hypercholesterolemia or mixed familial hyperglyceridemia (hyperlipemia) and hypercholesterolemia. It is distinguished by elevated beta lipoprotein and serum cholesterol as well as pre-beta lipoprotein and serum triglycerides. (3) *Type 4.* This is known as carbohydrate induced hyperglyceridemia (hyperlipemia) without hypercholesterolemia. It is marked by elevated pre-beta lipoprotein and serum triglycerides. (4) *Type 5.* This is referred to as fat and carbohydrate induced hyperglyceridemia (hyperlipemia). It is relatively rare and characterized by mixed biochemical features particularly elevated pre-beta lipoprotein levels.

Favorable biochemical responses to dietary adjustments have been recorded in these lipid metabolic disorders. Presumably deceleration of the atherosclerotic process then ensues. For example, the increase in beta lipoprotein and serum cholesterol in familial hypercholesterolemia, apparently due to hepatic overproduction of cholesterol and other constituents of beta lipoproteins, may respond to increased intake of polyunsaturated fat. Similarly, control of carbohydrate intake may correct Type 3 and Type 4 lipoprotein abnormalities.

Although hyperuricemia and gout are commonly believed associated with an increased incidence of coronary heart disease, recent epidemiologic studies suggest that this relation applies only to patients with actual gouty arthritis.

Endocrine dysfunction has been related to an increase in the incidence and severity of clinical atherosclerosis, particularly coronary heart disease. Accumulated data clearly indicate that the incidence of atherosclerotic heart disease increases significantly after menopause and the cessation of ovarian function. Furthermore, coronary heart disease is said to be four times as common in women who have undergone bilateral oophorectomy before menopause.[9]

The mechanism whereby gonadal function in the female influences atherogenesis may be related to lipid metabolism since the concentration of low density beta lipoprotein increases materially after the menopause and when the ovaries are removed. Administration of estrogens not only reverses coronary atherosclerosis induced experimentally but causes a reduction in atherogenic serum lipids in premenopausal and postmenopausal women and in individuals who have suffered a previous myocardial infarction.

The relation of thyroid function to atherosclerosis has been repeatedly documented. Experimentally, the induction of atherosclerosis by cholesterol feeding is greatly assisted by depressing thyroid function. On the other hand, administration of thyroid extract inhibits experimental atherosclerosis. Hyperthyroidism usually is associated with a diminished serum concentration of atherogenic lipids perhaps as a result of increased intestinal excretion. The same effect is observed after treatment with large doses of desiccated thyroid. Contrariwise, myxedema is generally associated with unusually high levels of circulating cholesterol and an increased incidence of clinical atherosclerosis.

The adrenal cortex is also concerned with regulation of lipid metabolism and hence, perhaps, with atherogenesis. Although experimentally induced cholesterol atherosclerosis is not augmented by administration of steroids, hyperglyceridemia and hypercholesterolemia may follow cortisone administration and at least hypercholesterolemia has been observed in Cushing's disease.

SUMMARY

Although the specific factors initiating atherogenesis have not been identified, it is clear that a number of diseases are responsible for accelerating the process. Most prominent among these are hypertension, diabetes mellitus, lipid metabolic disorders and endocrine dysfunction. These illnesses are believed to exercise their effect by influencing the mechanical issues involved in atherosclerosis, such as the force, velocity and turbulence of blood flow, or by exaggerating an existing lipid metabolic error.

REFERENCES

1. Maier, N., and Haimovici.: Oxidative Capacity of

Atherosclerotic Tissue, Circulation Res. *16*:65, 1965; Metabolism of Atherosclerotic Tissue of Rabbit and Dog, with Special Reference to Esterase and Lipase. Circulation Res. *17*:178, 1965.

2. Anitschkow, N.: Arteriosclerosis: A Survey of the Problem, New York, The Macmillan Company, 1954.

3. Olson, R. E., *in* Hurst and Logue, The Heart, New York, McGraw-Hill Book Company, Inc., 1966, pp. 622–627.

4. Texon, M.: A hemodynamic concept of atherosclerosis with particular reference to coronary occlusion, A.M.A. Arch. Int. Med. *99*:418, 1957.

5. Katz, N. N., and Stamler, J.: Experimental Atherosclerosis, Springfield, Ill., Charles C Thomas, 1953.

6. Dawber, T. R., and Kannell, W. B.: Susceptibility to coronary heart disease, Mod. Conc. Cardiovas. Dis. *30*:671, 1961.

7. Wahlberg, F.: The intravenous glucose tolerance test in atherosclerotic disease with special reference to obesity, hypertension, diabetic heredity and cholesterol values, Acta med. scandinav. *171*:1, 1962.

8. Stanbury, J. B., Wyngaarden, J. B., and Fredrickson, D. S.: The Metabolic Basis of Inherited Disease. New York, McGraw-Hill Book Company, Inc., 1960.

9. Higans, N., Robinson, R. W., and Cohen, W. D.: Increased incidence of cardiovascular disease in castrated women. New England J. Med. *268*:1123, 1963.

References

Metabolic Changes in Myocardial Infarction

Sigmundur Gudbjarnason and Richard J. Bing

Myocardial infarction is defined as ischemic necrosis of cardiac muscle caused by diminution of blood supply to a portion of the myocardium, below the critical level necessary for viability.

The death of a part of the working muscle sets in motion a chain of events in the heart which are aimed at repairing the damage and compensating for loss of active muscle. The reactions of the heart to myocardial infarction involve repair and replacement of necrotic muscle by connective tissue, and synthesis of new muscle protein in the noninfarcted area to compensate for the loss of contractile muscle.

The altered energy and metabolite requirements of the infarcted and noninfarcted tissue induce metabolic changes which differ, depending upon the biochemical environment and functional integrity of the tissue.

The alterations in metabolism of the infarcted heart include: (1) reversible changes in the ischemic muscle, (2) irreversible changes in infarcted, necrotic tissue, (3) changes in metabolism of noninfarcted muscle during compensatory hyperfunction, and (4) changes in lipid metabolism of energy-deficient muscle.

METABOLISM OF ISCHEMIC HEART MUSCLE

The metabolic changes occurring in an acutely ischemic heart muscle have been studied extensively[1,2,3] and a great deal has been learned about the regulation of myocardial glycolytic activity. The studies of Chance *et al.*[4] Williamson[5] and Wollenberger and Krause[6] indicate that the shift from aerobic to anaerobic metabolism in the myocardium occurs in an oscillatory fashion. The principal control sites in the oscillating glycolytic system of anaerobic muscle have been identified as phosphorylase and phosphofructokinase with additional potential control sites at the level of glyceraldehyde-3-phosphate dehydrogenase and pyruvate kinase.[6] Ischemia of the myocardium causes a rapid diminution in tissue levels of ATP and creatine phosphate but a rise in inorganic

orthophosphate and in the end products of glycolysis, lactate and alpha-glycerophosphate.[6,7] The beating warm-blooded heart cannot tolerate ischemia and the ensuing hypoxia of its tissue for more than a minute without serious impairment of its function. The energy utilized by the contractile apparatus is derived from ATP and creatine phosphate (CP), which represents the pool of high energy phosphate that can be drawn upon to supply the free energy to perform mechanical work. The rapid changes in tissue content of energy rich phosphate following coronary artery occlusion reflect the

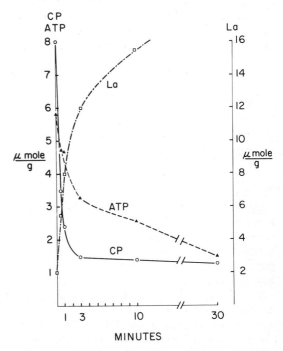

CHANGES IN MYOCARDIAL ENERGY METABOLISM FOLLOWING CORONARY OCCLUSION

FIG. 1. Changes in tissue content of ATP, creatine phosphate (CP) and lactate (La) in ischemic heart muscle following coronary occlusion.

deficiency in synthesis of ATP in ischemic muscle while the accumulation of lactate and alpha-glycerophosphate illustrates the accelerated anerobic carbohydrate metabolism[7] (Fig. 1).

In heart muscle, entry of glucose into the cell is restricted by a permeability barrier, which is relieved wholly or partially by drugs or humoral factors such as insulin,[8] epinephrine,[9] glucagon,[10] ouabain,[11] by anoxia,[12] or by an increase in the work load on the heart.[13] The fact that the state of mechanical activity of the heart affects the glucose transport system, implies some form of functional feedback, so that when more glucose is required, more is supplied to the glycolytic enzymes. Since the myocardial free glucose pool accounts for only a minor portion of glycolysis in the muscle during ischemia, glycogen constitutes the major source of the glycolytic products formed in this condition. Glycogen phosphorrylase is usually present in the aerobic mammalian heart in the b form and its activity is probably curtailed by the inhibitory aerobic concentration of ATP, glucose-6-phosphate and on account of the low aerobic concentration of one of its substrates, orthophosphate. Moreover, the concentration of 5'-AMP, the cofactor of phosphorylase b, is lowest in the aerobic state. The b→a transformation is thus of decisive importance in increasing the rate of breakdown of cardiac glycogen in early myocardial ischemia.[6] The equilibrium between these two forms of phosphorylase can be expressed as follows:[14]

$$2 \text{ phosphorylase b} + 4 \text{ ATP} \xrightarrow[\text{Mg}^{2+}]{\text{phosphorylase b kinase}} \text{phosphorylase a} + 4 \text{ ADP}$$

$$\text{phosphorylase a} + 4 \text{H}_2\text{O} \xrightarrow{\text{phosphorylase phosphatase}} 2 \text{ phosphorylase b} + 4 \text{ Pi}$$

The first of these reactions, the phosphorylase b → a conversion is commonly spoken of as "phosphorylase activation." It is the acceleration of this reaction rather than the slowing of the phosphatase reaction which is responsible for the increase in phosphorylase a caused by catecholamines,[15] muscular activity[16] and anoxia.[17]

Phosphorylase b kinase may exist in cardiac muscle,[18,19] as it does in skeletal muscle[20] in a non-activated form and an activated form. Activation of the nonactivated enzyme has been achieved by incubation of cell-free fraction of heart muscle with Ca[++] or with ATP plus cyclic 3', 5'-AMP.[21] Drummond *et al*[22]. observed an activation of the kinase in the perfused rat heart treated with epinephrine, an effect which probably was mediated by stimulation

of adenyl cyclase[15] and the resulting increase in the formation of 3', 5-AMP.[23]

The second rate-controlling site in the glycolytic sequence in ischemic heart muscle is phosphofructokinase which is rapidly activated in heart muscle by lack of oxygen.[6]

In the aerobic heart muscle phosphofructokinase appears to be normally in a highly inhibited state due to relatively large tissue levels of ATP. This inhibition is removed in the ischemic muscle by increases in 5'-AMP, 3', 5'-AMP, ADP, orthophosphate, fructose-6-phosphate, and fructose-1, 6-diphosphate.[24] Among these compounds only orthophosphate and fructose-diphosphate were found to activate PFK significantly within the first 20 seconds following arrest of the coronary flow.[6]

The experiments of Williamson[5] indicate that the glycolytic flux in heart muscle is mainly limited by the activity of phosphofructokinase. When the energy demand on the heart is increased, as with epinephrine, or when oxidative phosphorylation is diminshed, as in ischemia, the production of glycolytic ATP is increased by increased phosphofructokinase activity as a result of the fall in the phosphate potential, (ATP)/(ADP) (Pi). On the other hand, when noncarbohydrate fuels are present in abundant supply and oxidative processes are unimpaired, phosphofructokinase is inhibited by an increase in the level of citrate.[5] There is thus multiple feedback control between energy-producing steps in the mitochondria, and energy producing steps in the cytoplasm.

An increase in PFK activity, in response to increasing energy demands, was observed in the nonischemic left ventricular muscle adjacent to an ischemia area[7] produced by ligation of coronary arteries supplying a limited region of the left ventricle. Following coronary occlusion the nonischemic muscle is called upon to perform additional work compensating for the nonfunctioning ischemic myocardium. The additional work load requires increased energy production in nonischemic muscle, which in turn must be met by increased substrate flux. This increased metabolic activity of the nonischemic muscle was illustrated by a 75 per cent increase in the activity of PFK observed 5 minutes after coronary occlusion. The increase in activity of PFK was followed by an increase in activity of other glycolytic and some oxidative enzymes.[7]

The contractile apparatus of cardiac muscle appears to be able to utilize ATP with equal efficiency for any given work performance regardless of whether the ATP was supplied by oxidative phosphorylation or by anaerobic glycolysis.[8,25] The beating mammalian heart can, however, only for a very short time rely on its anaerobic metabolism to carry it through an ischemic stress.[26] Although the mammalian myocardium may not be able to sustain mechanical activity on anaerobic energy metabolism, the glycolytic metabolism may play a significant role in preserving myocardial function and structure and promote recoverability of the anoxic heart.[27] In a recent study Weissler *et al.*[27] observed that anaerobic metabolic support by glucose permitted a higher level of electrical and mechanical performance of the isolated rat heart during and after recovery from a 30-minute exposure to anoxia than it did in hearts perfused aerobically for 90 minutes. Anaerobic metabolic support by glucose also prevented the ultrastructural changes induced by anoxia in the absence of anaerobic support.

METABOLISM OF INFARCTED TISSUE

The energy metabolism of irreversibly damaged, infarcted muscle differs fundamentally from the reversible metabolic changes of temporarily ischemic heart muscle, where the ultrastructural and metabolic alterations return to normal if coronary circulation is re-established within 15 to 20 minutes following coronary artery occlusion.

The cells within an ischemic area stop contracting shortly after occlusion. The loss of contractility is, however, not necessarily permanent and the ischemic cells regain their contractility if the arterial flow is restored. If the ischemia is prolonged beyond 15 to 20 minutes, some of the affected cells become irreversibly injured. Complete structural disorganization or necrosis follows the onset of irreversible injury.[28,29,30]

Information concerning the energy metabolism of the infarcted tissue is scarce, but the analysis of the enzyme profile and the analysis of tissue levels of energy rich phosphates and glycolytic metabolites permit certain assumptions regarding the role of the various metabolic pathways in the metabolism of living cells active in the necrotic area of infarcted muscle.

Alterations in Enzyme Profile

The irreversible damage to heart muscle cells affected by the occlusion of coronary arteries supplying a limited area of the myocardium is accompanied by significant alteration in the biochemical machinery; i.e., the enzyme profile of the tissue. The interpretation of the changes observed in the enzyme profile and metabolism of the damaged heart muscle is difficult because the destruction of muscle cells and replacement of the necrotic muscle

by connective scar tissue generates an ill-defined, heterogeneous tissue consisting of various cell types performing different tasks.

The metabolism of the infarcted tissue can therefore not be ascribed to one specific cell population, but must be attributed to the collective effort of the various cell types involved in the repair and replacement of the damaged muscle.

It must also be pointed out that alterations observed in enzyme activity, as measured in tissue extracts in vitro, do not necessarily reflect accurately the alterations in the tissue in vivo since numerous factors can influence the activity of an enzyme, such as concentrations of the substrate, product, cofactors and coenzymes, allosteric regulators, inhibitor, activator, conformational changes, etc. Our procedure differs thus from the histochemical staining procedure in so far as it measures the optimal attainable activity under most favorable conditions, whereas the histochemical staining procedures used for evaluation of myocardial damage may often reflect the depletion of labile substrates and cofactors from the infarcted muscle.[31,32]

Despite these difficulties, significant changes in the enzyme profile of a tissue suggest alterations in metabolism, possibly induced by altered substrate availability, altered energy requirements, altered biochemical environment or even induced by the proliferation of different cell types such as fibroblasts and leukocytes.

Hexosemonophosphate-Shunt Activity. The alterations in enzyme profile of infarcted heart muscle observed during tissue repair following sudden coronary occlusion are characterized by a significant increase in activity of the hexosemonophosphate shunt and by a rapid decrease in the activity of oxidative and glycolytic enzymes.[33,34,35] The increase in hexosemonophosphate shunt activity was illustrated in a continuous increase in the activity of glucose-6-phosphate dehydrogenase (G-6-PDH) and 6-phosphogluconate dehydrogenase (6-PGDH) for at least 10 days following coronary artery occlusion.[33,34,35] Ten days after infarction the activity of G-6-PDH had increased 34-fold in the center of infarct and 23-fold in the periphery of infarct[35] (Fig. 2). The activity of 6-PGDH was similarly elevated in the infarcted tissue.[35] Nine months after coronary occlusion, the activity of G-6-PDH was still significantly higher in the scar tissue of the healed infarct than in normal cardiac muscle.[33] This increase in hexosemonophosphate-shunt activity may in part be due to phagocytosis and the earliest appearance of G-6-PDH and 6-PGDH in the periphery rather than in the center of the infarct provides some biochemical evidence that these enzymes

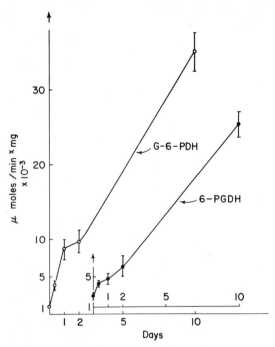

INDUCTION OF HEXOSEMONOPHOSPHATE-SHUNT ENZYMES DURING TISSUE REPAIR

FIG. 2. Changes in the specific activities of G-6-PDH and 6-PGDH in infarcted heart muscle as a function of time after coronary occlusion.

may be carried by leukocytes. However, the persistent elevation of G-6-PDH as late as nine months after the infarction suggests that the elevated hexosemonophosphate-shunt activity in the affected area is not due to phagocytosis alone, but may reflect the fibroblastic proliferation in the developing scar tissue.

Further evidence for the increased activity of the hexosemonophosphate shunt was obtained by the enhanced formation of $^{14}CO_2$ from glucose-1-C^{14} in infarcted tissue. The magnitude of change in oxidation of glucose-1-C^{14} to $^{14}CO_2$ in infarcted tissue compared to noninfarcted muscle lends additional support to the observed increase in activities of the hexosemonophosphate-shunt enzymes. The increase in C_1/C_6 ratio (from the oxidation of glucose-1-C^{14} and glucose-6-C^{14} to $^{14}CO_2$) from 3.5 in normal muscle homogenate to 9.8 in homogenate from infarcted tissue is of significance because both tissue samples were obtained from the left ventricle of the same heart and reflect alterations due to the coronary occlusion.[34]

The increased activity of this shunt may be of importance for several reasons. For instance, an increasing supply of glyceraldehyde-3-phosphate (GAP) could be delivered by the hexosemonophos-phate shunt since the activity of G-6-PDH continues to increase for at least ten days after infarction. This might facilitate additional ATP formation. In addition, the hexosemonophosphate-shunt is essential for the formation of ribose-5-phosphate required for nucleic acid synthesis and for NADP-dependent synthesis.

An important role of the HMP-shunt in cell proliferation and accumulation of specific cell products has been observed in developing organs. Studies on the development of pig heart,[36] sea urchin embryo,[37] and chick brain[38] indicate that the development of an organ and the increased demand for specific substrates for RNA and DNA synthesis and cell proliferation require a high level of HMP-shunt activity. A high level of the HMP-shunt was observed here in the irreversibly injured necrotic heart muscle, when connective scar tissue is called upon to replace necrotic muscle cells.

The increased HMP-shunt activity in the infarcted heart muscle may, however, not be due to tissue repair and fibroblastic proliferation alone. De-differentiation and degeneration of heart muscle cells may also play an important part in the increased HMP-shunt activity. Fujimoto and Harary[39] have observed significant enzyme changes associated with dedifferentiation and loss of function of heart cells in tissue culture. The authors observed a diminution in malate dehydrogenase and isocitrate dehydrogenase activity but an increase in G-6-PDH activity when nondividing beating rat heart cells were grown in a lipid-free medium and subsequently ceased beating. The shift from lipid to carbohydrate oxidation and the loss of beating could be correlated with a decrease in oxygen uptake.

The increase in HMP-shunt activity of injured heart muscle is not limited to the infarcted area but also extends to noninfarcted areas of the left ventricle, although to a much smaller degree.[34] The increase in HMP-shunt activity of noninfarcted muscle probably reflects the development of compensatory cardiac hypertrophy in the surviving muscle. The adjustment of the muscle to the increased workload requires, according to Meerson,[40] an increased activity of the HMP-shunt facilitating nucleic acid and protein synthesis providing the necessary building blocks for development of cardiac hypertrophy. An increase in fibroblastic proliferation in cardiac muscle has also been observed in cardiac hypertrophy.[41] It is therefore not possible to ascribe the increased HMP-shunt activity exclusively to heart muscle cells, since the increase in number of fibroblasts in the hypertrophied heart might also be responsible for the increased HMP-shunt activity.

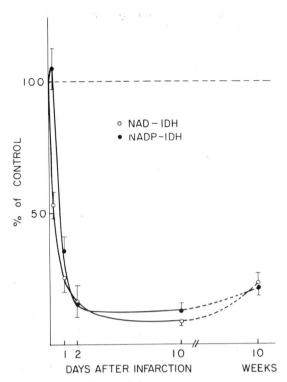

FIG. 3. Relative changes in the activities of NAD and NADP specific isocitrate dehydrogenases (IDH) in infarcted heart muscle compared to uninfarcted tissue of the left ventricle.

Glycolytic and Oxidative Enzymes. In contrast to the marked increase in activity of the HMP-shunt, there was a significant decline in the activity of both oxidative and glycolytic enzymes in infarcted cardiac muscle.[33] Mitochondrial enzymes, such as NAD-and NADP-specific isocitrate dehydrogenase (Fig. 3), malate dehydrogenase and glutamate oxaloacetate transaminase reached the lowest level in the center of the infarcted tissue ten days after infarction with 8-12 per cent of normal activity. Ten weeks after infarction, there was some recovery of enzyme activities with an increase to 17-40 per cent of the control.

The activity of glycolytic enzymes was also significantly decreased. Aldolase and lactate dehydrogenase (LDH) decreased to 14 and 21 per cent of original activity, respectively, whereas the activity of GAPDH was reduced somewhat less or to 32 per cent of control ten days after infarction.[33,34] The periphery and center of the infarct showed similar enzyme activity 24 hours after infarction, but ten days and even ten weeks after infarction the periphery had about two to three times higher activity than the center of the infarct.[33,34] The relatively high activity of GAPDH remaining in infarcted tissue indicates that anaerobic substrate phosphorylation of ADP to ATP can continue at relatively high levels in the ischemic and infarcted area if the substrate GAP can be provided. As mentioned above, an increasing supply of this substrate could be delivered through the hexosemonophosphate shunt.

The quantitative decrease in LDH activity of infarcted muscle was accompanied by qualitative changes in the isoenzyme pattern as well[42] (Fig. 4).

LDH is a tetrameric molecule made up of four subunits of the two principal molecules, H (heart) and M (muscle) type. The isozymes of LDH repre-

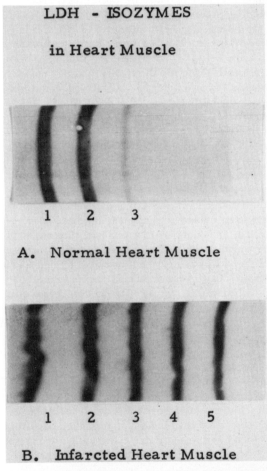

FIG. 4. Qualitative changes in LDH of infarcted heart muscle. (*A*) In normal dog heart muscle LDH displays three isoenzymes, with two strong bands representing isoenzyme I (H_4) and II (H_3M), and one weak band representing isoenzyme III (H_2M_2). (*B*) In infarcted heart muscle all five isoenzymes can be observed illustrating an increase in isoenzyme III and the appearance of isoenzyme IV (HM_3) and V (M_4).

sent the combination of these two subunits into five distinct molecular forms: H_4, H_3M, H_2M_2, HM_3 and M_4.[43] These molecular forms can be separated and are classified as isozymes, I, II, III, IV and V. The synthesis of the H and M subunits appears to be regulated independently[43] and an example of the independent regulation of H and M genes is provided by alterations in oxygen tension, both in vivo and in vitro. The changes in the synthesis of LDH subunits with changes in oxygen tension are in line with the proposed physiological role of M and H proteins. The low oxygen tension favors synthesis of M-LDH, the form best suited for anaerobic metabolism. High oxygen tension favors synthesis of the H enzyme, the form which predominates in aerobic tissues.[43]

In normal dog heart muscle LDH displays only three isozymes, with two strong bands representing isozyme I (H_4) and II (H_3M), and one weak band representing isozyme III (H_2M_2).[42] In the infarcted tissue all five isozymes can be observed, and in this tissue the relative strengths of bands III, IV (HM_3) and V (M_4) are similar to those of bands I and II.

The diminution in LDH activity of infarcted heart muscle is in part due to a release of LDH into the coronary sinus blood and in part due to inactivation of the enzyme or altered enzyme kinetics accompanying the changes in isozyme pattern. The release of LDH and other myocardial enzymes into the blood has been utilized to aid in the diagnosis of myocardial infarction.[28,44] The presence of recent myocardial infarction is characterized by a gross increase in the activity of isozyme I (or isozyme I and II) in serum, due to necrosis and increased permeability of ischemic heart muscle.[44] The decrease in isozymes I and II in the infarcted, necrotic muscle is paralleled by a relative increase in isozymes III, IV and V and probably reflects the replacement of the necrotic muscle by connective tissue. The processes of tissue repair and proliferation of fibroblasts take place in an ischemic area where a new tissue develops, equipped with an enzyme pattern that must fit into the biochemical environment in which it will operate. The ischemic environment of the infarcted tissue, with its low oxygen tension, may thus favor synthesis of M-LDH, the form best suited for anaerobic metabolism,[43] and this increase in synthesis of M-LDH is illustrated in the increase in isozyme IV (HM_3) and isozyme V (M_4) in the infarcted heart muscle.

ALTERATIONS IN TISSUE CONTENT OF ENERGY-RICH PHOSPHATES AND GLYCOLYTIC METABOLITES

The changes in the energy level of infarcted

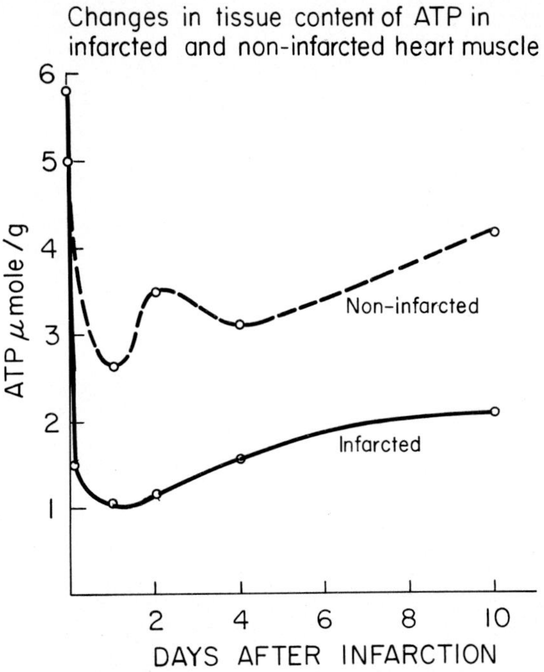

FIG. 5. Changes in tissue content of ATP in infarcted tissue and noninfarcted muscle after coronary occlusion.

muscle were illustrated in an immediate decrease in the tissue content of ATP and creatine phosphate (80-90% diminution), followed by a slow increase in tissue content of these substances after 48 hours. The tissue content of ATP increased from 1.05 μmole/gm. 24 hours after coronary occlusion to 2.1 μmole/gm. on the tenth day (Fig. 5). The CP level increased from 1.4 μmole/gm. 30 minutes after coronary occlusion to 3.0 μmole/gm. on the tenth day (Fig. 6). The diminution in tissue content of energy rich phosphates was accompanied by a marked increase in tissue content of lactate (Fig. 7). The initial burst in glycolytic activity was illustrated in the 10-fold increase in lactate levels observed immediately after coronary occlusion. These changes were followed by a second rise in lactate levels 48 hours after infarction and a subsequent diminution in lactate levels approaching normal tissue content of lactate after the fourth day.

The increase in tissue level of ATP and the diminution in lactate level of infarcted tissue, observed ten days after infarction, parallel the increase in HMP-shunt activity, but at this time there was no increase in the activity of mitochondrial enzymes.[34,45] The increased ATP formation ten days after infarction could be related to an increase in substrate phosphorylation at the level of GAPDH despite the

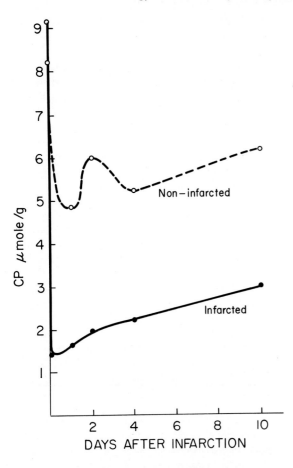

FIG. 6. Changes in tissue content of creatine phosphate (CP) in infarcted tissue and noninfarcted muscle following coronary occlusion.

infarcted tissue where the dead myocardial cells are replaced by more primitive connective tissue cells. These cells proliferate rapidly and require energy for numerous synthetic processes, among these protein and nucleic synthesis.

ENERGY METABOLISM OF NONINFARCTED MUSCLE AND MYOCARDIAL PERFORMANCE

The coronary occlusion and irreversible damage to a portion of the left ventricle is accompanied by significant changes in the energy metabolism of the noninfarcted muscle as well. The tissue content of energy-rich phosphates (ATP and CP) diminishes rapidly in the noninfarcted muscle, reaches a minimum 24 hours after coronary occlusion and increases subsequently. The ATP level diminished from 5.8 μmole/gm. to 2.65 μmole/gm. 24 hours after infarction, increased to 3.5 μmole/gm. on the second day and reached 4.2 μmole/gm. on the tenth day (Fig. 5). Creatine phosphate levels fell from

diminution in lactate content of the tissue. The relatively high activity of GAPDH in infarcted tissue indicates that anaerobic phosphorylation of ADP to ATP can continue at a relatively high rate in the ischemic area, if the substrate GAP can be provided. This could be accomplished in part by way of an increase in HMP-shunt activity during tissue repair, which would supplement the diminished output of the glycolytic pathway.[34] Calculations of the quantitative role of the HMP-shunt in energy metabolism of infarcted tissue have not been attempted, but considerable recycling of F-6-P to G-6-P[46] must be assumed if this process could be expected to have any significance for the formation of GAP and ATP in the infarcted tissue.

The possible role of GAPDH as a regulatory enzyme in the glycolytic metabolism of myocardial cells has been pointed out above. This enzyme may even have a greater role in the energy production of

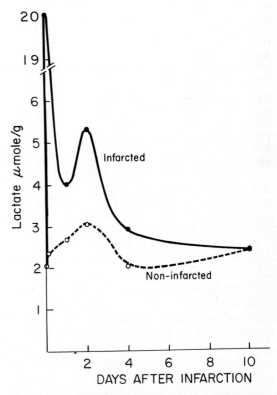

FIG. 7. Changes in tissue content of lactate in infarcted tissue and noninfarcted muscle following coronary occlusion.

9.2 μmole/gm. to 4.85 μmole/gm. on the first day and increased subsequently reaching 6.2 μmole/gm. on the tenth day (Fig. 6). The decrease in tissue levels of energy-rich phosphates was followed by a 50 per cent increase in lactate levels two days after infarction, returning to normal on the fourth day (Fig. 7).

These changes in energy metabolism of the noninfarcted tissue probably reflect the compensatory hyperfunction of the surviving muscle, observed when the energy requirements of the heart exceed the energy production. The loss of functioning muscle results in an increased load on the intact muscle which may lead to impaired function. The decrease in energy level of the noninfarcted muscle was accompanied by corresponding changes in hemodynamics. Changes in stroke output, stroke work and power, ejection rate and rate of pressure rise (dp/dt) correlated well with changes in ATP after the first day of infarction.[47] In animals with normal myocardial ATP values (5.6—5.8 μmole/ gm.), these hemodynamic parameters were slightly diminished and fell within the first or second standard deviation (SD) of their normal mean value. Those with ATP below 71 per cent but above 48 per cent of normal fell in the third standard deviation and those with ATP less than 48 per cent fell in the fourth standard deviation of the mean of normal hemodynamic values.

Correlation with CP content was evident only if CP levels had declined to less than 54 per cent of normal.[47] This may be due to the role of CP as an energy reservoir, which means that a considerable portion of CP may be consumed before the ATP level, available for contractile processes, would be affected.

These observations indicate that the reversible changes in energy-rich phosphates, occurring in the nonischemic myocardium, have an important bearing on left ventricular performance in the postinfarction period.

The increase in tissue content of energy-rich phosphates ten days after infarction is paralleled by the development of compensatory hypertrophy in the noninfarcted muscle. During the development of hypertrophy the rate of protein synthesis has increased significantly in the noninfarcted muscle and reached a level of 88 per cent above normal ten days after infarction.[48] These observations suggest that with progressive increase in synthesis of protein and a subsequent increase in the mass of intact muscle, the aerobic energy formation is enhanced and thereby the ability of the myocardium to handle the additional work load.[48]

LIPID SYNTHESIS AND FAT ACCUMULATION IN INFARCTED TISSUE

The biochemical regulation of lipid synthesis in heart muscle has received relatively little attention. The major site of fatty acid biosynthesis in heart muscle is located in mitochondria.[49] Mitochondrial synthesis of fatty acids occurs in large part by chain elongation in contrast to the cytoplasmic system, which results in de novo synthesis and involves the formation of a malonyl intermediate.[50]

The physiological significance of the mitochondrial chain elongation system has been recently explored by Whereat et al.,[51] and their studies indicate that the rate of fatty acid synthesis is regulated by the NADH/NAD ratio. The mitochondrial fatty acid synthesis-oxidation system can be viewed as a complex of enzymes with bidirectional capability regulated by the NAD oxidation-reduction state.[51] The functional significance of this fatty acid cycle may be related to the problem of storage of acetyl-units. Fatty acid oxidation would be maximal in the heart when there was a need for high-energy compounds, such as during exercise. There has to be abundant phosphate acceptor and ready access to oxygen so that acetate can be oxidized to CO_2 and phosphorylation can proceed rapidly. Synthesis of fatty acids would occur physiologically when oxidizable substrate was abundant but phosphate acceptor limited. Physiologically, such circumstances might occur during sleep, during anesthesia, or in the resting postabsorptive state. It might also occur during prolonged exercise, when phosphate acceptor is not limited but a high NADH/NAD ratio might be imposed by limitation of oxygen delivery. These elongated and newly synthesized fatty acids would be available for oxidation when there is a fall in the NADH/NAD ratio. During hypoxic states this mechanism of fatty acid synthesis might be an important mechanism for the reoxidation of NADH.[51]

An increase in myocardial neutral fat in ischemic heart muscle has been observed on histochemical examination by several investigators.[52,53] The increase in fat droplets was observed one to three hours after coronary artery occlusion and increased steadily for 18 hours. The fat was deposited diffusely through the sarcoplasm of injured ischemic fibers but not in cells that died rapidly. Similar intracellular accumulation of lipid has been observed in viable muscle at the margin of myocardial infarcts in humans.[54] The increase in intracellular lipid in the ischemic tissue has been explained as being the result of degeneration of structural components of the cell or due to increased esterification of extracted fatty acids.[55] The anaerobic glycolysis observed in ischemic or hypoxic heart muscle is accompanied by increased formation of α-glycerophosphate, which has been shown to augment incorporation of fatty acids into glycerolipids via the phosphatidic acid pathway. This mechanism has been suggested to explain the increased phospholipid synthesis in the hypoxic isolated heart.[55,56]

The relative importance of increased esterification of extracted exogenous fatty acid or increased de novo synthesis of fatty acids in the genesis of lipid accumulation in the hypoxic heart muscle may be difficult to evaluate, but in the infarcted heart muscle, the extraction of exogenous fatty acids is markedly diminished because of the reduction of coronary blood flow.[57]

We have examined the correlation between changes in energy metabolism of infarcted heart muscle and the rate of lipid synthesis in infarcted and noninfarcted tissue at various intervals after coronary occlusion.[34,45] The incorporation of acetate-1-C[14] into lipids of normal and infarcted heart muscle was studied in vivo by injecting the labeled acetate intravenously (30 μc/kg.) into the animals 46 hours and 10 days after infarction. Two hours after injection of the tracer the thorax was opened under pentobarbital anesthesia and biopsy samples were obtained rapidly from the normal and infarcted myocardium, quickly frozen and analyzed for ATP, lactate, lipids, etc.

The increase in glycolytic metabolism of infarcted and noninfarcted muscle, described above, was accompanied by a significant increase in lipid synthesis in the energy-deficient muscle. The incorporation of acetate-1-C[14] into lipids was increased 2-4 fold in infarcted as well as noninfarcted energy-deficient tissue.[34,45] The increase in lipid synthesis was also associated with an alteration in the fractional distribution of acetate-1-C[14] in the various lipids.[45] In infarcted tissue the relative incorporation of labeled acetate was significantly increased in the triglyceride fraction, whereas the relative incorporation into phospholipids was markedly diminished.[45]

A correlation between the ATP content of the tissue and the rate of lipid synthesis was established illustrating an ATP-dependent incorporation of acetate-1-C[14] into lipids. The acetate-1-C[14] incorporation into lipids reached a maximum in infarcted muscle at an ATP level of 1-2 μmole/gm. The incorporation diminished significantly with increasing ATP content of the tissue and reached the lowest level in the normal heart muscle not subjected to myocardial infarction (Fig. 8). The same relationship

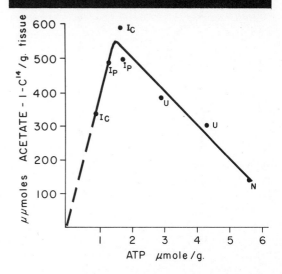

FIG. 8. The relationship between in vivo incorporation of acetate-1-C[14] into lipids of normal and infarcted heart muscle and the ATP content of the tissue (μmole/g). Biopsy samples were obtained 2 and 10 days after infarction. N = normal left ventricle; U = uninfarcted muscle; Ip = periphery of infarct; Ic = center of infarct.

was observed in vitro in heart muscle homogenates and in isolated mitochondria.[45] The in vitro studies suggest that the rate of fatty acid synthesis may be regulated by the concentration of ATP. ATP might thus be an inhibitor of fatty acid synthesis at higher ATP levels (ATP > 6 mM) and prevent fatty acid synthesis in response to momentary or oscillatory fluctuations in the NADH/NAD ratio. When the ATP concentration diminishes below 6 m—the rate of fatty acid synthesis increases and aids in the reoxidation of NADH.

The regulation of lipid synthesis in infarcted, necrotic tissue is not known at the present time, but it might follow a similar mechanism. The increase in fatty acid and glyceride synthesis seems to serve two functions: (1) to regenerate NADP required for continued operation of the HMP-shunt, and (2) to remove the product of the Embden-Meyerhof pathway, i.e., pyruvate via acetyl-CoA, and to convert it into fatty acids and triglycerides. In this way the increase in fatty acid synthesis serves to substitute for oxygen and facilitates continued operation of both the HMP-shunt and the Embden-Meyerhof pathway in the ischemic tissue[34] (Fig. 9).

METABOLISM OF INFARCTED TISSUE

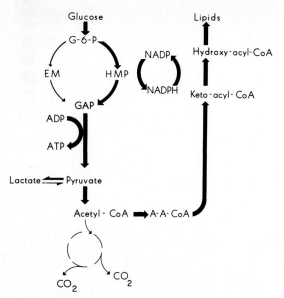

Fig. 9 Metabolism of infarcted heart muscle. The heavy lines indicate metabolic pathways that have increased in activity in the infarcted tissue during tissue repair [hexosemonophosphate-shunt (HMP) and lipid synthesis]. The thin lines indicate diminished activity of the Krebs cycle and a segment of the Embden-Meyerhof pathway.

REFERENCES

1. Michal, G., Naegle, S., Danforth, W. H., Ballard, F. B., and Bing, R. J.: Metabolic changes in heart muscle during anoxia, Am. J. Physiol. *197*:1147, 1959.
2. Furchgott, R. E., and De Gubareff, T.: High energy phosphate content of cardiac muscle under various experimental conditions which alter contractility, J. Pharmacol. & Exper. Therap. *124*:203, 1958.
3. Bing, R. J.: Cardiac metabolism, Physiol. Rev. *45*: 171, 1965.
4. Chance, B., Williamson, J. R., Jamieson, D., and Schoener, B.: Properties and kinetics of reduced pyridine nucleotide fluorescence of the isolated and in vivo rat heart, Biochem. Ztschr. *341*:357, 1965.
5. Williamson, J. R.: Metabolic control in the perfused rat heart, *in* Chance, B., Estabrook, R. W., and Williamson, J. R. (Eds.), Control of energy metabolism, New York, Academic Press, 1965, p. 333.
6. Wollenberger, A., and Krause, E. G.: Metabolic control characteristics of the acutely ischemic myocardium, Am. J. Cardiol. *22*:349, 1968.
7. Braasch, W., Gudbjarnason, S., Puri, P. S., Ravens, K., and Bing, R. J.: Early changes in energy metab-

8. Bleehen, N. M., and Fisher, R. B.: The action of insulin in the isolated rat heart, J. Physiol. (London) *123*:260, 1954.
9. Williamson, J. R.: Metabolic effects of epinephrine in the isolated, perfused rat heart, J. Biol. Chem. *239*:2721, 1964.
10. Kreisberg, R. A., and Williamson, J. R.: Metabolic effects of glucagon in the perfused rat heart, Am. J. Physiol. *207*:721, 1964.
11. Kreisberg, R. A., and Williamson, J. R.: Metabolic effects of ouabain in the perfused rat heart, Am. J. Physiol. *207*:347, 1964.
12. Morgan, H. E., Henderson, M. J., Regen, D. M., and Park, C. R.: Regulation of glucose uptake in muscle, J. Biol. Chem. *236*:253, 1961.
13. Morgan, H. E., Neely, J. R., Brineaux, J. P., and Park, C. R.: Regulation of glucose transport, *in* Chance, B., Estabrook, R. W., and Williamson, J. R. (eds.) Control of Energy Metabolism, New York, Academic Press, 1965, pp. 347–355.
14. Krebs, E. G., and Fischer, E. H.: Molecular properties and transformations of glycogen phosphorylase in animal tissues, Advances Enzymol. *24*:263, 1962.
15. Sutherland, G. W., and Rall, T. W.: The relation of adenosine-3', 5'-phosphate and phosphorylase to the actions of catecholamines and other hormones, Pharmacol. Rev. *12*:265, 1960.
16. Danforth, W. H., Helmreich, E., and Cori, C. F.: The effect of contraction and of epinephrine on the phosphorylase activity of frog sartorius muscle, Proc. Nat. Acad. Sc. *48*:1191, 1962.
17. Krause, G. G., and Wollenberger, A.: Uber die Activierung der Phosphorylase-b-kinase im akut ischämischen Myokard, Acta Biol. Med. Germ. *19*:381, 1967.
18. Chance, B., Higgins, J., Holmes, W., and Conelly, C. M.: Localization of interaction sites in multicomponent transfer systems: Theorem derived from analogues, Nature *182*:1190, 1958.
19. Drummond, G.I., Duncan, L., and Friesen, A.J.D.: Some properties of cardiac phosphorylase b kinase, J. Biol. Chem. *240*:2778, 1965.
20. Krebs, E. G., Delang, R. J., Kemp, R. G., and Riley, W. D.: Activation of skeletal muscle phosphorylase, Pharmacol. Rev. *18*:163, 1966.
21. Hammermeister, K. E., Yunis, A. A., and Krebs E. G.: Studies on phosphorylase activation in the heart, J. Biol. Chem. *240*:986, 1965.
22. Drummond, G. I., Duncan, L., and Hertzman, E.: Effect of epinephrine on phosphorylase b kinase in perfused rat heart, J. Biol. Chem. *241*:5899, 1966.
23. Robinson, G. A., Butcher, R. W., Oye, J., Morgan, H. E., and Sutherland, E. W.: The effect of epinephrine on adenosine-3, 5'-phosphate levels in the isolated perfused rat heart, Molec. Pharmacol. *1*:168, 1965.
24. Lowery, O. H., and Passonneau, J. V.: Phosphofructokinase and the control of glycolysis, Abstract 6th Internat. Congr. Biochem. IUB Vol. 32, IX, p. 705, New York, 1964.
25. Reeves, R. B.: Energy cost of work in aerobic and anaerobic turtle heart muscle, Am. J. Physiol. *205*:17, 1963.
26. Coffman, J. D., and, Gregg D. E.: Oxygen metabolism

and oxygen debt repayment after myocardial ischemia, Am. J. Physiol. *201*:881, 1961.

27. Weissler, A. M., Kruger, F. A., Baba, N., Scarpelli, D. G., Leighton, R. F., and Gallimore, J. K.: Role of anaerobic metabolism in the preservation of functional capacity and structure of anoxic myocardium, J. Clin. Invest. *47*:403, 1968.

28. Bing, R. J., Castellanos, A., Gradel, E., Lupton, C., and Siegel, A.: Experimental coronary infarction: Circulatory, biochemical and pathological changes, Am. J. M. Sci. *232*:533, 1956.

29. Jenning, R. B., Kaltenbach, J. P., Sommers, H. M., Bahr, G. F., and Wartman, W. B.: Studies of the dying myocardial cell, *in* James, T. N., and Keyes, J. W., (eds.): The Etiology of Myocardial Infarction, Boston, Little, Brown and Company, 1961, p. 189.

30. Bing, R. J., Castellanos, A., Gradel, E., Siegel, A., and Lupton, C.: Enzymatic and pathological studies in myocardial infarction, Tr. A. Am. Physicians *69*:170, 1956.

31. Nachlas, M. M., and Shnitka, T. K.: Macroscopic identification of early myocardial infarcts by alterations in dehydrogenase activity, Am. J. Path. *42*:379, 1963.

32. Kaltenbach, J. P., and Jennings, R. B.: Metabolism of ischemic cardiac muscle, Circulation Res. *8*:207, 1960.

33. Gudbjarnason, S., Cowan, Ch., Braasch, W., and Bing, R. J.: Changes in enzyme patterns of infarcted heart muscle during tissue repair, Cardiologia *51*: 148, 1968.

34. Gudbjarnason, S., Braasch, W., Cowan, Ch., and Bing, R. J.: Metabolism of infarcted heart muscle during tissue repair, Am. J. Cardiol. *22*:360, 1968.

35. Gudbjarnason, S., Cowan, Ch., and Bing, R. J.: Increase in hexosemonophosphate-shunt activity during tissue repair, Life Science *6*:1093, 1967.

36. Jolley, R. L., Cheldelin, V. H., and Newburgh, R. W.: Glucose catabolism in fetal and adult heart, J. Biol. Chem. *233*:1289, 1958.

37. Krahl, M. E.: Oxidative pathway for glucose in eggs of the sea urchin, Biochim. et Biophys. acta *20*:27, 1956.

38. Burt, A. M., and Wenger, B. S.: Glucose-6-phosphate dehydrogenase activity in the brain of the developing chick, Develop. Biol. *3*:84, 1961.

39. Fujimoto, A., and Harary, J.: The effect of lipids on enzyme levels in beating rat heart cells, Biochem. Biophys. Res. Commun. *20*:456, 1965.

40. Meerson, F. Z., Spiritchev, V. B., Pshennikova, M. G., and Djachkova, L. B.: The role of the Pentose-phosphate pathway in adjustment of the heart to a highload and the development of myocardial hypertrophy, Experientia *23*:530, 1967.

41. Meerson, F. Z., Alekhina, G. M., Alexandrov, P. N., and Bazardjan, A. G.: The dynamics of nucleic acid and protein synthesis of the myocardium in compensatory hyperfunction and hypertrophy of the heart, Am. J. Cardiol. *22*:337, 1968.

42. Gudbjarnason, S., and Priver, D. M.: LDH-iso-

enzymes in infarcted heart muscle, Life Sciences *7*: 623, 1968.

43. Dawson, D. M., Goodfriend, T. L., and Kaplan, N. O.: Lactic dehydrogenases: Functions of the two types, Science *14*: 929, 1964.

44. Van der Helm, T. J., Zondag, H. A., Hartog, A. H., and Van der Kool, M. W.: Lactic dehydrogenase isoenzymes in myocardial infarction, Clin. Chim. Acta *7*:540, 1962.

45. Gudbjarnason, S., Braasch, W., and Bing, R. J.: Defective energy metabolism and fatty degeneration in heart muscle, *in* Reindell, H., Keul, J., and Doll, E. (eds.): Herzinsuffizienz. Pathophysiologische Grundlagen und pharmakologische Beeinflussung. Stuttgart, Georg Thieme Verlag, 1968, pp. 253–258.

46. Wood, H. G., Katz, J., and Landau, B. R.: Estimation of pathways of carbohydrate metabolism, Biochem. Ztschr. *338*:809, 1963.

47. Puri, P. S., Gudbjarnason, S., and Bing, R. J.: Postinfarction sequential correlation between changes in energy-rich phosphates in non-ischemic myocardium of left ventricle and its dynamic performance, Circulation *28*, Supplement 4, p. 159, 1968.

48. Gudbjarnason, S., Braasch, W., and Bing, R. J.: Protein synthesis in cardiac hypertrophy and heart failure, *in* Reindell, H., Keul, J., and Doll, E. (eds.): Herzinsuffizienz. Pathophysiologische Grundlagen und pharmakologische Beeinflussung. Stuttgart, Georg Thieme Verlag, 1968, pp. 184–189.

49. Christ, E. J., and Hulsman, W. C.: Synthesis of long-chain fatty acids by mitochondrial enzymes, Biochim. et Biophys. acta *60*:72, 1962.

50. Wakil, S. J.: Mechanism of fatty acid synthesis, J. Lipid Res. *2*:1, 1961.

51. Whereat, A. F., Hull, F. E., and Orishimo, M. W.: The role of succinate in the regulation of fatty acid synthesis by heart mitochondria, J. Biol. Chem, *242*:4013, 1967.

52. Caulfield, J., and Klionsky, B.: Myocardial ischemia and early infarction, an electron microscopic study, Am. J. Path. *35*:489, 1959.

53. Wartman, W. B., Jennings, R. B., Yokoyama, H. O., and Clabaugh, G. F.: Fatty change of the myocardium in early experimental infarction, Arch. Path. *62*:318, 1956.

54. Reiner, L., Wittels, B., Barnett, R. J., and Rutenburg, A. M.: Histological profile of the human myocardium in coronary artery disease, J. Histochem. *3*:409, 1955.

55. Evans, J. R.: Importance of fatty acid in myocardial metabolism, Circulation Res. Suppl. II. Vol. 14 and 15, p. 96, 1964.

56. Scheuer, J., and Brachfeld, N.: Myocardial uptake and fractional distribution of palmitate-1-C^{14} by the ischemic dog heart, Metabolism *15*: 945, 1964.

57. Evans, J. R., Bunton, R. W., Baker, R. G., Beanlands, D. S., and Spears, J. C.: Use of radioiodinated fatty acid for photoscans of the heart, Circulation Res. *16*:1, 1965.

Collateral Circulation and Myocardial Infarction

Donald E. Gregg

In this presentation we shall consider the day to day compensatory responses to controlled coronary insufficiency and abrupt coronary artery occlusion in the unanesthetized and unrestrained dog, with each animal serving as its own control.

The experimental model is basically similar to that employed for studying the normal coronary circulation with the addition that either an ameroid cuff or an adjustable constrictor was placed around the circumflex coronary branch distal to the pneumatic cuff.[1,2]

Following recovery from surgery, the state of the left circumflex and left descending coronary beds, and of the systemic circulation and their responses to certain test conditions were observed almost daily during a two- to three-week control period, and then for 2 to 6 weeks during partial and complete coronary occlusion. The tests were performed with the dog resting and lying on its right side.

Coronary insufficiency was achieved in two ways. In the first, the circumflex artery was abruptly occluded by the pneumatic cuff for at least 24 hours and then released. In the second, coronary flow was initially controlled by means of an ameroid cuff placed around the artery distal to the occlusive cuff. This, however, was not very satisfactory because it was impossible to be sure that the ability of this bed to dilate and/or the actual coronary flow was not compromised to some degree by artery constriction within the first ten days or so after operation, and while the dog was still recovering. Thus it was difficult to be sure of control values. Accordingly, an adjustable reversible coronary constrictor device which could be controlled externally was placed on the left circumflex artery beyond the zeroing cuff so that flow could be controlled and reduced as desired. The rate of constriction of the coronary artery was designed to induce coronary insufficiency and electrocardiographic evidence of myocardial ischemia but with minimal or no infarction. With a little practice, it was found that coronary flow could be reduced to any desired fraction of the flow level of the dog at rest, and held at this level for hours, days or weeks. In different dogs, coronary flow was decreased abruptly to and held at 20, 40, and 60 per cent of the resting flow for periods of days and weeks. It was then decreased further to zero flow.

The major indices used to detect coronary insufficiency and compensation are change in myocardial contractility; increase in flow in a nonoccluded coronary artery, the descending branch; decrease in reactive hyperemia or the peak coronary flow response following release of a 10-inch circumflex occlusion; rise of residual pressure in the circumflex distal to the point of its temporary and permanent occlusion; rise in the clearance of Xe^{133} following its injection into the circumflex branch after its temporary and permanent occlusion. For clarity, examples of the estimation of the two collateral indices, the peripheral coronary pressure (PCP) and Xe^{133} clearance that are obtained from the indwelling coronary tube are illustrated below.

Figure 1 (top) shows typical recordings of phasic pressure in the aorta, and of phasic pressure and flow in the circumflex coronary artery before and after occlusion. At 4 second occlusion, mean PCP is 2 mm. Hg. In different dogs, this varies and at times is as high as 15 mm. Hg.[1]

Figure 1 (bottom) shows that the clearance of Xe^{13} approximates 12 ml./100 Gm/min. following its injection into the normal left circumflex coronary artery beyond the point of its temporary occlusion for about 60 seconds. In different dogs with nonconstricted coronary arteries, this normal clearance varies from 0 to 16 ml./100 Gm./min.[3]

Figure 2 illustrates that as coronary insufficiency develops, reactive hyperemia or dilatability following a 10 second occlusion of the circumflex branch disappears but the level of coronary flow is unchanged.[3] The first derivative of the left ventricular pressure curve, used here as an index of contractility, drops progressively. Left ventricular end-diastolic pressure is not elevated. However, further artery constriction beyond this point leads to a precipitous fall in coronary flow.

The temporal relation and order of magnitude of these internal compensations of the microcirculation are indicated in Figure 3, which is a somewhat

COLLATERAL   INDICES

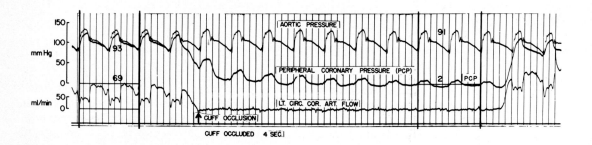

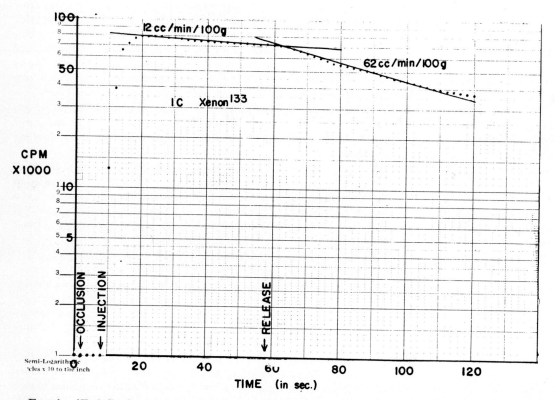

FIG. 1. (*Top*) Sections from resting dog before left circumflex constriction showing phasic curves of aortic blood pressure, coronary pressure and circumflex flow before and during 4 second circumflex occlusion and after artery release. Vertical time lines 0.1 sec. (Modified after Elliot, et al[2].) (*Bottom*) Clearance curve of Xe[133] injected into the left circumflex coronary branch of resting dog about 10 seconds after its temporary occlusion for 50 seconds.

idealized graph of a typical experiment in a dog with chronic cardiac insufficiency.[4] With vessel constriction and development of a small pressure gradient, reactive hyperemia or ability of the bed to dilate, starts to fall, while PCP and xenon clearance, initially about zero, both start to rise. The important point is that these indices of collateral development reach quite significant levels before there is any change in the metered coronary inflow. The level of coronary flow is maintained and does not start to fall until

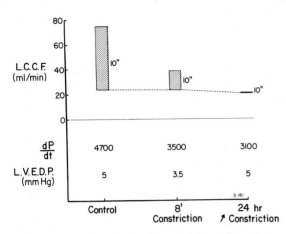

FIG. 2. Maintenance of flow and loss of reactive hyperemia in left circumflex coronary branch during its progressive constriction.

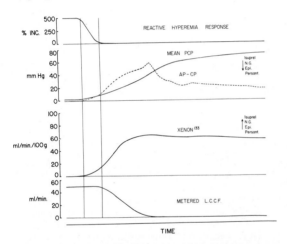

FIG. 3. Composite chart showing changes in microcirculation of left circumflex coronary branch during its progressive occlusion and the effect of intracoronary drugs. Based on work of Khouri, et al.[1]; Elliot, et al.[2][3] PCP, peripheral coronary pressure. AP-CP, mean pressure difference in mm. Hg between aortic and coronary sinus pressures. LCCF, left circumflex coronary flow. Modified after Gregg.[4]

reactive hyperemia is essentially zero. The major portion of the rise in xenon clearance and PCP occurs during the decline in coronary flow and not after zero coronary flow is reached. Actually, Xe^{133} clearance appears to reach a maximum before coronary inflow is reduced to zero. The rate of rise of PCP is directly related to the level of PCP before coronary artery constriction. The mean PCP $_{max}$ rise-time is 6 mm. Hg/24 hours with an initial PCP of 2-3 mm. Hg; the mean PCP $_{max}$ rise-time is 15 mm. Hg/24 hours with an initial PCP of 15 mm. Hg.

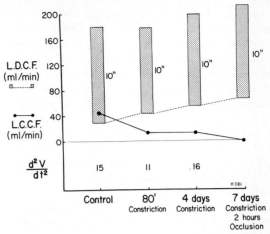

FIG. 4. Maintenance of reactive hyperemia and increase of flow in left descending coronary branch at different periods during sustained reduction and removal of left circumflex flow.[1]

The preceding points out the rapidity of development of the microcirculation of the coronary insufficient bed. This bed is now able to undergo further dilatation from drug injection. The fact that intracoronary injection of Isuprel, nitroglycerin, epinephrine and Persantin (presumably without contact with the collateral vessels) markedly decreases PCP and greatly increases capillary clearance strongly suggests that the bed has developed a large dilating capability, that the dilatation is within the vascular bed of the occluded coronary artery and not in the collaterals.

Most of the blood now supplying the microcirculation of the insufficient left circumflex coronary bed must come from the other non-occluded coronary arteries. I should like to consider briefly the compensatory changes in the left descending bed. Figure 4 illustrates the changes in the left descending bed after circumflex coronary flow was reduced abruptly by about 75 per cent from 46 ml. to 14 ml./min. This did not cause myocardial infarction. Descending flow progressively rises from a control of 35 ml./min. to reach 43 ml. at 80 minutes, 53 ml. at 4 days, and 66 ml./min. at 7 days partial and 4 days total occlusion. This increase in descending flow is about 70 per cent of that lost through circumflex closure. The reactivity or reserve ability of this bed to dilate following a 10 second occlusion is well maintained, approximating 500 per cent before and 400 per cent after vessel constriction.

Let us now consider the changes in the coronary collateral circulation after abrupt and complete occlusion of the circumflex branch for 24 hours.[5] This procedure was carried out in 7 dogs. Of these,

6 survived the 24 hours of occlusion while the remaining dog underwent ventricular fibrillation at 10 to 11 hours after circumflex occlusion. At present, it is not possible to explain why fibrillation did not occur in these dogs while circumflex occlusion in the anesthetized open chest dog causes almost 100 per cent mortality. About 15 to 20 minutes after occlusion, all 7 dogs were slightly restless, especially if there was a temporary and mild increase in sinus rate. However, there was no evidence of pain, whining or crying out throughout the occlusion period. Classical changes in the electrocardiogram were observed with some elevation of the S-T segment within the first 10 minutes, and later depression of the S-T segment. At autopsy massive infarction was present.

Control values obtained on the same day and prior to circumflex occlusion were similar to those observed almost daily during the previous 3 to 4 weeks. During occlusion, sinus rhythm and a low heart rate were maintained through the first 3 to 4 hours. Thereafter, the rhythm gradually became entirely ventricular with the heart rate increasing to about 200. Aortic pressure remained relatively stable or decreased. The mean peripheral circumflex pressure, initially 5 to 15 mm. Hg., rose gradually to reach values 4-6 times the control. The amplitude of the phasic peripheral pressure more than doubled. The Xe133 clearance, initially 5-20 ml./100 gm./min. rose progressively to 60 ml./min. The arterial and coronary sinus creatine phosphokinase (CPK) values and potassium (K) values did not start to rise for 3 to 4 hours. Then the K values rose moderately and the CPK values reached very high levels. The coronary bed retained its ability to dilate even after 24 hours' occlusion; the increase in coronary flow after release of a 10-20 second occlusion could be as large as before occlusion.

Finally, the systemic and coronary responses to abrupt 24 hour circumflex occlusion have been studied in the chronic dog whose nerve connections to the heart had been interrupted by a stripping technic.[6] The clinical symptoms and anatomic findings were similar to those in dogs with intact cardiac nerves. The physiological findings were also characterized by a long delay in the onset of arrhythmia and ventricular tachycardia, in the rise of CPK and K values, without evidence of pain and with maintenance of reactive hyperemia after release of the occlusion.

In summary, the observations presented indicate massive, early and timely compensations in the microcirculation of the coronary insufficient bed when coronary inflow is reduced in stages or abruptly to zero. In addition, the fact that abrupt circumflex coronary occlusion does not cause ventricular fibrillation for at least 24 hours permits this preparation to serve as an experimental model for study of the natural history of development of the coronary collateral circulation.

REFERENCES

1. Khouri, E. M., Gregg, D. E., and Lowensohn, H. S.: Flow measurements in the major branches of the left coronary artery during experimental coronary insufficiency in the unanesthetized dog, Circulation Res. *23*: 99, 1968.
2. Elliot, E. C., Jones, E. L., Bloor, C. M., Leon, A. S., and Gregg, D. E.: Day-to-day changes in coronary hemodynamics secondary to coronary artery constriction in dogs, Circulation Res. *22*: 237, 1968.
3. Elliot, E. C., Bloor, C. M., Jones, E. L., and Gregg, D.E.: Xe133 measurement of coronary collateral flow in chronic dogs, Fed. Proc. *26*: 771, 1967.
4. Gregg, D. E.: The microcirculation of the heart in reduced flow states, *in* D. Shepro and G. P. Fulton (eds.) Microcirculation as Related to Shock, New York, Academic Press, 1968, p. 51.
5. Pasyk, S., Bloor, C. M., and Gregg, D. E.: Myocardial Xe133 clearance and its response to vasodilators before, during and after coronary artery occlusion, Fed. Proc. *27*: 632, 1968.
6. Gregg, D. E., Khouri, E. M., Donald, D. E., Pasyk, S., and Lowensohn, H. S.: The coronary circulation in the conscious dog with cardiac neural ablation, Circulation *38*:vi-88, 1968.

The Natural History of Coronary Atherosclerosis*

Henry I. Russek and Burton L. Zohman

Knowledge of the natural history of disease enables the physician to estimate its relative severity, probable course, residual effects, and ultimate outcome in the individual case. Moreover, it is only with a background of such knowledge that the physician can hope to weigh the possible benefits and hazards of any form of therapy, old or new, against the risks attending the natural course of the disease in a given patient. This is particularly true in coronary heart disease in which the clinical course is remarkably variable and almost every form of treatment is associated with dangers arising from the therapy itself.[1,2] Although it is axiomatic that good medical practice can be achieved only by individual consideration of patients and treatment of each case according to its own merits, routine procedures regrettably have gained wide popularity in the management of coronary syndromes. In many instances, such indiscriminate therapy has arisen from the enthusiasm that attends the introduction of new methods, but more often it has been the consequence of a serious lack of understanding of the natural history of coronary artery disease. Even at present, clinical determinations of the proper place for anticoagulant therapy, cardioversion, "intensive coronary care," corrective surgery, and a host of other technics continue to suffer from this weakness. The conclusion is, therefore, inescapable that without adequate insight into the fundamental characteristics of this formidable disease, the potential benefit from any therapeutic measure and the specific indications for its use cannot be logically assessed.

PREVALENCE OF CORONARY ATHEROSCLEROSIS

It is generally recognized that even in populations subject to a high risk of ischemic heart disease, the presence of intimal involvement, fibrous plaques, complicated lesions, and calcified lesions is greater among those dying from coronary disease than among those suffering accidental deaths. These and

*Portions of this article have appeared *in* Brest, A.N., and Moyer, J.H.: Cardiovascular Disorders, Philadelphia, F. A. Davis, 1968.

other observations support the hypothesis that coronary atherosclerosis is the most significant factor in determining the risk of fatal ischemic heart disease in any given population. Although grossly visible lesions are rare in the first decades of life and, when found, are composed primarily of fatty streaks, atherosclerotic plaques are encountered in almost all adults in the United States.[3] Indeed, in white males it would be virtually impossible to delineate a control group "without atherosclerosis" after age 20. In females, on the other hand, the onset and progression are markedly delayed so that fibrous plaques not only appear two decades later but the extent of total intimal surface involvement up to the age of 60 remains appreciably less than in white males.

Although the natural history of coronary atherosclerosis is reflected, in general, in the clinical course of coronary heart disease, the time relationships are at variance. Thus, while the most rapid development of coronary lesions in white men is encountered in the fourth decade of life, it is not until middle age, approximately 20 years later, that the peak incidence of clinical coronary disease is observed. It seems clear therefore that it is only after several decades of silent evolution that mural arterial lesions commonly give rise to clinical manifestations of myocardial ischemia. While the unfolding spectrum of diverse coronary syndromes is often closely correlated with the underlying pathologic disease, the anatomic lesions alone do not consistently afford an accurate means of evaluating clinical manifestations or prognosis in individual cases. The increasing use of selective coronary angiography for such purposes, therefore, has very definite limitations since the technic tells little about coronary arterial flow, the status of small coronary arterioles, or exchanges at the cellular level. Consequently, evaluations based on coronary angiographic findings may be misleading in some instances, just as a change in such findings after surgical intervention may be deceptive in suggesting significant clinical and functional improvement.

Since it has been established that the pathologic lesions responsible for the staggering morbidity and mortality from coronary heart disease in middle-aged American men arise several decades prior to the onset of symptoms, any search for etiologic factors or application of prophylactic measures must be directed to the early period of adult life.

MODE OF ONSET IN CLINICAL CORONARY DISEASE

While the first clinical manifestation of coronary artery disease may be sudden death or the incidental finding of electrocardiographic abnormalities, in most instances the disease is expressed initially either as the anginal syndrome or as frank myocardial infarction. Available data appear to indicate that approximately equal numbers of patients present with angina pectoris as with myocardial infarction.[4,5] However, since it has been estimated that more than one half million persons in the United States sustain silent infarctions each year,[6] a significant but unknown number of this total group undoubtedly manifest as their first symptom either an arrhythmia, congestive heart failure, or a thromboembolic incident.

CLINICAL COURSE OF CORONARY ARTERY DISEASE

When analyzed on a long-term basis, coronary artery disease presents striking variability in its symptomatology. The clinical disease does not progress inexorably from its inception to death but rather is punctuated by periods of quiescence and exacerbation. Thus, the course of coronary heart disease is characterized predominantly by angina pectoris, acute coronary insufficiency, major infarctions, and asymptomatic intervals. Although the clinical events and prognosis have been analyzed separately in patients who were first seen because of the onset of angina pectoris and in those whose first manifestation was acute myocardial infarction, with the passage of time these disorders so frequently coexist that initial differentiation in this manner yields limited predictability of course and outcome. Most reports suggest that the onset as angina is more favorable to longevity than the onset as myocardial infarction. Thus, in a study of long survivors, Pader and Levy[5] found that angina pectoris was the first clinical manifestation more than twice as often as myocardial infarction (67.5% compared with 32.5%). This finding assumes greater significance when viewed in the light of the approximately equal incidence reported for angina pectoris and myocardial infarction as initial manifestations of clinical coronary disease.[4,5] The distinctly higher survival rates found in patients with angina pectoris followed

for 25 years than in patients with infarction studied for a similar interval[7] also attests to the more favorable prognosis with angina pectoris.

In some cases the disease begins with angina pectoris that subsides after a variable period of time leaving the patient asymptomatic for many months or years. Some who start with angina pectoris sustain myocardial infarction in the course of time while others appear "immune" to this complication. The anginal syndrome develops in some in whom the underlying disease presented initially as myocardial infarction while others of this group remain symptom-free. By far the most common clinical course is that of intermittent angina, often with long periods of complete freedom from pain, and often without the development of a myocardial infarction or without a second infarction in those patients whose disease presented as infarction. One-half of all the long-term survivors in a carefully studied series manifested this "benign" clinical pattern.[5] Among those with angina at onset only about one-fourth subsequently developed infarction and only about one-fourth of those whose disease was heralded by myocardial infarction developed a second infarction. In the combined series, only 12 per cent exhibited persistent angina. On the other hand, 10 per cent of those enjoying long survival after an onset with infarction experienced complete and persistent absence of all cardiac symptoms. From these findings, obtained in retrospect, it is clear that even in the more favorable cases the clinical course in an individual patient is unpredictable. Indeed, the multiplicity of factors which influence morbidity and mortality not only render the choice of established methods of treatment most difficult but also hinder accurate appraisal of new forms of therapy for this disease. The magnitude of the problem is amply reflected in the striking differences in duration of life and mortality statistics reported by different groups of investigators for relatively limited series of patients with apparently similar coronary syndromes. From the diversity of findings, it appears likely that closely comparable series can be obtained only by random selection of groups comprising at least 1,000 patients or more.

CLINICAL COURSE WITH ANGINA AT ONSET

Angina pectoris takes an extremely variable course, from the mildest short attacks occurring at long intervals over many years, with death not infrequently the result of a noncardiac cause, to severe, prolonged and frequent attacks terminating in myocardial infarction or sudden death within a few days or weeks of the onset of the symptom. In the majority of instances, anginal episodes continue intermittently for many years often punctuated by periods of quiescence especially if severe stresses are curtailed. In these patients the pattern of angina is relatively stable and often predictable so that adjustments are possible to permit fairly normal existence. This is particularly true when nitroglycerin and related drugs are used prophylactically to their full advantage. Often, however, without apparent reason the need for these agents greatly diminishes or disappears. Recurrence of mild episodes for brief periods is not uncommon in these patients as a consequence of seasonal changes, disturbances in other organ systems, emotional influences, and unknown factors. Consequently, for the majority of patients a clinical course characterized by variability in the dimensions of the pain experience, often with periods of freedom from angina, continues for many years until coronary occlusion, sudden death, or unrelated disease provokes fatal termination. The danger of sudden death is an ever present threat for patients with angina pectoris since it eventually occurs in about 10 to 15 per cent of cases. Furthermore, the lack of definite correlation between such fatality and antecedent clinical features dictates caution in any attempt at prognostication. In some instances, a cerebrovascular accident, congestive heart failure, or renal insufficiency due to associated hypertension and generalized atherosclerosis may account for the patient's demise. In still others, angina pectoris is tolerated well without serious complication until death ensues from malignancy, intercurrent infection, or unrelated disease.

In about one-third of the patients with angina pectoris the clinical course is complicated by an episode of acute myocardial infarction from which approximately 40 per cent succumb either suddenly at onset or in the weeks that follow. In many instances, even without positive evidence, acute coronary occlusion may be presumed to have occurred from the sudden sharp increase in the frequency and severity of anginal episodes or from the unexpected development of congestive heart failure. If angina pectoris has been present for several months prior to infarction, it generally recurs after convalescence. Occasionally, however, such symptoms may actually disappear so that the patient's capacity for exercise increases. Improvement of this type was observed in less than 10 per cent of a series of patients in whom the onset of clinical coronary disease was heralded by angina pectoris. On the other hand, it is not uncommon for angina to subside or disappear completely with the development of congestive heart failure or permanent atrial fibril-

lation subsequent to infarction.

In about 15 to 25 per cent of patients who experience angina pectoris as the first clinical manifestation of coronary heart disease, the pain becomes more intense and of greater frequency. Episodes are provoked more readily with considerable variability in the pain experience from day to day and week to week. Not infrequently this unstable pattern of angina pectoris may persist even for months causing moderate to severe disability and may eventually terminate in fatal myocardial infarction or sudden death. Nevertheless, the frequency of remissions even when symptoms have been regarded as "intractable" make it possible to treat such patients with optimism. Moreover, as Friedberg[8] has emphasized, these cases do not represent a distinct clinical entity (acute coronary insufficiency, coronary failure, intermediate syndrome) since some are associated with significant myocardial necrosis while others are related only to reversible myocardial ischemia.

SURVIVAL PERIOD AFTER ONSET WITH ANGINA PECTORIS

In assessing data on duration of life after the onset of symptoms, it is essential to avoid the distortion that arises from inclusion of persons whose angina pectoris is due to a noncoronary cause or in whom death is unrelated to the underlying coronary disorder. Most important for a true picture of survival is the necessity of differentiating series of cases in which all patients had died at the time of study from those in which many patients were still alive. The average duration of life has ranged from 4.2 to 9.4 years in various published reports[4,7,9-12] (Table 1). In Sigler's series,[4] in which the average survival was only 4.6 years, more than half of the total had had a coronary occlusion and somewhat more than 60 per cent were still alive at the time of the report. The relatively poor outlook reflected in the series of Zoll and associates[11] may be ascribed in part to the inclusion of 37 patients with angina due to valvular heart disease but also suggests the presence of relatively more severe disease in their patients. One-third of their subjects were dead within one year after the onset of angina, almost half (47 per cent) were dead within two years, and the 5-year and 10-year mortality rates were 72 and 92 per cent respectively. In sharp contrast, Paul[13] has reported a most favorable prognosis for 24 subjects discovered to have unrecognized angina pectoris during the routine screening of 2,000 men 40 to 55 years of age. After an average follow-up of 5.4 years from the onset of symptoms, there have been no deaths and only two clinically recognized infarcts. Almost all

TABLE 1
Survival After Onset of Angina Pectoris

Author	Date	Number of Cases Followed		Average Age at Onset	% Survival Rates After Onset Symptoms (Yrs.)		Av. Duration Life (Yrs.) From Onset Symptoms
		Total	To Death		5	10	
White et al.[9]	1943	497	445	56.5	—	—	7.9
Parker et al.[10]	1946	2827	—	57.1	69	43	—
Sigler[4]	1951	1700	679	55.8	—	—	4.6
Zoll et al.[11]	1951	177	117	58.0	28	8	4.2
Block et al.[12]	1952	5945	—	56.3	58	37	—
Richards et al.[7]	1956	456	445	—	—	—	9.4

published data pertains to patients whose symptoms have aroused sufficient concern to lead to a search for medical aid at the physician's office, clinic or hospital. Yet there are many who undoubtedly experience angina but never consult a physician because of the mildness of their pain or simply because the discomfort disappears for months or years. Consequently, if over all prognosis were considered, the outlook would probably be far more favorable than available data suggest. But, even the average span of 9.4 years reported by Richards and associates[7] would indicate a common survival to approximately 65 years since the onset of angina pectoris is usually in the mid-fifties (Table 1). While such data, used with discretion, may be informative and useful, each patient presents a separate problem with individual features determining prognosis.

The duration of survival in angina pectoris is influenced unfavorably by a variety of factors, most important among which are cardiac enlargement, congestive heart failure, hypertension, atrial fibrillation, valvular heart disease, diabetes, and a history of infarction. Francis and associates[14] have recently reported significantly shorter survival for patients who have had angina pectoris prior to myocardial infarction than for those without antecedent angina. Inasmuch as this symptom-complex arises only with advanced occlusive changes or with inadequate compensation for reduction in the internal caliber of major branches, the anginal patient, as Likoff[15] has emphasized, is predictably in a less favorable position to withstand the complication of a myocardial infarction. In our experience the outlook for the obese patient has appeared better than for the normal or thin subject. The benefit to ischemic myocardium which follows successful weight reduction in the obese patient with angina pectoris can seldom be matched by responses obtainable from other forms of treatment in the nonobese. Moreover, because of the increased cardiac load in overweight subjects, it seems probable that angina pectoris may surface to clinical view at an earlier stage of coronary circulatory impairment, thus permitting greater

opportunity for therapeutic success. Unfavorable heredity is often associated with a brief and ominous course manifested by early complications and death. Age and sex also appear to exert an influence on prognosis. Thus an onset of angina before the age of 40 generally suggests an underlying hereditary vascular weakness and an unfavorable outlook for survival.[10] Women appear to have longer survival periods after the onset of angina than do men.[9,10]

Despite such determinants of longevity, most patients live at least 5 to 10 years after the onset of angina pectoris. Five-year survival or longer was achieved by 58.4 per cent of the 5,945 patients followed by Block and associates[12] as compared with a rate of 86.9 per cent for the normal population. In the same study, a 10-year survival of 37.1 per cent was recorded compared to an expected 70.4 per cent. It is not uncommon for patients to live more than 15 or 20 years after the onset of angina pectoris. Pader and Levy[5] observed 167 coronary patients for 15 years or more and 10 patients for 25 years or more and among these a higher percentage had had their onset with angina pectoris than with myocardial infarction. In the long-term studies of White et al.,[7] 6 patients had actually survived for an average of 31.7 years.

ACUTE CORONARY INSUFFICIENCY

The syndrome of coronary insufficiency characterized by prolonged attacks of angina pectoris at rest, or on slight provocation, without the usual signs of myocardial infarction has been ascribed by various authors to an intermediate form of ischemic heart disease. Hudson[16] has found that the hearts from patients with "coronary insufficiency" almost invariably show widespread coronary artery stenosis or occlusion, with scattered small lesions of various ages, and often one or more large scars. He believes that the active lesions are too small to be recorded by the electrocardiogram as definitive lesions or to produce any of the usual clinical or blood changes. Others contend that sudden narrowing of a major coronary vessel as a result of acute edema or subintimal hemorrhage within an atherosclerotic plaque may be the commonest cause of the syndrome. Clinically, the episode is generally produced by a sudden inadequacy of coronary blood flow which may occur spontaneously or may be precipitated by a variety of aggravating factors. Wood[17] considered that the sudden onset of symptoms was evidence of coronary artery thrombosis, not severe enough to cause infarction but capable of producing almost total incapacity from pain, day and night, with or without the usual provocation in a patient previously suffering only mild attacks, or none at all. In his experience, the attacks of pain lasted 10 to 30 minutes and recurred for days, weeks or months, often leaving the patient quite well between these periods. One quarter of the patients had had a previous infarction and 87 per cent had an "ischemic" electrocardiogram. In 50 per cent the course was acute (less than 6 weeks), in 45 per cent it was subacute (2 to 6 months) and in 5 per cent the condition was chronic. In 80 per cent the electrocardiogram showed depression of the S-T segment at rest, but there was no fever, no leukocytosis and no rise in serum enzymes. In 22 per cent of untreated cases the picture merged into that of myocardial infarction. The average age of the patients in Wood's series was 56 years, with three times more men than women; the duration of previous ischemic symptoms averaged 3.7 years. Since the clinical picture of acute coronary insufficiency may represent the impending phase of acute myocardial infarction, prognostication is difficult or impossible. Cutts and associates[18] have shown that such cases are not always mild in their subsequent course. In a series of 69 patients admitted to hospital, there were 24 deaths of which 14 were known to be due to heart disease, chiefly myocardial infarction. Of the cardiac deaths, 7 occurred in the first year of follow-up. Frequently, such cases are treated for a "mild" coronary with complete disappearance of pain and electrocardiographic changes and discharged after one or two weeks, only to suffer another episode of pain this time due to transmural infarction. Although some have claimed that anticoagulants greatly improve prognosis in such cases of "impending" infarction, the validity of all published data is open to question. Friedberg,[8] moreover, has convincingly maintained that cases of "acute coronary insufficiency" form a "motley group," some of which are best classified clinically as angina pectoris (more or less severe or prolonged) and others as acute (subendocardial) myocardial infarction. Persistence of deep inversion of T waves for more than a day or two after the pain has subsided indicates that some myocardial necrosis

has probably occurred. Consequently, angina pectoris, subendocardial ischemia, coronary occlusion without infarction, subendocardial infarction, and transmural infarction are all consequences of coronary insufficiency. Obviously, the clinical course, outlook, and treatment are largely determined by the presence of only reversible myocardial ischemia or significant myocardial necrosis.

The term "acute coronary insufficiency" has also been applied to a group of cases in which cardiac pain may or may not be present but in which there are predisposing or precipitating factors, such as pulmonary embolism, shock, hemorrhage or tachycardia and electrocardiographic changes indicating myocardial ischemia. The clinical course and prognosis in such cases are dependent on a wide variety of factors in addition to those concerned primarily with the heart.

COURSE AFTER ONSET WITH ACUTE MYOCARDIAL INFARCTION

Although this form of clinical onset is encountered as frequently as the onset with angina pectoris[4,5] the incidence of infarction probably exceeds that of the latter disorder. This is largely because approximately 1 in 10 infarcts occurs silently and 1 in 5 results in sudden death within minutes.[19] Since few of these cases are included in the statistics of hospital and clinic series, the morbidity and mortality of myocardial infarction may be easily misjudged.

Prolonged symptom-free periods are much more frequent in patients whose clinical disease begins with an acute myocardial infarction than in those with angina at the onset. More than two-fifths of 500 patients who suffered a coronary occlusion and were studied by Master and associates[20] made a complete functional recovery. Of those who sustain a first attack of acute myocardial infarction and recover, at least 80 per cent resume their occupation, although occasionally on a slightly restricted level.[8] Among those disabled, angina pectoris, dyspnea on effort or at rest, and weakness or easy fatigability constitute the major impediments.

In many cases, recovery from the acute attack is followed by disturbing symptoms, limited activity or appreciable disability. Bland and White[21] found that one-third of their patients were restricted in their activity by angina pectoris alone. Palmer[22] reported the occurrence of angina pectoris in about 60 per cent of the patients who had recovered from an acute infarct, an incidence higher than that observed before the attack. Friedberg[8,23] maintains that angina pectoris develops after recovery in about one-half of the patients with myocardial infarction at onset although it is usually absent during the first year. Moreover, even among those remaining symptom-free following the attack, angina frequently becomes manifest with increasing age of the patient. Confirming this view is the finding that only 10 per cent of a group of long survivors actually experienced complete and persistent absence of all cardiac symptoms after an onset with infarction.[5]

Although the subsequent course in those who develop angina pectoris after acute myocardial infarction is that described for patients whose onset is with angina pectoris, the outlook in general is distinctly less favorable. Whether or not angina pectoris develops after infarction, the risk of one or more recurrent attacks remains high, with each additional episode increasing the probability of a fatality or the development or intensification of disabling angina or congestive heart failure. Although clinical studies suggest that recurrent coronary occlusion develops in about 30 per cent of cases, usually within 2 years after the first attack, postmortem observations indicate a much higher frequency of additional episodes. New attacks often remain undetected because associated symptoms either are not as characteristic as those of the first attack or are obscured by the clinical features of congestive heart failure. In addition, electrocardiographic diagnosis is often more difficult when new alterations are superimposed on previous abnormalities.[8] Congestive heart failure and serious arrhythmias are important complications in many patients, leading to the expectation of serious disability and decreased survival. Postinfarctional angina itself appears to indicate a distinctly less favorable prognosis than exists in the absence of this complication. This was clearly shown in the study of Bland and White[21] in which only one-third of a group of patients with this complaint survived for 10 years or longer as compared with more than one-half of those remaining symptom-free.

SURVIVAL PERIOD AFTER ONSET WITH ACUTE MYOCARDIAL INFARCTION

The mortality rate from the acute attack of myocardial infarction, among patients admitted to hospital, has been reported by many investigators as averaging about 30 to 50 per cent. Since the highest mortality occurs in the first few hours following the onset of the attack, hospital statistics are markedly influenced by the relative frequency of early admissions. It also appears likely that the status of general health and incidence of concomitant disease are important factors in determining coronary disease mortality in any patient population. The frequency with which nutritional deficiency, chronic alcoholism, untreated diabetes, tuberculosis, and other local and systemic disease accompany acute myocardial infarction in patients admitted to county or city hospitals may explain, in part, fatality rates of about 50 per cent which have been reported for such institutions.[24,25] Among patients seen in private practice and treated at home or in voluntary hospitals, the mortality rate is undoubtedly less than half this figure. Master *et al.*[26] recorded a death rate of 16.5 per cent in 267 patients with a rate of only 8 per cent among those of the series suffering their first episode. Moreover, in the uncomplicated first attack, Russek and Zohman[28] reported the mortality rate to be only 3.3 per cent among 1,000 "good risk" patients.

Despite these findings, it is clear that all reports of hospital series underestimate the immediate mortality of first attacks. Of a total of 229 initial episodes of coronary heart disease in the Framingham study,[19] approximately 45 per cent were not hospitalized, in most instances because of sudden death. Of those who were hospitalized, 17 per cent died in the early phase despite treatment. Of those not hospitalized, 46 per cent died suddenly within minutes and another 21 per cent of first infarcts were silent having been detected by routine electrocardiograms. Combining the hospitalized and nonhospitalized series, it becomes evident that in about 20 per cent of the cases the initial episode of coronary heart disease will result in sudden death, another 10 per cent will be silent, and about 14 per cent will die despite treatment.

Considerable data indicate that, exclusive of sudden immediate death or death within an hour of onset, approximately 50 per cent of the deaths occur within the first 24 hours. Thus, the prognosis for immediate survival markedly improves after the first 24 hours and continues to become even more favorable with each passing day. Indeed, if the patient remains asymptomatic and without complication after the first week, the outlook for survival may be assumed to be excellent despite the occasional occurrence of sudden unexpected death at any point during subsequent convalescence. Moreover, even in the early hours following the onset of an attack, fairly accurate prognostication appears possible in a large proportion of cases from a consideration of the history and physical findings alone. Thus, in the absence of the following poor prognostic signs at the time of the first examination, the outlook appears most favorable:[27,28] (1) Previous history of myocardial infarction, (2) intractable pain, (3) severe or persistent shock, (4) significant

TABLE 2

Mortality and Incidence of Thromboembolism in Good-Risk Cases of Acute Myocardial Infarction

	No. Cases	Overall (%)	After 48 Hrs. (%)	Preventable* (%)	Thromboemb. (%)
		Mortality Rate in 1,000 Cases			
Group 1	489	3.1	1.7	1.0	0.8
Group 2	511	3.5	1.8	0.8	3.7
Average		3.3	1.7	0.9	2.3

*Percentage of deaths theoretically preventable with anticoagulants
Group 1, Retrospective study
Group 2, Prospective study

TABLE 3

Analysis of Causes of Death in 1000 Good-Risk Patients

Within 48 hours	16
Noncardiac	4
Rupture of ventricle	4
Recurrent infarction	3
Cerebral embolism	1
Unknown causes	5
Total	33

enlargement of the heart, (5) congestive heart failure, (6) gallop rhythm, (7) auricular fibrillation or flutter, ventricular tachycardia or intraventricular block, (8) diabetic acidosis, (9) varicosities in the lower extremities, (10) other states predisposing to thrombosis.

We have observed a mortality rate of only 3.3 per cent among 1,000 patients who were classified as "good risk" on the basis of these criteria.[27,28] Although an increase in the severity of symptoms does occasionally occur with attacks considered as "mild" at onset, such changes in the clinical picture almost invariably make their appearance during the first 48 hours. This is reflected by the finding that approximately half of the few deaths that do occur in this mild group, develop during the first 48 hours of observation (Table 2). It is apparent, therefore, that only 1 or 2 out of every 100 patients classified in this manner are apt to die during the acute phase of the attack if survival has extended beyond the first two days of admission to hospital. Similarly, the risk from thromboembolic complications is relatively small in this selected group. Certainly, from an analysis of the causes of death in the 33 fatalities among the 1,000 "good risk" patients in our series (Table 3), it is evident that anticoagulant therapy, with its attendant dangers from hemorrhage, is

unlikely to improve the prognosis in such cases.

In sharp contrast, we have found a mortality rate of 60 per cent and a thromboembolic complication rate of 10.6 per cent among 558 "poor risk" patients manifesting one or more of the unfavorable prognostic signs enumerated above.[29] As indicated, factors which greatly add to risk include severe shock, serious arrhythmias, heart block, congestive heart failure, previous infarction, and diabetic acidosis. From the consistent finding that there is a greater mortality rate among patients over the age of 60 than in younger patients, it has been erroneously assumed that age *per se* is a determinant of prognosis in the individual case. The studies of Russek and Zohman[30,31] have pointed up the fallacy in this concept. Thus, it was shown that the higher mortality rate in the latter decades of life stems from the appreciably higher prevalence of initially severe attacks in old-age groups (Table 4). Among those 60 years or over, almost two-thirds qualified as "poor risk" at onset as compared with less than one-half under 60 years of age. When allowance was made for variations in the severity of the attack by comparing similar groups of cases, no differences whatever were noted in mortality rates as a consequence of age (Table 5). It seems clear, therefore, that in the individual case the age of the patient does not add a further dimension by which immediate prognosis may be determined from the clinical picture.

The prognosis after recovery from the acute attack is much more favorable than was previously realized (Table 6).[32-40] With modern diagnostic methods mild cases of infarction are now freely identified and as a consequence survival statistics more accurately reflect overall prognosis. It now appears certain that more than 70 per cent of patients survive for more than 5 years and at least 40

TABLE 4

Analysis of 1047 Cases of Acute Myocardial Infarction According to Age and Severity of the Attack

Age of Patients	Total	Good Risk		Poor Risk	
		No.	Per Cent	No.	Per Cent
All ages	1047	489	46.7	558	53.3
Under 60 years	618	331	53.6	287	46.4
60 years or over	429	158	36.8	271	63.2

TABLE 5

Mortality Rate in 1047 Cases of Acute Myocardial Infarction According to Age and Severity of Attack

Age of Patients	Total (%)	Good Risk (%)	Poor Risk (%)
All ages	33.4	3.1	60.0
Under 60 years.......	28.8	3.0	58.5
60 years or over	40.1	3.2	61.6

TABLE 6

Survival After Recovery From Acute Myocardial Infarction

Author	Year	Cases No.	5 Years (%)	10 Years (%)	15 Years (%)
Cole et al.[32]	1954	285	67	44	10
Richards et al.[33]	1956	162	49	31	14
Biorck et al.[34]	1957	389	66	—	—
Helander & Levander[35]	1959	286	58	—	—
Beard et al.[36]	1960	503	69	—	—
Juergens et al.[37]	1960	224	55	29	—
Dimond[38]	1961	202	83	—	—
Pell & D'Alonzo[39]	1964	932	74	—	—
Little et al.[40]	1965	120	79	—	—

per cent for 10 years or more. Little et al.[40] reported a 5-year survival rate of 79 per cent in 120 men with coronary occlusion compared with 91 per cent in 120 healthy controls. Similarly, the 5-year survival rate in 932 patients studied by Pell and D'Alonzo[39] was 74 per cent compared with 95.8 per cent in apparently normal persons free from infarction. Among Metropolitan Life Insurance policy holders with a history of coronary occlusion, the 5-year survivorship was 77 per cent as compared to 94 per cent for standard insured males of corresponding ages.[40] For those under the age of 50, the mortality ratio was six times that of standard insured risks while for those 50 years or older it was only three times the standard risk. In general, the milder the attack the more complete is the recovery and the older the age of the patient at the time of the infarction the more favorable is the long-term outlook in relation to normal life expectancy. Obviously the prognosis is considerably more favorable if analysis is limited to patients who have fully recovered after an acute myocardial infarct without subsequent angina pectoris, congestive heart failure, hypertension, or diabetes. Indeed, the outlook of those who survive five or ten years with no functional disability or symptoms and who are of standard risk otherwise has been sufficiently favorable to warrant the issuance of life insurance to such patients by many American life insurance companies.

Among all factors that reflect long-term prognosis, the best index of survival and a return to normal life is the degree of completeness of recovery after the first month of convalescence.[42] Likoff[15] regards the ability of the patient to resume his pre-infarction degree of activity without angina pectoris

as the best clue to longevity. Paradoxically, however, he has reported in a five-year survival study that recurrences and ultimate death rates for individuals with mild infarctions resembled those encountered in patients with advanced coronary atherosclerosis. Since the greatest functional recovery is, in the main, observed in patients sustaining relatively mild attacks, the conclusions drawn from these prognostic indices appear incongruous. Although it is true that in some instances the "mild" coronary may be merely an initial but incomplete manifestation of a major event which is yet to follow, this sequence is generally far more characteristic of the clinical syndrome which has been described as "acute coronary insufficiency" rather than of classical infarction. In our experience, the long-term prognosis has been excellent for "good risk" survivors, i.e., patients surviving a relatively mild first attack of acute coronary occlusion. Among factors exerting an adverse influence on prognosis are cardiac enlargement, arterial hypertension, congestive heart failure, serious arrythmias, thromboembolic complications, and recurrent myocardial infarction. Rupture of the interventricular septum or of a papillary muscle is usually associated with a rapid downhill course. Ventricular aneurysm poses the threat of congestive heart failure and systemic embolism with unfavorable prospects for survival.

Although diabetes mellitus in the absence of acidosis does not appear to influence immediate prognosis in acute myocardial infarction, prospects for long survival are materially reduced.[32] In accord with this finding, the 5-year survival in 127 diabetics with acute coronary occlusion was observed to be only 38 per cent.[43] As noted clinically, therefore, diabetes mellitus frequently causes progressive and relentless atherosclerotic disease.

Younger patients have been reported to enjoy longer survival after myocardial infarction than older patients. Nevertheless, the percentage of normal life expectancy is much less in the young. Thus, although the duration of life was generally one to four years longer when the age of onset was at 45 years than at 55 years, the average age at death was substantially higher in the persons with a later onset of the infarct.[41] Among patients in the older group with minimal symptoms and little or no functional incapacity, average survival extended beyond 71 years of age and was only 4 or 5 years less than normal longevity. In contrast, comparable patients sustaining a first myocardial infarct at age 45 survived to an average age of only 63. These findings do not confirm the impression that the disease is more benign in the young.

REFERENCES

1. Russek, H. I.: Hazards in the treatment of acute myocardial infarction, Am. J. M. Sc. *232*:403, 1956.
2. Russek, H. I.: Medical perspectives in the treatment of coronary heart disease, Angiology, *18*:15, 1967.
3. Strong, J. P., and McGill, H. C., Jr.: The natural history of coronary atherosclerosis, Am. J. Path. *40*:37, 1962.
4. Sigler, L. H.: Prognosis of angina pectoris and myocardial infarction, Am. J. Card. *6*:252, 1960.
5. Pader, E., and Levy, H.: The natural history of coronary artery disease of long duration, J. Chron. Dis. *15*:1083, 1962.
6. Master, A. M.: Silent Coronary Artery Disease, *in* Medical Tribune, April 29, 1964.
7. Richards, D. W., Bland, E. F., and White, P. D.: A completed twenty-five year follow-up study of 456 patients with angina pectoris, J. Chron. Dis. *4*:423, 1956.
8. Friedberg, C. K.: Diseases of the Heart, Philadelphia, W. B. Saunders Company, 1966, pp. 726–731.
9. White, P. D., Bland E. F., and Miskall, E. W.: The prognosis and insurability in coronary artery disease, J.A.M.A. *123*:801, 1943.
10. Parker, R. L., Dry, T. J., Willius, F. A., and Gage, R. P.: Life expectancy in angina pectoris, J.A.M.A. *131*:95, 1946.
11. Zoll, P. M., Wessler, S., and Blumgart, H. L.: Angina pectoris. A clinical and pathologic correlation, Am. J. Med. *11*:331, 1951.
12. Block, W. J., Crumpacker, E. L., Dry, T. J., and Gage, R. P.: Prognosis of angina pectoris. Observations in 6882 cases, J.A.M.A. *150*:259, 1952.
13. Paul, O.: The Prognosis of Angina Pectoris, Coronary Heart Disease, New York, Grune and Stratton, 1963, pp. 469–471.
14. Francis, R. L., Achor, R. W. P., and Brown, A. L. Jr.: Angina pectoris preceding initial myocardial infarction, Arch. Int. Med. *112*:226, 1963.
15. Likoff, W.: The Prognosis of Myocardial Infarction, Coronary Heart Disease. New York, Grune and Stratton, 1963, pp. 472–477.
16. Hudson, R. E. B.: Cardiovascular Pathology, Baltimore, Williams and Wilkins, 1965, p. 668.
17. Wood, P.: Acute and subacute coronary insufficiency, Brit. M. J. *1*:1779, 1961.
18. Cutts, F. B., Merlino, F., and Easton, F. W.: Chest pain with inverted T waves, predominantly in precordial leads, as the only electrocardiographic abnormality, Circulation *16*:599, 1957.
19. Kannel, W. B. *et al.*: Risk factors in coronary heart disease, Ann. Int. Med. *61*:888, 1964.
20. Master, A. M., Jaffe, H. L., Teich, E. M., and Brinberg, L.: Survival and rehabilitation after coronary occlusion, J.A.M.A. *156*:1552, 1954.
21. Bland, E. F., and White, P. D.: Coronary thrombosis (with myocardial infarction) 10 years later, J.A.M.A. *117*:1171, 1941.
22. Palmer, J. H.: Prognosis following recovery from coronary thrombosis with special reference to the influence of hypertension and cardiac enlargement, Quart. J. Med. *6*:49, 1937.
23. Friedberg, C. K.: The natural history of coronary heart disease, atherosclerotic heart disease, Hahnemann Symposium, June, 1966.
24. Malach, M., and Rosenberg, B. A.: Acute myocardial infarction in a city hospital, clinical review of 264 cases, Am. J. Cardiol. *1*:682, 1958.
25. Griffith, G. C., Leak, D., and Hegde, B.: Conservative anticoagulant therapy of acute myocardial infarction, Ann. Int. Med. *57*:254, 1962.
26. Master, A. M., Jaffe, H. L., and Dack, S.: Treatment and the immediate prognosis of coronary artery thrombosis (267 Attacks), Am. Heart J. *12*:549, 1936.
27. Russek, H. I.: Current myths and realities in anticoagulant therapy for coronary heart disease, M. Clin. North America, *48*:355, 1964.
28. Russek, H. I., and Zohman, B. L.: Prognosis in the uncomplicated first attack of acute myocardial infarction, Am. J. M. Sc. *224*:496, 1952.
29. Russek, H. I., and Zohman, B. L.: Evaluation of anticoagulant therapy in acute myocardial infarction, Am. Heart J. *43*:871, 1952.
30. Russek, H. I., and Zohman, B. L.: Age and survival in cases of acute myocardial infarction, J. A. M. A. *147*:1731, 1951.
31. Russek, H. I., and Zohman, B. L.: Chances for survival in acute myocardial infarction, J. A. M. A. *156*:765, 1951.
32. Cole, D. R., Singian, E. B., and Katz, L. N.: Long-term prognosis following myocardial infarction and some factors which affect it, Circulation *9*:321, 1954.
33. Richards, D. W., Bland, E. F., and White, P. D.: A completed twenty-five year follow-up study of 200 patients with myocardial infarction, J. Chron. Dis. *4*:415, 1956.
34. Biorck, G., Blomquist, G., and Sievers, J.: Studies on myocardial infarction in Malmo 1935 to 1954. Morbidity and mortality in hospital material, Acta med. scandinav. *159*:253, 1957.
35. Helander, S., and Levander, M.: Primary mortality and five-year prognosis of cardiac infarction, Acta med. scandinav. *163*:289, 1959.
36. Beard, O. W., Hipp, H. R., Robins, M., Taylor, J. S., Ebert, R. V., and Beran, L. C.: Initial myocardial infarction among 503 veterans. Five-year survival, Am. J. Med. *28*:871, 1960.
37. Juergens, J. L., Edwards, J. E., Achor, R. W. P.,

and Burchell, H. B.: Prognosis of patients surviving first clinically diagnosed myocardial infarction, Arch. Int. Med. *105*:444, 1960.

38. Dimond, G. E.: Prognosis of men returning to work after first myocardial infarction, Circulation *23*:881, 1961.

39. Pell, S., and D'Alonzo, C. A.: Immediate mortality and five-year survival of employed men with a first myocardial infarction, New England J. Med. *270*:915, 1964.

40. Little, J. A., Shanoff, H. M., Roe, R. M., Csima, A., and Yano, R.: Studies of male survivors of myocar-

dial infarction. IV. Serum lipids and five-year survival, Circulation *31*:854, 1965.

41. Statistical Bulletin, Metropolitan Life Insurance Co. Dec. 1963, p. 5; Oct., 1965, p. 1.

42. White, P. D., Bland, E. F., and Levine, S. A.: Further observations concerning the prognosis of myocardial infarction due to coronary thrombosis, Ann. Int. Med. *48*:39, 1958.

43. Partamian, J. O., and Bradley, R. F.: Acute myocardial infarction in 258 cases of diabetes. Immediate mortality and five-year survival, New England J. Med. *273*:455, 1965.

Panel Discussion: Can We Prevent Ischemic Heart Disease?

CHAIRMAN CORDAY: Our distinguished panelists who have dedicated much of their life to the problem, will discuss "Can We Prevent Ischemic Heart Disease?" Doctors Meyer Friedman, Wilhelm Raab, and Ancel Keys have already been introduced to you earlier today, but Campbell Moses, Medical Director of the American Heart Association, has just joined the panel. As Chairman, I have the privilege of stirring up controversy in order to seek scientific truth. We must seek a way of preventing dreaded occlusive vascular disease which is killing over six hundred thousand Americans each year.

There is a very excellent pamphlet printed by the American Heart Association which reviews the risk factors in coronary disease, and another pamphlet reviews diet and heart disease. Among the predisposing factors listed are a familial history of coronary disease, the presence of hypertension, and electrocardiographic abnormalities, and these were all discussed earlier today. The other factors include diabetes mellitus, lipid abnormalities, obesity, gout, and certain personality behavior patterns. The environmental factors listed include cigarette smoking, lack of physical activity, emotionally stressful situations, serum cholesterol elevations of more than two hundred sixty milligrams, a fasting triglyceride of greater than two hundred fifty milligrams percent, or a prominent electrophoretic beta prebeta lipoprotein band, sustained blood pressure of one hundred sixty over ninety-five and body weight thirty percent or more above standards listed in the tables of desirable weight prepared by the Metropolitan Life Insurance Company. I believe a history of gout or uric acid levels over 7.5 mg., fasting blood sugar of more than 120 mg. or a casual blood sugar of 180 mg., electrocardiographic abnormalities and habitual cigarette smoking are all significant factors.

From the discussions this morning, we might be led to believe that if we could grade the patient according to his risk factors and then treat him according to his category that we might be able to prevent ischemic heart disease. Many of us are becoming a little discouraged with the prevention and treatment of coronary artery disease because we continue to see individuals who develop early serious coronary disease despite the fact that they have avoided the risk factors religiously by following a careful diet, abstaining from smoking, and maintaining a normal blood pressure and cholesterol level. I wonder if Campbell Moses would care to comment on the present methods of preventing ischemic heart disease.

DR. MOSES: I think we would be foolish to believe that there is any magic uniquely in the things that we now identify as risk factors. They are steps along the way, but only steps along the way and I'm sure, as Dr. Raab has mentioned earlier, that there are many etiologic factors both known and unknown. In any case, it is apparent that generally we devote our attention to controlling the coronary risk factors after the process in the vessels is fairly well developed. I submit that after twenty years of exposure to high cholesterol and triglycerides or hypertension and the like, it may take as long to reverse atherosclerosis as it did to develop it in the first place. Consequently, we are usually trying to "prevent" atherosclerosis after the fact. The time to pay attention to the prevention of this disease is in the twenties. In this regard, we might learn from the example of one of my laboratory technicians. She lost her first husband and was about to marry her second. I came back to the laboratory late one Saturday night and happened to meet him. He was about fifty-five and she was about thirty-five. She was doing a cholesterol on him before getting married and she said "Well, that's more important than a Wasserman in this particular case".

CHAIRMAN CORDAY: That's a very interesting approach. Do you personally follow a low cholesterol diet?

DR. MOSES: I'm usually on some experimental program and I don't think it's very fair to take what I might do personally as a model. In addition I have a unique advantage over some of the rest of you. I believe that exercise is a very important thing and one of the ways I like to get my exercise is by doing it constantly so I carry twenty or twenty-five pounds extra weight around in a very soft pliable container molded to my underlying bone structure.

CHAIRMAN CORDAY: This morning we heard from Dr. Raab, who expressed the opinion that exercise will not prevent atherosclerosis; in his view it has a beneficial effect on the myocardium itself. Is this your opinion?

DR. MOSES: I think that this is the only way in which the available data can be interpreted. There's no evidence which is applicable to man. With animal data you can prove a lot of things one way or the other about exercise, but so far as the process of human atherosclerosis is concerned, if you're exercising it's not to modify that particular process. It may be to modify some of the sequelae, some of the things that may happen in the myocardium or in combination with atherosclerosis, but it doesn't directly effect what happens in those middle sized vessels of the coronary circulation.

CHAIRMAN CORDAY: Well, now I've seen patients who religiously follow the principles of diet that we are stressing, they exercise and follow the prescribed regimen. With their bad family history, they soon develop a coronary and pass away in the usual fashion. I know Dr. Keys that you have some new studies along this line concerning the significance of exercise. Would you like to tell us about them now?

DR. KEYS: My main point is this: We have found major differences between population groups in the incidence of coronary heart disease but those differences are not explicable on the basis of differences between the populations in physical activity. Among the men we have studied the world over, there is one outstanding group of people who don't exercise, who are physically indolent, nonenergetic; these are the majority of American men of practically any occupation at the present time in the United States. The other population samples of men around the world are a good deal more comparable. When we compare those other men around the world, we don't find any parallelism between the amount of exercise they get and their susceptibility to coronary heart disease. This doesn't mean that exercise is a bad thing. All I say is that a great deal of exercise doesn't prevent the Finns, for example, from having more coronary heart disease than we have. I don't know about the amount of atherosclerosis. Today we've said a lot of loose things about how much atherosclerosis is present, but there aren't any figures that are statistically valid on the extent of atherosclerosis in any population group. We can, however, count bodies and that's what I've been doing the last ten years.

CHAIRMAN CORDAY: Could we see some of your figures?

DR. KEYS: I have three slides that might be interesting. The differences we find between population groups in the death rate from coronary heart disease— and we are sure that this is coronary heart disease and can prove it also by total death rate— cannot be explained entirely by differences in serum cholesterol. For example, in Greece, Dalmatia and East Finland, there are about three thousand men whom we have followed for five years; they are comparable in smoking habits, physical activity, obesity and so on. They differ markedly on the average, however, in their serum cholesterol values— 200 mg/dl for the Greeks and Dalmatians versus 265 for the East Finns. Put these figures in grams per liter to make the next calculations easier. We know in this country from followup studies that the likelihood of developing coronary heart disease increases roughly at the third power, the cube, of the cholesterol level. So take these figures and cube them—2^3 versus $(2.65)^3$; the result is 8 versus 18.61. From this result we would say, "Well, the Finns ought to have about two-and-a half times as much coronary disease as the Greeks and the Dalmatians." Then I said "No wait a minute; we've got to adjust for the fact that there's a little more hypertension in Finland." We also have follow-up studies to tell us what we should expect from this. When we correct for hypertension, we are led to conclude that the East Finns should have something like three times more coronary heart disease than the Greeks and Dalmatians. Actually, the difference is over ten to one instead of three to one. The point of this is simply that in our large-scale follow-up material we confirm the importance of blood lipids and blood pressure, but there is obviously something else or perhaps it's the combination of the two that increases the effect. Is that clear?

CHAIRMAN CORDAY: Yes, Dr. Raab, would you like to comment on Dr. Keys' remarks?

DR. RAAB: Not specifically. I would like to make one point which is a sort of obsession with me. Although it didn't originate in my brain, the term "pluricausal" coined by Selye who is a great man for inventing appropriate terms, is particularly applicable to this disease. Not only myocardial infarction, but degenerative heart disease in general, to use a neutral term, is a pluricausal condition. I don't think there is the slightest doubt anymore that there are several factors involved and several very different factors among which coronary atherosclerosis is obviously one of the most important predisposing and contributing factors. But there are a number of others which have been almost completely disregarded. If we are to develop any deeper understanding of this entire problem it is absolutely necessary to consider, analyze and discuss those other factors involved. As an example, let's say in a kitchen or in an office, plumbing is very important. It may be under certain circumstances all important, but is not so all the time. There are many other things which can completely mess up the situation in a kitchen or in an office or industry. We are, at long last, out of the era of completely one-sided vascular interpretation of degenerative heart disease. No longer can we assume that all cases arise solely from a deficient blood and oxygen supply. Certainly there are many instances of so-called "coronary" heart disease in which coronary atherosclerosis, even if it's there, is far below any noxious degree. I think there exists a mental block causing a constant return to the term "coronary". This is best illustrated in the present illogical use of the term "coronary care unit." Nobody does a single thing for the coronaries in the coronary care unit. Instead, something is actually being done, fortunately, with great intelligence and considerable success, for an object that hardly anybody talks about, the myocardium and its metabolism. What do people die from? From disturbances in the myocardial metabolism which is very largely affected by the coronaries but by many other correlated things as well, for example, the nervous system and the hormonal system. Very much more is known about these fundamental principles than meets the average and frequently also the expert eye. The trouble is that during our information explosion, masses of very valuable and at times vital information fly out into space never to reach the minds of those who need it most.

CHAIRMAN CORDAY: Dr. Raab, we hadn't planned to go into a different direction right now, but I'd like to come back to that. Let us focus our attention on the studies that Ancel Keys is presenting for the first time. Dr. Friedman, would you like to discuss these statistics? Are you happy about them?

DR. FRIEDMAN: What do you mean by happy?

CHAIRMAN CORDAY: I know that you usually don't agree on everything. Do you agree with his conclusions?

DR. FRIEDMAN: Well, I'd like to see similar data on the West Finns. How about that Dr. Keys?

DR. KEYS: I have just taken the extremes here.

DR. FRIEDMAN: No. I want data concerning West Finns because their diet is the same as the East Finns.

DR. KEYS: No, it's not I'm sorry to say.

DR. FRIEDMAN: Oh I'm sorry, but you have said this in the literature. You analyzed their diets twice. You studied them in the summer and also in the winter. Their blood cholesterols were about the same, yet the Eastern Finns had twice as much coronary disease.

DR. KEYS: No. Cholesterol levels are not the same. The cholesterol figure is about two hundred fifty in the West Finns instead of two sixty-five. There's also a major difference in the frequency of hypertension between East and West Finland. This is one thing we do know.

DR. FRIEDMAN: There's also the possibility that there may be a major difference in the origin of the East Finn as compared with that of the West Finn. You've counted bodies, but how many bodies did you count who were born in the Karelian Peninsula and who were expelled from Russia in 1940?

DR. KEYS: I'm sorry. You're getting into technicalities. I can assure you that there are just as many deported Karelians in West Finland as there are in East Finland.

DR. FRIEDMAN: There is one thing that is very certain, Dr, Keys, and that is that the immigration of any race whether it's the Japanese, the Yemeni or the Irish from Ireland to Boston increases coronary disease. So it's not inconsequential particularly when the San Francisco Finnish Consul has told me, "Of course the East Finns might have more heart disease; many of them are immigrants from the Karelian Peninsula. Also the way of life in Eastern Finland is a more difficult one." I'd like to see your West Finns' statistics.

DR. KEYS: Well, I'm sorry. I think you should go to Finland and spend a few years, as we have, and find out about the matter.

DR. FRIEDMAN: Didn't Dr. Roine who was your collaborator go back to see if the difference in morbidity was due to more colloid goiters in the East Finns? Does that explain the difference? That's what he intimated because I have just reviewed the literature.

DR. KEYS: Roine is a nutritionist. He has nothing to do with pathology.

DR. FRIEDMAN: And you're not familiar with the fact that he studied the East Finns and said that they had a higher goitrigenic index?

DR. KEYS: No, the question is whether the difference in iodine intake might be interesting. We're studying that now.

CHAIRMAN CORDAY: Gentlemen, I think we'll jump off that topic.

DR. FRIEDMAN: Well, I am not very happy about the data.

CHAIRMAN CORDAY: Well, as you see, in assessing all these factors it's very difficult to get agreement. Every time Ancel Keys comes back with new statistics he meets with loyal opposition. It just seems that we're far away from the solutions and that we're all walking down the same investigative pathways that have now become ruts. We have to fan out in different directions in our attack on the problem of occlusive vascular disease. Every little lead might mean something. Now let's go on to the next problem that of high blood pressure. As you all know, Dr. Wilbur from Georgia has emphasized that there is need to detect and treat the patients with hypertension, to prevent atherosclerosis. We're all paying attention to diet and psychological factors and things like that; but there are so many people that seldom see their doctor, or maybe not at all. Wilbur detected the hypertensives by his mobile clinics and later proved fairly conclusively that if these hypertensives are earmarked and then ushered into their doctor's office for treatment, that this will reduce the incidence of ischemic heart disease. Campbell, what do you think of this approach? Is it worthwhile?

DR. MOSES: It's worthy of a study. We really don't know what the survival times are going to be when previously unrecognized modest degrees of hypertension are effectively treated. I don't think the data permit us to give very accurate predictions of how much we're going to help a person with a 160 mm. systolic blood pressure effectively treated for ten years. There's some suggestive data, but I'm not so sure it's the kind of data to permit us to pound the table firmly.

CHAIRMAN CORDAY: Have we any studies at our local chapters of the Heart Association that are involved in a similar survey?

DR. MOSES: Local chapters of the Heart Association and I hope every doctor in the room is engaged in hypertension screening programs. The practicing physician is performing this task daily whether he's doing health examinations or illness examinations. I know that there's a good deal of enthusiasm for treating modest degrees of hypertension with drug therapy of one sort of another. I'm familiar with the data that indicate that even modest degrees of hypertension put people at increased risks. I do think we need more data, however, before assuming that correcting such degrees of hypertension will in the long run effectively change the incidence of coronary disease or stroke.

CHAIRMAN CORDAY: Dr. Keys, would you comment on that?

DR. KEYS: Yes. I just wanted to ask Dr. Moses a question. In these same data, wasn't it true that roughly half of all persons who had known hypertension were doing nothing about it?

DR. MOSES: Yes, that's true. I don't know whether it was half but it was certainly a large percentage.

CHAIRMAN CORDAY: Say we have fifty percent of our afflicted population who know they have elevated blood pressure and fifty percent who don't. It's quite obvious that screening processes might bring those unaware patients in for treatment and this could be just as important as diet and the other factors mentioned. Now at what pressure level should the practitioner start treating the patient with hypertension?

DR. MOSES: Well I'd like to define what I would mean by treating it first. The first step in therapy is determining, if you can, why he has the 160 over 90. Sometimes this can be identified as arising from a situational circumstance or from some specific problem, but let's assume that the cause can't be identified. Then I'd suggest that the initial way to approach management is with sodium restriction, dietary induced and not drug induced, as a first step around in order to see what happens in three or four months. I think Dr. Friedman has more accurate data on this specific subject.

CHAIRMAN CORDAY: Dr. Friedman, what's your opinion?

DR. FRIEDMAN: I pretty much agree with what has been said. I think in our thirty-two hundred man study—I don't know how many hundreds have hypertension—the thing that struck us as most desolatingly discouraging was that in every man who had a history of hypertension under therapy it didn't seem to make much difference as far as his blood pressure was concerned. When we took it, it was elevated. This is very discouraging. In other words, if a man said he was being treated with drugs for hypertension, when the technician took his blood pressure, his blood pressure always seemed to be up. I don't mean that it was strikingly high, but above 90 mm. diastolic and above one hundred fifty systolic which are our cut off points. To us there is no question whatsoever that hypertension, just as indicated in the Framingham study, carries a great risk. It's probably the greatest risk of all, considering the number of people. I don't know of any study, as Dr. Moses said, in which half of the hypertensive subjects have been treated vigorously to see if the incidence of coronary disease could be materially influenced. I think it should be done.

DR. MOSES: Just so we don't leave this on too pessimistic a note, I'm not so sure I know the reason for it and some of the results may be unrelated to proven techniques or treatment, but since 1950 there has been a very substantial decrease in the death rate from hypertensive heart disease and I don't think it's simply a matter of reclassifying the cause of death. It's down some sixty-five percent in sixteen years from 1950 to 1966. I wish I was as glib about the reasons that might be responsible for this as I am in reporting the fact that this decrease has occurred.

CHAIRMAN CORDAY: Dr. Keys, have you any comment?

DR. KEYS: Yes, I think that Dr. Moses is wrong in minimizing the effect of reclassification. I think a very large amount of the change in death rates can be traced very directly to reclassification. Now that doesn't mean that there isn't something substantial there as well, but a lot of it at certain times is reclassification.

CHAIRMAN CORDAY: Dr. Raab, have you any comment on this problem? Would you care to state whether the patient with hypertension should be treated vigorously and at what level?

DR. RAAB: I prefer not to express any opinions on practical questions because I do not have enough experience of my own. I prefer to indulge in pathophysiological reasoning which I do think does have it's place and there too hypertension obviously plays a role. Now we heard today from Dr. Moyer that hypertension does contribute to atherogenesis, but I'm not speaking about this simply because I don't feel competent. On the other hand, we do know that high blood pressure does interfere with myocardial metabolism in a way which is certainly not favorable. In hypertrophic hearts from hypertension, we have found abnormal electrolyte distributions which are qualitatively the same as observed in a number of other cardiac conditions. In human hearts after myocardial infarction there is a severe electrolyte derangement for a week or ten days which must be functional, and hypertension acts in a similar direction.

CHAIRMAN CORDAY: Dr. Friedman, I want to ask several questions submitted by the audience. There is some interest concerning the treatment of patients with diabetes and hyperuricemia. When these patients are treated, does this influence the morbidity and mortality from coronary artery disease?

DR. FRIEDMAN: I don't know from my own practical experience in treating diabetic patients. My suspicion has been that the more vigorously you treat the blood glucose level perhaps the more violently you may accelerate the coronary disease. No, I'm not saying that jokingly, I say it tragically. Now whether that means by having a urine free of sugar you are subjecting the patient day in and day out to episodes of catecholamine excess and thereby damaging arteries day in and day out, I don't know. Maybe the sloppy way is the best. There is one more thing I would like to say. I want to make a comment on the influence of reclassification. I'm a simple soul and

thirty years ago when I went to my hospital at least three to four times a week we would have a subarachnoid hemorrhage due to hypertension. This is very rare in our hospital today and I don't think it is a result of reclassification. I believe that vigorous treatment of hypertension accounts for the rarity of catastrophic cerebral vascular hemorrhages and also congestive heart failure and uremia. I just don't see those conditions in our hospital and I'm very simple; what I don't see, I don't believe exists.

DR. MOSES: I wanted to comment on the diabetic problem that Dr. Friedman referred to. I couldn't agree with him more that the degree of disturbance of carbohydrate metabolism and the correction we invoke probably have little to do with the effective control of the vascular disease. He commented about the possibility of hyperglycemia and catecholamine release. I'd like to call attention to something else. Many of the important problems in diabetes, vascular problems, are microvascular lesions and the immunology people now are showing us with increasing emphasis the importance of anti-insulin antibodies. It may well be that, to quote an old expression of Doctor Katz stated some twenty years ago at an atherosclerosis meeting, "Perhaps this insulin is causing all this atherosclerosis". It could well be that the insulin that we administer contributes in some very important ways to the microvascular lesions of diabetes. I think this is consistent with some of the data and the early problems of diabetes as in persons with the disease who show increased amounts of circulating insulin. The answers aren't clear but at least we know less for certain about diabetes and atherosclerosis than we did five years or ten years ago.

DR. KEYS: Yes, I think this is very important. That means that we should distinguish sharply between the high insulin level and the low insulin level diabetics and this of course is one thing that hasn't been done in the past in following up the outcome in terms of vascular disease. Even Dr. Friedman agrees with me.

CHAIRMAN CORDAY: Here is a question from the audience: "The Framingham study and also the studies conducted by Gofman indicate that after the age of fifty-four there is no correlation between the incidence of myocardial infarction and the lipid level. If this is so, is there any need to place patients after the age of fifty-four on anti-lipemic diets and anti-lipemic medication?"

DR. KEYS: I wouldn't say anything about the need, but there is certainly this much that we can say in a strictly actuarial sense. The predictability of the outcome, the future, goes down with advancing age if you're using any of these measures—blood pressure, serum cholesterol and probably even personality. Eventually you arrive at the point of no return. Now, of course, you don't tell your patients that, but I don't know what age this is. I think fifty-four, Gofman suggested something like age fifty-four, was the cut off point several years ago. I think that the later figures from all of our studies actually show that some predictive value from all of these factors, including serum cholesterol, extends well into the sixties.

CHAIRMAN CORDAY: Dr. Friedman, would you also answer the question as to whether or not there is any need to place these patients after that age on a rigid diet and on anti-hyperlipemic medication?

DR. FRIEDMAN: Well, I'm pretty biased and I prescribe a low cholesterol, low fat diet for every patient regardless of how old he is, particularly emphasizing the fat after fifty-five. I'm going to quote Parry. He said in 1797 that a patient having angina should be kept on a diet low in fat. I think an acute fat load whether it's of vegetable or animal origin may kill a patient not because it damages the coronary vessels necessarily but because it damages in some manner the sustenance of myocardial function. I don't know how it does so.

CHAIRMAN CORDAY: Doctor Friedman, is it not true that the Framingham study found stress did not affect the incidence of coronary artery disease? I think the Bell Telephone Company study also questioned whether stress was such an important factor.

DR. FRIEDMAN: Do you mean the Bell Telephone or the American Cancer Society study of coronary artery disease? Let me say that we're very sorry that Dr. Hinkle can't go on with his Bell Telephone study. We couldn't agree with him more. We have never said that position determines coronary heart disease prevalence. We want to know by what arrogance an epidemiologist sets up standards to determine emotion. What makes him think the president of a concern becomes more emotionally charged because he has more responsibility. Since when is responsibility synonomous with emotion? What we say is "What does the individual respond to in his particular setting"? Dr. Hinkle has asked to observe our study and to learn our technique. We have told the people at Framingham 3 years ago that if they want to learn our technique we would be glad to have their representative visit us. They have not attempted to learn our technique for classification of behavior patterns. We don't have a questionnaire that we depend on. We're interested, as Dr. Ernest Friedman of Cleveland indicated, in the stylistics of the interview. It's not what an individual says in

response to our questions, it's how he says it and detection of stylistics may be subtle, but if it's subtle, this is no reason it shouldn't be included in an epidemiological study. I'd like to point out just one thing. If in the nineteenth century they did an epidemiologic study on hypertrophy of the left ventricle, they would have found rheumatic heart disease to be a very important cause, syphilitic heart disease too, but they would have completely missed hypertension because there was no decent way to measure hypertension. Therefore, hypertension didn't exist, I presume. Because we can't measure an entity is no sign that it does not exist.

CHAIRMAN CORDAY: Well, gentlemen, our time is moving very quickly and I would like to bring up for discussion the anti-hyperlipemic drugs, particularly Atromid-S. I note that there are funds provided for a large cooperative study across the nation. It hasn't been implemented yet. Would Atromid be of benefit in reducing the incidence of coronary artery disease? Should patients receive it from childhood on to prevent atherosclerosis? What is your impression, Dr. Moses?

DR. MOSES: I don't like to single out Atromid-S from dextrothyroxin, the other drug that I've had experience with and I wish I could tell you in advance which patients will uniquely fail to respond to dietary restrictions of various kinds, but successfully respond to Atromid-S or to dextrothyroxin. Despite some of the recent pronouncements from NIH, I don't think we do know exactly how to classify everybody with hyperlipemia. I think there are mixed types and I wish it was as simple as the five types popularized even though even that gets pretty complicated in clinical practice. As to whether everybody from the cradle to the grave should be on Atromid-S, I think we have need for prospective studies, dietary as well as drug. I think it's very important that we do implement these prospective programs because to base our recommendations or lack of recommendations only on experiences in people who have had myocardial infarction restricts our perspective to a very special kind of problem. I wouldn't want you to be at all left with the feeling, and I don't think anybody is anymore, that cholesterol and triglycerides are the only factors. The things Dr. Raab has referred to, the stress factors and other influences are desperately important. We're only going to effect a specific segment with hypercholesterolemic problems and I wish I could tell you exactly which ones will be benefited.

CHAIRMAN CORDAY: Dr. Friedman, would you like to comment upon the same question?

DR. FRIEDMAN: I am in complete agreement with Dr. Moses. I wish the American Heart Association also shared this view. I think it's a pity that the American Heart Association in the last ten years has consistently neglected the "emotional" and "stress" factors. Secondly, I also agree, and I think Dr. Keys will too, with what has been said concerning the so-called phenotyping of the various kinds of lipoproteinemia. When you really do this in the laboratory, gentlemen, what you end up with is a mess. Now let's take types 1, 2, 3, 4 and 5. Type 1 is a straight triglyceride increase and there are about several hundred recognized patients in the United States who have this. Type 2 is the betalipoproteinemia group which Gofman has already exploited. They constitute no more than ten to twenty per cent of the population. Types 3, 4 and 5 are mixtures, of prebeta, beta and triglycerides. Isn't that about right? So a pre-beta syndrome as a pure entity is not too frequently seen. There's another thing that is all through the literature; people are saying "If the fasting plasma triglyceride is under one hundred fifty mg./100 ml. that's normal". Not in our book! We would want to know how long has that patient fasted. If the patient has fasted twelve hours or more, a triglyceride of over 100 mg./100 ml. is abnormally high. It must be below 100. Now in our WCGS study, our fasting triglyceride is around one hundred fifty, but the men only omit one meal, breakfast. They may have eaten at 10 or 11 p. m. the night before, in other words, they had only a nine or ten hour fast. One fat meal may take 15 to 24 hours to clear in a behavior pattern A individual.

CHAIRMAN CORDAY: Well, gentlemen, our time is almost up. It would appear that there is no sure way of treating atherosclerosis at the present time. We had hoped that with a drug like Atromid-S, we could tell our patients to disregard their diet. We've heard from the experts and we learned that there is no uniformity of opinion at the present time. We're still facing a deplorable mortality rate. It's quite obvious that we require much more research. Possibly different approaches to the investigation of this disease are needed. Every little clue counts. For instance, the transplantation people found that the heart which was transplanted into the atherosclerotic recipient developed atherosclerosis within a very short period of time. The intima became thick and swollen and within two months occluded the arteries. We might look upon this as a new research model that might help us out of this dilemma.

Diagnosis of Ischemic Heart Disease

Part One
Chairman
Burton L. Zohman, M.D.

Diagnostic Value of an Adequate History
Paul D. White, M.D.

Tests for the Diagnosis of Latent (Silent) Coronary Artery Disease
Arthur M. Master, M.D.

Detection by Monitoring Devices in Native Environment
Tzu-Wang Lang, M.D.
Eduardo Rosselot, M.D.
Eliot Corday, M.D.

Atypical Angina Pectoris
John F. Briggs, M.D.

Part Two
Chairman
Louis F. Bishop, M.D.

Value and Limitations of the Electrocardiogram in the Diagnosis of Coronary Syndromes
David Scherf, M.D.

Apex Cardiography in Ischemic Heart Disease
E. Grey Dimond

Clinical Application of New Cardiac Enzymes
John S. LaDue, M.D.

Terminal Arteriole, Capillary or Cellular Dysfunction
William Likoff, M.D.

Papillary Muscle Dysfunction
George E. Burch, M.D.
John H. Phillips, M.D.
Nicholas P. DePasquale, M.D.

Panel Discussion: Prognosis in Myocardial Infarction; Yesterday and Today
Moderator: Paul D. White, M.D.
Panelists: Arthur M. Master, M.D.
Henry I. Russek, M.D.
William B. Kannel, M.D.
Eliot Corday, M.D.
Pavl Lukl, M.D.

Diagnostic Value of an Adequate History

Paul D. White

Forty years ago in preparing the first edition of my book on heart disease I made the statement that in my own experience an accurate history of a cardio-vascular patient made up in importance about 50 per cent of the total examination. I rated the physical examination as 30 per cent, the electrocardiogram as 10 per cent, X-ray study as 5 per cent, and all other technics as the remaining 5 per cent. Technical advances in the intervening years require some reappraisal and I would add 10 per cent or more in a few cases to other technics such as cardiovascular catheterization and angiocardiography when they are essential. In cases where they are necessary they would reduce the relative importance somewhat and about equally of both the physical examination and the history. But in the majority of my patients I would still rate history as having the priority. This may not be agreed to by all physicians, even including cardiologists, but this is, I believe, due to a failure to appreciate the finer nuances of clues from history that may seem obscure.

I speak to you of course as a consultant and realize that the general practitioner and even the internist cannot, or at least does not, have the time that I have myself felt necessary for any patient, but that is one major reason why there is such a specialty as ours. I do think, however, that what I shall say does apply pretty much to all cardiovascular consultants.

PRESENT ILLNESS

Let me now take up the various facets of the patient's history in the order of the interview. Since he or she comes to us because of present concern or symptoms we shall discuss this part of the history first. Very important at the outset is the source of the reference of the patient to the consultant. Is it the family doctor or some other physician whose active concern is responsible? If so, we are likely to find important abnormalities unless the reference is because the doctor would like confirmation of the relative unimportance of some symptom or sign which unduly worries the patient or his family. Now and then the consultant acts as an umpire between two doctors who have disagreed, especially in the case of a patient or his family who have "shopped around." Not rarely I have had patients, especially from overseas, who may have started with consultations in their own communities and countries and then gone on to check these opinions in, say, Switzerland, Paris, London, and New York. They have arrived in my office utterly confused, often not so much by gross differences of opinion as by trivial differences of diagnosis or treatment, especially where neither of two drugs under debate is in my opinion either necessary or harmless. And, of course, I too may be wrong. And finally there are patients who come to me referred by wife or husband or other member of the family or by the patient himself or herself, with a letter from the family doctor who is acquiescent. It is important to know when this happens, and incidentally in such instances I find it very helpful to have the family member responsible on hand, since this saves a lot of trouble later.

Another preliminary comment that I consider of great importance is the time that I devote to the history taking, never less than a half hour and sometimes a full hour with a new patient and about half that time with an old patient, whose back history I have already recorded. I find that many patients have never had such attention paid to them before and not only are they appreciative, but they are much more likely to become friendly and co-operative, and to follow up the advice that finally results at the end of the total examination. In closing this paragraph I would add that I record in longhand the history which I take myself, which leaves me and the patient unhurried and unhampered by an assistant taking notes by dictation. Incidentally I believe that the major importance of the history requires the concentrated attention of the cardiologist himself: if for any reason he must delegate part of the examination to others, it should never be the history.

Another advantage of the cardiologist's meeting the patient at the start for the history taking is that he observes his demeanor as he enters the office or as he looks up from his hospital bed. His composure or lack of it, his facies, any asymmetry of body motion, his handshake, a sigh or two, hesitation or slurring of speech, and early fatigue are all clues that singly or in combination should be noted by the physician during his history taking to be added to the findings of the total examination.

Now let us take up section by section the history itself. What brings the patient to the doctor? A sign or a symptom or a question mark? Is it because there has been much heart disease or hypertension or diabetes or hypercholesterolemia in the family? Has there been doubt about the electrocardiogram either in a first record taken or in a serial tracing? Is there doubt about the x-ray film or fluoroscopy? Are his blood lipids abnormal? Here I would add the important advice to secure, in order to study, not just the reports of the electrocardiograms and x-ray films but at least representative tracings and films themselves, especially those taken at critical times. We should receive reports of previous blood and urine tests and it goes without saying that we should know what drugs and diet and special procedures, investigative, electrical, and surgical have been administered.

SYMPTOMS

Since we are concerned in this volume with coronary or ischemic heart disease, we shall now discuss the symptoms thereof although it should be noted that any other kind of heart disease may also be present, either superimposed or already present when ischemia is added. Although dyspnea, palpitation, and snycope, faintness, vertigo, and edema should, of course, be asked about and noted as complications, as well as their degrees and circumstances, it is the characteristic symptom of ischemic muscle in which we are now preponderantly interested.

Angina Pectoris

It certainly would not be necessary to quote Heberden again if it were not for the fact that errors of commission or omission are still not rare in the diagnosis of angina pectoris as the characteristic symptom of the ischemic myocardium. Angina pectoris described by Heberden in 1768 is never sharp or burning itself or long in duration unless the exciting factor continues owing to the continuation of effort or excitement or the presence of the status anginosus resulting from paroxysmal tachy-cardia or acute coronary thrombosis. If none of these factors supervenes, the symptom of angina pectoris usually subsides in two or three minutes. Another important point about angina pectoris is that so far as I know it never occurs at physical, emotional, or gastrointestinal rest at a normal heart rate without occurring more readily on exercise, excitement, or hearty eating.

The symptom is that of an uncomfortable high or low substernal or anterior chest oppression or heaviness of any degree from a hardly noticeable sensation to an unbearable strangling (which the Greek word angina literally means). There is rarely any feeling of impending death, even though it may soon occur, except in highly emotional or neurotic persons or when it is overwhelmingly severe. I speak not only from experience with some thousands of patients with the symptom but also from personal experience with a minor degree of angina pectoris which can be induced by hurry and fast walking after a hearty meal especially in cold and windy weather. However, I regard its occurrence in my own case as more or less normal since it didn't begin till three months before my eighty-first birthday and I consider any longevity after eighty as "borrowed time," nature not having planned that the world should be too full of very aged people. As a matter of fact I consider as a distinct possibility the idea that my collateral circulation can still outdistance my coronary atherosclerosis to allow me to outgrow my angina.

There are a few more things to be said about the symptom of angina pectoris. It may or may not radiate as a numbness to the arms and even to the hands, more often or more heavily to the left, or to the front of the neck or to the jaws, especially if there is trouble with the teeth and gums, but it rarely goes to the back unless there is something wrong there or with the gallbladder or the spine, and it rarely goes down to the abdomen and never to the legs. Angina abdominalis is, I am sure, a definite entity but due rather to ischemia of the gut from atherosclerotic obstruction of the aorta or of the aortic branches going to the viscera. On occasion the radiation of the pain is reversed, starting for example in the arms (even in the injured right wrist of a patient of mine, which I might call angina brachialis or manus) and radiating back to the substernal area. This atypical myocardial ischemic pain is very interesting and can be an important though overlooked clue. It has the same duration and occurs under the same circumstances as ordinary angina pectoris; I call it sympathetic.

Another item of much importance is that angina pectoris never can be pinpointed in one area on the chest the size of a finger tip. Its area requires at least the palm of one hand or more often the palms of both hands to cover it and it is also not tender unless we are dealing with another factor, a sore chest wall or skin, or a neurocirculatory asthenic person. Also it is not changed by respiration, though the slowing of the heart rate by carotid sinus pressure may shorten its duration.

If angina pectoris is prolonged so that it continues at rest, without tachycardia, for more than a quarter of an hour, one must think of the probability of acute coronary thrombosis, especially if nitroglycerin or amyl nitrite does not clear it. Incidentally a good test which helps to establish the diagnosis of this symptom and of myocardial ischemia is the oral absorption of the quick acting nitrites.

Complications of myocardial ischemia, usually only when it is severe, are faintness or syncope, pallor, sweating, and, from the use of nitroglycerin, headache and more faintness.

Differential Diagnosis of Angina Pectoris. Let me complete the discussion of angina pectoris with a few words about differential diagnosis. I suppose that the most common confusion is with cardiospasm involving the esophagus and upper end of the stomach, with or without a hiatus hernia so popular in older persons, but there are differences that many patients themselves recognize. Cardiospasm is more likely to be burning or sharp and to be accompanied by gas, which may or may not seem to relieve the discomfort when belched. Also cardiospasm lasts longer and is not quickly relieved by the nitrites— hot water swallowed is more helpful. But a very important point is that the geographic and neurologic relationships of angina pectoris and cardiospasm are so close that they often occur together, the one symptom precipitating the other. The angina due to the myocardial ischemia may be so brief and relatively mild that it is quickly masked by the burning or sharper pain of the cardiospasm which it induces; as a result the pain of the cardiospasm may be wrongly called angina pectoris. It may take five or ten minutes of a careful interview to untangle these particular clues.

Other symptoms which may be confused with angina pectoris, brief or prolonged (as when ushering in acute coronary thrombosis), include those especially of neurocirculatory asthenia, with left breast aching and tenderness, often prolonged, and sighing dyspnea; muscular and rib tenderness from strain or trauma; neuralgia which is sharp; peptic ulcer and cholecystitis; acute pericarditis, aggravated by breathing; and mediastinal emphysema and pneumothorax.

Complicating cardiovascular symptoms due to coronary heart disease superimposed on myocardial ischemia are few except for the arrhythmias which include premature beats, the paroxysmal atrial and ventricular tachycardias, flutters, and fibrillations, and the A-V and bundle branch blocks. These are not common accompaniments of angina pectoris but, like vascular collapse and myocardial weakness and failure with the symptoms of pulmonary and systemic edema, they are common in serious myocardial infarction, acute and chronic. Adams-Stokes attacks can also accompany infarction of minor extent but of critical areas of the A-V conduction system in coronary heart disease, but I have followed many cases of symptomless A-V or bundle branch block for a good many years before they succumbed to further episodes of coronary artery and heart involvement or died noncardiac deaths.

FAMILY HISTORY

Having completed this story of the present illness I turn to the often helpful family history. I enquire about the ages and causes of death, so far as they are known by patient or his doctor, of the parents, siblings, and of the grandparents too if possible. Now and then in the case of an older coronary patient I find that a young or middle aged son has acquired the disease at a much younger age than either his father or mother acquired it. Coronary deaths of parents or siblings under the age of 60 should be carefully noted as well as the occurrence of diabetes or hypercholesterolemia in either family or the patient.

PAST HISTORY AND HABITS

The past history of the patient comes next. Besides the diseases asked about, the rich fat feeding for tuberculosis or peptic ulcer should also be noted. The discovery in earlier life of congenital, rheumatic, syphilitic, or hypertensive disease and follow up findings are important, as is also the occurrence of the symptom complex of neurocirculatory asthenia or nervous prostration, knowledge of which can be very helpful in the analysis of important clues. The maximal and minimal body weights as well as the current weight should be ascertained, for in my own experience a considerable percentage of my coronary patients have been grossly obese although at the time they come to me they may have reduced by 20, 30 or even 40 pounds.

And, finally, the habits should be recorded. They are helpful clues when added to other findings. The amount of tobacco, coffee, and alcohol, the number of years exposed to these materials, and the dates they were omitted are all to be noted. And finally the kinds and degrees of physical exercise through the years and the stress of life need appraisal, the stress to include that of family, business, and social and political nature. These are all environmental factors which in combination may well outweigh genetic factors in the etiology of ischemic heart disease.

Thus, in conclusion, I have attempted to evaluate in considerable detail information of various sorts and of various importance in securing a comprehensive history of a patient with coronary, that is ischemic, heart disease. It is doubtless more comprehensive than any of us achieve, myself included, but even so I have probably omitted items that others consider important clues and if so I shall be glad to add them.

Tests for the Diagnosis of Latent (Silent) Coronary Artery Disease

Arthur M. Master

What is silent coronary artery disease? It is completely asymptomatic disease in which anginal equivalents and other symptoms of heart disease, such as dyspnea, palpitation, and weakness, are absent. That this entity exists has been demonstrated not only by epidemiologic surveys but also by pathologists who have discovered myocardial infarctions at post-mortem examination of patients who had never had a complaint, been sick or lost a day of work because of illness. The existence of this silent form of coronary artery disease has been substantiated further in reports on "sudden deaths" by medical examiners.

In my own private practice I encounter almost a score of such patients weekly. Usually, the patient is referred because routine electrocardiograms show unexpected but definite abnormalities. Some tracings may even show evidence of previous transmural myocardial infarction; e.g., Q waves and QS patterns. In some patients the resting electrocardiogram may be normal and the exercise electrocardiogram (two-step test) abnormal; in such cases the patient is referred for consultation because he has no complaints.

INCIDENCE

Silent coronary artery disease is encountered daily by physicians during routine examinations of patients and in medical surveys of executives, by the military medical corps even in apparently healthy men in the armed forces, and by industrial physicians. What has not been realized is the ubiquity of asymptomatic coronary disease. In previous reports, my colleagues and I have demonstrated that from 3 to 5 million people, 35 years of age or more have silent significant coronary disease without infarction and that approximately 1,000,000 men have silent acute myocardial infarctions yearly.

Some revealing figures on silent coronary disease are given in Tables 1, 2 and 3. The post-mortem studies of healed myocardial infarction by three groups of investigators from 1946 to 1955 are summarized in Table 1. The incidence of recognized clinical disease, 48, 50, and 61 per cent, is compared with the incidence of completely silent disease, 52, 50, and 39 per cent respectively. In all instances the investigators delved very deeply into the patients' past history to confirm the fact that the disease was genuinely silent.

TABLE 1

Post-Mortem Studies of Healed Myocardial Infarction Incidence of Clinical Recognition

Investigator	Period of Study	No. Cases	No. Recognized	% Presumably Silent
Achor, Futch Burchell & Edwards	1946—50	227	108 (48%)	52
Johnson, Achor, Burchell & Edwards	1953—54	113	57 (50%)	50
Gould, S. E., & Cawley, L.P.	1945—55	452	277 (61%)	39

Table 2 reveals the clinical incidence of myocardial infarction ascertained in three studies from 1956 to 1959. If the percentages are weighted, we find that 30 per cent of these patients never had a single complaint.

Table 3 disclosed the prevalence of silent coronary disease for the years 1960 to 1963. The first column describes the type of coronary disease, the second column the number of cases in the sample, the third the percentage assumed to be silent, and the fourth the actual number of people with asymptomatic coronary disease. Let me attempt to clarify these data further.

It has been found that approximately 2,000,000 people a year have a myocardial infarction. As my colleagues and I have already established, in 30 per cent of these people the attacks are silent. Thus, approximately 600,000 people a year have silent coronary disease.

In our articles on silent coronary disease, we have shown that according to the literature, 56 per cent of those in whom myocardial infarction developed gave no history of preceding angina. Since a coronary occlusion is not a de novo process but one that develops over a period of time, it is obvious that for some months at least, if not years, these people had serious coronary disease without any symptoms at all. Thus, of the 2,000,000 people a year who suffer myocardial infarction, 56 per cent or 1,120,000 have silent coronary artery disease without infarction.

At least 4 to 6 per cent of the people in this country over the age of 35 have latent (silent) coronary artery disease. This would mean that in 1963, when there were 80,000,000 people in this country 35 years of age and over, 3,200,000 to 4,800,000 people had significant but silent coronary disease without infarction. Of course, all these figures overlap but from them we can get an idea of the great number of people who suffer from this condition.

TABLE 2
Clinical Incidence of Silent Myocardial Infarction

Investigator	Year of Report	Total No. Myocardial Infarction	% Silent*
Snow, Jones & Daber	1956	32	36%
Stokes, J., & Dawber, T. R.	1959	87	33%**
Price, L.	1959	414	30%

*Weighted average of the 3 series 30.8%
**Actual plus probable cases

TABLE 3
Estimated Prevalence of Silent Coronary Disease 1960—1963

Manifestation	Total Number	% Silent	Number Silent
1. Myocardial infarction	2,000,000	30	600,000
2. Projecting death certificates			563,000 to 840,000
Myocardial infarction without preceding angina	2,000,000	56	1,120,000
Coronary Disease without Infarction	80 million persons-35 years & over	4—6	3.2 to 4.8 million

HISTORIC BACKGROUND OF DIAGNOSTIC TESTS

As far back as 1889, and up to 1964, it was re-ported that systolic blood pressure and heart rate increased during and directly after muscular work, and then gradually returned to normal. In these early tests (and in the original two-step procedure) blood pressure and pulse rate were determined at certain time intervals after measured exertion and compared with the pre-exercise blood pressure and pulse rate. If these values did not differ significantly, myocardial function was considered to be normal.

Functional tests of the heart usually included some form of body movement, such as flexing and extending the arms, flexing the trunk, knee bending, hopping and jumping, or stair climbing. Stair climbing was in vogue for many years and is still in use. In 1901, Brittingham and White used dumbbell swinging, from the floor to an arm's length overhead. For essentially quantitative tests, the stationary bicycle, ergostats, and ergometers were used, calling into play the muscles of the fingers, arm or leg. These have been described by Mendelsohn, Graupner, Benedict and Carpenter, Krogh, Cathcart, Wishart and McCall, and Gillespie, Gibson and Murray.

One of the criticisms of such tests was that the workload required was the same for all subjects regardless of sex, age or weight. In addition, since valid standards for normal subjects had not been established, the results could not be meaningfully assessed.

Two-Step Test

The original two-step procedure, the results of which were also interpreted initially on the basis of the response of the blood pressure and pulse rate to standardized exercise, was devised by Enid Tribe Oppenheimer and the author, at the Cornell University Medical College between 1925 and 1929. After four years of trial, the "two-steps," each 9 in. high, were made the basis for the test. It was observed that age, sex and weight were important factors in work performance efficiency. Trial tests revealed that the efficiency of work in foot-pounds per minute decreased with increasing age, that the maximum work capacity for women was less than for men, and that efficiency declined with increasing weight. Hundreds of tests performed on normal persons substantiated this effect of age, sex and weight. Mathematically formulated tables recorded the number of trips on the two-steps according to these variables (Table 4).

Two-Step with Electrocardiograms

In 1940, we turned empirically to the routine employment of the electrocardiogram in conjunction

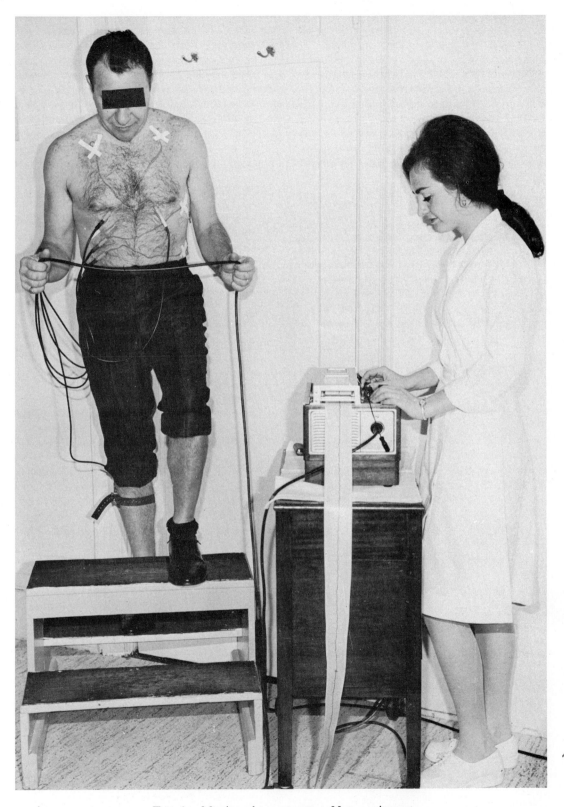

Fig. 1.   Monitored two-step test. Note equipment.

with the same standardized two-step in use since 1925. By this time the visual writing machines had become quite practical. Our first paper giving the results obtained with this new method was published in 1941. Since then we have found the electrocardiographic responses to be more objective and practical than the original blood pressure and pulse rate criteria.

In 1951 Robb, and in 1954 Mattingly, Fancher, Bauer and Robb published their observations on a large number of patients in whom the two-step electrocardiographic test was performed essentially in accordance with our methods.

Monitored Two-Step Test

Our experience with the "monitored two-step test," using several radiotelemetric devices as well as a direct hardwire hookup system, has been reported in detail (Fig 1). The key to obtaining a successful tracing lies in the selection of the electrode and the technic of its application (Fig 2).

Monitoring the two-step test by either radiotele-

metry or direct connection consumes much recording paper, usually requires the help of two people, and involves a great deal of marking, cutting, and mounting if a permanent record is desired. However, the electrocardiogram may be shown on an oscilloscope screen. We have found the regular postexercise test to be more valuable in making a diagnosis than the monitoring. Both are equal when searching for arrhythmias.

The Anoxemia Test

This test was popularized in this country by Robert Levy. It was in vogue for some years but has been replaced by more accurate diagnostic tests. It yielded almost 20 per cent each of false-positive and false-negative results. Moreover, vasomotor collapse occurred in normal persons.

Ballistocardiogram

The ballistocardiogram demonstrated too many abnormalities in healthy people, particularly in those over 50 years of age. Hence, it is of value only if negative in those over 50 years of age or positive in those under 45 years of age. Results will be abnormal whenever peripheral blood flow is obstructed, even though the coronary arteries are intact; e.g., in PVD, diabetes, amputees. Despite these obstacles, I think its potential is good.

Coronary Angiography

We are gradually depending on coronary angiog-

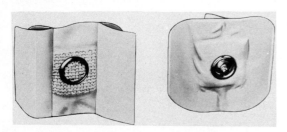

FIG. 2.   Electrodes for two-step test.

TABLE 4
*Trips Performed in Master Double (3 Minute) Two-Step Exercise Test**
Males and (Females)

Weight lb.	15—19	20–24	25–29	30–34	35–39	40–44	45–49	50–54	55–59	60–64	65–69	70–74	75–79
50–59	64 (64)												
60–69	62 (60)												
70–79	60 (58)												
80–89	58 (56)	58 (56)	58 (56)	56 (54)	54 (52)	54 (48)	52 (46)	50 (44)	50 (42)	48 (42)	46 (40)	46 (38)	44 (36)
90–99	56 (52)	56 (54)	56 (52)	54 (50)	54 (48)	52 (46)	50 (44)	50 (44)	48 (42)	46 (40)	44 (38)	44 (38)	42 (36)
100–109	54 (50)	56 (52)	56 (52)	54 (50)	52 (48)	50 (46)	50 (44)	48 (42)	46 (40)	44 (38)	44 (36)	42 (36)	40 (34)
110–119	52 (46)	54 (50)	54 (50)	52 (48)	50 (46)	50 (44)	48 (42)	46 (40)	46 (38)	44 (36)	42 (36)	42 (34)	40 (32)
120–129	50 (44)	52 (48)	54 (48)	52 (46)	50 (44)	48 (42)	46 (40)	46 (38)	44 (38)	42 (36)	40 (34)	40 (32)	38 (30)
130–139	48 (40)	50 (46)	52 (46)	50 (44)	48 (42)	46 (40)	46 (38)	44 (38)	42 (36)	40 (34)	40 (32)	38 (30)	36 (30)
140–149	46 (38)	48 (44)	50 (44)	48 (42)	48 (40)	46 (38)	44 (38)	42 (36)	40 (34)	40 (32)	38 (32)	36 (30)	36 (28)
150–159	44 (34)	48 (42)	50 (40)	48 (40)	46 (38)	44 (38)	42 (36)	40 (34)	40 (32)	38 (32)	36 (30)	36 (28)	34 (26)
160–169	42 (32)	46 (40)	48 (38)	46 (38)	44 (36)	44 (36)	42 (34)	40 (32)	38 (32)	36 (30)	36 (28)	34 (26)	34 (24)
170–179	40 (28)	44 (38)	46 (36)	46 (36)	44 (34)	42 (34)	40 (32)	38 (32)	36 (30)	36 (28)	34 (26)	34 (26)	32 (24)
180–189	38 (26)	42 (36)	46 (34)	44 (34)	42 (34)	40 (32)	38 (32)	38 (30)	36 (28)	34 (28)	32 (26)	32 (24)	30 (22)
190–199	36 (24)	40 (34)	44 (32)	42 (32)	42 (32)	40 (30)	38 (30)	36 (28)	34 (26)	32 (26)	30 (24)	30 (24)	28 (22)
200–209		38 (32)	42 (30)	42 (30)	40 (30)	38 (28)	36 (28)	34 (26)	32 (26)	32 (24)	30 (22)	28 (22)	28 (20)
210–219		36 (30)	42 (28)	40 (28)	38 (28)	36 (26)	34 (26)	34 (26)	32 (24)	30 (22)	28 (22)	28 (22)	26 (20)
220–229		34 (28)	40 (26)	40 (26)	38 (26)	36 (26)	34 (24)	32 (24)	30 (22)	28 (22)	26 (20)	26 (20)	24 (18)

*Master, A.M., & Rosenfeld, I.: The "two-step" exercise test brought up to date, New York J. Med. *61*:1850, 1961.

raphy more and more when the diagnosis is in doubt and surgery for coronary heart disease is contemplated. Coronary angiography is not an office procedure and should not be attempted unless resuscitative apparatus is at hand. An image intensifier is necessary. In expert hands this procedure is very dependable. Sones and his co-workers have obtained positive results in 95 per cent of those with typical angina and in 99 per cent of those with myocardial infarction. (However, in the November 2, 1968, issue of the Canadian Medical Association Journal, 8 cases of myocardial infarction were reported in which the coronary arteries were found to be normal by angiography.)

Dangers. As for the danger involved in coronary artery visualization, fatalities have occurred in 1/10 to 1/3 of 1 per cent of the patients subjected to this procedure. Since vascular damage to the brachial artery may ensue, it has been suggested that the catheters be inserted via the femoral artery. The coronary intima may be injured and signs of coronary occlusion may result. Transient episodes of cardiac arrhythmias, hemorrhage, or vascular thromboses have been reported in approximately 1 to 7 per cent of patients.

At times the angiocardiograms are false-negative, that is, they are negative when the clinical signs indicate that they should be positive.

In many of the recorded cases in which a clinical diagnosis of coronary heart disease was made, usually because of chest pain, the angiocardiogram was normal. Cited as explanations for a "false-negative" angiocardiogram, if it can be called that, are the following: The presence of myocardiopathy, an anomalous hemoglobin oxygen dissociation curve, and cardiac vein thromboses or involvement of vessels less than 100μ. Likoff has reported instances of a normal angiocardiogram with abnormal exercise tests predominantly in women. It is his belief that in these cases either microcirculation is involved or oxygen diffusion is impaired. For want of a better term, Likoff has temporarily designated this condition "syndrome X."

Richard Gorlin and his associates have observed normal coronary angiocardiograms in 10 to 15 per cent of their patients who have a good history of angina pectoris. They believe that this is due to either abnormal lactic acid metabolism or disease in the smaller vessels rather than in the coronary vessels themselves.

Many angiographers have observed signs of coronary spasm on the angiocardiogram and have found them to disappear following the administration of nitroglycerin. This would account for a normal angiocardiogram in patients with angina

pectoris. Others deny the existence of coronary spasm.

Apex Cardiogram

Clinically useful information can be gained from an analysis of the low frequency spectrocardiogram, that is, the recording of the low frequency precordial vibration put in motion by the cardiac beat. The time may come when this will be done after exercise and it may prove useful.

Atrial Pacing

In carrying out this procedure, Sowton and his associates pass a bipolar catheter into the right atrium of the patient, who is in a supine position. They then increase the heart rate steadily until the patient has pain in the chest. Ischemic changes in the RS-T segment are then observed. According to Sowton *et al.* pain occurs in the same patient always at the same rate of atrial pacing. In performing right atrial pacing Lau and his colleagues increase the heart rate until the monitored ECG reveals changes in the RS-T segment, not until pain appears. The latter investigators have compared their results with the Master two-step test results and have found that they are very similar. However, Lau *et al.* find that right atrial pacing yields a little higher percentage of positive results in patients with angina.

STANDARD TWO-STEP TEST

Recent reports have suggested that in stress electrocardiography the amount of exercise performed should be determined by the maximum heart rate attained rather than predetermined on the basis of age, sex and weight, as in the standardized Master two-step test. Optimum exercise is said to be that which induces 85 per cent of the maximum "age-predicted rate," as determined by Robinson in 1938 in his physical fitness studies of healthy subjects. In other words, it has been implied that the two-step exercise induces less than adequate increments in heart rate. Thus, Sheffield, Holt and Reeves, although maintaining that "standardization of an exercise electrocardiographic test for myocardial ischemia is desirable," advocate a "graded" exercise test in which the amount of stress performed will induce 85 per cent of the maximum age-predicted heart rate. The fallacy of this, however, is that the maximum age-predicted heart rate set as the standard was calculated in healthy subjects and is undoubtedly excessive for patients with cardiac disease. Sheffield, Holt and Reeves claim that graded exercise results in greater sensitivity in the diagnosis of ischemic heart disease than does the conventional two-step test. Use of a graded exercise test requires some type of monitoring device, since the heart rate achieved is determined during exercise, not after its completion. At present, we believe that their type of exercise test, going up and down a 12-inch step, may be dangerous for the patient with angina if it is given by the unskilled.

Rowell, Taylor, Simonson and Carlson, after evaluating 14 male subjects, concluded that the "physiological load imposed by the double Master two-step test fails to provide a physiologically equivalent workload for individuals differing in body weight." These investigators suggest the use of a treadmill to effect the same oxygen consumption per kilogram for all individuals of the same sex. The validity of these conclusions is open to question since the data are derived from a study of only 14 persons between the ages of 12 and 27, with four of them actually 12 to 14 years old! Ischemic heart disease does not develop in youngsters. In addition, the *treadmill* is a much bulkier and costlier device than the simple two-step apparatus and some older persons, particularly those with arthritis or neuromuscular disorders of the back, may find it difficult to maintain the tilt of the body required to walk along the inclined treadmill.

As already stated, the maximum age-predicted heart rate used by both Rowell and by Sheffield, and their respective co-workers, is derived from a single study carried out in 1938 which dealt with physical fitness in healthy boys and men, not with the detection of ischemic heart disease.

Some investigators reported the results of exercising subjects well beyond the upper limits of the two-step table. For example, Doan *et al.* had their subjects continue the treadmill exercise until they reached the point of virtual exhaustion; they suggested that the electrocardiographic abnormalities that occur after such maximum stress may be of prognostic significance even in apparently healthy volunteer subjects. Whether or not the expected prognostic implications materialize will depend on the results of long-term follow-up, and on the incidence of morbidity and mortality from coronary heart disease in subjects with an "abnormal" response after maximum exercise. As we have already intimated, strenuous exertion may lend itself to epidemiologic surveys of vigorous, young adults but its use in clinical medicine is limited and apt to be hazardous.

We sincerely believe that the Master two-step test is adequate for the detection of ischemic heart disease. Evidence in support of our belief is the following.

We conscientiously reviewed 100 male patients with classic angina successively. Half of these patients had a normal resting electrocardiogram and the other half had an abnormal but stable tracing. Their heart rates were studied continuously, at rest, during the two-step test and after completion of the test. The recording was maintained until the tracing indicated a return to the resting state, which was determined by the contour of the waves on the electrocardiogram and the original heart rate.

A "steady state" was attained in 92 per cent of the men who performed the two-step test. We considered a "steady state" had been reached when the rates during the last 30, 45, 60, 75 or 90 seconds of exercise did not differ by three beats per minute. The heart rate was recorded every 15 seconds during the two-step test. The "maximum rate" reached and the "steady state" coincided. Since this took place in the last 30 to 75 seconds of the two-step exercise, it may be stated that maximum rate, the plateau rate and the steady state coincided.

In the 50 men with angina who had a normal resting electrocardiogram following the two-step exercise, the depression in the RS-T segment did not correlate with age, resting rate, highest rate attained or with the percentage increase in the latter. The maximum depression was 2.25 mm.

In 50 men who had an abnormal but stable tracing on the electrocardiogram the degree of depression in the RS-T segment did not correlate with age, resting rate, maximum heart rate attained, or with the percentage increase of the latter over that of the resting rate. The RS-T depressions ranged from 0.6 to 7 mm. in depth.

That the highest rate attained in the two-step test, as revealed by our monitored technics, is adequate for diagnosis, is confirmed by the fact that positive ischemic responses in all 100 patients were obtained just as often with an actual maximum rate of 110 beats per minute or even less, as with the highest rate of 150 to 170 beats per minute. This is true whether the percentage increase in the maximum heart rate during exercise was 72 over the rate at rest, e.g., 90 to 155 beats per minute, or whether it was 142 per cent, e.g., from 60 to 145 beats per minute.

Standardization of the two-step test makes it possible to compare results all over the world, regardless of the heart rate attained during exercise. Drug effects can be studied easily and physiologic experiments performed readily with the two-step test. The results obtained with this test are comparable whether studied by more than one investigator or performed in different geographical areas.

We have insisted that the two-step procedure

remain standardized for many reasons. Some of these follow. The limits of exercise were established on the basis of physiologic study of a large number of healthy men and women and corrected for age, sex and weight. There is virtually no risk of over-exercising the subject; when properly performed, the test has been shown to be completely safe. Over-exercising a normal person may cause abnormal responses on the ECG. Forcing a patient to continue exercising indefinitely until pain or other symptoms appear may be followed by serious consequences, especially when the subject is sick, and even more especially if he does not know or sense that he is ill. In addition to the safety factor, standardization permits comparable and reproducible data, be it clinical, physiologic or pharmacologic.

The two-steps, the nurse-technician, and the patient being monitored during the two-step test are shown in Figure 1. The electrodes are depicted in Figure 2.

Use of the published table ("standardization" of the test) limits the exercise to the number of trips called for on it (Table 4). Overexertion even by normal people, may induce "ischemic" RS-T segment depressions, and in people with coronary disease injury may result. Standardizing or limiting exercise to the number of trips indicated in the table is a safety feature. In previous publications we have given illustrations of the harmful results when physicians, for example, have the patient walk on the two-steps until exhausted.

Illustrations Demonstrating the Value of Standardization

A 49-year-old man (P.V.) with severe angina and hypertension (Fig. 3), was very neurotic and his psychoanalyst considered all his complaints functional. A single (1-minute) test was negative but the regular double (3-minute) test disclosed ischemic RS-T depression in lead V5 of the 2-minute tracing. One year later this patient died while driving a car. The medical examiner discovered an acute transmural infarction.

The full number of trips, that is, the 3-minute exercise, is required to establish the diagnosis of coronary disease. Even in patients with severe angina pectoris, "understressing" often may not produce any change in the exercise ECG.

Another benefit that may be derived from standardization of the test is shown in Figure 4. In this case the patient, a 63-year-old man (H.K.), had a very severe anginal syndrome. The resting electrocardiogram revealed a sinus bradycardia but it was essentially normal. He was treated with iproniazid (Marsilid), a monoamine oxidase inhibitor. After a week all the pain disappeared. Regardless of what he did physically he had no symptoms or pain.

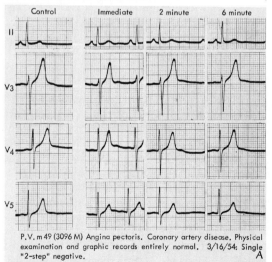

P.V. m 49 (3096 M) Angina pectoris. Coronary artery disease. Physical examination and graphic records entirely normal. 3/16/54: Single "2-step" negative.   A

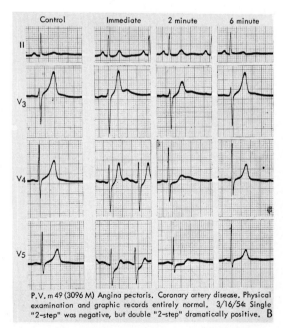

P.V. m 49 (3096 M) Angina pectoris. Coronary artery disease. Physical examination and graphic records entirely normal. 3/16/54: Single "2-step" was negative, but double "2-step" dramatically positive. B

FIG. 3. P. V., a 49-year-old man, had a severe angina pectoris. The resting ECG was normal. (*Left*) Since the patient was in status anginosus, it was thought safer to do only a single two-step test. It was negative. (*Right*) Therefore the regular double two-step test was performed. "Ischemic" RS-T changes appeared, particularly evident in the 2-minute Leads V4-V5. The "immediate" Lead V5 revealed an abnormal "j" depression, more than 3 mm. deep.

The patient developed a severe myocardial infarction 2 months later and died.

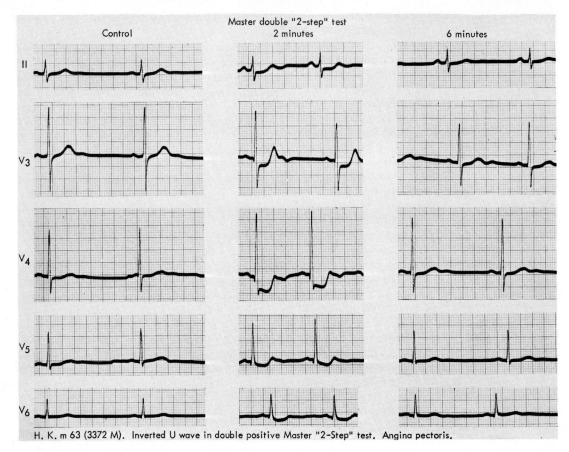

H. K. m 63 (3372 M). Inverted U wave in double positive Master "2-Step" test. Angina pectoris.

FIG. 4. H. K., a 63-year-old man with a severe anginal syndrome, almost "status anginosus." His pain was completely relieved by iproniazid (Marsilid) but his coronary disease was unchanged as indicated by the two-step test. The control tracing showed sinus bradycardia, 37 beats per minute. Following the regular 3 minute two-step test, dramatic RS-T depressions and inversion of the U-wave appeared. With the cessation of drug thereapy, the angina returned.

However, the 2-step test remained dramatically positive. Deep depressions of the RS-T segment and also inversion of the "u"-wave can be seen in the 2-minute tracing of leads V3 and V4. Thus, despite the complete loss of symptoms and a sense of well-being, the course of the severe coronary disease had not been altered by the drug.

With a standardized test, comparable physiologic and pharmacologic results anywhere in the world can be accepted and compared.

The need for standardization was revealed in still another way in a 36-year-old man with an anginal syndrome (J.F.) (Fig. 5). His 2-step test was monitored. Ischemic depressions did not appear until the very end of the test (42nd trip). In many cases of angina the full number of trips must be made before depressions in the RS-T segment are observed. The regular post-exercise ECG is shown in Figure 5(*bottom*); both significant "J" and

ischemic depressions are visible.

The value of the standardized two-step test in a patient with atypical chest pain and the significance of an ischemic depression of only 0.5 mm. in the RS-T segment are shown in another case (Fig. 6). This patient, a man of 51 (G.G.), gave a six-week history of substernal ache on exertion or under tension. It was not relieved by the ingestion of nitroglycerin. Furthermore, the episodes lasted as long as an hour. For these reasons the family physician excluded angina.

The control tracing was negative but the 2-step exercise test disclosed ischemic depressions although only 0.5 mm. (see 2 minute tracing of lead V6). Nevertheless, these were considered proof of angina. Three months later the patient had a fatal heart attack; an electrocardiogram a few hours before death showed massive diaphragmatic wall infarction.

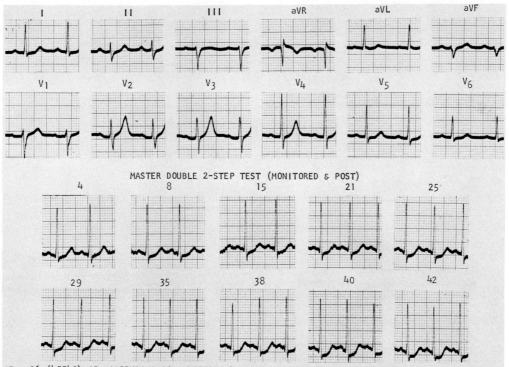

MASTER DOUBLE 2-STEP TEST (MONITORED & POST)

JF m 36 (45549) AP. IMPENDING CO. <u>RESTING</u> LAD, SLIGHT ST DEPRESSION V_5, V_6. D2S <u>MONITORED</u> "J" BECOMES "ISCHEMIC" 42ND TRIP. <u>POST</u> "ISCHEMIC" ST DEPRESSION, MAXIMAL $^5_2(V^6_5)$.

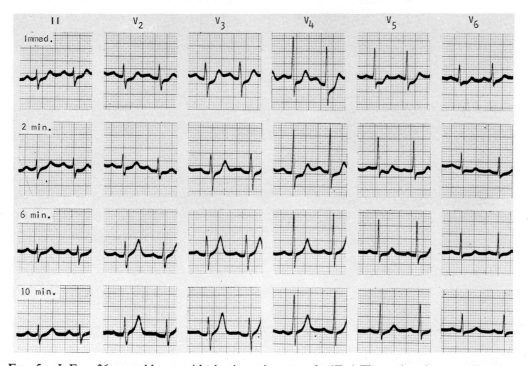

Fig. 5. J. F., a 36-year-old man with classic angina pectoris. (*Top*) The resting electrocardiogram was normal. The monitored two-step test at first showed "j" (junctional) depressions; these became more pronounced as the exercise continued until they became ischemic at the very last trip, the 42nd. (*Bottom*) The regular postexercise tracing showed ischemic depressions, maximum at two minutes in V5. The monitored test showed then ecessity of performing the full number of trips indicated in the published tables, since the tracing became ischemic only at the very end of the exercise. In other words, it is essential that exercise tests be standardized for age, sex, and weight.

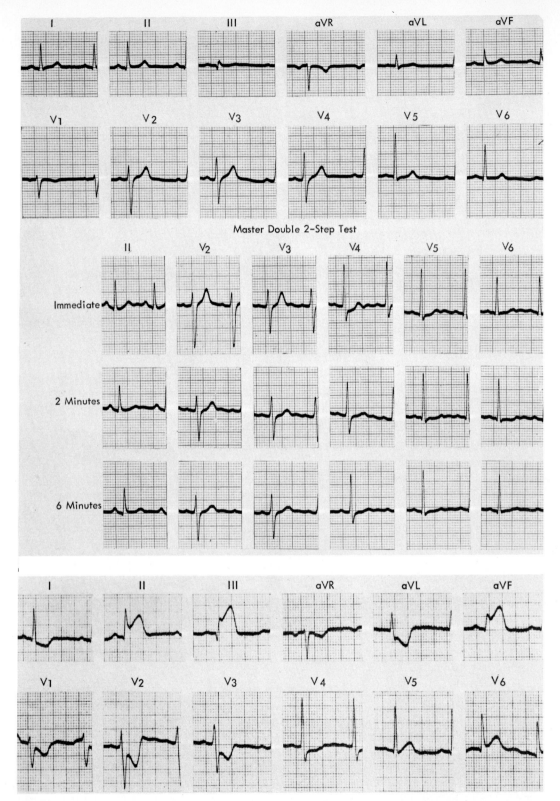

Fig. 6.   G. G., a 51-year-old man with a six-week story of substernal pressure on exertion. (*Top*) The resting electrocardiogram (upper two rows) was negative. At two minutes, the double two-step test revealed only 0.5 mm. ischemic ST depression in V6, but three months later, the patient experienced a severe pain. (*Bottom*) The electrocardiogram now disclosed monophasic curves characteristic of acute inferior infarction. The patient died five minutes later. The degree of ST depression correlates with the severity of the coronary disease only in a general way, but occasionally an "ischemic" ST depression of only 0.5 mm. is significant.

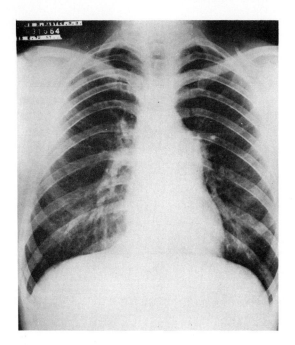

FIG. 7. F. M., a 22-year-old man with idiopathic dilatation of the pulmonary artery. (*Left*) A very harsh systolic murmur was heard in the pulmonary area. He was completely asymptomatic. (*Below*) The resting electrocardiogram (upper row) and the double two-step test were negative. On the strength of this, he was accepted by the Army and served in Korea.

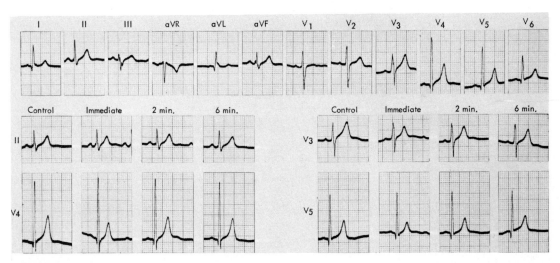

Congenital Heart Disease

The 2-step test is also of value in congenital heart disease as illustrated in another example. The patient, a 22-year-old man (F.M.) with congenital idiopathic dilatation of the pulmonary artery was in perfect health (Fig. 7). In fact he was an athlete. Because of a loud harsh systolic blowing murmur in the 2nd left intercostal space, he had been rejected for service by the draft board at the close of the Korean War. The resting electrocardiogram was normal (upper row, Fig. 7). The 2-step test was entirely negative.

On the strength of the negative 2-step test, the young man was accepted into the U.S. Army despite the loud basal murmur. He served his regular

three-year tour of duty without the slightest incident. At this writing he is still well.

Arrhythmias in the 2-Step Test

Figure 8 shows that a significant arrhythmia indicates a positive 2-step test. In this patient, a 62-year-old man with angina pectoris (B.Z.), the resting electrocardiogram was normal. The monitored test was negative except for a run of 3 consecutive premature contractions at the 25th and 27th trips.

The regular postexercise ECG showed ischemic depressions of the RS-T segment in the "immediate" lead II.

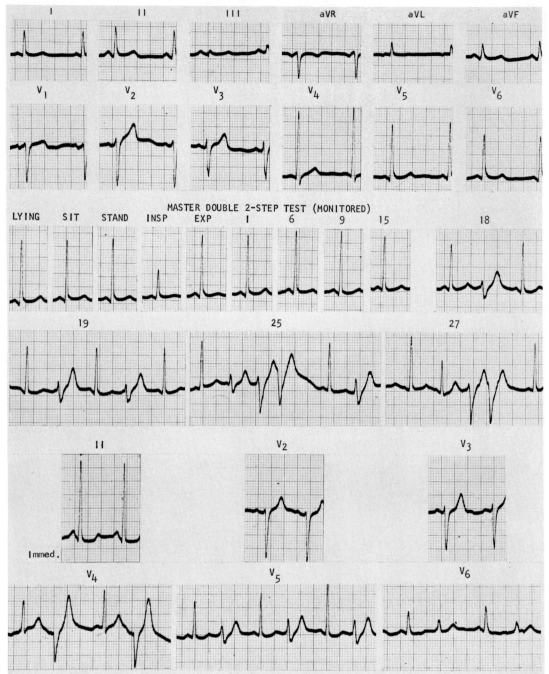

BZ m 62 (45986) EFFORT ANGINA 2 YEARS. RECENT ONSET SPONTANEOUS CHEST "PRESSURE". RESTING WNL. PARTIAL D2S MONITORED FUSION VPC'S AT 18TH AND 19TH TRIP. IN 25TH TRIP, NOTE RUN OF 3 CONSECU- TIVE VPC'S (NEVER MORE THAN THREE). 1ST BEAT IN THE SERIES IS A FUSION BEAT. POST IN IMMEDIATE V4, V5 AND V6, BIGEMINY DUE TO VPC'S, NONE CONSECUTIVE. ARRHYTHMIA ONLY IN "IMMEDIATE" TRACING, NONE LATER. NOTE ISCHEMIC ST DEPRESSIONS.

FIG. 8.   B. Z., a 62-year-old man, had had effort angina for 2 years. The chest pressure had become worse and recently had occurred spontaneously. The resting ECG (upper two rows) was within normal limits. The monitored double two-step test showed fusion ventricular premature contractions (VPC's) at trips 18 and 19. On trip 25, there were three consecutive VPC's; the first contraction was a fusion beat. On trip 27, chest pressure appeared and the exercise was terminated.

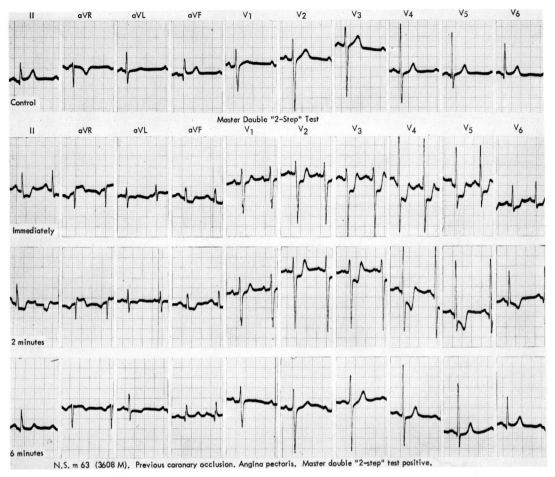

N.S. m 63 (3608 M). Previous coronary occlusion. Angina pectoris. Master double "2-step" test positive.

FIG. 9. N. S., a 63-year-old man, had had a previous coronary artery occlusion. The patient was first seen in 1955, when he presented himself with a classical anginal syndrome. However, he was free of symptoms for the following 11 years, no matter what he did. The patient has been examined regularly every 6 months. The resting ECG always showed Q waves in Leads II, III, and aV_F, the remains of the old coronary occlusion. It was essentially negative. The two-step test was always positive. In the beginning of 1967, a classical syndrome reappeared. Ten leads are shown in the two-step test to illustrate the point that the most marked electrocardiographic changes are usually observed in Leads II, V3, V4, V5, or Leads II, V4, V5, and V6. The case is also presented as one of completely asymptomatic but significant coronary disease for 11 years. Nevertheless, the two-step test demonstrated active coronary artery disease.

The 2-Step Test in Silent Coronary Disease

The 2-step is of value in silent coronary disease as illustrated in another example. This patient, (N.S.) had been under observation since 1955. In that year he had angina pectoris, almost a status anginosus. The control illustration, showing 10 leads, was normal (Fig. 9). After the 2-step test, "ischemic" changes were noted in the S-T segment, as usual best seen in leads V4 and V5. "J" or junctional depressions were observed in the 6 minute tracing of leads V3, V4 and V5 and in the "immediate" tracing of leap V6.

In 1956 the patient's complaints ceased. He remained entirely asymptomatic for 11 years despite his physical activities and an enlarged heart. His ECG following the 2-step test was always dramatically positive. This patient directed a large business but he paced his activities. In 1967 his anginal syndrome returned.

Negative 2-Step Test

A negative two-step exercise test is as valuable as a positive one. It practically excludes atherosclerotic

Fig. 10.   J. C., a 46-year-old man, who had been a "cardiac cripple" for 20 years. He had been in bed six weeks for two episodes of "coronary occlusion." Each time, he received morphine for severe chest pain. *(Below)* A single (1½-minute) two-step test was negative and the next day the regular double (3 minute) two-step test was also negative. Obviously, the patient had no heart disease at all. *(Right)* X-ray examination showed a hiatus hernia which accounted for the pain. After reassurance, the patient returned to work and has led a normal life for the past ten years.

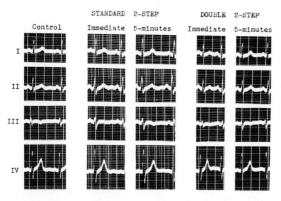

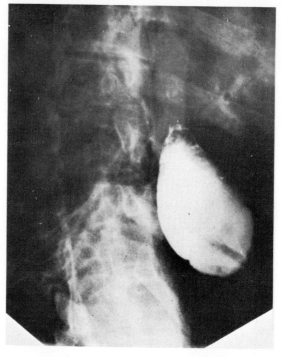

involvement of coronary arteries or inadequate coronary blood flow.

In the case illustrated in Figure 10, the patient, a 46-year-old man (J.C.) had been a "cardiac cripple" for 20 years. A diagnosis of coronary occlusion was made twice. On each occasion he had received morphine for pain and had been kept in bed for 6 weeks.

The control ECG was normal. The single 2-step test (1½-minute) was negative and on the following day the double or 3-minute test was negative. This convinced us more than ever that this patient had never had a myocardial infarction. X-ray examination revealed a hiatus hernia which was the cause of the patient's pain. Once the patient was reassured and convinced that he had no heart disease, he returned to work. He has been well ever since.

Confirmation of the value of the 2-step test has come from many sources. At the Walter Reed Hospital, Mattingly *et al.*, and at the Metropolitan Life Insurance Company, Robb and his associates have confirmed the value of a negative 2-step test. In persons in whom the exercise ECG is negative, coronary occlusions and deaths occur no more frequently than in healthy normal persons or in those considered as "standard risks" by insurance company doctors. By contrast, in those with "ischemic" depressions in the RS-T segment the number of heart attacks and deaths greatly increased.

Franco, Medical Director of the Consolidated Edison Company of New York, has also confirmed the value of a negative 2-step test. In 408 workers in whom the test was negative, follow-up disclosed infarctions in only 6, an incidence of barely 1½ per cent. By contrast, in those with positive 2-step tests, follow-up revealed coronary occlusion in fully 15 per cent and if we include all heart attacks, 20 per cent.

SUMMARY

After more than 40 years of experience with the standardized two-step test we have found it to be a safe, simple and reliable procedure for aiding in the discovery and evaluation of coronary heart disease and for evaluating the adequacy of the coronary circulation on exercise in people with other forms of heart disease.

"Ischemic" depression of the RS-T segment is the chief finding of a "positive" response, but "junctional" type depressions may also occur in patients who have compromised coronary artery circulation. A positive test suggests myocardial ischemia, and carries with it increased risk of cardiac morbidity or death, even in asymptomatic persons. A negative response has statistically been proved to indicate a favorable prognosis. The test may be performed in the presence of an abnormal control ECG provided it is stable and does not represent "impending" myocardial infarction.

Monitoring the ECG during exercise is also feasible, but it does not appear to increase the over-all diagnostic yield. It is worthwhile, however, in detecting arrhythmias which may appear only in the exercise period. Monitoring technics, both electronic and hardwire, depend on careful and secure application of electrodes, the most convenient of which are commercially available band-aid types. Various bipolar leads or conventional unipolar leads V4, V5, or V6 can now also be recorded.

In conclusion, any person whose work makes him responsible for the life of another, e.g., a pilot, bus driver, train engineer, or policeman, should have his heart function tested. In fact, every person in this country, 35 years of age or more, should annually undergo a physical examination, and have an x-ray picture of the chest and an ECG taken. If the latter is negative, the two-step test or an equivalent test should be performed.

Detection by Monitoring Devices in Native Environment

Tzu-Wang Lang, Eduardo Rosselot and Eliot Corday

The clinical value of the electrocardiogram in diagnosis of cardiovascular disease is still fundamental. However, the conventional electrocardiogram recorded in the doctor's office or hospital samples only a brief interval representing one five-hundredth of a patient's day.

We have found that more than 50 per cent of patients with cardiac arrhythmias are not aware of any disordered rhythm, and yet evanescent arrhythmias may cause obscure cardiovascular symptoms or remote neurologic,[1,2,3,4] renal,[5,6] and gastrointestinal[7,8,9] syndromes. Therefore, there is need for better diagnostic methods to detect these evanescent cardiac disorders and to correlate them with patients complaints. The diagnosis in many cases with angina pectoris cannot be made with certainty by the conventional electrocardiogram, particularly if episodes are transient and only occur in the native environment.[10,11,12]

A special electronic device which is capable of providing a continuous electrocardiographic record was devised by Holter.[13,15] This portable monitoring system appears to be an ideal diagnostic instrument because it permits a ten-hour period of continuous data recording in the patient's normal environment where he is exposed to provocative physical and emotional stress.

EQUIPMENT

The system developed by Holter, now commercially produced, consists of two major electronic units: a portable tape recorder, the electrocardiocorder, and a composite electrocardioscanner-electrocardiographic analyzer.

The portable 4-lb. electrocardiocorder is a small, transistorized unit, which can be carried in a camera-like leather case on a shoulder strap or a waist band. The 3-in. reel, magnetic recording tape which runs at $7\frac{1}{2}$ in. per minute, can provide electrocardiographic monitoring continuously for a ten-hour period. Two light, comfortable and liquid coupling electrodes are used: one placed over the manubrium sternum and the other over the rib inferior to the cardiac apex are connected by an inconspicuous thin wire to the electrocardiocorder. This bipolar lead along the long axis of the heart resembles an intermediate pattern between Lead I and Lead II of the standard electrocardiogram.

If the ill patient needs longer monitoring, a DC powered unit can record for longer intervals up to 24 hours at bedside without changing the tape or electrodes.

The composite electrocardioscanner-electrocardiographic analyzer actually consists of two parts: (1) electrocardioscanner and (2) electrocardiocharter. The electrocardioscanner has two display screens. The cathode-ray oscilloscopic screen at the left side called the AVSEP (audiovisual superimposed electrocardiographic presentation) portrays segmental PQRST complexes which are rapidly superimposed on one another, so that any change in configuration of P, QRS complex, T, or the isoelectric ST segment (elevated or depressed) can be easily detected. The cathode-ray screen of the arrhythmiagraph presents the RR interval in a picket-fence arrangement. Simultaneous changes in heart rate are represented by an audible signal. Any change in heart rhythm becomes immediately apparent by changing RR interval of the picket-fence or change in pitch of the sound.

A 12-hour time clock, mounted in the front of this unit, can depict the time that abnormalities appeared on either of the cathode-ray oscilloscopes, or in the audible signal. Thus, by setting the clock to the time that the monitoring process started, the patient's diary of events and experiences can be correlated temporally.

The electrocardiocorder tape can be played back on the scanner at precisely 60 times the recording speed so that the entire ten-hour tape record can be reviewed on the display screens in 10 minutes. If any abnormal event is noted during the rapid scanning, the observer pushes a bottom switch; then the electrocardiocharter, which is the other part of this unit prints out any desired segment of the ten-hour recording tape in real time on standard conventional electrocardiographic paper, or even in faster paper speed. These printed electrocardiograms can be used for final detailed analysis and reporting.

METHODS AND MATERIALS

The electrodes are applied to the patient's chest by the method described above and connected to the portable electrocardiocorder. The patient is then advised to keep a complete diary while carrying the electrocardiocorder on a shoulder or a waist strap. Because it is important to have a detailed record of all activities and symptoms incurred during the ensuing ten hours, a standard diary form is recommended as illustrated in Chart 1.

The patient is allowed to do any work which will not interfere with the course of testing, especially performing the daily activity in the circumstances which had previously provoked his symptomatology, with emphasis on the time of their occurrence. All facts, such as any change in position, character (including the volume) of foods ingested, special environment, physical and emotional events should be recorded in detail.

The tape is then fed into the composite electrocardioscanner-electrocardiographic analyzer and significant portions are chosen for read-out in conventional ECG paper. Each of the diary entries is carefully correlated with the electrocardiographic recordings.

Since 1960, we have studied over 2,000 patients in their natural environment. We have classified the symptoms into four categories:

1. The patient without heart disease whose presenting symptoms are due to cardiac arrhythmias.
   i. Chest pain or precordial distress
   ii. Dyspnea
   iii. Palpitation
   iv. Mesenteric vascular insufficiency
       a. Abdominal pain
       b. Flatulence or distention
       c. Paralytic ileus
       d. Nausea, vomiting and diarrhea
       e. Gastrointestinal bleeding
   v. Cerebral vascular insufficiency
       a. Vertigo
       b. Syncope
       c. Hemiparesis
       d. Paresthesias
       e. Visual disturbances

Chart 1.

NAME _____ AGE _____ SEX _____ DATE _____

TIME	ENVIRONMENT	ACTIVITY	SYMPTOMS

Office use only:

Name _____ Age _____ Sex _____ Date_____

Ref. _____ , M.D.

Clinical Diagnosis: _____

Statement of Conventional ECG _____

Patient Diagnosis _____

f. Psychoses

g. Seizures

2. The patient presenting symptoms which are related to cardiac disease.

3. Postprandial syndromes induced by arrhythmias or coronary insufficiency.

4. Evaluation of drugs such as antiarrhythmic agents and coronary dilators.

5. Arrhythmias due to myocarditis or myocardiopathies.

CLINICAL EXPERIENCES

Differential Diagnosis of Chest Pain[16]

It is often difficult to determine the origin of chest pain. The Holter monitor is of benefit in detecting the cause of evanescent chest pain which appears in the patient's home or office environment. Often patients who complain of chest discomfort will also have known coronary artery disease, hiatus hernia, aortic aneurysms, or anterior chest wall syndromes such as a tender rib cage.

Figure 1 illustrates recordings in a patient who was awakened almost each night with a severe precordial distress which was not relieved by nitroglycerin. This patient had a known hiatus hernia, coronary arteriosclerosis, aneurysm of the ascending aorta and also a costochondritis of the anterior chest wall. The resting electrocardiogram was within normal limits. The Master two-step test revealed marked S-T segment depression, diagnostic of coronary artery disease. However, the attending

physicians were of the opinion that the chest pain might be due to the aneurysm of the aorta. The Holter monitor was applied on three successive occasions. On two occasions, while the patient was awakened around 4:00 or 5:00 A.M., the monitor demonstrated marked S-T segment depression. This confirmed the cause of the nocturnal chest pain as due to coronary insufficiency. The patient died four months later and autopsy revealed severe arteriosclerosis of the anterior descending circumflex and right coronary artery.

Patients Unable to Perform the Exercise Test[17]

Because of orthopedic problems such as fusion of the knee or hip joint, the patient might not be able to perform exercise electrocardiographic testing to determine if the chest pain is ischemic in origin. Often the physician might fear exercise testing because the patient has severe coronary artery disease. The Holter monitor is of great value in eliciting myocardial ischemia in such situations.

Figure 2 illustrates tracings taken in a patient with a past history of coronary occlusion who had severe chest pain almost each day. His physician feared that exercise testing might precipitate an acute episode of coronary insufficiency. When we had the patient perform the usual physical maneuvers which precipitated the chest pain, as walking up stairs or lifting a child, the monitor revealed marked S-T segment depressions indicating that the pain was due to angina pectoris.

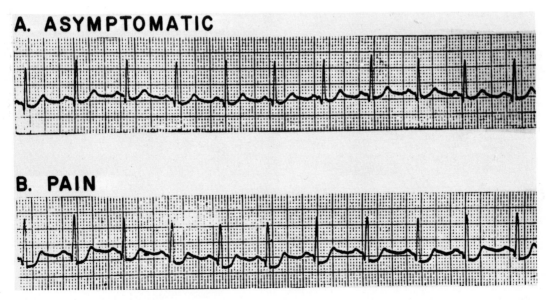

FIG. 1.   Monitored tracings. *A,* resting ECG, and *B,* tracing during pain, confirming the opinion that it was caused by coronary insufficiency.

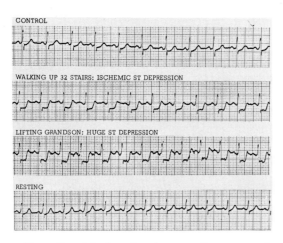

FIG. 2. Monitored electrocardiograms of patient with past history of coronary occlusion who had severe chest pain almost daily.

Angina in a Patient with a Negative Master Two-Step Test

Patients may have a normal exercise electrocardiographic stress test but because of their excellent muscular development and familiarity with the 2-step exercise maneuver, the test will not reveal significant changes. Performance of a particular maneuver while wearing a Holter monitor may reveal the cause of the chest pain as myocardial ischemia.

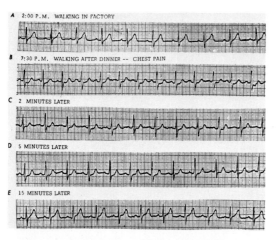

FIG. 3 Monitored electrocardiograms confirming diagnosis of ischemic heart disease.

Figure 3 illustrates the findings in a patient who complained of severe chest pain when walking after dinner. His Master two-step test was normal.

However, when he experienced chest pain while walking after dinner, S-T segment depressions occurred. This confirmed the diagnosis of ischemic heart disease and indicated that symptoms could only be elicited upon walking postprandially.

Postprandial Angina[18]

Patients with known coronary artery disease often complain of precordial distress after meals.

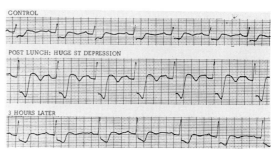

FIG. 4. Electrocardiograms of 64-year-old man with history of old myocardial infarction and recurrent angina pectoris. Postprandially he complained of severe chest pain on numerous occasions. Monitoring apparatus showed huge ST-T segment depressions during one of these episodes.

Figure 4 demonstrates the records in a patient with severe chest pain which occurred following meals. The marked S-T segment depression correlated with the clinical symptoms indicating the pain was due to ischemic heart disease.

Angina Pectoris Due to Cardiac Arrhythmias[19]

Very rapid supraventricular and ventricular tachycardias and frequent premature ventricular systoles may cause coronary insufficiency.

Figure 5 demonstrates findings in a patient with the Wolf-Parkinson-White syndrome who experienced severe angina. The Holter monitor clearly indicated that the cause of the angina was recurrent arrhythmia. Thus, angina was experienced during episodes of ventricular premature systoles and supraventricular tachycardia and was not relieved by nitroglycerin. When the patient was treated with quinidine, however, there was no recurrence of the angina for a follow-up period of three years.

Figure 6 shows the Holter monitor electrocardiogram of a patient with recurrent chest pain without apparent precipitating cause and without relief from nitroglycerin. He was not aware of any irregularity or rapid action of the heart. Holter monitor recordings demonstrated that a paroxysm of

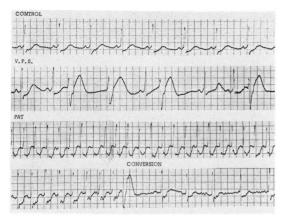

FIG. 5. Electrocardiograms of patient with Wolf-Parkinson-White syndrome who experienced severe angina. Holter monitor clearly indicated cause of angina was recurrent arrhythmia.

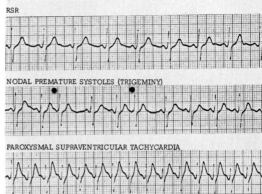

FIG. 6. Patient was a 68-year-old male who complained of recurrent chest pains without apparant precipitating cause. He was not aware of any irregularity of heart beat. Long-term monitoring demonstrated a paroxysmal supraventricular tachycardia associated with his symptoms.

supraventricular tachycardia was associated with his symptoms. Treatment with quinidine prevented further episodes. However, in the fourth month when the patient stopped his quinidine, the precordial distress recurred. When the quinidine therapy was reinstituted, he had no further episodes of angina, again proving that the angina was caused by the arrhythmia.

Detection of a Cause of Palpitation

Patients might not be aware that they are having a cardiac arrhythmia and also, they might complain of palpitation when they really are not experiencing an arrhythmia.

Figure 7 reveals findings in a patient who complained of palpitation but the Holter monitor only revealed sinus rhythm with S-T segment depression. When the monitoring was continued, she developed frequent premature ventricular systoles and runs of ventricular tachycardia. At that time, she was not aware of any cardiac arrhythmia. Subsequent examination revealed that the patient had a pheochromocytoma which was removed surgically. This illustrates that the Holter monitor is of value in demon-

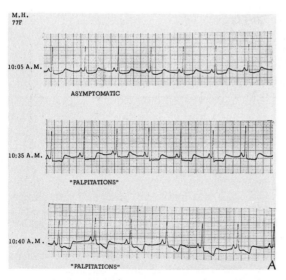

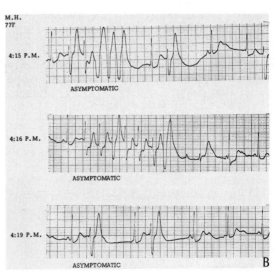

FIG. 7. (*Left*) Patient who complained of palpitation but in whom Holter monitor revealed only sinus rhythm with S-T segment depression. (*Right*) Continued monitoring demonstrated frequent premature ventricular systoles and runs of ventricular tachycardia.

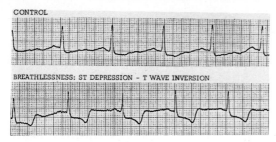

CONTROL

BREATHLESSNESS: ST DEPRESSION - T WAVE INVERSION

FIG. 8. An 88-year-old woman hospitalized for congestive heart failure was doing well clinically when she complained of bouts of dyspnea without evidence of failure. Holter monitor revealed marked depression and T wave inversions. An example of coronary insufficiency presenting itself with air hunger.

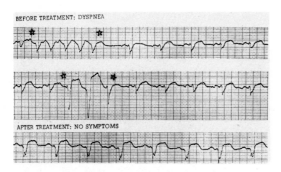

BEFORE TREATMENT: DYSPNEA

AFTER TREATMENT: NO SYMPTOMS

FIG. 9. Patient showing no evidence of congestive heart failure yet complaining of repeated episodes of dyspnea. Holter monitor recordings showed dyspnea to be due to paroxysms of ventricular tachycardia, and multifocal ventricular premature systoles. Treatment with procaine amide over four-year period prevented recurrence, suggesting episodes were due to cardiac arrhythmias.

strating the cause of the patient's palpitation and of detecting cardiac arrhythmias of which the patient is not aware.

Cause of Dyspnea

Ischemia of Myocardium. Patients might complain of dyspnea which is precipitated by ischemia of the myocardium. In the patient whose tracings appear in Figure 8, clinical examination did not reveal any signs of congestive heart failure. However, evanescent electrocardiographic changes of ischemia were detected by the Holter monitor, suggesting that the air hunger was due to coronary insufficiency.

Phantom Cardiac Arrhythmias. On numerous occasions we have found that the dyspnea might be due to cardiac arrhythmias and yet the patient was completely unaware of their presence.

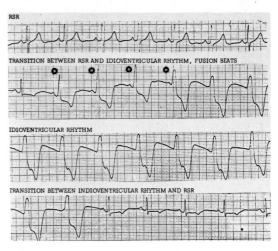

RSR

TRANSITION BETWEEN RSR AND IDIOVENTRICULAR RHYTHM, FUSION BEATS

IDIOVENTRICULAR RHYTHM

TRANSITION BETWEEN INDIOVENTRICULAR RHYTHM AND RSR

FIG. 10. A 58-year-old man who complained of air hunger with exertion and emotional stress. During such an episode, the monitor demonstrated an unsuspected arrythmia followed by classical ischemic ST-T changes.

Figure 9 illustrates the records of a patient who was observed in the hospital. Chest x-ray and clinical findings did not reveal any evidence of congestive heart failure, yet the patient complained of repeated episodes of dyspnea. Holter monitor recordings revealed that the dyspnea was due to paroxysms of ventricular tachycardiaand multifocal ventricular premature systoles. Treatment over a four-year period with procaine amide prevented any recurrence of the dyspnea, suggesting that the episodes were due to cardiac arrhythmias.

The tracings in Figure 10 are those of a patient with repeated episodes of air hunger. Holter electrocardiographic recordings revealed that they were due to a ventricular arrhythmia of which the patient was completely unaware.

SUMMARY

The Holter monitor is of benefit for detecting the actual cause of precordial pain, dyspnea, postprandial syndromes, epigastric pain, palpitation, phantom arrhythmias and ischemic heart disease, etc. The apparatus has great versatility in that it can monitor the electrocardiogram in the patient's native environment where the particular symptoms occur. A closely kept diary will permit correlation of symptoms with cardiac arrhythmias or coronary insufficiency. The technic is also of value for demonstrating the effect of drugs in the treatment of cardiac arrhythmias.

REFERENCES

1. Corday, E., and Irving, D. W.: Disturbances of Heart Rate, Rhythm and Conduction, Philadelphia, W. B. Saunders Company, 1961.
2. Corday, E., Rothenberg, S. F., and Putnam, T. J.: Cerebral vascular insufficiency: An explanation of some types of localized cerebral encephalopathy, Arch. Neurol. & Psychiat. *69*:551, 1953.
3. Corday, E., Rothenberg, S. F., and Weiner, S. M.: Cerebral vascular insufficiency: An explanation of the transient stroke, A.M.A. Arch. Int. Med., *98*:683, 1956.
4. Corday, E., and Rothenberg, S. F.: Primary cerebral angiospasm, *in* Myers, J. S. (ed.): Monograph of Cerebral Hypoxia, Springfield, Illinois, Charles C Thomas, 1961.
5. Galbraith, B. T.: Lower nephron nephrosis associated with prolonged shock from ventricular tachycardia, Am. Heart J. *42*:766, 1951.
6. Irving, D. W., and Corday, E.: Effect of the cardiac arrhythmias on the renal and mesenteric circulations, Am. J. Cardiol. *8*:32, 1961.
7. Corday, E., Irving, D. W., Gold, H., Bernstein, H., and Skelton, R. B. T.: Mesenteric vascular insufficiency: Intestinal ischemia induced by remote circulatory disturbances, Am. J. Med. *33*:365, 1962.
8. Sedlacek, R. A., and Bean, W. B.: Abdominal "angina": The syndrome of intermittent ischemia of mesenteric arteries, Ann. Int. Med. *46*:148, 1957.
9. Kilpatrick, Z. M., Farman, J., Yesner, R., and Spiro, H. M.: Ischemic proctitis, J.A.M.A. *205*:74, 1968.
10. Corday, E., Bazika, V., Lang, T. W., Pappelbaum, S., Gold, H., and Bernstein, H.: Detection of phantom arrhythmias and evanescent electrocardiographic abnormalities. (Use of prolonged direct electrocardiocording), J.A.M.A. *193*:417, 1965.
11. Corday, E., and Lang, T. W.: Cardiac arrhythmias and conduction defects, *in* Hurst, J. W., and Logue, R. B. (eds.), The Heart, New York, McGraw-Hill Book Company, 1966, pp. 286–290.
12. Shumak, K. H., and Brown, K. W. G.: Continuous portable electrocardiography, Canad. M. A. J. *98*: 139, 1968.
13. Holter, N. J.: New methods for heart studies, Science, *134*:1214, 1961.
14. Gilson, J. S., Holter, N. J., and Glasscock, W. R.: Continuous electrocardiograms, electrodes and lead systems, Am. J. Cardiol. *8*:212, 1961.
15. Gilson, J. S., Holter, N. J., and Glasscock, W. R.: Clinical observations using electrocardiocorder. AVSEP continuous electrocardiographic system, Am. J. Cardiol. *14*:204, 1964.
16. Utsu, F., Lang, T. W., Enescu, V., and Boszormenyi, E.: The detection of evanescent changes of myocardial ischemia, The New Physician *14*:341, 1965.
17. Perlman, L., Kohn, K. H., Neumann, M., and Ho, E.: Cardiac evaluation in consideration of prostheses for geriatric amputees, J. A. M. A. *199*:532, 1967.
18. Boszormenyi, E., Kivowitz, C., Vyden, J. K., and Bernstein, H.: Detection of postprandial coronary insufficiency by the Holter monitor system, The New Physician *15*:48, 1966.
19. Boszormenyi, E., Utsu, F., Lang, T. W., Enescu, V., and Bernstein, H.: Coronary insufficiency due to paroxysmal supraventricular tachycardia, The New Physician, *14*:299, 1965.
20. Corday, E., Bernstein, H., Lang, T. W., and Boszormenyi, E.: Dyspnea, an unusual manifestation of cardiac arrhythmias (in press).

Atypical Angina Pectoris

John Francis Briggs

Heberden described angina pectoris as a disorder of the breast associated with a sense of anxiety, distress and the fear of impending death.

There are many causes of angina pectoris but this discussion will be limited to those who have coronary atherosclerosis. For the purpose of this discussion it will be defined as any type of distress that occurs on physical exertion or emotional excitement which is relieved by rest or nitroglycerin. It occurs because there is a disproportion between the oxygen needed and the oxygen available to the heart muscle. It is a clinical syndrome.

ABDOMINAL ANGINA

Abdominal angina is not unusual. In certain individuals the pain of coronary insufficiency is referred entirely to the upper abdomen. The pain may simulate gallbladder disease or peptic ulceration. In the individuals with abdominal angina the condition may not be recognized unless attention is directed to the patient's complaint; namely, that the pain occurs in the abdomen on exercise or under emotional excitement and is relieved by rest or nitroglycerin. Should an associated gastrointestinal disease exist it must be treated as though angina pectoris did not exist.

ALCOHOLIC ANGINA

Alcohol is often recommended in the treatment of angina pectoris. Alcohol has no significant effect on the physiology of the coronary circulation and the relief obtained is due to the sedative action of the alcohol. Alcoholic angina is not uncommon. When the individual takes an excessive amount of alcohol, he performs excessive activities or becomes involved in emotional events that would under ordinary circumstances not precipitate an attack of pain. While under the effect of alcohol he may not recognize the seizure. The individual's enthusiasm for his treatment may become so great the treatment must be changed from that of angina pectoris to the treatment of alcoholism.

ANGINA SINE DOLORE

This term is a paradox because it means angina without distress. There are individuals who have attacks of angina in which pain is absent. As a result of physical exertion or emotional excitement the patient will be distressed but have no specific pain. This discomfort is relieved by taking nitroglycerin or by resting.

ANEMIA ANGINA

This angina occurs when the person develops anemia. It is relieved when the blood returns to normal.

ANOREXIC ANGINA

Certain individuals suffer great anginal pain either while eating or shortly after eating. Some develop a conditioned reflex in which the mere sight of food will produce an attack of angina pectoris. Frequent, small feedings may relieve this type of angina pectoris.

ANNIVERSARY ANGINA

Some patients find they experience few attacks of angina pectoris unless they are involved in an anniversary celebration. In these instances, the emotional excitement and physical effort incidental to developing the anniversary or participating in it will often cause very severe and repeated anginal attacks. See Figure 1.

BLADDER ANGINA

It is possible that the somatic expression of coronary insufficiency may involve reflex pathways

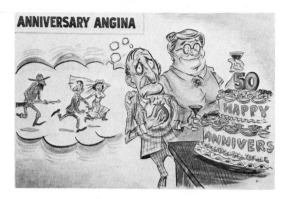

FIG. 1.

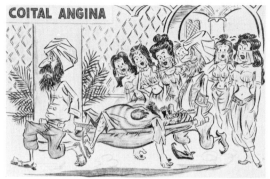

FIG. 2.

associated with urination. In bladder angina the patient may have chest pain but the predominant feature is the desire to void. This urgency may be extreme and may dominate the entire clinical picture. In such instances, patients may recognize that urgency to void comes with exertion and emotional excitement.

BOWEL ANGINA

In bowel angina the mechanism is similar to that of bladder angina. Here the somatic expression is through the bowel and the patient has an urgent desire to defecate. This may be associated with abdominal distension.

BURPING ANGINA

In burping angina the patient experiences very little pain in the chest, but rather has a feeling as though gas is present either in the abdomen or under the sternum. Relief is obtained by belching or by taking anti-acids as well as nitroglycerin. Burping angina is not uncommon.

COITAL ANGINA

Certain individuals suffer anginal pain either preliminary to coitus, during the act, or following it. This is a serious complication in that it often produces reactive depression, psychic impotence, and marital discord. It is suggested that the prophylactic use of nitroglycerin assists in decreasing the number of seizures. Frank discussion with the partners concerning the problem and educating them to adjust to it often relieves the situation. See Figure 2.

COLD ANGINA

Some individuals experience pain only when they either eat or drink something cold or hold something cold in their hands. In such patients holding an ice cube may produce electrocardiographic changes.

CONDITIONED ANGINA

Many individuals can carry on a full program of activities without having an anginal seizure. If, however, they eat before performing these activities, they develop angina pectoris. In conditioned angina, the anginal pain is conditioned by some other event in the patient's activity. In one individual smoking a cigarette before carrying on his routine would result in angina, but if he omitted smoking, he could perform these activities without pain.

CONSULTING ROOM ANGINA

In consulting room angina the patient is free of his anginal attacks until he is in the doctor's consulting room to be examined. I believe these attacks result from apprehension concerning the physician's verdict.

ELECTROCARDIOGRAPHIC ANGINA

In electrocardiographic angina the patient will sustain an anginal seizure when his electrocardiogram is being taken. This, like consulting room angina, I believe, represents the patient's apprehension.

GLANDULAR ANGINA

Chest pain may be completely absent in glandular angina. The somatic expression is through the glandular system. The somatic result is cold sweats or marked salivation. Glandular angina is not common.

HAPPINESS ANGINA

Most recognize the depressing effects of certain emotional patterns and associate angina with such events as anger. Happiness can also produce anginal seizures.

HABITUATING FACTORS IN ANGINA

There are individuals who have a basic compulsive and obsessive type of personality. Such patients take an excessive amount of nitroglycerin, constantly popping the tablets into their mouths, or are oxygen dependent. They will not go anywhere without carrying a tank of oxygen.

IATROGENIC ANGINA

Iatrogenic angina is the angina produced by the physician. This occurs when improper evaluation of the history or overemphasis on certain minor electrocardiographic changes has influenced the physician to misinterpret the nature of the chest pain. The treatment is very difficult.

INTRACTABLE ANGINA

I do not believe that such a condition exists. I believe that in these cases it is an intractable patient who has angina.

NOCTURNAL ANGINA

Nocturnal angina is rare. It occurs in certain individuals who experience angina pectoris when they go to bed at night. They are able to sleep or nap through the day without having the attack. I have no explanation for this.

PRURITIC ANGINA

In pruritic angina the somatic expression of pain is in the form of itching. This may occur in the usual sites of referred pain.

RAYNAUD'S ANGINA

In Raynaud's angina the chest pain may be associated with secondary Raynaud's phenomena involving either the left hand or both the right and left hands.

RECUMBENT ANGINA

In recumbent angina the patient sustains the attack when he lies down but never has an attack when he sits up in a chair or is propped up in bed. There are a number of explanations for this type of angina, none of which is satisfactory.

REFERRED ANGINA

The chest pain may be absent or minimal in nature. In many of these individuals, however, maximum pain is at the point of reference, so the patient has severe pain in the angle of the jaw, or severe pain in the upper abdomen, or severe pain in the left wrist, etc.

REMUNERATIVE ANGINA

Remunerative angina exists when the patient receives so much psychologic and/or financial reward from his angina pectoris he cannot be rehabilitated. There is no successful treatment.

SHOULDER-HAND SYNDROME

In certain individuals the anginal pain is referred to the left shoulder. These attacks may be so severe that either through disuse of the left shoulder and arm or because of internuncial reflexes the shoulder girdle becomes fixed. This may lead to atrophy of the left hand and even to Dupuytren's contracture.

TELEVISION ANGINA

When radio first appeared some patients experienced attacks while listening to prize fights, ball games, and the like. The advent of television now combines visual as well as auditory excitement and many patients sustain severe seizures when watching television See Figure 3..

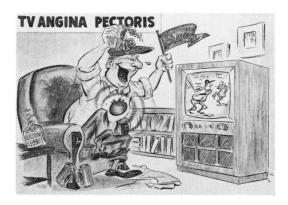

FIG. 3.

WEEKEND ANGINA

The victim of coronary sclerosis may have very few attacks during the week. On the long weekend he increases his alcoholic intake, eats excessively, and during this period of alcoholic intake is not aware of the anginal attacks and often exceeds his physical limits. On Monday he notices he has anginal attacks during the morning, but these gradually subside during the day and by Tuesday, he returns to his usual pain pattern. This weekend type of angina may be associated with a gain of five or six pounds in weight over the weekend. This is the result of increased fluid, food and sodium intake. The treatment is obvious, Mercurial diuretics on Monday often hasten the recovery. See Figure 4.

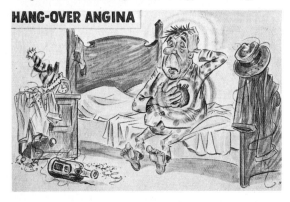

FIG. 4.

CONCLUSION

A description of the atypical in angina pectoris has been given.

Regardless of where the pain is or where it goes, in atypical angina, the diagnosis is made by the patient when he says the pain comes with physical or emotional excitement and is relieved by rest or by nitroglycerin.

Angina pectoris is a disease diagnosed by history. The diagnosis is made by paying more attention to what you hear from the patient than what you hear through your stethoscope and what you see in the patient than what you see in his electrocardiogram.

Value and Limitations of the Electrocardiogram in the Diagnosis of Coronary Syndromes

David Scherf

CORONARY SCLEROSIS

It seems that beyond the age of 49 the average man exhibits at the time of death a rather severe degree of arteriosclerosis in both coronary arteries.[1] In much younger men, killed in action in the Korean War, coronary artery sclerosis was found in 77.3 per cent.[2] This abnormality cannot be diagnosed, even with coronary angiography, as long as no narrowing of the coronary arteries is present. The electrocardiogram of these patients is often normal. The diagnosis can be suspected only in the rare case in which calcified plaques are seen in the area of the coronary sulcus in the radiogram. For the diagnosis of coronary artery stenosis one has to rely mainly on the history of angina on effort. When anginal pain is absent the appearance of signs of myocardial involvement, such as dilatation of the heart or congestive heart failure, may be due to coronary artery disease. This speculative diagnosis is often correct, particularly in the middle aged or elderly patient in the absence of myocarditis; occasionally, however, another lesion is the cause of the myocardial disease. Aortitis with narrowing of the coronary ostia, while much less common than in the past, should always be considered.

MYOCARDIAL INFARCTION

Obviously it is not necessary today to stress the value of the electrocardiogram for the diagnosis of myocardial infarction. Myocardial infarction has been diagnosed clinically before the characteristic electrocardiographic patterns became known. However, the recognition of the changes of the QRS complex and of the RS-T segments helped immensely in the diagnosis of doubtful and atypical cases and was, in turn, of great value in the development of new clinical signs useful in the diagnosis of infarction. At the present time the diagnosis is rarely missed in typical cases with large infarctions, caused by the occlusion of one of the main coronary arteries; however, smaller infarctions, which we prefer to call, in analogy with the little strokes of Alvarez, "little infarctions," are usually not diagnosed. In such patients severe chest pain may repeatedly occur, without or with only slight fall in blood pressure, without or with slight changes of the blood enzymes, and without fever and leukocytosis. Such attacks are caused by occlusion of one of the small coronary arteries. This may be caused by fibrosis without thrombosis. The clinical diagnosis often is "coronary insufficiency" because pathologists and clinicians alike consider only occlusions of the main coronary arteries and not the pathology of the smaller intramural ones.[3] Fibrous narrowing or occlusions were described in the tertiary branches of the coronary artery tree in patients between 50 and 60; fatty infiltrations and arteriosclerotic plaques were seen in 30- to 40-year-old patients.[4] Donomae *et al.*[5] found fibrotic occlusions of the intramural coronary arteries often in men over 40. Vessels with a diameter of 40–80 micra are obliterated.[6-8] These changes are particularly common in patients with hypertension. The occlusion of such small vessels induces patchy myocardial necrosis and finally fibrosis. It is our firm conviction, based on clinical observations, that these little infarctions may cause severe anginal pain not responding to nitroglycerin and lasting for several hours.[3,9] Such attacks cause no change in the electrocardiogram or only a transient lowering or inversion of the T waves.

Not rarely one sees a patient with the complaint of a typical chest pain lasting half an hour or more, but thorough examination, including repeated electrocardiograms, does not reveal any abnormality. Some of these patients developed months or years later an easily diagnosable myocardial infarction. We believe that the first episode of chest pain experienced by these patients was due to an occlusion of a small coronary artery leading to no, or very limited, necrosis of the myocardium which is not diagnosed with currently available laboratory methods. We learned to take more seriously such pains with negative findings.

In recent times patients were described who had a typical angina pectoris but a normal coronary arteriogram. It is possible that here also we are dealing with patients in whom a small coronary artery is involved. It is not yet established whether narrowing of intramural coronary arteries cannot initiate anginal pain. We do not know how large an ischemic area of the myocardium must be in order to induce pain.

Coronary insufficiency is a useful term to designate the discrepancy between blood supply and blood requirement. It occurs in a great variety of conditions even with normal coronary arteries (carbon monoxide intoxication, acute blood loss, excessive tachycardias). Coronary insufficiency is therefore not a diagnosis but a description of a certain state which may or may not be accompanied by anginal pain.[9] It causes occasionally an inversion of the T waves without depression of the RS-T segments.

In the classical myocardial infarction caused by the occlusion of a main coronary artery, the electrocardiogram may remain normal in about 2 per cent of cases. Well known is the difficulty encountered in the diagnosis of a true posterior or lateral wall infarction. Typical changes in the electrocardiogram may appear several days after the onset of chest pain. Intramural infarctions do not usually alter the electrocardiogram. It must be stressed that in some cases of myocardial infarction although the electrocardiogram is not normal the characteristic changes fail to appear. The tracing shows nonspecific abnormalities of the RS-T segments and the T waves. Determination of the age of an infarction from one electrocardiogram alone is impossible once the acute displacement (high take-off) of the RS-T segments disappears, Only when several electrocardiograms, obtained within a few days, show progressive changes can the process be diagnosed as an acute or an evolving one.

The same electrocardiograms as in an acute thrombosis of a main coronary artery may occur in coronary embolisms, tumor metastases, occlusions of a coronary artery by a tumor (bronchogenic carcinoma), or rarely in myocarditis with massive circumscribed foci of inflammation.

Multiple infarctions may cancel out the electrocardiographic changes and make the diagnosis difficult or impossible. As in rheumatic pericarditis, shortly after the development of the infarction for a day or two, in rare cases, characteristic T wave changes may disappear and even a normal electrocardiogram may be found. A complicating focal pericarditis is perhaps responsible.

It is well known that in the presence of bundle branch block the diagnosis of a myocardial infarction may be very difficult. In right bundle branch block the activation of the left ventricle occurs first, as in the normal heart, and infarctions will change the QRS complexes in a recognizable way, making the diagnosis possible. In most cases of left bundle branch block, on the other hand, only in the acute stage with displacement of the RS-T segments can the diagnosis be made with certainty. In myocardial infarction a pattern similar to left ventricular hypertrophy may occur (subendocardial infarctions). Left as well as right ventricular hypertrophy may cause changes in the electrocardiogram imitating those of acute infarction.[10] In subendocardial infarctions the characteristic depression of the RS-T segments may imitate the changes seen in digitalis therapy, where the subendocardial layers of the myocardium are also mainly altered. Even the shortening of the Q-T interval may be identical in both conditions. Patients with acute pancreatitis, intracranial hemorrhage or acute cor pulmonale may exhibit electrocardiograms as seen in acute myocardial infarction.

Within a few months or years the changes of a myocardial infarction may disappear completely, owing to contraction of the scar. This happens most frequently in an anterior wall infarction.[12] Even in inferior infarctions the Q waves may disappear, or become borderline, or may be present only in lead III and not in lead aVF.[13–15] The diagnostic Q waves disappeared or became borderline after 3.5 years in 30 per cent of cases.

In one study comprising 134 instances of an old infarction examined at autopsy, the diagnosis from the electrocardiogram was equivocal in 34 per cent and in 31 per cent no diagnostic evidence of an infarction was seen in the electrocardiogram. However, only 2 per cent had a normal electrocardiogram.[17] In another study, after 4 years a normal electrocardiogram was found in 20 per cent of the cases.[18]

To conclude from changes in more than one chest lead that an extensive infarction is present is not justified. Configuration of the chest and position of the heart have to be considered.

The opinion that a lesion of the subendocardial layers alone does not cause Q waves was not confirmed[19]

In some patients the configuration of extrasystoles can help in the diagnosis. In a patient with bundle branch block, Dressler described characteristic changes of the RS-T segments of ventricular extrasystoles which permitted the diagnosis.[20] Very common is the presence of deep Q waves in the chest leads in ventricular extrasystoles in patients with myocardial infarction. These Q waves are seen normally in leads over the right atrium and may be seen in healthy individuals in leads VI and V2. In the other chest leads a QS wave appears in a normal person only when the extrasystole originates just beneath the electrode, for obvious reasons. It has been stated that only QR waves or QRs and Qrs waves seen in extrasystoles in chest leads V2-V6 are typical for infarction and not QS waves.

The extrasystoles in Figure 1, showing a Q wave in VI and a rSR wave in lead V2, are not indicative

of an old myocardial infarction. They were found in a healthy 50-year-old man.

In large clinical material[22,23] as well as in single observations[24] the value of the form of the ventricular extrasystoles for the diagnosis of myocardial infarction has been demonstrated, but sometimes the diagnosis based on this sign is not correct.[25]

LONG Q-T(U) INTERVAL

In patients with bradycardia usually induced by an incomplete or a complete A-V block, a very pronounced prolongation of the Q-T(U) interval may be found. Figure 2 shows such a tracing, with a Q-T(U) interval of 0.76 second, obtained from a 62-year-old woman with coronary sclerosis. On the following day, with disappearance of the 2:1 block, the Q-T interval was normal (Fig. 3). The changes of Figure 2 may persist for days or weeks. They were attributed by Holzmann to changes of the cardiac metabolism (Stoffwechselsyndrom).[26] The similarity to the electrocardiogram seen in hypokalemia, where giant U waves also appear, is great.[27]

ELECTROCARDIOGRAPHIC EXERCISE TEST

In 1932 we began to investigate the electrocardiogram after exercise in patients with angina pectoris and on the basis of these studies the electrocardiographic exercise test for the diagnosis of coronary stenosis was introduced.[28–30] We recommended in our first publications and recommend today adaptation of the amount of work required to be performed by the patient to the history and his clinical condition. In patients with syphilitic stenosis of the coronary orifices we found marked alterations of the T waves after the patient had been sitting up in bed a few times. In some patients with angina pectoris due to coronary sclerosis alterations appeared in the electrocardiogram only after they climbed quickly several flights of stairs.

The two-step test as recommended by Missal[31] and later intensively propagated by Master[32] is often referred to as a "standardized" exercise test. Tables developed for another test were adapted and used to indicate the amount of work the patient should perform. These tables arranged the workload according to sex, age and weight. The arrangement according to weight has no solid basis.[33] Furthermore, a woman of 50 may have the same degree of coronary stenosis as a man of the same age, and there is no justification whatsoever to demand from her less exercise than from a man. Therefore the arrangement of the amount of work according to sex

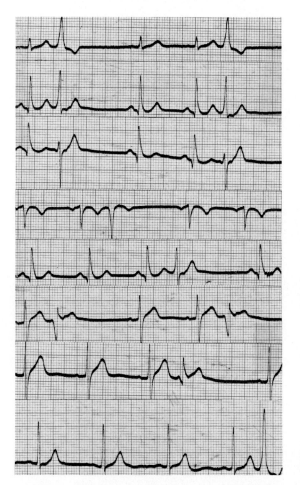

Fig. 1. The electrocardiogram was obtained from a 50-year-old healthy man. Leads I, II, III, aVR, V1, V2 and V6 are reproduced. In each lead ventricular extrasystoles are seen which are conducted reversedly to the atria. The extrasystoles reveal a broad and deep Q wave in lead VI.

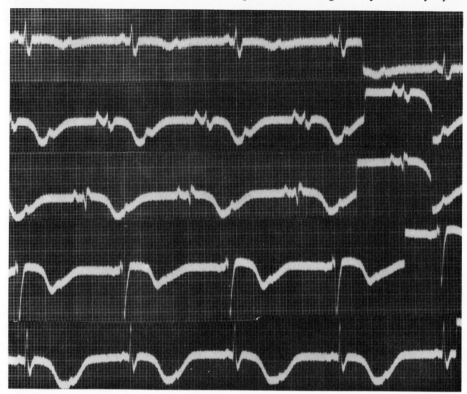

FIG. 2.   This electrocardiogram, taken from a 62-year-old woman on October 11, 1948 shows a 2:1 A-V block, with giant inverted T-U waves in each lead. The Q-T(U) interval is 0.76 second. The patient had clinical evidence of coronary sclerosis. The leads are lead I, II, III, V2 and V5.

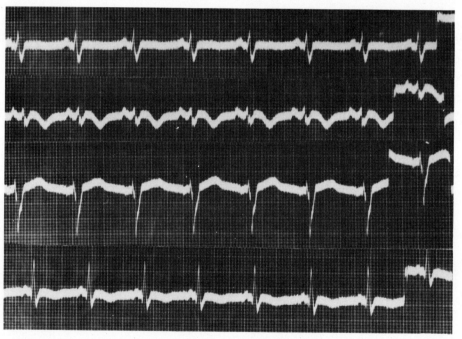

FIG. 3.   Leads I, II, III, V2 and V6 from the same patient, obtained on the following day (October 12, 1948). The 2:1 block and the prolongation of the Q-T(U) interval had disappeared.

does not make sense. With regard to age, what physician does not know a 50-year-old man with more advanced stenosis than one who is 70 years old?

The test does not consider the physical fitness of the patient, his mental attitude to the test and often not even the speed with which the exercise is performed. All these factors influence the outcome of the test.

The results of the standard test were so unsatisfactory that a "double standard" test has been recommended, a very curious phenomenon in standardization. The statement that the standard test only permits comparison of the results obtained on different occasions is of course not justified, because whatever the work load is, whether it consists in sitting up exercise, walking in a treadmill, knee bends, bicycle riding, ergometer or dumbbell exercises, if the same patient repeats the same exercise under similar conditions the results are comparable. To demand the same workload from all patients with the same age, sex and weight for comparison is unphysiologic and unreasonable.

Differences of opinion exist with regard to the criteria for an abnormal test. They were often so loose that a "positive" test, speaking for coronary stenosis, has been found in the healthy or in psychoneurotic individuals. The spilling of catecholamines in a tense individual may lead to a tachycardia with a depression of the RS-T segments of 0.5 mm. or more. In order to avoid false positive tests with all the dire consequences for the patient, we proposed much stricter criteria, namely a depression of the RS-T segments of 1.5 mm. in the standard leads and 2 mm. in the chest leads. This will give us some false negative tests but this is unavoidable since, even with "negative exercise tests," that is when only the physiological changes appear after exercise in the electrocardiogram, coronary stenosis cannot be ruled out. The statement that a negative exercise test proves the absence of coronary sclerosis is not justified.

The opinion that the appearance of abnormal changes of the RS-T segments in several leads speaks for a more extensive process is not correct. As in myocardial infarction, several factors are responsible for the presence of changes in more than one chest lead. A patient with a negative test may develop a myocardial infarction caused by coronary thrombosis within a few days. A patient with a decidedly positive test may live for many years; therefore conclusions as to prognosis must be guarded in the individual case.

Abnormal tests appear in patients with myocarditis and in some patients with mitral stenosis and are seen in healthy persons after an unusually severe exercise. The depression of the RS-T segments has been said to be more marked when a depletion of K is present.[34] Therefore, and because of the depression of the RS-T segments induced by digitalis, in patients who received this drug different criteria must be used. The degree of changes in the electrocardiogram does not run parallel to the degree of pain induced by the exercise. The test is not an exercise "tolerance" test, as often stated.

REFERENCES

1. White, N. K., Edwards, J. E., and Dry, T. J.: The relationship of the degree of coronary sclerosis with age in man, Circulation *1*:645, 1950.
2. Enos, W. F., Holmes, R. H., and Beyer, J.: Coronary disease among United States soldiers killed in action in Korea, J. A. M. A., *152*:1090, 1953.
3. Scherf, D., and Boyd, L. J.: Cardiovascular Diseases, ed. 3, New York and London, Grune and Stratton, 1958, p. 460.
4. Wolkoff, K.: Ueber die Atherosklerose der Koronararterien des Herzens, Beitr. path. Anat. *82*:555, 1929.
5. Donomae, I., Matsumoto, Y., Kokubo, T., Koide, R., Kobayashi, R., Ikegami, R., Ueda, E., Fujisawa, T., and Fujimoto, S.: Pathological studies of coronary arteriosclerosis, especially of intramural arteries, Jap. Heart J. *3*:423, 1962.
6. James, T. N.: The coronary circulation and the conduction system in acute myocardial infarction, Progr. Cardiovas. Dis. *10*:410, 1968.
7. More, B. M., and Sommers, S. C.: Status of the myocardial arterioles in angina pectoris, Am. Heart J. *64*:323, 1962.
8. Okada, R., Harumi, K., Nomura, M., and Murao, S.: A case of coronary sclerosis in small arteries associated with diffuse myocardial fibrosis, Jap. Heart J. *1*:348, 1960.
9. Scherf, D., and Golbey, M.: An evaluation of the term "coronary insufficiency," Am. Heart J. *47*:928, 1954.
10. Meyers, G. B.: QRS-T patterns in multiple precordial leads that may be mistaken for myocardial infarction, Circulation *1*:844 and 860, 1950.
11. Pruitt, R. D., Dennis, E. W., and Kinard, S. A.: The difficult electrocardiographic diagnosis of myocardial infarction, Progr. Cardiovas. Dis. *6*:85, 1963.
12. East, T., and Oram, S.: Cardiac pain with recovery of the T wave, Brit. Heart J. *10*:263, 1948.
13. Malmcrona, R., Soederholm, B., Bjoerntorp, P., Thulesius, O., and Heyman, F.: Myocardial infarction in the younger age groups, Acta med. scandinav. *171*:59, 1962.
14. Pappas, M. P.: Disappearance of pathological Q waves after myocardial infarction, Brit. Heart J. *20*:123, 1958.
15. Woods, J. D., Laurie, W., and Smith, W. G.: The reliability of the electrocardiogram in myocardial infarction, Lancet *2*:265, 1963.
16. Kaplan, B. M., and Berkson, D. M.: Serial electrocardiograms after myocardial infarction, Ann. Int. Med. *60*:430, 1964.

17. Skjaeggestadt, O., and Molne, K.: Electrocardiogram in patients with healed myocardial infarction disclosed at autopsy, Acta med. scandinav. *179*:23, 1960.

18. Burns Cox, C. J.: Return to normal of the electrocardiogram after myocardial infarction, Lancet *1*:1194, 1967.

19. Durrer, D., Van Lier, A. A. W., and Bueller, J.: Epicardial and intramural excitation in chronic myocardial infarction, Am. Heart J. *68*:765, 1964.

20. Dressler, W.: A case of myocardial infarction masked by bundle branch block but revealed by occasional premature ventricular beats, Am. J. M. Sc. *206*:361, 1943.

21. Bisteni, A., Medrano, G. A., and Sodi-Pallares, D.: Ventricular premature beats in the diagnosis of myocardial infarction, Brit. Heart J. *23*:521, 1961.

22. Anttonen, V. M., Leskinen, E., Meurman, L., Oka, M., and Raunio, H.: The diagnosis value of unipolar precordial patterns of ventricular premature beats in myocardial infarction, Acta med. scandinav. Suppl. 387, 1962.

23. Soloff, L. A.: Ventricular premature beats diagnostic of myocardial infarction, Am. J. M. S., *242*:315, 1961.

24. Cohen, J.: Acute myocardial infarction, early and objectively diagnosed through ventricular extrasystoles, Am. J. Cardiol. *7*:882, 1961.

25. Benchimol. A., Lasry, J. E., and Carvallo, F. R.: The ventricular premature contraction: Its place in the diagnosis of ischemic heart disease, Am. Heart J. *65*:334, 1963.

26. Holzmann, M.: Klinische Elektrokardiographie, Ed. S. Stuttgart, Thieme, 1965.

27. Scherf, D., Cohen, J., and Shafiiha, H.: Ectopic ventricular tachycardia, hypokalemia and convulsions in alcoholics, Cardiologia *50*:129, 1967.

28. Scherf, D.: Fifteen years of electrocardiographic exercise test in coronary stenosis, New York J. Med. *47*:2420, 1947.

29. Scherf, D.: Development of electrocardiographic exercise test, Am. J. Cardiol. *5*:433, 1960.

30. Scherf, D., and Schaffer, A. I.: The electrocardiographic exercise test, Am. Heart J. *43*:927, 1952.

31. Missal, M. E.: Exercise tests and the electrocardiograph in the study of angina pectoris, Ann. Int. Med. *11*:2018, 1938.

32. Master, A. M., Friedman, T., and Dack, S.: The electrocardiogram after standard exercise as a functional test of the heart, Am. Heart J. *24*:777, 1942.

33. Simonson, E., and Keys, A.: The electrocardiographic exercise test, Am. Heart J. *52*:83, 1956.

34. Gubner, R.: An appraisal of the exercise electrocardiogram test, J. Occup. Med., *2*:57, 1960 and *3*:110, 1961.

Apex Cardiography in Ischemic Heart Disease

E. Grey Dimond

In this paper I will confine my discussion of ischemic heart disease to that transitory experience, angina pectoris. An acute myocardial infarction also is certainly an event of ischemic heart disease and some of the alterations that occur in precordial movement are identical in the evanescent event, angina, and in the fixed event, infarction.

However, the intermittent nature of angina, its dependable, provokable pattern, with a surprising degree of "safety" to the patient, its near-assured relief by rest or nitroglycerin, make it a reliable, faithful, clinical experiment.

Beginning in 1959, Alberto Benchimol and I carried out a series of experiments, correlating angina, precordial movements, and intracardiac pressure.[1-14] The purpose of this paper is to discuss the following suggestions which resulted from these studies plus related observations by others:

1. Angina pectoris is often associated with an elevated end-diastolic left ventricular pressure (LVEDP). If the alteration is not present at rest, it frequently can be produced by exercise (Figs. 1, 2).

2. This elevated LVEDP is a transitory event and does not seem similar to the elevated LVEDP typical of usual left heart failure.

3. Several other measurable circulatory events are associated with this rise in LVEDP: A rise in left atrial pressure, a rise in pulmonary vein pressure, a rise in capillary pressure (Fig. 3), an altered contour of the P wave of the electrocardiogram, an increased atrial component of the phonocardiogram and, pertinent to this paper, an altered chest wall movement usefully defined as a "large *a* wave" of the apex cardiogram (Fig. 4).

Pragmatically this can be expressed as an equation: A.P. $\cong \uparrow$ LVEDP $\cong \uparrow a$ACG in which

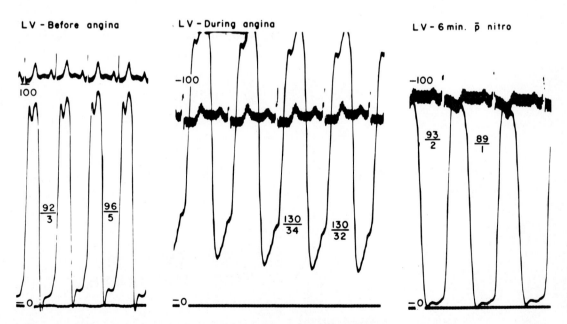

FIG. 1. Left ventricular pressure recorded at rest, during spontaneous angina, and after exercise. Note rise in LVEDP from 5 mm. Hg to 34 mm. Hg and return to 2 mm. Hg.

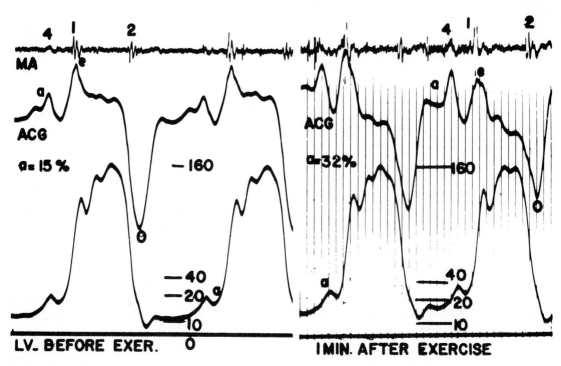

FIG. 2. Left ventricular pressure, apex cardiogram, phonocardiogram. LVEDP 18 mm. Hg at rest; 30 mm. Hg after exercise. (Brit. Heart J. *25:* 389, 1963)

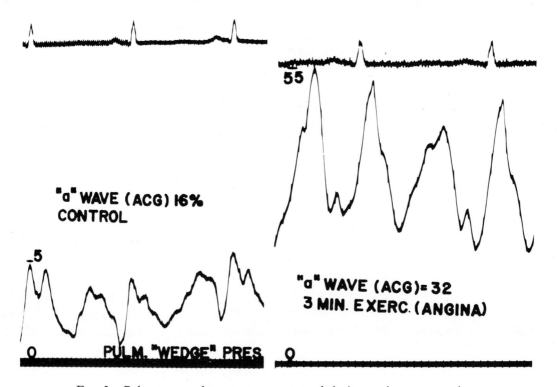

FIG. 3. Pulmonary wedge pressure at rest and during angina, postexercise.

FIG. 4. Phonocardiogram, apex cardiogram, carotid trace, recording during spontaneous angina pectoris. Note marked increase in "a" wave during angina. (Benchimol, A., and Dimond, E.G.: Am. Heart J. *65:* 795, 1963)

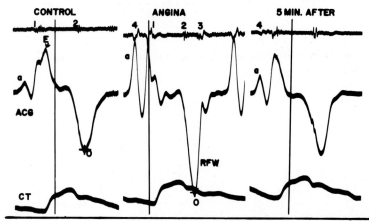

A.P. = angina pectoris, ↑LVEDP = increased left ventricular diastolic pressure, ↑aACG = enlarged atrial wave of the apex cardiogram. And immediately, a footnote must be added to confirm that this equation does not mean 100 per cent of the time, nor does it mean that these events happen only in angina pectoris.

Other observations concerning this altered chest wall movement and LVEDP in patients with ischemic heart disease are of interest:

1. Nitroglycerin quickly removes these changes (Fig. 5).

2. Exercise provokes the changes (Fig. 6).

3. Exposure to cold provokes these changes (Fig. 7).

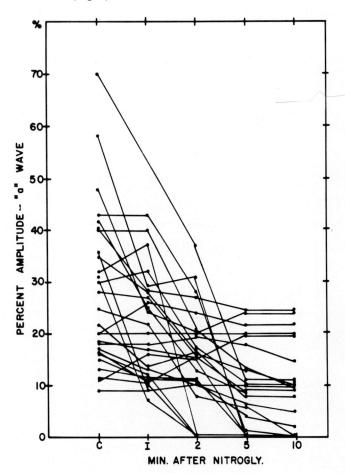

FIG. 5. Change in amplitude of atrial component of apex cardiogram (per cent amplitude "a" wave) at rest and after nitroglycerin in 26 patients with angina by history.

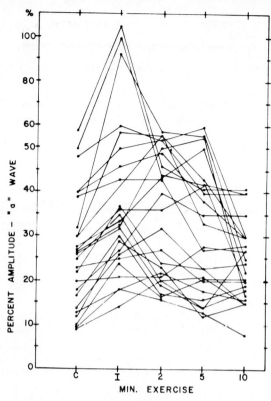

FIG. 6. Per cent amplitude of the "a" wave of the apex cardiogram in 25 patients with history of angina, recorded at rest, immediately, two, five, and ten minutes after completing a double Master two-step test.

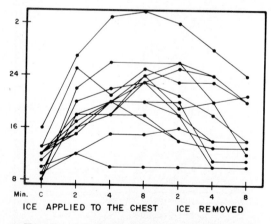

FIG. 7. Amplitude of "a" wave of apex cardiogram expressed as ratio of "a" wave to total ACG, measured in 7 patients with history of angina, at rest, during the application of an ice bag to the chest, and after removal of the ice.

4. Four limb venous tourniquets remove or lessen these changes (Figs. 8, 9).

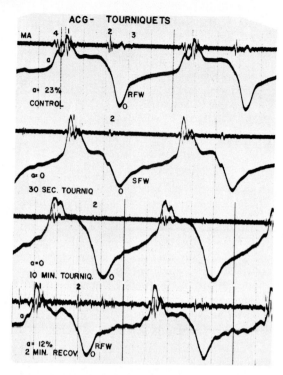

FIG. 8. Apex cardiogram recorded from patient with history of angina. Top tracing recorded during rest and demonstrates a prominent "a" wave. Recordings then made at 30 seconds and 10 minutes of application of tourniquets to limbs to occlude venous return. Note disappearance of "a" wave. Last record recorded two minutes after removal of tourniquets. Note beginning return of "a" wave.

5. A tight abdominal binder removes or lessens these changes (Figs. 10, 11).

6. In some patients, cigarette smoking provokes these changes (Fig. 12).

The apex cardiogram as used in most of the experiments cited here had two faults or limitations. First, the Sanborn crystal microphone, No. 374, did not have a linear frequency response. We were aware of this and called attention to this inconsistency in 1964 (Fig. 13).[10]

The second handicap with the technic was the necessity to record the ACG with the patient in the left lateral position, respiration suspended. The possible use of the ACG as a monitoring device obviously was lessened. However, Siegel[15] (Fig. 14), has made good progress in computer "averaging" of the ACG recorded from active subjects. Therefore, flat response transducers and averaged tracings may open up a wider range of usefulness.[15]

The apex cardiogram, similar to the electrocardiogram, can be studied at rest and after exercise. The

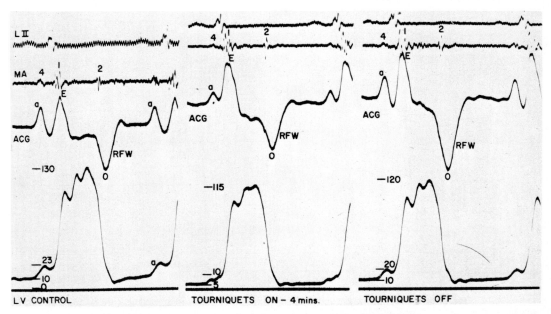

FIG. 9.   Left ventricular pressure, apex cardiogram, phonocardiogram, electrocardiograms recorded in patient with angina by history. Note marked lowering of LVEDP and "a" wave during application of tourniquets.

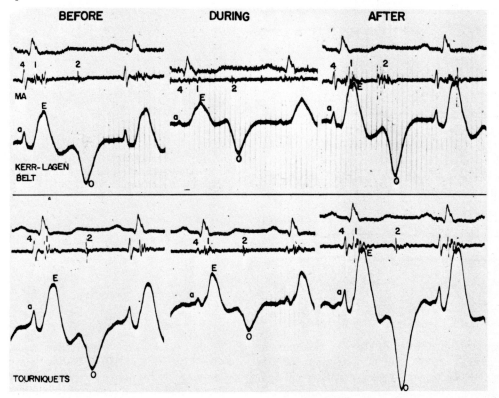

FIG. 10.   Marked diminution in amplitude of "a" wave of apex cardiogram in patient with history of angina; abdominal binder applied during upper tracing, venous tourniquets during lower recording. (Dimond, E. G., Li, Y., and Benchimol, A.: J. A. M. A. *187:* 981, 1964)

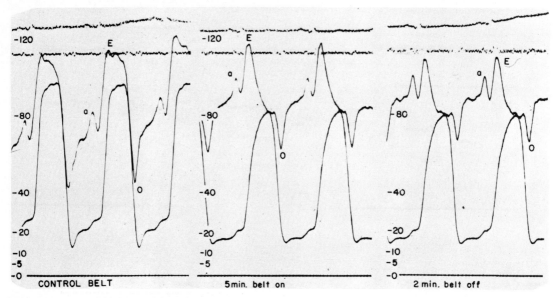

FIG. 11.   Decrease in LVEDP in patient with history of angina, during application of tight abdominal binder.

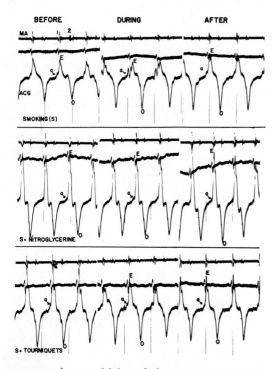

FIG. 12.   Change in amplitude of "a" wave in one patient with angina by history studied three times: smoking, smoking plus nitroglycerin, and smoking plus tourniquets.

comparative sensitivity of the two measurements, the postexercise ECG and the postexercise ACG, has been studied by Ginn, Ross, and Baker at Johns Hopkins.[16] Their conclusion, in a small series, was that ". . . the postexercise ACG appears to provide the better separation of normal and coronary heart disease groups."

Roos and Snellen[17] have further validated the authenticity of the ACG. During human heart surgery, "apex" cardiograms were recorded from various regions on the ventricular surfaces simultaneously with ventricular pressures. Regardless of the place on the epicardium from which the "ACG" was recorded, the tracing "showed a striking re-

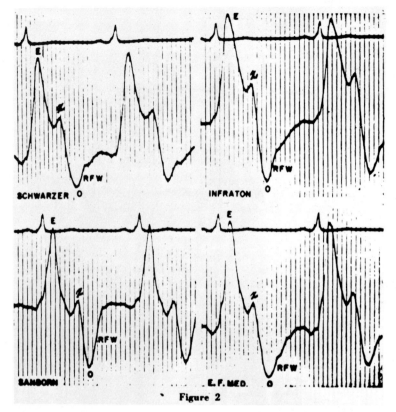

FIG. 13. Alteration in apex cardiogram due to pick-up device. Apex cardiograms obtained from the some patient but with four different pick-ups (Sanborn Infreton, Schwerzer, and Electronics for Medicine). Note particular contour with Sanborn crystal microphone No. 374. (Dimond, E. G: Circulation *30:* 285, 1964. with permission of the American Heart Association)

semblance with the precordial 'apex' cardiograms . . ."

These authors also studied in dogs the variations in heart circumference, using mercury filled elastic tubes. They concluded, "The mercury tube recording and the epicardial 'apex' cardiogram were virtually identical in shape as well as in time relations."

The diagnostic value of the atrial gallop both in angina and in myocardial infarction has had substantial validation.[18,19]

The atrial component of the abnormal ACG of ischemic heart disease usually can be seen, felt, and heard, in that order of frequency. In other words, the very low frequency nature of the vibration makes it difficult to hear, but the eye and hand may readily recognize the additional vibration. Occurring before the main systolic thrust of the heart or if not as a separate vibration, it often can be noted as a hesitancy or flicker on the ascending limb of the main systolic wave. Once *seen,* or *felt,* the chances of *hearing* the signal increase, especially as one learns to listen with the lightest touch of the bell endpiece,

and to listen with the patient on his left side, in varying phases of respiration.

SUMMARY

The literature on apex cardiography is 80 years old.[20] Angina pectoris, undoubtedly an ancient human experience, was put into the literature by William Heberdon. Cardiac catheterization has been a widely used diagnostic procedure since the mid-1940s.

We have the interesting paradox of a very common human, dolorous experience, angina, and a remarkably simple procedure, apex cardiography, coexisting for 80 years and no shared literature.

In the same vein, we have the elegant, complicated technic of cardiac catheterization, occupying the best of medical research talent from 1946 on—and no major literature as evidence of an understanding of the altered physiology which surely must accompany angina.

The two major English literature heart textbooks

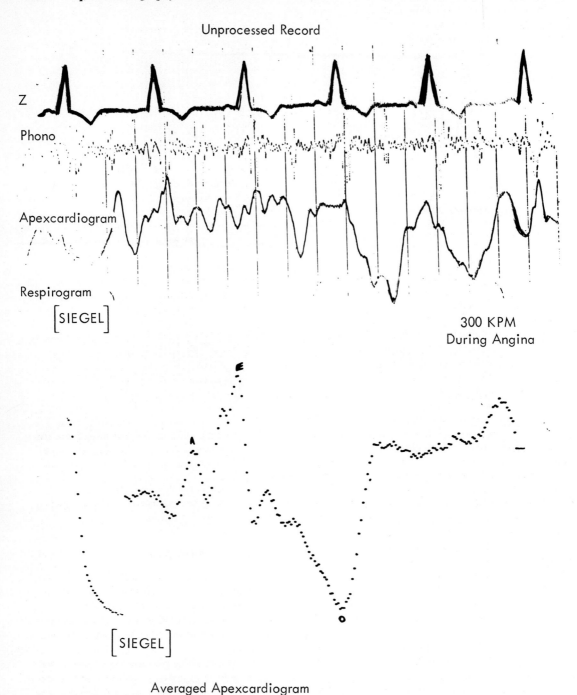

Unprocessed Record

Z

Phono

Apexcardiogram

Respirogram

[SIEGEL]

300 KPM
During Angina

[SIEGEL]

Averaged Apexcardiogram
300 KPM   During Angina

FIG. 14.   Tracings recorded from precordium during activity and angina. Upper record is actual tracing; lower tracing result of "averaging" through computer.

which were the standard references in the late 1950s and the early 1960s were those of Paul H. Wood and Charles K. Friedberg.[21,22]

In the index of these two books, the phrase "apex cardiography" does not appear. Under the heading "angina pectoris," neither cardiac catheterization nor apex cardiography appears. Under the heading, "cardiac catheterization," equally, there are no cross references. A careful reading of the entire sections of each book on ischemic heart disease reveals no suggestion that there is a correlation between angina pectoris, a precordial movement, and an intra-cardiac pressure dynamic. Wood, an acknowledged master of physical diagnosis, who must have thoughtfully, carefully, and critically examined the precordiums of thousands of patients with angina pectoris, does not describe a visible or palpable event occurring prior to the main apex thrust of the heart.

Why? In the answer to this must be a lesson. What other observations are obscured from our view because we are prepared *not to see?*

REFERENCES

1. Benchimol. A., Dimond, E. G., Waxman, D., and Shen, Y.: Diastolic movements of the precordium in mitral stenosis and regurgitation, Am. Heart J. *60*:417, 1960.
2. Benchimol, A., Dimond, E. G., and Carson, J.: The value of the apex cardiogram as a reference tracing in phonocardiography, Am. Heart J. *61*:485, 1961.
3. Benchimol, A., and Dimond, E. G.: The apex cardiogram in ischemic heart disease, Brit. Heart J. *24*:581, 1962.
4. Dimond, E. G., and Benchimol, A.: The exercise apex cardiogram in angina pectoris: Its possible usefulness in diagnosis and therapy, Dis. Chest *43*:93, 1963.
5. Benchimol A., and Dimond, E. G.: The apex cardio-gram in normal older subjects and in patients with arteriosclerotic heart disease. Effect of exercise on the "a" wave, Am. Heart J. *65*:789, 1963.
6. Benchimol, A., and Dimond, E. G.: Normal and abnormal apex cardiogram. Its physiologic varia-tions and its relation to intracardiac events, Am. J. Cardiol. *11*:368, 1963.
7. Legler, J., Benchimol, A., and Dimond, E. G.: The apex cardiogram in the study of the 2–OS interval, Brit. Heart J. *25*:246, 1963.
8. Dimond, E. G., and Benchimol, A.: Correlation of intracardiac pressure and precordial movement, Brit. Heart J. *25*:389, 1963.
9. Benchimol, A., Legler, J., and Dimond, E. G.: The carotid tracing and apex cardiogram in subaortic stenosis and idiopathic myocardial hypertrophy, Am. J. Cardiol. *11*:427, 1963.
10. Dimond, E. G.: Precordial vibrations. Clinical clues from palpation, Circulation *30*:284, 1964.
11. Dimond, E. G., Li, Y., and Benchimol, A.: Tourni-quets and abdominal binders in ischemic heart disease. Effects on the apex cardiogram, J.A.M.A. *187*:981, 1964.
12. Benchimol, A., Wu, T. L., and Dimond, E. G.: The apex cardiogram in the diagnosis of congenital heart disease, Am. J. Cardiol. *17*:63, 1966.
13. Dimond, E. G., Duenas, A., and Benchimol, A.: Apex cardiography, Am. Heart J. *72*:124, 1966.
14. Getzen, J., and Dimond, E. G.: The saga of the fourth heart sound, Am. J. Cardiol. *22*:609, 1968.
15. Personal communication from Wayne Siegel, Aug. 29, 1968.
16. Ginn, W., Ross, and R., Baker, B.: A study of the apex cardiogram and electrodcardiogram in ischemic heart disease, Clinical Research *10*:390, 1962.
17. Roos, J. P., and Snellen, H. A.: Hemodynamic origin of "apex" cardiograms, Circulation *38*:166 (Supplement VI) 1968.
18. Hill, J. C., O'Rourke, R. A., Lewis, R. P., and Mc-Granahan, G. M.: The diagnostic value of the atrial gallop in myocardial infarction, Circulation *38*:99 (Supplement VI) 1968.
19. Wayne, H. H.: Serial apex cardiograms, phono-cardiograms and carotid tracings in myocardial infarctions, Circulation *30*:203 (Supplement VI) 1968.
20. Marey, E. J., Lederer, L. G., and Mandes, J. C.: La Méthode Graphique dan les Sciences Expériment-ales, Ed. 2, Paris, Masson & Cie, 1885.
21. Wood, P. W.: The heart and Circulation. Second edition, Philadelphia, J. B. Lippincott Company, 1956.
22. Friedberg, C. K.: Diseases of the heart. Ed. 2. W. B. Saunders Company, Philadelphia and London, 1956.

Clinical Applications of New Cardiac Enzymes

John S. LaDue

ENZYMATIC ASSESSMENT OF MYOCARDIAL DAMAGE

The antemortem electrocardiographic diagnosis of myocardial infarction is a shaky 50 per cent for patients showing multiple infarcts at autopsy and only 80 per cent for single initial infarctions.

The nonspecific phase reactants such as leukocytosis (WBC), sedimentation rate (ESR), serum complement (C'), C'-reactive protein (CRP), temperature, fibrinogen levels, mucopolysaccharides, and trace metals are abnormal in up to 90 per cent or more of patients at some time after myocardial infarction but are nonspecific and may be altered by any infectious process as well as by myocardial infarction (Table 1).[2,3]

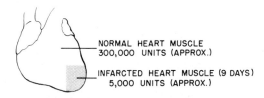

NORMAL HEART MUSCLE
300,000 UNITS (APPROX.)

INFARCTED HEART MUSCLE (9 DAYS)
5,000 UNITS (APPROX.)

Loss of GO-T from infarcted heart muscle results in increased transaminase activity in the serum:

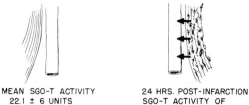

MEAN SGO-T ACTIVITY
22.1 ± 6 UNITS

24 HRS. POST-INFARCTION
SGO-T ACTIVITY OF
50 TO 600 UNITS

Fig. 1. See discussion in text.

The introduction of methods for analyzing muscle enzyme activity in the serum has increased the diagnostic accuracy in clinical and autopsy series to 95 per cent. The serum activity of these enzymes may increase as a result of acute damage to skeletal muscle, liver, brain, kidney, red blood cells and various other organs as well as to myocardium. The measurement of a spectrum of enzymes may pinpoint more accurately the specific site of injury. Unlike alterations in the nonspecific phase reactants, there is no evidence that these enzymes will rise in the serum without tissue breakdown. Furthermore, no qualitative or quantitative relationship exists between these enzyme changes and changes in the nonspecific phase reactants.

TABLE 1
Nonspecific Phase Reactants

Agent	Onset (days)	Duration (days)	% Abnormal
ESR	$\frac{1}{2}$–4	10–50+	90+
CRP	$\frac{1}{2}$–5	14–50+	90+
Fibrinogen	1–5	14–50+	90+
C'	$\frac{1}{2}$–3	3–50+	90+
WBC	$\frac{1}{2}$–3	3–20+	90+
Temp.	$\frac{1}{2}$–5	3–10+	90+[*]

Heart muscle is abundantly rich in enzymes which catalyze different biochemical reactions. The serum activity of these enzymes may be changed by various diseases and profoundly so by myocardial infarction. The discovery of high glutamic oxalacetic transaminase (GOT) activity in heart muscle led to the study of changes in the serum and muscle activity of this enzyme in heart disease.[15]

Acute transmural myocardial infarction is followed by an increase in the activity of numerous enzymes in the serum. Since the activity of GOT is approximately 5000 to 10,000 times greater in human heart muscle than in serum and the activity of LDH is 3000 and GPT is 1000 times greater (Table 2), release of these enzymes from the damaged myocardium with its rich enzyme content probably accounts for the major increase in serum activity following acute myocardial cell damage (Fig. 1).

Since the discovery of increased SGOT activity in the serum following acute myocardial infarction,[7] the activity of many enzymes other than those discussed here has been reported to increase after myo-

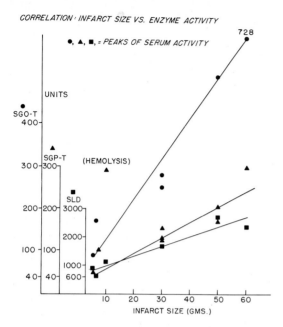

FIG. 2. Correlation of infarct size versus enzyme activity.

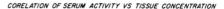

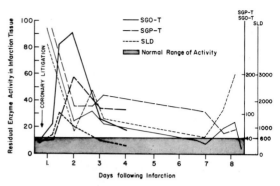

FIG. 3. Correlation of serum activity versus tissue concentration.

cardial cell injury including: phosphohexose-isomerase, isocitric dehydrogenase, alkaline phosphatase and cholinesterase. Because most of the myocardial enzymes studied have similar behavior, we will discuss SGOT in detail as the prototype and will elaborate significant differences of the other enzymes under appropriate headings.

After experimental myocardial infarction, the peak increase in SGOT activity is proportional to the size of infarction (Fig. 2). Furthermore, the changes in enzyme activity in the serum and in the infarcted muscle were inversely proportional (Fig. 3). The decrease in myocardial enzyme content after myocardial infarction is proportional to the age of the infarct.

Extreme experimental myocardial ischemia of 10 to 30 minutes' duration such as to produce profound T and ST changes without Q abnormalities failed to change the activity of either the serum or the ischemic myocardium (Table 3).[9]

CLINICAL CORONARY INSUFFICIENCY

Fifty patients with status anginosus or recurrent precordial or substernal pain of thirty minutes' duration or longer associated with definite T wave or ST abnormalities or both had serial transaminase determinations but without electrocardiographic evidence of evolution of recent transmural myocardial infarction. Thirteen showed electrocardiographic evidence of healed infarction. All had marked T and ST wave variations at some time during the attacks of chest pain without any new Q wave changes.

Sixteen of these 50 patients had elevations of SGOT activity at some time during the acute phase of their illness. Five who had congestive heart failure and two who had moderate shock at the time of hospital admission had normal transaminase levels throughout the period of observation. Six of 12 patients with increased SGOT activity and 8 of 27 without it revealed abnormalities in at least two of the following three determinations: WBC, ESR or temperature. In 8 patients, the transaminase did not become elevated until after the fourth day of observation. Figure 4 shows the SGOT levels of a patient who had status anginosus associated with T wave abnormalities as depicted. The rise of 56 probably represents the presence of a small infarct; this is characteristic of the type of curves seen in 16

TABLE 2
Range of Enzyme Activity in Humans and Dogs

Enzyme	GOT		GPT		LD	
	Human	*Dog*	*Human*	*Dog*	*Human*	*Dog*
Serum (Units/ml.)	5–40	5–40	5–35	5–40	100–600	100–600
Heart Muscle (Units/Gm.)	155,000–(?)	150,000–400,000	7,130–(?)	20,000–80,000	221,600–(?)	300,000–700,000

TABLE 3
Diseases Rarely Associated With Increased SGOT, LDH, SHBD or CPK Activity

	SGOT	LDH	SHBD	CPK
		Changes in activity from		
		0 to ±, +, + +, + + +, + + + +		
Angina pectoris	0	0	0	0
Coronary insufficiency without infarction	0	0	±	0
Rheumatic fever with carditis	±	±	0	0
Pulmonary infections	0	0	0	0
Peritonitis	0	0	0	0
Genitourinary infections	0	0	0	0
Other infections	0	0	0	0
Arthritis	0	0	0	0
Other bone diseases	0	0	0	0
Dermatitis	0	0	0	0
Uremia	0	0	0	0
Neoplasias without liver involvement	0	±	±	0
Leukemias	0	±	±	0
Anemias	0	0	±	0
Metabolic diseases	0	0	0	+
Allergic diseases	0	0	0	0
Pregnancy	0	0	0	0

0	= No change
±	= Variable
+	= Consistent mild
+ +	= Consistent moderate
+ + +	= Consistent severe
+ + + +	= Consistent marked

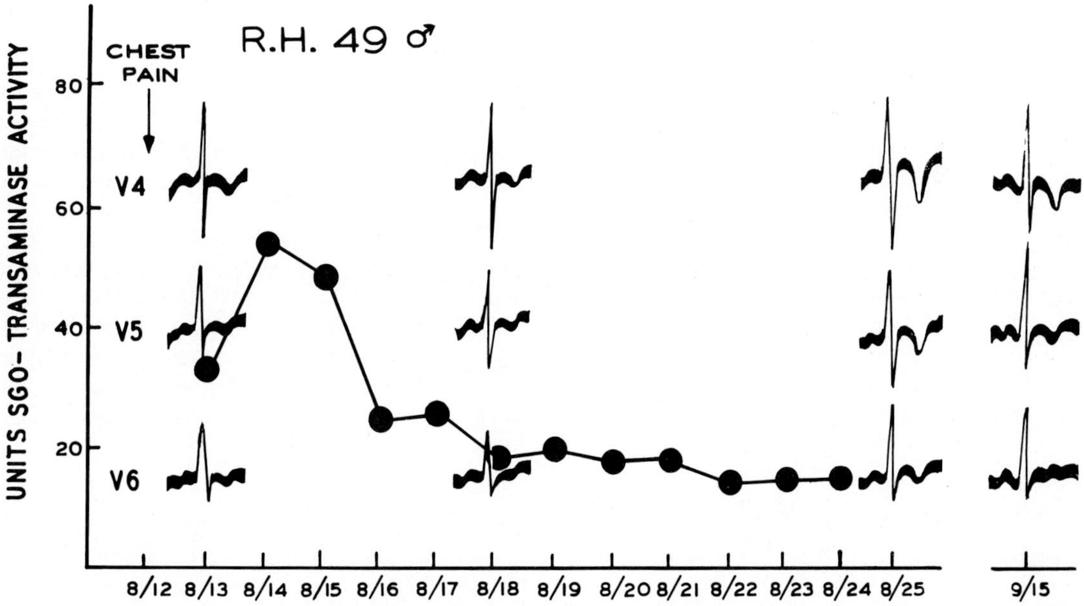

FIG. 4. See discussion in text.

among 50 patients with chest pain who showed elevations of transaminase at some time during the acute phase of their disease. Figure 5, in contrast, shows the SGOT levels of a patient who had similar pain and equally marked T wave abnormalities on his electrocardiogram but whose SGOT levels re-mained within normal limits throughout the period of observation.[10]

MYOCARDIAL INFARCTION

Acute transmural myocardial infarction has been

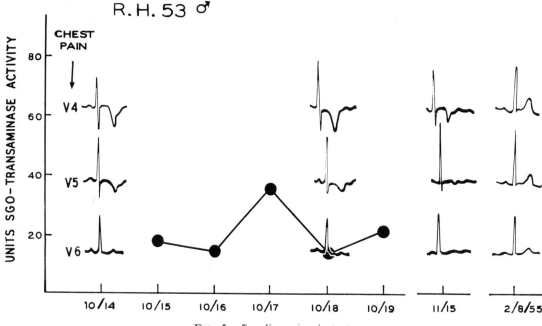

FIG. 5.   See discussion in text.

followed by increased SGOT activity in 96.9 per cent of 1255 cases reported in the world literature. The range and mean of SGOT activity in 300 patients with unequivocal transmural myocardial infarction are seen in Figure 6. Levels 1.5 to 20 times normal were found in 297 of these patients. The SGOT activity measured three to five days after myocardial infarction was within normal limits in 60 per cent emphasizing the importance of blood sampling 12 to 48 hours postinfarction. Secondary elevations were noted after recurrent chest pain due to extension or development of a new infarction in the same patient.

Lactic dehydrogenase (LD) is concerned with the reduction in the presence of DPNH, of alpha-keto and diketo acids to lactic acid. Maximum reduction by LDH has been shown to occur with pyruvic acid. The LDH activity is measured spectrophotometrically. Normal activity in human serum is 100 to 600 units[11] in cardiovascular disorders. LDH activity is present in all human serums and all whole blood hemolysates but in decreasing amounts in red blood cells, liver, heart, skeletal muscle, kidney, pancreas, spleen, brain and lung.

The diagnostic accuracy of LDH following myocardial infarction is somewhat lower than the 97 per cent reported for SGOT. Peak elevations developed after three to four days, falling off to normal by the eighth to fourteenth day in 85 per cent of the patients.[4]

Figure 7 compares the average changes in SGOT, SGPT, and LDH activity in 43 patients following acute transmural myocardial infarction. SGOT rises proportionately higher than LDH, but the activity falls off more rapidly. SGPT usually remains within normal limits unless SGOT levels are above 150 units.

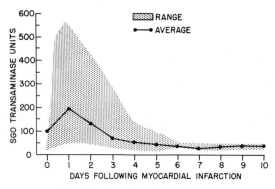

FIG. 6. See discussion in text.

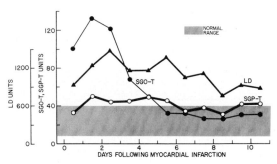

FIG. 7. See discussion in text.

LDH ISOENZYMES

The finding that total LDH activity consisted of several related but biologically different LDH components, the so-called isoenzymes, led to the search for methods to measure and separate the component in the serum derived from the myocardium. Electrophoretic studies have separated LDH into 5 components. The most rapidly migrating fractions are derived from the heart, red blood cells and kidney, while the slower moving components appear to originate from the liver and from the skeletal muscle tissue. It has been shown that increased LDH activity following myocardial infarction is primarily due to the rapidly migrating components.[12] It has also been shown that the LDH arising primarily from the myocardium is relatively heat stable, permitting partial differentiation between LDH activity due to liver and skeletal muscle damage from that following myocardial necrosis.[13] Preliminary studies of these two methods in the diagnosis of myocardial infarction have been promising, but too few patients have been studied to permit final evaluation of the role of isoenzymes in the diagnosis of myocardial infarction, despite reports that myocardial LDH remains elevated in the serum as long as five days after total LDH activity has returned to normal.

Alpha-hydroxybutyric dehydrogenase (SHBD) catalyzes the reduction of alpha-ketobutyrate to alpha-hydroxybutyrate. SHBD has its highest activity in heart, skeletal muscle and liver, and its normal range in human serum is 120 to 260 units.[14]

SHBD activity closely mimics that of the LDH isoenzymes following acute myocardial infarction (Fig. 8). Its activity peaks between 48 and 72 hours but persists for 11 to 16 days. The slow clearing rate of SHBD permits the detection of myocardial infarction in serum drawn at a time when SGOT and creatine phosphokinase (CPK) activities may have returned to normal.[15]

SHBD levels may be elevated in neoplastic diseases, liver disease, megaloblastic anemia and in polymyositis and some forms of muscular dystrophy. Hemolysis may cause marked increases in SHBD levels. SHBD activity is not increased in infectious diseases, including pericarditis or cholecystitis.[16]

The stated advantages of prolonged duration of activity of SHBD of 90 to 100 per cent accuracy and of greater specificity await confirmation. The high incidence of increased activity in ischemic heart disease without definite evidence of infarction should be confirmed.

Creatine phosphokinase (CPK) catalyzes the transfer of a phosphoryl group from adenosine triphosphate (ATP) to the acceptor creatine with the formation of phosphocreatine and adenosine diphosphate (ADP).[17]

CPK activity is high in skeletal muscle, myocardium, and brain but only traces of activity have been detected in the lung, liver, kidney and pancreas. This property makes measurements of CPK more specific in detecting the presence of heart muscle cell damage. The activities of the other enzymes already discussed must be judged in terms of the possibility of concomitant liver cell injury secondary to acute congestion, shock, drugs, anesthesia, hepatitis, obstructive jaundice and, to a lesser extent, with acute injury to the lung, kidney or pancreas. Another advantage of CPK is the negligible activity in red blood cells so that hemolysis does not give falsely high activities—a frequent technical problem in the assay of LDH and SHBD.

CPK activity begins to increase four to six hours following acute myocardial infarction with peak levels at 12 to 36 hours and falls to within normal limits in two to seven days.[18]

Figure 9 shows the usual CPK activity following acute myocardial infarction. Both the magnitude and duration of activity appear to be proportional to the size of the infarct.[19]

It is premature to compare the diagnostic accuracy

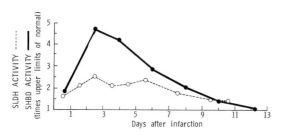

FIG. 8. See discussion in text.

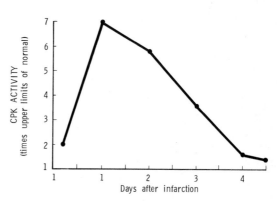

FIG. 9. See discussion in text.

of CPK or SHBD with that of SGOT or LDH because of limited experience with the former. However, myocardial infarction has been confined clinically to 60 to 100 per cent of series of reported instances of myocardial infarctions for both CPK and SHBD. Autopsy verification of the diagnostic accuracy of CPK, SHBD and the LDH isoenzymes in acute myocardial infarction is lacking at present. CPK has a basic advantage over the other enzymes of being relatively more specific.

More recent studies employing a modified method of analysis for CPK activity have shown much less specificity. For example, 75 per cent of patients who have delirium tremens, a third of the patients who have chronic liver damage, and a significant number of patients after electroshock therapy, episodes of epilepsy, cerebrovascular accidents, congestive heart failure, acute alcoholism and various forms of renal disease also exhibit significant elevation of the CPK.[20] Finally, CPK activity does not appear as reliable as SGOT or LDH in confirming the diagnosis of myocardial infarction.

INTERPRETATION

Table 4 lists the disease states associated with increased activity of enzymes commonly used in confirming the diagnosis of myocardial infarction, and Table 3 lists disease states uncommonly associated with altered enzyme activity. It is apparent that SGOT, SGPT, LDH and SHBD activities are altered by many diseases associated with acute damage of the liver, skeletal muscle, kidney, pancreas and, to a lesser extent, brain. However, the clinical setting will usually determine the interpretation. It is noteworthy that liver cell injury does not signif-

TABLE 4

Disease States Commonly Causing Variable Elevation of SGOT, LDH, SHBD and CPK Activity

	SGOT	LDH	SHBD	CPK
	Changes in activity from 0 to ±,+,++,+++,++++			
Myocardium				
Acute infarction	+++	++	+++	++++
Myocarditis (rheumatic)	±	+	±	0
Severe pericarditis	+	+	±	0
Hepatic				
Hepatitis	++++	++++	++++	0
Cirrhosis	±	±	±	0
Obstructive jaundice	++	++	++	0
Metastatic involvement	++	+	++	0
Mononucleosis	+	+	+	
Drug injury	+++	+++	+++	0
Cholecystitis	0	0	0	0
Central lobular injury	++	++	++	0
Shock (2+hours)	+++	+++	+++	0
Acute passive congestion	+++	+++	+++	0
Persistent rapid arrhythmias	+	+	+	0
Muscle cell damage				
Injury and burns	++	++	++	++
Dermatomyositis	++	++	++	+++
Muscular dystrophy	++	++	++	+++
Muscular atrophy	0	0	0	0
Infarction, kidney, spleen, bowel	++	++	++	0
Pancreatitis	+	+	+	0
Cholecystitis	0	0	0	0
Drugs (opiates in post-cholecystectomy syndrome)	++	++	++	0
Severe pulmonary infarction	±	++	±	0
Hemolysis	±	+++	+++	0
Cerebral				
Cerebral vascular accidents	±	±	±	+
Brain tumor	±	±	±	±
Degenerative diseases	0	0	0	0
Convulsive disorders	0	0	0	0

0	= No change
±	= Variable
+	= Consistent mild
++	= Consistent moderate
+++	= Consistent severe
++++	= Consistent marked

icantly alter CPK activity. The simultaneous measurement of SGOT and CPK activity in the first 24 hours following myocardial infarction will eliminate most of the difficulty in the early diagnosis of small or large infarcts. LDH and SHBD will help detect the probability of heart muscle cell damage 4 to 16 days following heart muscle cell necrosis of average degree.

Small infarcts are associated with minimal increased activity of short duration and large infarcts with high peak levels that persist much longer. There is a rough correlation between peak activity of SGOT and prognosis with mortalities of 80 per cent or more when SGOT rises to 200 units or more and 5 per cent or less with values below 80 units. Persistently increased CPK activity on the third day after myocardial infarction was associated with a 40 per cent mortality, whereas only 17 per cent succumbed when CPK was within normal limits on the third day.[21] Borderline elevations may not indicate myocardial necrosis. Variations within normal limits have no diagnostic significance. Care must be taken to collect blood without hemolysis, to separate serum from the red blood cells and to refrigerate promptly unless analyses can be done at once.

SUMMARY

Ischemia of several hours' duration does not result in loss of GOT and LDH into the circulation or alter the enzyme content of heart muscle. Necrosis is followed by rapid decrease in cellular GOT and increase in SGOT during the first four hours, the maximum reciprocal change usually developing within two days.

Leakage of enzymes from the necrotic myocardium (Fig. 9) is the most probable explanation of increased serum activity in the great majority of cases.

LDH[5] (probably identical with SHBD) appears to increase significantly in the serum after heart muscle cell injury but is much less specific than CPK. How tissue specific the isoenzymes of LDH and even CPK will prove to be awaits further study. The wide distribution of many enzymes in numerous cellular structures diminishes, but does not exclude, the possibility of discovery of enzymes whose presence in the serum will not only reflect more specific sites of cellular abnormality but also may give a more precise index of the degree of injury to heart muscle and other organs.

On the basis of our present knowledge, it seems hazardous to rely on variations of the serum levels of one enzyme alone for verification of myocardial necrosis. If early confirmation is necessary, SGOT and CPK activities rise more rapidly after myocardial infarction, with CPK proportionately higher than any other enzyme studied to date. If prompt laboratory analysis is not possible, SGOT is much more stable. Should the clinician see the patient two or more days after infarction, LDH or SHBD activities will be higher and persist for 4 to 16 days. When complicating factors such as acute congestion of the liver, shock of two or more hours' duration, liver disease or pancreatitis are present, CPK must be the choice except in the presence of skeletal muscle injury. Ideally, SGOT, SHBD or LDH and CPK activities should be determined. CPK activity would provide greater specificity and LDH or SHBD improve late diagnosis.

REFERENCES

1. Melichar, F., Jedlicka, V., and Haulik, L.: Study of undiagnosed myocardial infarctions, Acta med. scandinav. *174*:761, 1963.
2. Kroop, I. G., and Schackman, N. H.: C-reactive protein determination as an index of myocardial necrosis in coronary artery disease, Am. J. Med. *22*:90, 1957.
3. Losner, C. S., Volk, B., and Aronson, S.: Test aids in acute myocardial infarction: Clinical and experimental, Am. Heart J. *54*:225, 1957.
4. Agress, C. M.: Evaluation of the transaminase test, Am. J. Cardiol. *3*:74, 1959.
5. Cohen, P. P., and Hekhuis, G. L.: Rate of transamination in normal tissues, J. Biol. Chem. *140*:711, 1941.
6. LaDue, J. S., Nydick, I., and Ruegsegger, P.: The Etiology of Myocardial Infarction. Boston, Little, Brown & Company. 1963, pp. 207–223.
7. LaDue, J. S., Wroblewski, F., and Karmen, A.: Serum glutamic oxaloacetic transaminase activity in human acute transmural myocardial infarction, Science *20*:497, 1954.
8. Nydick, I., Wroblewski, F., and LaDue, J. S.: Evidence for increased serum glutamic oxaloacetic transaminase (SGO-T) activity following graded myocardial infarcts in dogs, Circulation *12*:161, 1955.
9. LaDue, J. S., Burckhardt, D., and Nydick, I.: Enzymatic assessment of myocardial damage, Geriatrics *22*:184–200, 1967.
10. LaDue, J. S., Nydick, I., Ruegsegger, P., and Streuli, F.: Measurement and significance of enzymes, *in* Coronary Heart Disease. W. Likoff and J. H. Moyer (eds.), New York, Grune & Stratton, Inc. 1963, pp. 256–272.
11. Wroblewski, F., Ruegsegger, P., and LaDue, J. S.: Serum lactic dehydrogenase activity in acute transmural myocardial infarction. Science *123*:1122, 1956.
12. Wroblewski, F., Ross, C., and Gregory, K.: Isoenzymes and myocardial infarction, New England. J. Med. *263*:531, 1960.
13. Latner, A. L., and Skillen, A. W.: Heat stability index of lactic dehydrogenase in cardiac infarction, Proc. Assoc. Clin. Biochem. *2*:100, 1963.

14. Rosalki, S. B., and Wilkinson, J. H.: Reduction of a-ketobutyrate by human serum, Nature *188*:1110, 1960.
15. Forster, G., and Feissli, S.: Zur diagnostischen Bedeutung der a-hydroxybutter-saeure-dehydrogenase aktivitaet des Serums. Helvet. med. acta *31*:389, 1964.
16. Konttinen, A., and Halonen, P. I.: Serum CPK and a-hydroxybutyric dehydrogenase activity compared with GOT and LDH in myocardial infarction, Cardiologia (Basel) *43*:56, 1963.
17. Sorensen, N. S.: CPK in the diagnosis of myocardial infarction. Acta med. scandinav. *174*:725, 1963.
18. Duma, R. J., and Siegel, A. L.: Serum creatine phosphokinase in acute myocardial infarction, Arch. Int. Med. *115*:443, 1965.
19. Konttinen, A., and Halonen, P. K.: Serum a-hydroxybutyric dehydrogenase (HBD) in myocardial infarction. Am. J. Cardiol. *10*:525, 1952.
20. Eshchar, J., and Zimmerman, H. J.: Creatine phosphokinase in disease. Am. J. M. Sc. *253*:272, 1967.
21. Bruce, R., Todd, J. K., and LeDune, L.: Serum transaminase: Its clinical use in diagnosis and prognosis. Brit. M. J. *2*:1125, 1958.

Terminal Arteriole, Capillary or Cellular Dysfunction: Angina Pectoris and Abnormal Resting and Exercise Electrocardiograms in Patients With Normal Patent Coronary Arteries

William Likoff

Cine coronary arteriography has made it possible to correlate the clinical manifestations of coronary heart disease with the distribution and severity of the vascular pathology in living patients. A number of these studies have indicated that in most patients with angina pectoris and abnormal resting or exercise electrocardiograms, atherosclerosis is widely distributed throughout the major coronary arteries and is seriously obstructive in at least two main vessels.

Obviously, this does not apply when a major anomaly of the coronary circulation, severe aortic valvular disease, idiopathic hypertrophic subaortic stenosis or a cardiomyopathy is solely responsible for the clinical problem. In each of these instances, a mechanism other than actual vascular obstruction accounts for the imbalance between coronary flow and the nutritional needs of the myocardium.

Recent reports have indicated that angina pectoris and electrocardiographic abnormalities at rest and after exercise may also be encountered in patients who have normally patent coronary arteries and no evidence of any other cardiovascular disorder.[6-9] The initial communication regarding this matter was based on a survey of a small group of patients whose chest pains and electrocardiographic patterns at rest and after exercise had, for some time, supported an unquestioned diagnosis of coronary heart disease.[6] The majority of these individuals had classical angina. For some the pain occurred at rest as well as exercise and was not uniformly relieved by nitroglycerin. However, the differences between typical and atypical pain were too small to suggest the latter was not angina.

Electrocardiographic abnormalities at rest consisted of S-T segment depressions in bipolar and unipolar limb and precordial leads often associated with flat or inverted T waves (Fig. 1). Exercise increased the magnitude of these changes even when chest pain did not develop simultaneously (Fig. 2).

A fresh appraisal of these patients was initiated because as normotensive, nondiabetic, nonhyperlipemic, normally menstruating females, they represented unlikely victims of advanced coronary atherosclerosis. The evaluation included clinical, electrocardiographic and hemodynamic responses to measured physical stress, ventriculography and coronary visualization.

Each subject tested had a normal hemodynamic response to exercise. Left ventriculography did not uncover any abnormality in chamber size or contractility. Coronary visualization disclosed normal main and peripheral arteries free of discernible atherosclerosis.

Subsequent independent reports provided additional examples of patients with angina pectoris and abnormal resting and exercise electrocardiograms in whom there was no objective evidence of cardiovascular disease.[7-9] The total experience which has now been documented indicates the incidence is small and limited almost entirely to females in the fourth and fifth decades of life. Electrocardiographic abnormalities in this group generally do not include the findings of transmural infarction, serious arrhythmias or major conduction defects. Although metabolic disorders are uncommon, abnormal glucose tolerance tests may be encountered occasionally.

There are a number of possible explanations for the appearance of cardinal manifestations of coronary heart disease, angina and electrocardiographic abnormalities involving the RST segment and T wave in bipolar and unipolar leads, in individuals in whom cine arteriography reveals normal coronary vessels. First among these is the possibility that arteriography does not disclose the full measure

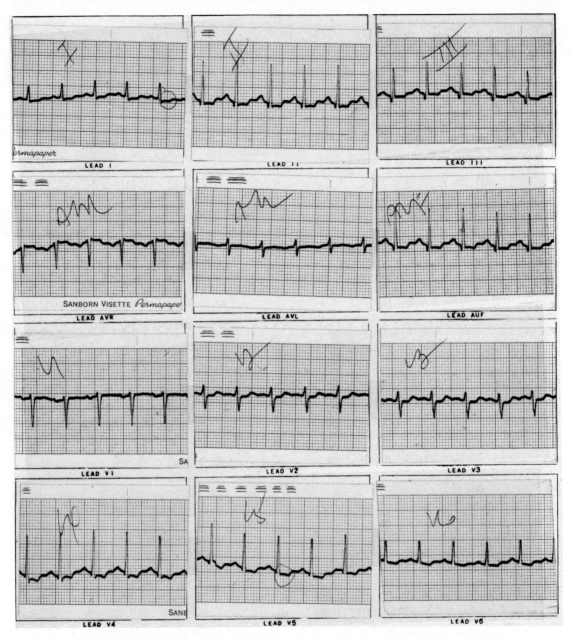

FIG 1.   Resting electrocardiogram of a 42-year-old white female. Note RST-T wave abnormalities in Leads I, II, III, avf, and V4 to V6 inclusive.

of existing pathology. Admittedly the visibility provided does underestimate the severity of coronary atherosclerosis. However, the failing is modest and cannot possibly account for the depiction, as morphologically normal, of diffuse, severe, visibilty discernible vascular changes usually present in individuals with angina pectoris and abnormal electrocardiograms.

In individuals in whom recanalization of obstructing lesions has been recorded by serial cine arteriog-

raphy, the residual hallmarks of the basic vascular abnormality are still readily seen. In view of the fact that the arteriograms of the patients under question are entirely normal, it does not seem reasonable to claim that significant vascular disease was present previously.

The possibility that functional constriction of the coronary arteries accounts for the clinical manifestations is exceptionally remote because, when present, unusual vasomotor activity is generally

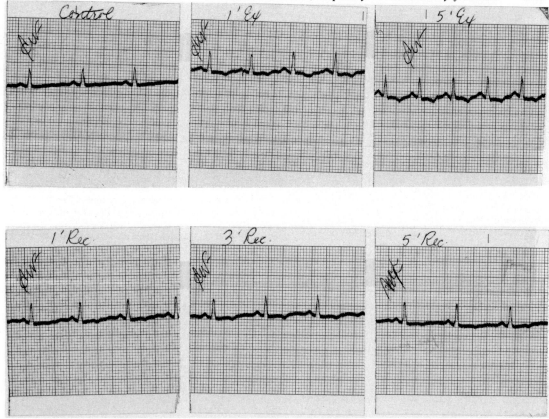

FIG. 2. Control and post-exercise electrocardiogram (lead avf) of 34-year-old white female patient. Note alterations in RST-T wave abnormalities with exercise.

recognized with ease at the time of coronary arteriography.

It is difficult to substantiate a claim that structural or functional disease of the peripheral coronary system is responsible for the clinical findings. These vessels are adequately revealed during cinearteriography and abnormalities in form or function should be recognized without difficulty. Furthermore, obstructive disease of peripheral vessels is exceptional unless major arteries are similarly involved.

Coronary arteriography does not appraise the status of the microcirculation. It is conceivable that the clinical manifestations result from an oxygen diffusion impairment at this vascular level or from inappropriate oxygen utilization by the myocardial cell. Eliot and Mizukani[7] have demonstrated what appears to be a physiochemical abnormality of hemoglobin and a resultant abnormal hemoglobin oxygen affinity in these patients. They suggest this could account for or contribute to the paradox of the occurrence of myocardial ischemia or necrosis in the presence of adequate arterial saturation and patent coronary arteries.

Neill, Kassebaum and Judkins[9] demonstrated

myocardial hypoxia and anaerobic metabolism during induced tachycardia in a female patient with angina pectoris, an abnormal exercise electrocardiogram and normally patent coronary arteries. They postulated that the myocardial hypoxia was responsible for the chest pain and the electrocardiographic changes. However, at least in this instance abnormal oxygen dissociation was not the cause of the hypoxia since a normal hemoglobin oxygen affinity was recorded. The authors suggested as possible alternative explanations for the myocardial hypoxia: inadequate size or distribution of normal coronary arteries; inappropriate coronary vasomotor reactivity to an increased metabolic need of the myocardium; obstruction of peripheral coronary vessels; a myocardial metabolic error.

In brief, there now resides, in the material collected to this point, ample documentation that angina pectoris and abnormal resting and exercise electrocardiographic patterns may be encountered in patients with normal coronary vessels and no other discernible form of cardiovascular disease. Myocardial hypoxia has been implicated as the underlying pathophysiology. The cause for the hypoxia, however, remains obscure. Among the explanations, that of a defective microcirculation and that of an abnormality in the enzyme activity of the myocardial cell are merely attractive hypotheses. Abnormal oxygen dissociation may be involved but apparently it is not a consistent default.

Neither the treatment nor the prognosis has been defined.

REFERENCES

1. Likoff, W., Kasparian, H., Segal, B. L., Novack, P., and Lehman. J. S.: Clinical correlations of coronary arteriography, Am. J. Cardiol. *16*:159, 1966.
2. Proudfit, W.: Symposium: Coronary Arteriography, presented at meeting of American Heart Association, Scientific Session, October, 1964.
3. Cohen, L. S., Elliott, W. G., Klein, M. D., and Gorlin, R.: Coronary heart disease: clinical cinearteriographic and metabolic correlations, Am. J. Cardiol. *17*:153, 1965.
4. Likoff, W., Kasparian, H., Segal, B. L., Forman, H., and Novack, P.: Coronary arteriography: correlation with electrocardiographic response to measured ercexise, Am. J. Cardiol. *18*:160, 1966.
5. Proudfit, W. L., Shirey, E. K., and Sones, M.: Clinical Features of Angina Pectoris, Related to Extent of Arterial Obstruction, Demonstrated by Selective Cinecoronary arteriography, presented at meeting of American Heart Association, Scientific Session, October, 1966.
6. Likoff, W., Segal, B. L., and Kasparian, H.: Paradox of normal selective coronary arteriograms in patients considered to have unmistakable coronary heart disease, New England J. Med. *276*:1063, 1967.
7. Eliot, R. S., and Mizukani, H.: Oxygen affinity of hemoglobin in persons with acute myocardial infarction and in smokers, Circulation *34*:331, 1966.
8. Eliot, R. S., and Bratt, G. T.: Paradox of myocardial ischemia and necrosis in young women with normal coronary arteriograms—relationship to anomalous hemoglobin-oxygen dissociation, Am. J. Cardiol. *21*:98, 1968.
9. Neill, W. A., Kassebaum, D. G., and Judkins, M. P.: Myocardial hypoxia as the basis for angina pectoris in a patient with normal coronary arteriogram, New England J. Med. *279*:789, 1968.

Papillary Muscle Dysfunction

George E. Burch, John H. Phillips, and Nicholas P. DePasquale

Although the physiologic significance of the papillary muscles in normal mitral and tricuspid valve function has been known for years, only recently has emphasis been given to disorders of papillary muscle function in clinical cardiology. Since various forms of papillary muscle dysfunction, at least in part, are among the most common causes of pathologic murmurs originating from the atrioventricular valves, it is important that facts and concepts regarding these disorders be placed in proper general perspective. This is the chief purpose of this presentation.

Only a brief review of the pertinent anatomy, physiology, pathology and clinical manifestations of papillary muscle dysfunction can be provided here. It should be noted that the orientation will be toward the mitral valve apparatus, but the concepts as elaborated may easily be applied to tricuspid valve function. Further, although papillary muscle dysfunction may arise from a number of disease processes, chief emphasis in this presentation will be toward that associated with coronary heart disease. For more detailed information covering various specific aspects of the problem of papillary muscle dysfunction, the reader is referred to earlier published reports from this laboratory.

ANATOMY

Structures of importance to normal mitral valve function range in spatial continuity from the atrial muscle to the ventricular muscle and include the valve ring, the valve leaflets, the chordae tendineae and the papillary muscles (Fig. 1). As will be evident, the vascular supply, the pacemaker system and the conducting system are other structures of importance to normal valve function.

The left ventricle has two groups of papillary muscles, the posteromedial group and the antero-

Supported by grants HE0-6769 from the National Heart Institutes of the U.S. Public Health Service, the Rudolph Matas Memorial Fund for the Kate Prewitt Hess Laboratory and the Rowell A. Billups Fund for Research in Heart Disease.

MITRAL VALVE APPARATUS
(Normal)

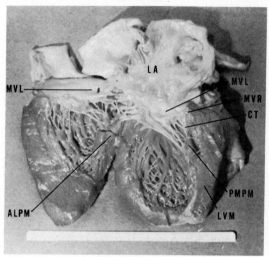

FIG. 1. Photograph of an open normal heart. Shown are the left atrium (LA), mitral valve leaflets (MVL), mitral valve ring (MVR), chordae tendineae (CT), anterolateral and posteromedial papillary muscles (ALPM and PMPM), and left ventricular muscle (LVM). (G.P. *11*:99, Non.1969)

lateral group. The former arises from the posterior wall of the left ventricle near the junction with the interventricular septum and receives its blood supply through tributaries from the circumflex branch of the left coronary artery and/or from the posterior descending branches of the right coronary artery. The anterolateral group arises from the free wall of the left ventricle and receives its blood supply from tributaries of the circumflex artery. The distribution of the blood supply to the papillary muscles is schematically presented in Figure 2. Details of the distribution of arterial vessels in these muscles are shown in Fig. 3, *A* and *B*. These small papillary arteries course longitudinally to the apex of the papillary muscles where they terminate in the arterioles, capillaries, venules and small veins. At

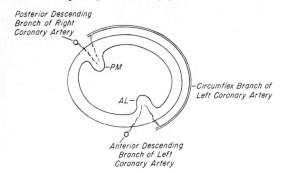

FIG. 2. Schematic representation of blood supply to the papillary muscles of the left ventricle. (Heart Bull. 17; 4, Jan.-Feb., 1968)

times the papillary arteries form arcuate anastomes near the distal ends of the muscle. From Figure 3, *B* it is evident that the arterial blood supply to the papillary muscles usually represents the most remote extensions of the coronary arterial system. Considering the extreme mechanical demands placed on these muscles and the relative remoteness of their vascular supply from the epicardial location of the main coronary vessels, it is not surprising that the papillary muscles are frequently the site of ischemic lesions.

Although not commonly conceived, the pacemaker system and the conducting system of the heart are structures of importance to normal mitral valve function. As endocardial structures, the papillary muscles are richly supplied with fibers of the Purkinje system. Along with the pacemaker

system, this assures co-ordinated and appropriate sequential activation of the various structures of the mitral apparatus and early activation of the papillary muscles in the time course of ventricular depolarization.

PHYSIOLOGY

It is obvious that the purpose of the mitral apparatus is to allow easy transfer of blood from the

FIG. 3. *Below. A*, Longitudinal section through the ventricles of a human heart. The arterial vessels have been injected and filled with a finely divided barium sulfate (Micropaque) suspension in 10 per cent formalin. The whitish globules represent areas of extravasation of the barium. Shown are left ventricular cavity (LVC), right ventricular cavity (RVC), interventricular septum (IVS), left ventricular free wall (LVFW), papillary muscle (PM), extravasated barium (Ba). The area enclosed by the rectangle represents that portion illustrated in B. *B*, Stereoscopic presentation of x-ray photographs of barium-filled vessels in the area of the left ventricle demarcated by the rectangle in A. This figure may be viewed stereoscopically by placing a card between the two portions of the illustration and slowly moving the illustration away or toward one's eyes until a threedimensional relationship is appreciated. With practice and adjustment of visual distance it is possible to obtain a three-dimensional image of this illustration with the unaided eyes. For those unable to do this, stereoscopic lenses may be employed. In this typical example, note the linear distribution of the arteries of the papillary muscle coursing longitudinally through the papillary muscle and also the arcuate anastomosis of some of these vessels near the muscle tip. With such a vascular distribution as illustrated here, one can readily appreciate with ischemia the vulnerability of the distal areas of the papillary muscle. (Am. Heart. J. *75:*399, 1968)

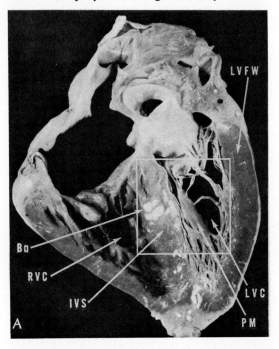

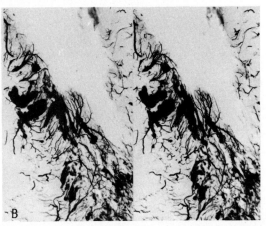

atrium to the ventricle during the diastolic ventricular filling period and to prevent regurgitation of blood from the ventricle to the atrium during ventricular systole and the protodiastolic phase and isometric relaxation phase of early diastole. The interrelationships of the time courses of changes in intracardiac pressure with valvular movements can be appreciated by careful study of the accompanying diagram (Fig. 4). It is in the prevention of regurgitation that the papillary muscles exercise their primary function, and this action is diagrammatically illustrated in Figure 5. For the purpose of simplification in this and other similar illustrations, a single chorda tendinea is depicted as supplying a single mitral leaflet. Actually, chordae tendineae from both papillary muscles supply the corresponding half of each mitral leaflet. Thus, the function of a papillary muscle is reflected in both valve leaflets, and any malfunction of a muscle would affect both leaflets to some degree.

Normal mitral valve function evidently begins

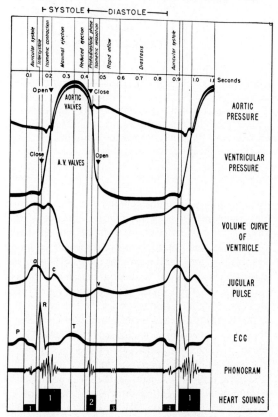

FIG. 4. Temporal relationship of the time-courses of various cardiac events during a cardiac cycle. In order to appreciate fully the temporal sequence of mitral valve function, this figure should be studied carefully. (*A Primer of Cardiology,* Philadelphia, Lea and Febiger, 1964.)

during atrial systole as the augmented ventricular filling and distention during this time bring the leaflets into loose apposition. Shortly after this period and during the initial inscription of the QRS complex of the surface electrocardiogram, the endocardial areas of the myocardium, including the papillary muscles, are excited, initiating mechanical ventricular systole. That the papillary muscles are among the myocardial areas to be activated earliest is important to the maintenance of valvular competence from the earliest rise of intraventricular pressure. The dynamic and finely co-ordinated nature of the function of the papillary muscles and chordae tendineae to restrain the movements of the mitral valve leaflets during the remainder of ventricular systole should be obvious.

Normal mitral valve function depends upon maintenance of the proper spatial relationships of the papillary muscles, chordae tendineae and mitral valve leaflets throughout the cardiac cycle. Of further importance is the fact that in the normal-sized heart, the long axis of the papillary muscles are oriented almost perpendicular to the atrioventricular ring. This orientation provides a mechanical advantage in that tension developed by the papillary muscles is applied almost perpendicular to the mitral valve leaflets. This mechanical advantage is of importance because the papillary muscles must support a large force acting upon the mitral valve. This force is equal to the intraventricular pressure times the cross-sectional area of the atrioventricular orifice. Theoretic considerations suggest that each papillary muscle of the left ventricle supports a total peak load of 19 tons during a 24-hour period for a heart rate of 70 beats per minute and an arterial blood pressure of 120/80 mm. Hg. In the dilated heart, however, the papillary muscles migrate laterally so that the tension developed by these muscles is applied tangentially to the mitral leaflets. The greater the lateral displacement of the papillary muscles, the greater the mechanical disadvantage.

During the isovolumetric phase of ventricular systole the rapid rise in intraventricular pressure (Fig. 4) causes the mitral valve leaflets to bulge towards the left atrium and to come into firm surface contact with each other, thus closing the atrioventricular orifice. This effect of intracavitary pressure upon closure of the mitral valve continues throughout systole (Figs. 5, 6). The movement of the mitral valve leaflets towards the atrium pulls the chordae tendineae taut. During the ejection phase of ventricular systole, the apex of the left ventricle moves toward the atrioventricular orifice. Since the moment-to-moment length of the chordae tendineae is relatively fixed, the papillary muscles must shorten

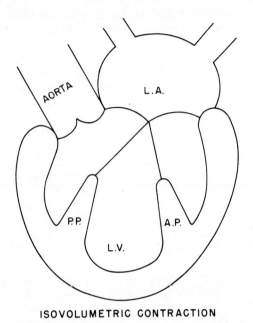

ISOVOLUMETRIC CONTRACTION

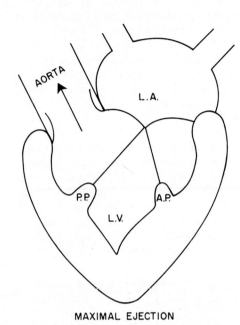

MAXIMAL EJECTION

FIG. 5.   Normal papillary muscle function. For purpose of simplification in this and other similar illustrations, a single chorda tendinea is depicted as supplying a single mitral leaflet. Actually, chordae tendineae from both papillary muscles supply the corresponding half of each mitral leaflet. During iso-volumetric contraction the mitral leaflets are in contact and bulge toward the atrium, pulling the chordae tendineae taut as intraventricular pressure increases. As the musculature of the ventricle shortens during ejection, contraction of the posteromedial (PP) and anterolateral (AP) papillary muscles maintains a proper distance between the papillary muscles and valve leaflets, thus keeping the mitral valve closed during systole.   (Arch. Int. Med. *112*:112, 1963)

during systole to maintain the proper distance between the base of the papillary muscles and the atrioventricular orifice in order to prevent eversion of a portion of the mitral leaflets into the left atrium. Thus, contraction of the papillary muscles takes up the slack which would have been created in the chordae tendineae as a result of the diminution in the size of the ventricular cavity.

PATHOLOGIC PHYSIOLOGY

Significant alteration in the normal spatial relationships of the papillary muscles, chordae tendineae and atrioventricular orifice at any time during ventricular systole may result in abnormal function of the mitral leaflets manifested by mitral valve incompetence with regurgitation. Such manifestation is the hemodynamic and thus the clinical expression of papillary muscle dysfunction. Regardless of the basic etiology or disease process, this dysfunction may result from a number of mechan-

isms including normal papillary muscle contraction but improper spatial orientation, proper spatial orientation but ineffective contraction, proper spatial orientation and contraction but improper temporal expression, or a combination of these. This triphasic dysfunction potential is diagrammatically depicted in Figure 7. Abnormally great tension or restraint exerted by the papillary muscles on the mitral leaflets may pull the leaflets into the ventricle so that firm apposition of the leaflets necessary for closure of the atrioventricular orifice cannot occur. In contrast, inadequate restraint of the leaflets allows a portion of each leaflet to evert into the atrium, again preventing satisfactory closure of the atrioventricular orifice. It is through such basic mechanisms that specific disease processes cause papillary muscle dysfunction and thus mitral regurgitation. The character and time course of this mitral regurgitation vary depending upon the nature of the disease process and the papillary muscle dysfunction induced. Thus, the character of the

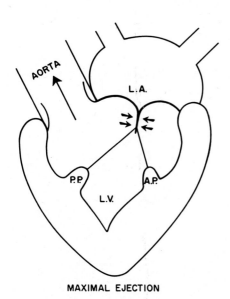

MAXIMAL EJECTION

Fig. 6. Sketch showing the effect of left ventricular intracavitary pressure in firmly sealing the
overlapping edges of the mitral valve leaflets.
(G.P.*11*:99,Nov.1969)

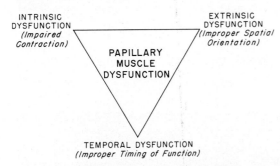

Fig. 7. The triphasic dysfunction potential of
the papillary muscle. Consult text for details.

clinical expression of this dysfunction (particularly
the associated murmur) may provide a clue to the
type of underlying specific etiology.

ETIOLOGY AND PATHOGENESIS OF PAPILLARY MUSCLE DYSFUNCTION

Dysfunction of the papillary muscles may arise
from one or more specific disease processes. A
classification of these various diseases is presented
in Table 1. The discussion to follow is purposely
limited to papillary muscle dysfunction secondary to
coronary heart disease. The concepts involved here,
however, may easily be extended by the reader to
understand dysfunction accompanying other disease
states.

TABLE 1
Etiology of Papillary Muscle Dysfunction

Circulatory insufficiency (ischemia)
  Angina pectoris
  Infarction of papillary muscle
    Acute
    Chronic (fibrosis)
  Systemic circulatory disturbances (hypotension,
    erythrocytosis, anoxia, hematometakinesia, etc.)
Left ventricular dilatation
  Generalized
  Localized (aneurysm)
Nonischemic atrophy of papillary muscle
  Senile
  Associated with cachexia
Defective development of papillary muscle apparatus
  Congenitally long or short papillary muscle or
    chordae tendineae
  Ectopic origin of papillary muscle
  Ectopic insertion of chordae tendineae
Endocardial disease
  Endocarditis
  Endocardial fibroelastosis
  Endomyocardial fibrosis
Heart muscle disease
  Inflammatory (myocarditis)
  Degenerative cardiomyopathy
  Infiltrative (metastatic carcinoma, amyloidosis)
  Neoplastic (primary tumor of myocardium)
Disturbances in the time course of papillary muscle
  activation and contraction
Rupture of papillary muscle or chordae tendineae

Circulatory insufficiency of one form or another
is probably the most common cause of papillary
muscle dysfunction. During episodes of ischemia
or following infarction of a papillary muscle, the
muscle is rendered completely or partially incapable
of contraction. Providing that the heart is not
enlarged, the normal spatial relationships of the
elements of the mitral valve apparatus are maintained during isovolumetric contraction and the
valve is competent (Fig. 8). During ventricular
ejection, however, the slack created in the chordae
tendineae by the apex-to-base movement of the left
ventricle is not compensated for because of failure
of the ischemic or infarcted papillary muscle to
shorten. Thus, a portion of each valve leaflet everts
into the left atrium and mitral regurgitation results.
If the ischemia is only transient, as during an episode
of angina pectoris, the clinical signs of mitral regurgitation rapidly subside as the ischemic papillary
muscle regains the ability to contract. Following
infarction of a papillary muscle, however, the clinical
signs are more persistent. The cardiac autopsy
findings from a patient with papillary muscle
dysfunction secondary to infarction of the papillary
muscle are illustrated in Figure 9.

When ischemic disease results in diffuse scarring,
degeneration or atrophy of a papillary muscle, the

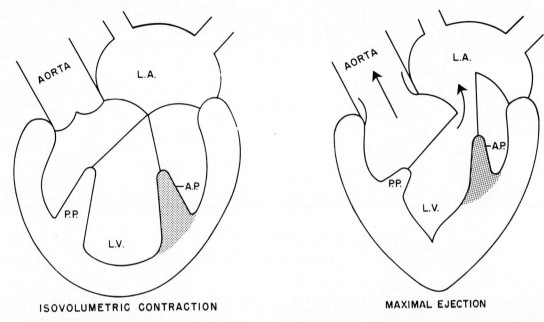

ISOVOLUMETRIC CONTRACTION   MAXIMAL EJECTION

FIG. 8.   Papillary muscle dysfunction following infarction or ischemia of the anterolateral papillary muscle. Although the papillary muscle cannot contract (shorten), the mitral valve leaflets remain closed during isovolumetric contraction. However, failure of the papillary muscle to shorten during ejection creates a situation in which the portion of each mitral leaflet supplied by chordae tendineae from the non-contracting papillary muscle everts toward the atrium. The murmur, in this instance, begins after iso-volumetric contraction. Ventricular dilatation may modify the characteristics of the murmur. (Arch. Int. Med. *112:*112, 1963)

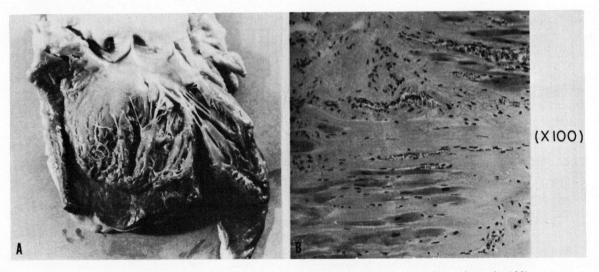

FIG. 9.   *A*, Recent gross photo of infarcted papillary muscle. *B*, Microscopic sections. (×100)

retracted muscle pulls a portion of each mitral leaflet into the ventricle so that the valve is incompetent even during isovolumetric contraction (Fig. 10). During the systolic ejection phase, the apex-to-base movement of the left ventricle may permit better apposition of the mitral valve leaflets

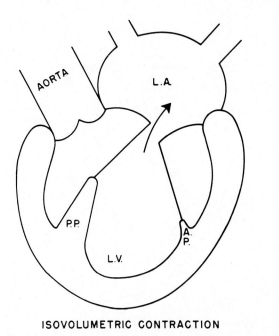 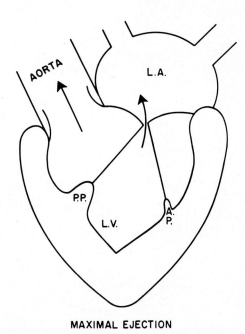

ISOVOLUMETRIC CONTRACTION   MAXIMAL EJECTION

Fig. 10.   Fibrosis and atrophy of the anterolateral papillary muscle are depicted as pulling a portion of the mitral valve into the ventricle during isovolumetric contraction and allowing a portion of the valve to evert into the atrium during ventricular ejection. The resulting murmur is variable depending upon the degree of fibrosis and the state of the myocardium. (G. P. *11*:99, Nov. 1969)

than during isovolumetric contraction, so that the degree of valve incompetence decreases.

Dilatation of the left ventricle is a frequent cause of papillary muscle dysfunction and its discussion is appropriate here since coronary artery disease, with or without infarction, is commonly the basic disease process. With uncomplicated dilatation the papillary muscles may contract normally but the spatial relationships of these muscles, the chordae tendineae and the atrioventricular orifice are altered by the downward and lateral migration of the wall of the left ventricle away from the A-V orifice. Thus, the valve leaflets are pulled downward into the ventricle so that they are incompetent (Fig. 11). In addition, as noted earlier, the oblique orientation of the papillary muscles to the atrioventricular orifice results in a mechanical disadvantage. Since the valve leaflets are pulled downward into the left ventricle in the dilated heart, the valve is incompetent during isovolumetric contraction. However, as the left ventricle contracts, the valve leaflets may be brought into better apposition so that the degree of mitral incompetence decreases as systole progresses (Fig. 11). Left ventricular dilatation is frequently complicated by a diseased papillary muscle with impaired contractility. How this

combination can result in mitral regurgitation throughout systole is illustrated in Figure 12.

At times, ventricular dilatation is not generalized but rather is localized to a given area of the myocardium, such as with a ventricular aneurysm. Frequently the base of a papillary muscle is incorporated into one of these aneurysms. The paradoxical movement of the aneurysm outwards during ventricular contraction in such a situation increases mitral incompetence throughout the course of systole (Fig. 13). Whether or not the incorporated papillary muscle is capable of contraction would influence the character of the associated mitral regurgitation.

Disturbances in the time course of papillary muscle activation and contraction may occur in the context of coronary heart disease through such mechanisms as premature ventricular contractions, bundle branch block, defective intrinsic intraventricular conduction and artificial extrinsic electrical cardiac pacing. It is clear that in order to maintain the proper spatial relationship of the various elements of the mitral valve apparatus, not only must the papillary muscles be structurally and functionally normal, but they must also be activated in proper time sequence relative to activation of the free wall and other parts of the left ventricle. Activa-

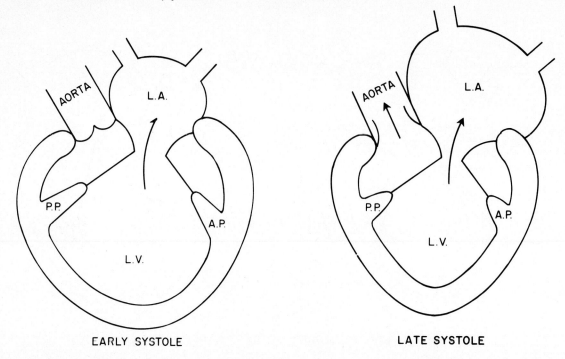

EARLY SYSTOLE   LATE SYSTOLE

FIG. 11.   Left ventricular dilatation results in centrifugal migration of the papillary muscle away from the atrioventricular orifice with retraction of the mitral leaflets into the ventricle. In addition, both papillary muscles are at a mechanical disadvantage because they must exert tension against intraventricular pressure more tangentially than they normally would. The murmur begins immediately after the first heart sound because the valve is incompetent during isovolumetric contraction. However, it may decrease in intensity during ventricular ejection because of better approximation of the valve leaflets. (Am. Heart J. *75*:399, 1968).

tion of a papillary muscle either too early or too late may result in some degree of mitral incompetence.

Although relatively rare, papillary muscle rupture is another type of papillary muscle dysfunction encountered in coronary heart disease. The posteromedial papillary muscle is the one that ruptures most frequently and the rupture is almost always secondary to myocardial infarction and necrosis. How this event would result in wide-open mitral regurgitation, should be obvious.

CLINICAL MANIFESTATIONS OF PAPILLARY MUSCLE DYSFUNCTION SECONDARY TO CORONARY HEART DISEASE

Symptomatology

In general, papillary muscle dysfunction does not produce any specific symptomatology. The associated symptoms are more related to the disease process responsible for the muscle dysfunction than to the dysfunction itself. It should be noted, however, that when papillary muscle dysfunction develops suddenly, and particularly when it is of marked degree (e.g., papillary muscle rupture), the symptoms of left ventricular failure are to be expected. Since ischemic heart disease is the most common cause of papillary muscle dysfunction, it is to be expected that symptoms of angina pectoris, myocardial infarction and congestive heart failure are frequently associated.

Physical Findings

The cardinal physical manifestation of papillary muscle dysfunction is the systolic murmur of mitral valve insufficiency. Considering the many possible basic mechanisms of papillary muscle dysfunction discussed earlier, it should be obvious that the associated murmur may present with many different characteristics. The murmur may be early or late in onset, short or long (even holosystolic) in duration, early, mid or late systolic in timing, and decrescendo, crescendo or crescendo-decrescendo in configura-

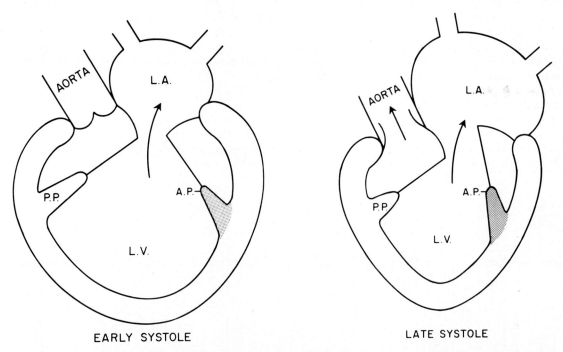

EARLY SYSTOLE LATE SYSTOLE

FIG. 12. Papillary muscle dysfunction secondary to both left ventricular dilatation and infarction of a muscle. Note how this combination results in regurgitation that starts with isovolumetric contraction and continues or even increases throughout the remainder of systole. (G. P. *11*:99, Nov. 1969)

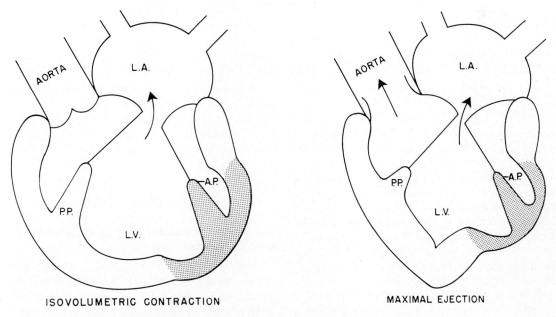

ISOVOLUMETRIC CONTRACTION MAXIMAL EJECTION

FIG. 13. Papillary muscle dysfunction resulting from the incorporation of the anterolateral papillary muscle into an aneurysm of the left ventricle. (Arch. Int. Med. *112*:112, 1963)

tion. Thus, relating the origin of any one murmur to papillary muscle dysfunction frequently has to be done in light of the entire clinical picture. There is one type of murmur, when present, however, which in itself should suggest the possibility of papillary muscle dysfunction. This is the murmur which occurs primarily because of failure of a papillary muscle to contract and it usually occurs in the absence of significant localized or generalized myocardial dilatation or other complicating factors. It is characterized by delayed onset in systole with a crescendo-decrescendo configuration (diamond shape) with mid-

and congestive failure. Under these circumstances the mitral valve leaflets would be retracted downward into the ventricle at the end of ventricular filling so that the murmur may not be delayed in onset and may actually begin with the first heart sound.

The constancy of the physical findings in any one patient with a noncontracting papillary muscle depends on the activity of the underlying disease process. The murmur accompanying healed infarction or fibrosis of the papillary muscles tends to be constant even over extended periods. However,

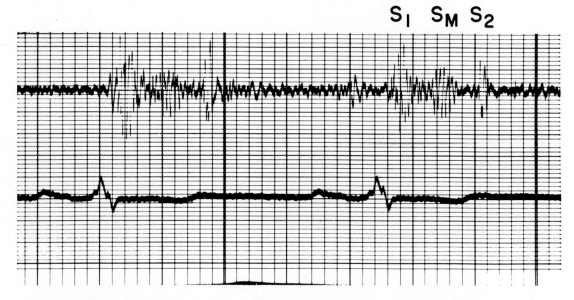

FIG. 14.   Phonocardiogram and electrocardiogram from a patient with papillary muscle dysfunction. Note the mid-systolic accentuation of the murmur. S_1 = first heart sound; S_2 = second heart sound; SM = systolic murmur of papillary muscle dysfunction. (G. P. *11:*99, Nov. 1969)

systolic accentuation (Fig. 14). Thus, it frequently appears to have the qualities of an "ejection" murmur. It is soft to moderately loud in intensity and tends to be somewhat "blowing" in quality. It is best heard at the apex, radiates somewhat to the axilla, and is only rarely associated with a thrill. The murmur is occasionally well transmitted to the aortic area which may cause confusion with aortic stenosis. The mechanism of the murmur as described is best understood in view of the time course of hemodynamic changes and spatial relationships of the elements of the mitral valve apparatus. It should be emphasized, however, that failure of a papillary muscle to contract is not invariably associated with such a murmur as described above. Myocardial infarction is a frequent cause of a noncontracting papillary muscle, and this combination of lesions is commonly accompanied by left ventricular dilatation

in instances where the underlying processes are changing, for example angina pectoris, coronary insufficiency, evolving acute infarction, and variable left ventricular dilatation, the associated murmur may change over periods of a few seconds to several days or longer.

LABORATORY DATA

Electrocardiogram in Coronary Heart Disease Involving Papillary Muscles

Ischemic disease with infarction and/or fibrosis of the papillary muscles of the left ventricle may be recognized by various alterations recorded in the surface electrocardiogram. Careful clinical and electrocardiographic study with follow-up autopsy correlation has been in progress in this laboratory for a number of years. Over this period it has become possible to recognize certain electrocardiographic features which show a high correlation with the presence of papillary muscle dysfunction clinically and with the subsequent autopsy demonstration of ischemic disease in the papillary muscles. In general and for the purposes of discussion, we have grouped these electrocardiographic changes into three types, but it should be clearly noted that this classification is somewhat arbitrary and there is considerable overlapping among these types. Type I consists of moderate depression of junction J with concavity-upward or slight convexity-upward deformity with depression of the ST segment (Fig. 15). Type II consists of slight-to-moderate depression of junction J with a prominent convexity-upward deformity of the ST segment and terminal inversion of the T wave (Fig. 16). Type III shows marked depression of junction J and marked depression of the ST segment (Fig. 17). Type III is frequently interpreted as "acute subendocardial infarction," but in our experience papillary muscle involvement is the rule in such

instances. It should be emphasized that prolongation of the QT interval along with abnormalities of the T-U segment or U wave is extremely common in each of the three types mentioned. Furthermore, any of the types may occur with or without Q waves of associated transmural infarction or evidence of ventricular aneurysm (Fig. 18). In general, with predominant involvement of the anterolateral papillary muscle group, the electrocardiographic changes described above are most pronounced in leads I, aV_L, V_5, V_6, whereas with predominant involvement of the posteromedial group, these changes are found especially in leads II, III, aV_F, and/or V_1 through V_4. Because simultaneous involvement of both muscle groups does occur, there may be some overlapping of the electrocardiographic findings.

Other Laboratory Data in Papillary Muscle Dysfunction Secondary to Coronary Artery Disease

Phonocardiography may aid in displaying the

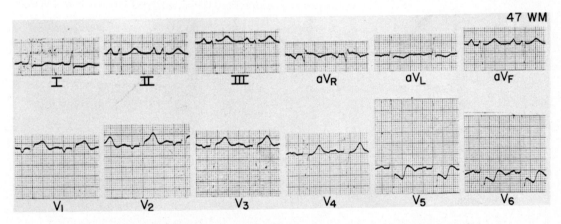

FIG. 15.   Electrocardiogram of Type I pattern. (G. P. *11*:99, Nov. 1969)

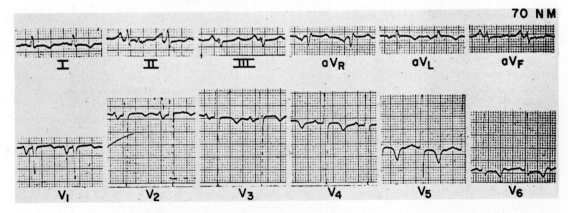

FIG. 16.   Electrocardiogram of Type II pattern. (G. P. *11*:99, Nov. 1969)

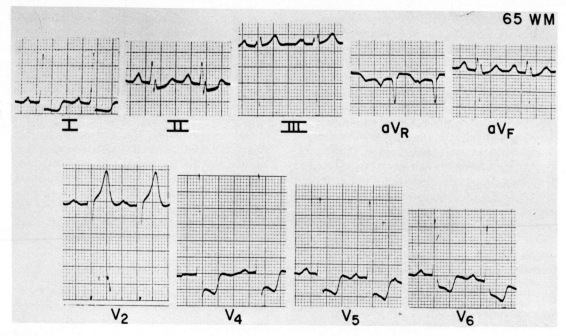

FIG. 17.   Electrocardiogram of Type III pattern.

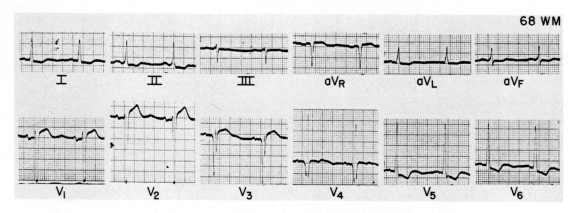

FIG. 18.   Electrocardiogram of a patient with a transmural infarct.

timing and configuration of the associated murmur of papillary muscle dysfunction and in confirming the auscultatory characteristics described above (Fig. 14). Cardiac catheterization with cardioangiography and dye-dilution techniques has confirmed the presence of mitral regurgitation in patients with papillary muscle dysfunction.

DIFFERENTIAL DIAGNOSIS

The murmur of papillary muscle dysfunction must be differentiated from systolic murmurs of other causes and origins. Chief among those for distinction are those of mitral valve leaflet deformity (e.g., rheumatic), valvular aortic stenosis, hyper-

trophic subaortic stenosis, rupture of a papillary muscle or chordae tendineae, rupture of the interventricular septum, and the late systolic murmur syndrome. Following are some clues helpful in differential diagnosis, but it should be clearly emphasized that these represent gross generalizations only and exceptions are common.

Because of mechanisms described above it should be clear that the murmurs of papillary muscle dysfunction may be extremely variable from one patient to another. In general, the murmur is blowing in quality, loudest at the apex, frequently radiates to the axilla and occasionally to the aortic area. The murmur becomes softer after amyl nitrite inhalation. Splitting of the second heart sound at the pulmonic area is usually normal and a thrill is infrequent. The electrocardiogram frequently, although certainly not invariably, shows evidence of papillary muscle disease with or without associated transmural infarction. The symptoms are generally those of ischemic heart disease and its complications. Long-term survival after diagnosis is not uncommon.

Systolic murmurs originating from deformity primarily of the mitral valve leaflets (e.g., rheumatic) are generally holosystolic with a plateau configuration. They are loudest at the apex, radiate well to the axilla and are blowing to moderately harsh in quality. They become softer with amyl nitrite inhalation. The two components of the second sound are frequently widely split. A diastolic rumbling murmur is a common accompaniment and a systolic thrill is frequent. Chest x-ray commonly shows left atrial enlargement; mitral calcification occurs in many. The electrocardiogram frequently shows left atrial overload or coarse atrial fibrillation along with left and/or right ventricular hypertrophy. There is frequently a history of rheumatic fever and a murmur from an early age. Long-term survival is certainly not uncommon.

The murmur of valvular aortic stenosis not infrequently is well heard or actually loudest at the apex and thus must enter into differential diagnosis. In general, the murmur is "ejection" in character, harsh in quality, loudest at the aortic area and radiates well into the neck. It becomes louder after amyl nitrite. The two components of the second sound are narrowly or even paradoxically split and an aortic insufficiency murmur is common. A systolic thrill at the aortic area and in the neck along with a narrow pulse pressure aid in diagnosis. X-ray demonstration of calcium in the aortic valve and aortic root dilatation is frequent. The electrocardiogram may show left ventricular hypertrophy with "strain." Angina and exertional syncope are frequent symptoms.

The systolic murmur of hypertrophic subaortic stenosis is frequently loudest near the cardiac apex and may mimic primary mitral regurgitation. It is generally late in onset and moderately harsh in quality. It becomes louder after amyl nitrite inhalation and during the Valsalva maneuver. The two components of the second sound are narrowly or paradoxically split and S_3 and S_4 gallops are very common. A pulsus biferiens is frequent as is a paradoxical change in the pulse volume after the compensatory pause of a premature beat. X-ray may show left ventricular enlargement but without aortic root dilatation. The electrocardiogram frequently shows left ventricular hypertrophy along with deep Q waves. Exertional dyspnea and syncope are common and may be worsened by digitalis therapy.

Papillary muscle or chordae tendineae rupture presents the sudden onset of a holosystolic murmur with mid-systolic accentuation. It is usually moderately harsh and loudest at the apex but may radiate quite well to the aortic area and neck. It becomes softer after amyl nitrite inhalation. Wide splitting of the second sound components, S_3 and S_4 gallops, and a systolic thrill are common. X-ray reveals cardiomegaly and pulmonary congestion and the electrocardiogram frequently shows a recent myocardial infarction. Distinction from papillary muscle dysfunction is usually not difficult since with rupture severe congestive failure and a rapid downhill course to death are expected.

Rupture of the interventricular septum accompanying acute myocardial infarction presents the sudden onset of a holosystolic murmur with mid-systolic accentuation which is usually loudest near the left lower sternal border, harsh in quality, and does not radiate well. A thrill is common. X-rays show cardiomegaly and pulmonary congestion and the electrocardiogram reveals a recent septal infarction. The clinical course is generally rapidly downhill with early death.

The late systolic murmur syndrome is a complex and interesting disorder of apparent congenital-familial origin. Prognosis for long life is excellent providing electrocardiographic QT prolongation and premature beats with repetitive firing are not present. The murmur is usually quite delayed in onset and is crescendo or crescendo-decrescendo in configuration. It is fairly well localized to the apex and is frequently musical in quality. A late systolic click is a common accompaniment. Routine chest x-rays are usually normal but the electrocardiogram may show Q waves, QT or ST abnormalities and premature beats.

TREATMENT OF PAPILLARY MUSCLE DYSFUNCTION SECONDARY TO CORONARY HEART DISEASE

Little need be said regarding the medical treatment of ischemic papillary muscle dysfunction since it is simply the treatment of ischemic heart disease and its complications. Mention should be made, however, concerning the place of cardiac surgery (prosthetic mitral valve replacements, aneurysmectomy, etc.) in management. At the present time it is our feeling that surgery has very little to offer in this regard. In spite of our experience with hundreds of patients with primary ischemic papillary muscle dysfunction, we have referred none for cardiac surgery to date. It would appear that in institutions where this has been done, an extremely high mortality rate is being encountered.

REFERENCES

1. Actis-Dato, A., and Milocco, I.: Anomalous attachment of the mitral valve to the ventricular wall, Am. J. Cardiol. *17*:278, 1966.
2. Barlow, J. B., Pocock, W. A., Marchand, P., and Denny, M.: The significance of late systolic murmurs, Am. Heart J. *66*:443, 1963.
3. Barlow, J. B.: Conjoint clinic on the clinical significance of late systolic murmurs and non-ejection systolic clicks, J. Chronic Dis. *18*:665, 1965.
4. Barlow, J. B., and Bosman, C. K.: Aneurysmal protrusion of the posterior leaflet of the mitral valve, An ausculatory-electro-cardiographic syndrome, Am. Heart J. *71*:166, 1966.
5. Bond, V. F., Jr., Wefare, C. R., Lide, T. N., and McMillan, R. L.: Perforation of interventricular septum following myocardial infarction, Ann. Int. Med. *38*:706, 1953.
6. Bowers, D.: An electrocardiographic pattern associated with mitral valve deformity in Marfan's syndrome, Circulation *23*:30, 1961.
7. Brock, R. C.: The surgical and pathological anatomy of the mitral valve, Brit. Heart J. *14*:489, 1952.
8. Brockman, S. K.: Mechanism of the movements of the atrioventricular valves, Am. J. Cardiol. *17*:682, 1966.
9. Burch, G. E., Ray, C. T., and Cronvich, J. A.: The George Fahr Lecture: Certain mechanical peculiarties of the human cardiac pump in normal and diseased states, Circulation *5*:504, 1952.
10. Burch, G. E., and Walsh, J. J.: Cardiac insufficiency in chronic alcoholism, Am. J. Cardiol. *6*:864, 1960.
11. Burch, G. E., DePasquale, N. P., and Phillips, J. H.: Clinical manifestations of papillary muscle dysfunction, Arch. Int. Med. *112*:112, 1963.
12. Burch, G. E., and Phillips, J. H.: Murmurs of aortic stenosis and mitral insufficiency masquerading as one another, Am. Heart J. *66*:439, 1963.
13. Burch, G. E., and DePasquale, N. P.: Viral myocarditis, *in* Ciba Foundation Symposium on Cardiomyopathies, London, J. & A. Churchill, Ltd., 1964, p. 376.
14. Burch, G. E., and DePasquale, N. P.: Time course of tension in papillary muscles of the heart, J. A. M. A. *192*:701, 1965.
15. Case records of Massachusetts General Hospital, New England J. Med. *267*:1033, 1962.
16. Chiechi, M. A., Lees, W. M., and Thompson, R.: Functional anatomy of the normal mitral valve, J. Thoracic Surg. *32*:378, 1956.
17. Davila, J. C., and Palmer, T. E.: The mitral valve, Arch. Surg. *84*:174, 1962.
18. DePasquale, N. P., and Burch, G. E.: The necropsy incidence of gross scars or acute infarction of the papillary muscles of the left ventricle, Am. J. Cardiol. *17*:169, 1966.
19. Durrer, D., and van der Tweel, L. H. Excitation of the left ventricular wall of the dog and goat, Ann. New York Acad. Sc. *65*:779, 1957.
20. Edwards, J. E., and Burchell, H. B.: Pathologic anatomy of mitral insufficiency, Proc. Staff Meet. Mayo Clin. *33*:497, 1958.
21. Estes, E. H., Jr., Dalton, F. M., Entman, M. L., Dixon, H. B., II, and Hackel, D. B.: The anatomy and blood supply of the papillary muscles of the left ventricle, Am. Heart J. *71*:356, 1966.
22. Harrison, R. J., Shillingford, J. P., Allen, G. T., and Teare, D.: Perforation of interventricular septum after myocardial infarction, Brit. M. J. *1*:1066, 1961.
23. Henke, R. P., March, H. W., and Hultgren, H. N.: An aid to identification of the murmur of aortic stenosis with atypical localization, Am. Heart J. *60*:354, 1960.
24. Holloway, D. H., Whalen, R. E., and McIntosh, H. D.: Systolic murmur developing after myocardial ischemia or infarction J. A. M. A. *191*:888, 1965.
25. Humphries, J. O., and McKusick, V. A.: Differentiation of organic and "innocent" systolic murmurs, Progr. Cardiovas. Dis. *5*:152, 1962.
26. Leatham, A.: Auscultation of the heart, Lancet *2*:703, 1958.
27. Leatham, A.: The value of auscultation in cardiology, Arch. Int. Med. *105*:349, 1960.
28. Lee, W. Y., Cardon, L., and Slodki, S. J.: Perforation of infarcted interventricular septum, Arch. Int. Med. *109*: 731, 1962.
29. Lev, M.: The normal anatomy of the conduction system in man and its pathology in atrioventricular block, Ann. New York Acad. Sc. *111*:817, 1964.
30. Levy, M. J., and Edwards, J. E.: Anatomy of mitral insufficiency, Progr. Cardiovas, Dis. *5*:119, 1962.
31. Mattingly, T. W.: Clinical features and diagnosis of primary myocardial disease. Mod. Concepts. Cardiovas. Dis. *30*:677, 1961.
32. McKusick, V. A. (ed.): Symposium on cardiovascular sound. II. Clinical aspects, Circulation *16*:414, 1957.
33. Osmundson, P. J., Callahan, J. A., and Edwards, J. E.: Mitral insufficiency from ruptured chordae tendineae simulating aortic stenosis, Proc. Staff Meet. Mayo Clin. *33*:235, 1958.
34. Payne, W. S., Hunt, J. C., and Kirklin, J. W.: Surgical repair of ventricular septal defect due to myocardial infarction, J. A. M. A. *183*:603, 1963.
35. Phillips, J. H., and Burch, G. E.: Selected clues in cardiac auscultation, Am. Heart J. *63*:1, 1962.
36. Phillips, J. H., Burch, G. E., and DePasquale, N. P.: The syndrome of papillary muscle dysfunction. Its clinical recognition, Ann. Int. Med. *59*:508, 1963.
37. Phillips, J. H., DePasquale, N. P., and Burch, G. E.: The electrocardiogram in infarction of the anterolateral papillary muscle, Am. Heart J. *66*:338, 1963.
38. Puff, von A., Barrenberg, M., and Goerttler, T.: Röntgenkinematographische Untersuchungen über den Bewegungsmechanismus der Mitralklappe, Fortschr. Geb. Röntgenstrahlen. *102*:607, 1965.
39. Reid, J. V. O.: Mid-systolic clicks, South African M. J. *35*:353, 1961.
40. Robinson, J. S., Stannard, M. M., and Long, M.: Ruptured papillary muscle after acute myocardial infarction, Am. Heart J. *70*:233, 1965.
41. Sanders, R. J., Kern, W. H., and Blount, S. G., Jr.: Preforation of interventricular septum complicating myocardial infarction, Am. Heart J. *51*:736, 1956.
42. Rushmer, R. F., Finlayson, B. L., and Nash, A. A.:

Movements of the mitral valve, Circulation Res. *4*:337, 1956.

43. Segal, B., Kasparian, H., and Likoff, W.: Mitral regurgitation in a patient with the Marfan syndrome, Dis. Chest. *41*:457, 1962.

44. Segal, B. L., and Likoff, W.: Late systolic murmur of mitral regurgitation, Am. Heart J. *67*:757, 1964.

45. Shapiro, H. A., and Weiss, D. R.: Mitral insufficiency due to ruptured chordae tendineae simulating aortic stenosis, New England J. Med. *261*:272, 1959.

46. Shone, J. D., Seller, R. D., Anderson, R. C., Adeams, P., Jr., Lillehei, C. W., and Edwards, J. E.: The developmental complex of "parachute mitral valve," supravalvular ring of left atrium, subaortic stenosis, and coarctation of aorta, Am. J. Cardiol. *11*:714, 1963.

47. Smith, H. L., Essex, H. E., and Baldes, E. J.: A study of the movements of heart valves and of heart sounds, Ann. Int. Med. *33*:1357, 1950.

48. Smith, J. C.: Rupture of a papillary muscle of the heart; report of two cases, Circulation *1*:766, 1950.

49. Tavel, M. E., Campbell, R. W., and Zimmer, J. F.: Late systolic murmur and mitral regurgitation, Am. J. Cardiol. *15*:719, 1966.

50. Van Buchem, F. S. P., Arends, A., and Schroder, E. A.: Endocardial fibroelastosis in adolescents and adults, Brit. Heart J. *21*:229, 1959.

51. Vogelpoel, L., Nellen, M., Swanepoel, A., and Schire, V.: The use of amyl nitrate in the diagnosis of systolic murmurs, Lancet *2*:810, 1959.

Panel Discussion:
Prognosis in Myocardial Infarction; Yesterday and Today

DR. HENRY RUSSEK: It is time for our panel discussion on "The Prognosis in Myocardial Infarction: Yesterday and Today." Volumes have been written about our moderator—Paul Dudley White—but who could possibly assess his worth as a cardiologist, a teacher, an international ambassador and friend. It is always an inspiration and a delight to see and to hear this roving world cardiologist and statesman. It is a pleasure and honor to present Dr. White.

CHAIRMAN WHITE: Thank you Henry Russek. Ladies and gentlemen; I appreciate very much this role that I've been asked to take today as a sort of senior historian, but first I'll tell you about the plans. When I was told that I was to be moderator of this Panel I decided that I would start the ball rolling and talk about my recollections and some facts that I had pulled out of my notes on the prognosis in myocardial infarction so far as it was known or recognized up to the 1930's. Arthur Master, who is quite a good deal younger than I am is to take the 1930's and Henry Russek has just volunteered at my invitation to take the 1940's. William Kannel will cover the 1950's while Eliot Corday will be our spokesman for the 1960's, right up to date, which is quite a job. The sixth member of the panel, who arrived at our house on Tuesday night, I've asked to summarize his viewpoint of what we've been saying and then to say perhaps a little more about what's going on in Czechoslovakia along with his own experience with respect to the prognosis not only of coronary heart disease, but of other things if he'd like to add them.

To set the stage I'd like to quote from the paper that I thought at the time was almost my last contribution: that was twenty-five years ago. It was entitled the "Reversibility of Heart Disease" and it was presented as the oration in medicine at the annual meeting of the Illinois State Medical Society in Chicago on May 16, 1944. Already I had been at it for thirty years and I thought that that might be my final oration. The quotation I'd like to present in

two or three paragraphs sets the stage and refers to the days before my time as well as during my early years. As I said then and as we still say "time marches on and with it there has come during the last twenty-five years, a truly extraordinary development in our understanding and therewith in our treatment of heart disease." The next sentence is italicized, about data just coming into evidence then. *"We have learned that heart disease of every single type is now often reversible."* Surgical operations for congenital heart disease were coming in and I referred to these and other things. "The thrill of being a doctor in these days and to have witnessed this one change alone has been worth more than all the other rewards that come to the medical worker. This will indeed go down in history as a golden age in cardiology."

That was twenty-five years ago. "We think every age is a golden age. Let me recount to you in summary from the history of this field of medicine and end with our present status and the promise of the future. Lest you regard medical history as a dry as dust preoccupation of the superannuated, I would hasten to say that it should be appreciated as a foundation of our medical instruction and a base on which our future progress must be built. We should seize upon the trends and methods of the past and present, that illuminate the path ahead and avoid the pitfalls and the errors, attractive or seductive as they may have at one time seemed in the medical fashions of the day."

"Heart disease was unknown before the year 1500" (and that I italicized). I think that's pretty well settled in history. "Damage of the heart from any cause was considered tantamount to death. Then autopsies on man, which began to be carried out with or without official sanctions of the church or state, revealed old scars of all parts of the heart that had not prevented long and active lives. Slowly heart disease came into more than it's own. By the turn of the eighteenth into the nineteenth century, heart disease was regarded by some, Corvisart for example (he was

Napoleon's physician), as more common than all other ills put together. This was his view in the early 1800's—as more common than all other ills put together and responsible for innumerable symptoms, most of which were trivial. You will quickly realize that some of these patients didn't have heart disease, but some did have who were carrying out very important activities, for example some of Napoleon's marshalls had rheumatic heart disease as proved at autopsy. Yet they carried through."

"But although much work was done and published by workers in pathology through the nineteenth century in the field of heart disease, there was astonishingly little correlation of all this with clinical observations or study of the natural history or evolution of heart disease in the living patient." The next sentence is italicized. *"In fact little progress had been made along these lines as recently as thirty years ago,"* which would now be fifty-five years ago. "When I was a medical student, intern and hospital resident, we were still being taught and believed that coronary heart disease was final and fatal; that the coronary arteries were forever 'end arteries' and that at best we could simply delay a little the day of dissolution and make a bit more comfortable the remaining hours of the victims. This is what we were taught, and now begins the exciting drama of the changes in our point of view and of our active attack on what had seemed so hopeless. A scant twenty years ago," this would now be in the nineteen twenties, "begins the exciting drama. A scant twenty years ago, the procession began with a clear cut proof of the reversibility of the effects of thyroid disease on the heart of both major types: thyrotoxicosis and myxedema. That's about the first time that operations began to be done for thyrotoxicosis and thyroid given for myxedema." Then I skip a few paragraphs and we come chronologically to the most important consideration of all, namely, coronary heart disease. This paper of mine was in 1944.

"It's an astonishing fact that despite all the work and writings of the pathologists during the nineteenth century on the structural changes in the heart associated with serious coronary artery disease including myocardial infarction old and new, that so little was known clinically about coronary heart disease prior to Herrick's classical paper in 1912. Some of his patients survived the attack. Indeed during my medical school days it was still perennially fresh, i.e., the old dispute, between those who thought that angina pectoris was due to disease of the aorta and those who blamed it on coronary insufficiency. Prior to Herrick it was currently believed that occlusion of a large coronary artery meant early death. As a matter of fact even after 1912 for a good

many years a long survival was not thought possible. If a man lived long after acute myocardial infarction or got rid of angina pectoris decubitus, it was a common opinion that the diagnosis had been wrong. So we missed all the favorable cases. During recent years, actually about ten," that carries us back into the thirties, "as a result of growing experience, clinical and electrocardiographic, and particularly of the fundamentally significant observations of Schlesinger and Blumgart"—I'm treading on Arthur Master's decade now—"we have become aware of the large number of cases of coronary heart disease that do well for many years after acute occlusion or the very first attack of angina pectoris. When the realization that this might be true dawned on us a decade or two ago, we began excitedly to report record survivals." One long survival I reported not long ago was thirty-nine years in a patient that I'd seen at the age of fifty-one who died at ninety and whose heart showed an old scar thirty-nine years old. But now such cases are commonplace.

"The answer is of course the development, in major part spontaneously, of a collateral coronary circulation to bypass the point or points of block and so to maintain an adequate circulation to all parts of the myocardium. Thus no longer were the coronary arteries 'end arteries' though functionally they started as such. Under the increasing head of pressure through the years, smaller coronary twigs and their branches become larger and able eventually to transport to the myocardium, when needed, increasing amounts of blood. With ordinary luck this is what happens to the average person as he or she grows older. There may actually be a complete slow occlusion of a major coronary trunk with no heart disease at all due to this spontaneous adjustment and we learned something about this, even before Schlesinger and Blumgart's notable work, from Timothy Leary of Boston who was Professor of Pathology at the Harvard Medical School and who taught us about coronary disease from his pathological experience in the 1920's. I'll never forget an evening that some of us—Sam Levine, Howard Sprague, Herman Blumgart and others— spent with Timothy Leary in the middle 1920's to learn about coronary heart disease. Thus coronary artery disease is not to be confused with coronary heart disease."

"The various measures medical and surgical that have been carried out to stimulate the development of this vital collateral circulation have not been at all outstanding in their successful results"—this was 1944—"Dame Nature still does the best job. It's tremendously important in our treatment to realize this, while not omitting our efforts at therapy. We are writing as to how we might help nature, but they are pretty primitive methods. They may, however, be the best after all."

I'd like to end my notes with reference to a paper that I gave in Memphis, Tennessee, published in the Memphis Medical Journal in 1932 and also in the Emanuel Libman Anniversary Volumes, Volume three, page 1205, that same year based on our experience largely in the 1920's. The title of that paper was "Optimism in the Treatment of Heart Disease." We were just beginning to realize that reversibility in coronary heart disease was possible, that you could have serious angina pectoris decubitus and be perfectly well in a few years or you could survive a moderately large myocardial infarct and be perfectly well, but this hadn't been thought possible in the middle of the 1920's. Now I shall call on Dr. Master who will carry on with the 1930's and give us his views from past experience.

DR. ARTHUR MASTER: Although I'm only forty, I'm sure you won't mind if I reminisce a little. I remember in my third or fourth year in Cornell Medical School, I was so inspired by Carl Wiggers that I went up to him and said: "Professor, I've decided to specialize in heart disease." "What, Master? As soon as you hear a murmur, as soon as you make a diagnosis of heart disease you know the man's going to die." That's how pessimistic he was and of course every time we were on a panel together for years after I would bring up that story. That's changed. Now one other thing I'd like to reminisce on that hasn't changed. In thirty years from now I expect to be a multi-millionaire. I'll tell you how. Paul White always writes to you in his beautiful handwriting. I've been saving those letters and as I say in thirty years I expect to get a lot of money for them.

Now to be a little serious the topic is prognosis in myocardial infarction. There are a lot of variables in myocardial infarction. We used to say in the thirties or forties that the mortality rate in hospitals was forty to fifty or sixty per cent. In private practice, it also varied. We reported papers where we said in private practice in the first attack the mortality was only five per cent. But here's what we didn't know. We're learning now from the coronary care units, from the automobile coronary care units that forty to sixty per cent of patients die of myocardial infarction before they get to a hospital. How are you going to get prognosis from hospital statistics or your own private statistics? Then there's a sign of myocardial infarction about which I talked a little. In 1930 you still expected the patient to have severe pain and Sam Levine in his book, a 1928 edition, wrote that he's often seen excruciating pain. The

patient would writhe in pain and so he did. It wasn't a dissecting aneurysm. We saw patients much later than we do now.

As to diagnostic skill—in the thirties and forties people still died of "acute indigestion"—a great many, although it was heart disease. Then you know the Public Health Service some six years ago said that the worst problem as to prognosis was in New York City and for frequency of myocardial infarction, New York State. But Ed Lew who is the statistician for the Metropolitan Life Insurance Company answered that by saying that it wasn't actually so. He said that we were sicker in New York City but that we had better diagnosticians. There were eight medical schools in the neighborhood and therefore the doctor had more opportunity to learn by experience. In the thirties or forties we had no serum enzyme tests. We only had three leads in electrocardiography, not four let alone twelve and if a patient had pain and any T wave change, we called it coronary occlusion. In other words, we didn't distinguish at all between subendocardial necrosis or ischemia and infarction from transmural involvement. But there is a big difference. Looking back now we mistreated patients. Think of giving patients in shock or very sick patients in heart failure without shock three to five thousand calories of a liquid diet of fruit juices. We gave glucose because the specialized tissue of the heart had glucose and for some reason it was always thought that fluids didn't have to be digested and we really hastened patients on. We mistreated them and that's why my colleague and I came out with the eight hundred calorie diet for the first two days. It doesn't make any difference whether it's four hundred or twelve, but you certainly don't give tremendous amounts. I remember two cases where the doctor ordered one to two ounces of whiskey every hour and as somebody said this morning this is another good way to die.

We had no anticoagulants and though I'm not all out for anticoagulants, there is still a tremendous indication for them if there's a history of thrombophlebitis, a family history, or a patient with a serious arrhythmia, a patient in shock and so on. I can well remember in New York Hospital, when I was still active there, two of my patients died while they were dressing to go home and I'm sure that was from an embolism from phlebitis in the leg. We used to see a great deal of nausea, vomiting, and hiccup. We didn't have the anti-motion drugs. We didn't have Dramamine, Bonamine and Marezine which have worked wonders in these patients and we didn't have sense enough to do away with fruit juices and milk which add to nausea; hiccup was also a very serious complication. It used to be intractable and now you don't see it and I think you don't see it because we're reassuring our patients. The doctor doesn't get alarmed and I think that's the reason it's disappeared. For shock in those days we only had epinephrine. In pulmonary edema we did phlebotomies and we gave morphine. We didn't know about rotating tourniquets and we didn't know about these wonderful diuretics like ethacrynic acid, chlorothiazide, and so forth.

We kept patients in bed six weeks still in 1930 to 1940 because of the work by Sutton. He took dogs and produced a coronary occlusion and one group he let lie around to heal by themselves. The other group he made run on a treadmill and, of course, those on the treadmill did worse. As a result we kept our patients in bed six weeks since the pathologists also said there was myomalacia for this period of time and only after six weeks would a scar develop. Now, of course, we use chair treatment and we get them up and if we don't give anticoagulants we have them move their toes and their legs and turn over and take breathing exercises and so on. We didn't know the difference between subendocardial infarction, as I said, and transmural, and about this great difference my colleagues and I began to write in 1937. As I said, any chest pain at all we called coronary occlusion. We know better now. The outlook, the prognosis in subendocardial involvement is much better than in transmural. We wrote of many multiple attacks of coronary occlusion. One, two, three, four, five. We looked back to 1937. Well, I don't believe anybody survives a third transmural infarction, but we never made that distinction then. We have been patient. I'm glad to say that my colleagues and I were always in the forefront of getting the patient back to work and you have no idea how difficult it was. The patient was scared; the family was even more apprehensive; the family doctor thought you were crazy and then there was the security of the insurance policy. The patient valued the annuity that he got by being completely disabled. So it was very difficult in the thirties and forties, let alone the twenties to get patients back to work, but we always did it.

We used to say in the thirties and forties that after the first year in severe cases there was a ten per cent mortality a year. So you can figure out how many survivors you would have. In five or ten years you certainly wouldn't have anybody left. In the milder cases we said five per cent. In our last cases, we found that after the first year or two, it's just a two per cent mortality a year for years and it's only when a patient gets old that the curve drops, but from two to fourteen years it's just about a two per cent mortality. I think I've covered everything I

want to say. Thank you.

CHAIRMAN WHITE: Thank you very much, Arthur. Now Dr. Russek will carry on. I've suddenly asked him to do this.

DR. HENRY RUSSEK: Thank you, Dr. White. When I first came to the U. S. Marine Hospital in 1938 as a second year intern, I volunteered for the cardiology service since no one else wanted the assignment. The "old crocks" as they were called on the 5th floor were considered beyond hope. Some of them had been there for years, distressed and despondent. There were syphilitic aneurysms of every description, rheumatic valvular deformities with congestive heart failure and anasarca, hypertensive cardiovascular disease in the malignant phase, status anginosus and a variety of other than disabling disorders. In 1940 I had the privilege of being a student of Dr. White so it's rather easy to talk about the treatment and prognosis for myocardial infarction in those days. I think the medical profession was under the influence of the teachings of Sir Thomas Lewis who believed that all patients should be kept at strict bed rest, regardless of the severity of the attack, and nursed by day and by night for six to eight weeks even in the mildest cases. The whole concept in those days was one of "masterful inactivity." The physician, it was felt, should be little more than "an attentive spectator to nature's processes of healing and repair." It was thought desirable to leave things alone and to avoid overtreating the patient. Most of us embraced this view, but we've had to change a good deal and become more aggressive with the passage of time as Dr. Corday will reveal.

In the early 1940's I wrote a paper on the "Hazards of Treatment in Acute Myocardial Infarction" in which I pointed out that just about everything that we do for a patient may be a double edged sword. "One man's meat is another man's poison" and thus we must always consider the possible hazards of the treatment against the potential benefits from therapy for any patient with myocardial infarction. This is still true insofar as almost every drug that we use—for example morphine and nitroglycerin—may be dangerous with an acute myocardial infarct. Anticoagulants and other agents have their dangers too. Then in the later forties through the efforts of Samuel Levine, William Dock and Tinsley Harrison, the dangers of immobilization in bed became evident. It was just about the time that we were beginning to use anticoagulants, that we were also beginning to move our patients around reducing their bedfast time and permitting them to feed themselves and to get out of bed earlier. So I believe that many of the benefits which have been attributed to anticoagulant therapy have been in reality a direct result of the change in our management of our patients with acute myocardial infarction. In those days we made our patients have long periods of convalescence and they had a great loss of time from work.

It took President Eisenhower's illness to demonstrate for our patients all over the world how active a life the coronary patient can actually lead, but the whole concept in the 1940's was dominated by the thought that if you do too much to the patient when ill, or if you excite him the least bit even when well, you might precipitate a fatal arrhythmia. To this day we have this fear, but the coronary care unit has done a lot to dispel it. Some of you may have read the letter in the American Journal of Cardiology recently from Dr. Grace who reports on a patient who went beserk in the coronary care unit. He broke up all the chairs and he ripped off the sheets from the beds of some of the patients in the coronary care unit yet continuous monitoring of all of these patients showed that none of them turned a hair. Nobody had an attack of any kind and everything went just fine. Only the nurses and the orderlies suffered arrhythmia. So apparently our great fear and our precautions of the past may have been to some extent overprotective toward the patient. Nonetheless I am sure that there are hypersensitive subjects who can be harmed by an atmosphere of tension and anxiety such as exists in the average coronary care unit. So with these remarks I will turn the discussion back to Dr. White.

CHAIRMAN WHITE: Thank you very much. Now Doctor Kannel will take over. As you all know, he has been working at Framingham and has much to say.

DR. WILLIAM KANNEL: Well, I hate to interrupt this rosy glow of optimism with a few facts, but I'm afraid we must face the facts. Each year now about two million deaths occur in the United States. An examination of the proportion of these deaths ascribed to various causes reveals that diseases of the heart and blood vessels constitute the major force of mortality. They are in fact responsible for every second death. Beyond age forty-five coronary heart disease is responsible for more than half the deaths attributed to disease of the circulatory apparatus making this the foremost killer of adults beyond age forty-five. Now, if you examine life expectancy from birth comparing 1920 and 1960 (the period under discussion) this reveals a substantial lengthening of the span of life from birth—from fifty-six years to sixty-seven. Beyond age forty-five in men, however, the improvement is a scant one year—from twenty-two to twenty-three years. We've

evidently not made a major impact on the degenerative or the neoplastic and cardiovascular diseases which are responsible for deaths after the age of forty-five. An examination of the natural history of coronary disease, the foremost killer beyond age forty-five, reveals why this has been so and why it may continue to be so. A reasonably undistorted picture of the manner in which this disease evolves and terminates fatally is obtained from an investigation of it's occurrence in a general population including all cases, particularly those too mild and those dying too suddenly to reach medical attention. Such an examination of it's natural history as has been done at Framingham and elsewhere in the 1950's suggests that further innovations in the management of symptomatic disease no matter how ingenius or how sophisticated are not likely to make a major impact on mortality due to coronary disease. In this community, where even suspected heart attacks are routinely hospitalized, as many as forty per cent of attacks do not reach the hospital. Exploring the reasons for this reveals that sudden death and silent or unrecognized infarctions are responsible for seventy-five per cent of the non-hospitalized attacks.

It is clear from this that a substantial proportion of attacks will not reach the hospital where they can receive the benefits of modern medical technology. An examination of the case fatality rates in those reaching the hospital alive in the 1950's in Framingham reveals that 17 percent failed to survive their initial myocardial infarction, a rate I want to point out to you virtually identical with that observed in those who did not receive the benefits of hospital care if one excludes the sudden deaths. This is hardly a therapeutic triumph. Now it's likely that the case fatality rate in those hospitalized will be halved through improved care in the coronary care units. However, while many individual lives will be saved, the overall impact on coronary mortality, regrettably, will be quite modest. An examination of all deaths in initial coronary attacks reveals that fully sixty-five per cent are sudden and unexpected and out of reach of medical care, no matter how sophisticated the therapeutic approach. One in every five myocardial infarctions presents with sudden death as its initial manifestation. Most sudden deaths in myocardial infarctions occurred without warning. Only twenty-four per cent were preceded by angina. In addition, a surprising proportion of myocardial infarctions never reached the clinical horizon. At least one in every five myocardial infarctions were either silent or clinically unrecognizable. Moreover, these attacks were not innocuous. Persons with this deceptively mild disease had a subsequent survival experience just about the same as those who survived symptomatic attacks.

So we are faced with a disease which is extremely common; which is highly lethal; which attacks without warning and in which the first symptom all too often is also the very last. Also, it's a disease in which an actual myocardial infarction can be silent. In addition, should the victim manage to survive the critical first few minutes and the hazardous first forty-eight hours, his troubles are far from over. He now runs a high risk of coronary recurrences. This is from five to ten times that of his cohorts depending on age. In five years, one in three can be expected to recur and half of these recurrences will be fatal and incidentally, he runs a three-fold increased risk of a stroke. Now it's difficult to see how mortality from a disease of this nature will be substantially reduced by management which focuses simply on symptomatic cases. Only a more comprehensive approach involving primary and secondary prophylaxis is likely to make a major impact. We must find a way to prevent sudden death; to detect unrecognized infarctions and other occult coronary disease; to detect precocious coronary atherosclerosis; to delay recurrences and to retard atherogenesis. We may find that coronary atherosclerosis is a pediatric disease and that we must begin its management then.

CHAIRMAN WHITE: That was lovely. I was going to say this at the end, but I'll say it now in case I don't have time at the end. In 1919 I came to New York City to visit the Friday evening heart clinic, at Bellevue Hospital, of Dr. John Wyckoff and at that time the New York Heart Association was called the New York Association for the Prevention and Relief of Heart Disease and perhaps we had better go back to that original name. It's quite obvious that our priority must be the prevention of serious atherosclerosis. Now Eliot Corday, will you carry on with the present problem, the 1960's.

DR. ELIOT CORDAY: The most dramatic development for the first eight years of the decade was the introduction of a new aggressive approach for management of coronary occlusion.

At the present time we're losing six hundred thousand Americans each year from coronary occlusions. Two hundred and fifty thousand die outside of a hospital. It's estimated that by 1970 we will save fifty thousand lives each year because by that time the nation will have 4,000 coronary care units which will provide a new aggressive management of myocardial infarction. But we still are losing about two hundred and fifty thousand each year from power failure of the heart after coronary occlusion.

The coronary care concept was first started about

1962 when Day and Meltzer independently set up coronary care units which signalled a warning to the nurse or the attending staff that heart arrest had occurred. Essentially it alerted the emergency staff to institute resuscitative measures. Seven thousand hospitals across the nation should have coronary care units, but at this time only twelve hundred have been established.

A Bethesda Conference conducted by the American College of Cardiology in 1965 contributed greatly when the conferees concluded that there was no sense in having a coronary care unit unless electric countershock was used promptly. They concluded that, because the doctor is with the patient only a few minutes of the day, the nurse must be authorized to use countershock. Therefore, to permit the nurse to perform these tasks the conferees recommended training her "razor sharp" in electrocardiography, electrical defibrillation and in the other new concepts of the aggressive management of myocardial infarction. Fortunately, Senator Lister Hill was receptive to the Bethesda Conference recommendations and convinced Congress to appropriate the funds to establish special training programs across the nation.

It soon appeared that the nurse was often better trained than the physician in management of the coronary patient, so that a further appropriation was voted for training programs for the Medical Directors of Coronary Care Units.

The next major breakthrough in the field of coronary care was provided by Lown when he showed that the early treatment of the irritable heart with antiarrhythmic drugs could prevent more serious arrhythmias and arrest. He showed that the prompt intravenous administration of procainamide or lidocaine can often quickly correct premature systoles and prevent more serious tachycardias and cardiac arrest. In a series of three hundred cases so treated Lown and Killip noted only three cardiac arrests. According to national statistics they might have anticipated 36. In other words, the coronary care units which were first set up as resuscitative units have now advanced to prevent cardiac arrest.

A study published in the December issue of the Archives of Internal Medicine compared the mortality rate of treating patients in two neighboring hospitals in Denver, Colorado—one with, and one without a coronary care unit. The same physicians provided care at both hospitals. In the "poor risk" group of patients with cardiac arrest the coronary care unit reduced the mortality from twenty-nine per cent to six per cent. In the "good risk" patients with cardiac arrest they reduced the mortality from fifty-seven per cent down to twelve per cent. They also compared their mortality statistics with other coronary care units across the nation. At Colorado General Hospital the mortality rate was 19 per cent; Lown reported a rate of 16.9 per cent in Boston; Day and Averill 20 per cent in Kansas; Meltzer and Kitchell 15 to 18 per cent in Philadelphia. But other figures were not as good and varied considerably. Brown had a 36 per cent mortality in his coronary care unit; Spann 27 per cent, and Goble 31 per cent. But we realize as we look at the bibliography that these higher mortality rates were reported earlier in 1963 and 1964 before it was understood that the nurse be trained to perform the tasks formerly reserved for the cardiologist.

The mortality in this nation has been reduced from thirty per cent down to about twenty per cent in this decade by applying the new aggressive techniques for treatment in acute coronary care. But we still have to do something about the 250,000 coronary patients in the USA who succumb to shock or heart failure. To reduce this terrible mortality rate, the National Heart Institute has set up eight myocardial infarction research units (MIRU) for the study of the basic pathophysiology of myocardial infarction. They reason that we must understand more about basic pathophysiology before we can determine new principles of treatment.

I agree with Dr. Kannel that we must do something to reduce the formidable mortality rate of 250,000 coronary patients who die each year before they reach the hospital. The American College of Cardiology and the Heart Disease Control Unit of HEW have scheduled a Bethesda Conference for January 1969 to see what might be done to reduce this deplorable mortality. Can the principles learned in the coronary care unit be applied for the care of the ambulatory coronary patient? For instance, should all patients with known coronary artery disease receive anti-arrhythmic agents, and if so, what drugs would be beneficial? It's entirely possible that proper prophylactic agents might prevent ventricular fibrillation in the ambulatory patient. Secondly, can we bring the defibrillator closer to the patient? Shouldn't we have defibrillators on all our ambulances? Shouldn't we arrange to have defibrillators where we have a large congregation of people over forty-five years of age, for example, at football games? In Ireland they saved nine out of twelve patients who had a cardiac arrest while being transported in the ambulance. Can we apply the Belfast experience of mobile coronary care ambulances to our urban or rural settings?

Doctor White asked me to comment on revascularization surgery. I know there are many that intimate they can reduce the mortality rate by various surgical procedures, but it is too soon to say if these have long-or even short-term benefit.

There is another topic which will be discussed at the Bethesda Conference and that is how to manage the patient with an impending coronary occlusion. We know by the course of events that these are patients whose angina has suddenly changed in character; instead of having ordinary recurrent anginal episodes on effort, it comes on more severely and at rest. The T waves tip over but return to normal within a few days. They are discharged from the hospital. Then one day soon they sustain a very severe episode of chest pain and develop the typical pattern of transmural myocardial infarction. Can we do anything about preventing a coronary occlusion in these patients, an event which is often fatal. We wonder if it shouldn't be attacked aggressively by the surgeon. If a patient has one particular coronary artery that is narrowed, can this artery be reconstructed? The worst that could happen as a result of surgery and this is rather provocative thinking—is that the artery will occlude. We find that after these arteries occlude, patients are often free of chest pain and they do very well afterwards. If, as a result of surgery, occlusion does occur, it develops under the controlled conditions of a coronary care unit and with considerably less hazard than attends its development in an ambulatory patient. Now this is very provocative thinking, but it's something that we may face in future years.

CHAIRMAN WHITE: Thank you very much. Now, I'm very happy to introduce Pavel Lukl, an old friend, who will end the discussion of the panel with his experiences in Czechoslovakia.

DR. PAVEL LUKL: Paul White, ladies and gentlemen. One of my old teachers, Sir John Parkinson, coined the phrase that when a patient with a coronary attack is seen by a doctor, he has a fifty per cent chance to survive. Today the chance is much better—about six to one. The prognosis seems to be markedly improved. It must be said that it remains difficult to analyze all facts, all components, as we have to deal with a dynamic subject and a steadily changing scene conditioned by progress in medicine and a number of other factors. Certainly the final outcome and prognosis are the result of an interplay of factors, some of them improving and others aggravating prognosis. Our diagnostic ability has improved with refined electrocardiographic chest leads and enzyme studies. This is a feedback for better bedside diagnosis so that we now detect more and more cases of the so called intermediary coronary syndrome. This certainly has something to do with the final outcome. Not only that, but the majority of cases previously labelled as angina are now considered either impending or past mild infarctions and are included in the infarction compartment.

To be sure myocardial infarction is overdiagnosed today and perhaps some of these unfounded diagnoses may distort for the better our statistics. There is no doubt that our treatment has had a definite role in improving prognosis. Early diagnosis with bed rest, the prevention of thromboembolism, diminished fear in the use of digitalis, shock therapy with catecholamines, and all the new antiarrhythmic drugs so necessary in the first days of infarction have had a favorable influence. Twenty to thirty years ago, everybody, at least in our country, was afraid to be admitted to the hospital. Now nearly all cases are coming there and coming quickly, which was also not the case before, in order to receive special care in coronary units with strict personnel and monitoring equipment.

It is well known that this coordinated effort has decreased early mortality as we have heard from Eliot Corday. The life span on the other hand has increased and this is certainly an aggravating prognostic factor as indicated by our own experience with a thousand observed cases in men. Myocardial infarctions seem nevertheless to affect more and more often the younger age group. There is no satisfactory explanation for that. Perhaps we are dealing with different body resistance and a more fragile generation from the cardiovascular point of view, a generation which has been protected from danger and death from infectious disease. Anyway, when we consider the strikingly low mortality of 3.5 per cent in the group under the age of forty-five, we must admit that age is a most decisive factor in prognosis. Factors like hypertension, angina, shock, and ECG changes may be present in all age groups but the single age factor can radically change the prognosis. What then is the powerful protector of the young? We don't know, but very probably the state of the myocardium.

Another interesting problem is the worse prognosis in women which is generally accepted. Why a woman with a better outlook for a longer life span should have here a worse prognosis is not quite fully understood. It is not the higher age for the attack, nearly ten years higher, because the prognosis is much the same at all ages, even in the young. There are perhaps some associated factors at play and of these obesity seems to be the most important. There is also another difference. Cardiac rupture is much more frequent in women: thirty-two per cent of fatal cases against twenty-three per cent in men. Cardiac rupture is correlated with late bed rest and late admission to the hospital; both are more pronounc-

ed in women. Smoking does not seem to aggravate prognosis. Of course the proportion of smoking women is only six per cent in our country so that in the future this may be altered by the present generation. Surprisingly also hypertension does not worsen the prognosis.

Much more important for prognosis are the objective signs at the beginning of the attack as was stated already by Dr. Corday; circulatory shock is a well known factor and has a high mortality of about thirty-one per cent; when we find a pressure of eighty mm. we have a seventy per cent mortality. It is most important to prevent very early such hypotension and there is an outstanding role for antiarrhythmic drugs especially for lidocaine. The same is true for the prevention and treatment of congestive failure. Mortality here is up to thirty-eight per cent and again we must not forget the importance of the early use of digitalis; the danger of arrhythmia from it is not as great as has been claimed.

Laboratory tests give in my experience very little aid for prognosis. Take the ECG. It is generally accepted that the so-called intermediary coronary syndrome has a better prognosis as mentioned by Dr. Master. In our material there was about a 12 per cent mortality against 20 per cent in the so-called transmural infarction cases. The difference is of course not so great and we must remember that we are speaking only in electrocardiographic terms. For instance, three of our so-called "non-transmural" infarctions, the intermediary syndrome without Qs, had ruptured hearts; so the non-transmural ECG may mean a very transmural lesion.

A very important matter is that most of the early deaths occur on the first day, seventy per cent in the first week, and practically no deaths after the twenty-first day. What that means for early care and observation is evident. It is much more difficult to assess later causes of death. Generally speaking, about 7 per cent of the survivors die every year so that the five-year survival is around sixty per cent in our material. It may be said that after the third year after a coronary attack the death rate is not much different from the age adjusted rate in the population. The cause of death in the majority of cases is heart failure and the recurrence of infarction. The prognosis includes not only death rate but also invalidism and crippling. Return to work may be some measure of this. Of course, a great portion of the cases are already in the retirement age. Of those still working, only fifty-two per cent of our cases have returned to their original or lighter work, but only five per cent are without complaints. I know that there are better results and more favorable statistics depending on social structure. Nevertheless

I am quite sure that ischemic heart disease remains in spite of improved prognosis a killing and crippling disease. We cannot achieve much more without effective prevention as has already been said.

The whole world, rich or poor, is adopting the American way of seeking happiness. I have many, many friends over here and know the real nature of American friendship which is here part of the way of life. It is very efficient and helpful friendship and is still not justly appreciated in the world. But as everybody now is adopting this American way I must say that there is too much concentration in it on the present moment, so that we are always more prepared to take than to give in behalf of future generations. There is planning without break or inhibition in unnecessary and useless competition bringing with it all the evils of overeating, sexual license, and overexcitement, and at the far end apprehension, crime, and violence. I am seriously doubtful whether in such an atmosphere just striking the saturated fats out of our diet or smoking out of our habits will be enough. Some profound change is needed in our hurried and often aimless lives to re-establish moral values and to provide time for contemplation and insight. Such change could afford a more effective means of prevention with regard to the complex phenomena involved in ischemic heart disease. Thank you.

CHAIRMAN WHITE: Thank you very much. I can see that this is a wonderful closing moment. I would like to add that in addition to the prevention of coronary heart disease and atherosclerosis, we need to keep a cardiological current flowing between the heart of Czechoslovakia and the hearts of the U.S.A.

Long-Term Management of Ischemic Heart Disease

Chairman
George E. Burch, M.D.

Current Status of Cholesterol Lowering Agents
William B. Abrams, M.D.

Zane N. Gaut, Ph. D., M.D.

A Critical Appraisal of the Use of Anticoagulants
Irving S. Wright, M.D.

New Dimension in Angina Pectoris Therapy: Propranolol-Nitrate Synergism
Henry I. Russek, M.D.

Management of Refractory Angina Pectoris
Louis F. Bishop, M.D.

Rationale for the Use of Beta Blockade as Therapy for Angina Pectoris
Steven Wolfson, M.D.

Ezra A. Amsterdam, M.D.

Richard Gorlin, M.D.

Rationale for Treating Coronary Patients with Psychotherapeutic Agents
J. Campbell Howard, M.D.

Emotional Rehabilitation of the Coronary Patient
John F. Briggs, M.D.

Programs for the Rehabilitation of the Coronary Patient
Jerome S. Tobis, M.D.

New Methods of Work Prescription for the Coronary Patient
Lenore R. Zohman, M.D.

Laboratory and Clinical Experience in Orthotopic Cardiac Allotransplantation
Adrian Kantrowitz, M.D.

Jordan D. Haller, M.D.

Yasunori Koga, M.D.

Eduard Sujansky, M.D.

Jose Caralps Riera

Hans E. Carstensen, M.D.

Howard A. Joos, M.D.

William Neches, M.D.

William Pomerance, M.D.

Marcial M. Cerruti, M.D.

The Current Status of Cholesterol Lowering Agents

William B. Abrams and Zane N. Gaut

Cholesterol and other lipids have been implicated in the pathogenesis of atherosclerosis by a variety of clinical, pathologic, epidemiologic and investigational evidence. For this reason, the major attack on atherosclerosis involves dietary measures and drugs designed to reduce the cholesterol content of blood and, hopefully, arteries.

Studies of cholesterol metabolism in man, however, are fraught with uncertainties. In clinical studies one samples a small and "laaile" pool,

namely serum. Figure 1 depicts the major body pools of cholesterol, their relative sizes and exchangeabilities via the serum. Heavy arrows indicate rapid exchange and light arrows, slower exchange. For example, cholesterol equilibration between serum, blood cells, liver and the intestinal lumen occurs within hours, whereas that between the abdominal aorta and serum requires weeks.[1] Since cholesterol in atheromas is exchangeable with that in serum, there is hope that a prolonged decrease in

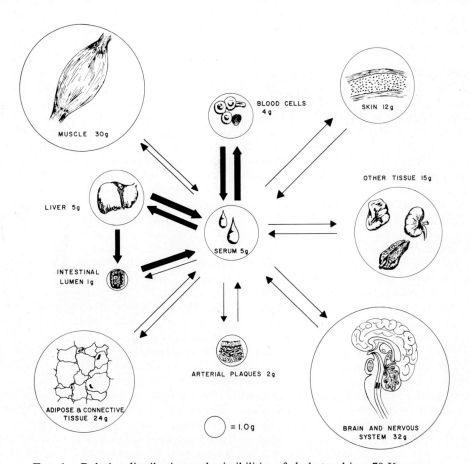

FIG. 1.   Relative distribution and miscibilities of cholesterol in a 70 Kg. man.

the serum concentration would result in a net efflux of cholesterol from these arterial lesions and thus reverse atherosclerosis. As will be noted later, decreases in the size of xanthomas have been associated with drug induced reductions of serum cholesterol levels in man. It is not yet possible to be certain that this applies to atheromatous plaques as well.

Dietary measures comprise the use of low caloric, low cholesterol, low fat, carbohydrate restricted and low saturated, high unsaturated fat diets. Although the role of diet in atherosclerosis is discussed elsewhere in this book and this chapter is concerned with drugs, dietary measures are mentioned here to emphasize their importance in the management of this disease.

The cholesterol-lowering drugs which are currently in use or in broad clinical trial act by reducing cholesterol absorption from the intestinal tract, by inhibiting its biosynthesis, by increasing its excretion or by mechanisms which are currently unknown.

Interest in the blockage of cholesterol absorption as a means of combating hypercholesterolemia followed the observations that certain plant sterols, chiefly the sitosterols, are nonatherogenic and compete for absorption with both exogenous and endogenous cholesterol.[2] Alpha-sitosterol is the main sterol of soybean and beta-sitosterol is the main sterol of cottonseed oil. Corn oil also contains sitosterols, and these may contribute to its cholesterol-lowering effect. Administration of sitosterols to humans has produced falls in serum cholesterol levels in the range of 15 to 17 per cent.[3-5] Unfortunately, very large doses must be used and prolonged treatment is expensive. According to most reports, the effects are variable. Sitosterols are available commercially as Cytellin.

Another agent which reduces blood cholesterol by intestinal action is cholestyramine.[6-8] This is a strongly basic, bile acid binding, ion exchange resin. It forms a nonabsorbable bile acid complex in the intestine which prevents the normal enterohepatic circulation of the bile acids. Fecal excretion is therefore increased.[9] Since the bile acids fail to return to the liver, the oxidation of cholesterol is increased in an attempt to produce more bile acids. The result is a lowering of the serum cholesterol. Some doubts have been introduced by a study in pigs. Cholestyramine increased bile acid excretion tenfold in these animals; however, cholesterol biosynthesis increased nineteen-fold and plasma cholesterol levels did not decline.[10] The efficacy of cholestyramine[6-8] suggests this does not occur in man. Cholestyramine may be more effective in Type II hyperlipoproteinemia than in other forms[11] but was reported to be ineffective

in patients with homozygous familial hypercholesterolemic xanthomatosis.[12] In another study, daily doses of 20 Gm. per day over a six-month period was associated with a reduction in the cutaneous lesions in patients with this disorder.[13] The major limitations of cholestyramine are that large doses are required and administration is unpleasant.

Neomycin has been under study as a cholesterol-lowering agent since 1958.[14] Doses of 0.5 to 2.0 Gm. daily can produce a 14 to 33 per cent reduction in this sterol.[15-17] The oral use of neomycin has been free from serious toxicity, but a significant incidence of gastrointestinal side effects has been encountered. Studies employing tritium-labeled cholesterol were reported to show that the neomycin-induced fall in serum cholesterol is associated with a reduction in the rapidly miscible pool of this sterol which includes serum, red blood cells and liver cholesterol[16] (Fig. 1). Some of the plaque cholesterol may have participated in this process. The mechanism of action of neomycin was originally linked to its antibiotic activity since intestinal organisms are involved in the metabolism of bile acids in the gut.[15,18] However, it now appears that neomycin reduces cholesterol by forming nonabsorbable precipitates with bile acids.[19,20] The mechanism of action, then, is like that of cholestyramine.

Studies in animals suggested that certain polysaccharides, such as pectin, chondroitin sulfate and dextran may have cholesterol-lowering effects. These substances also act in the intestine, inhibiting cholesterol and/or bile acid absorption.[21-26] In humans, daily doses of 6 to 15 Gm. of pectin significantly reduced blood cholesterol levels.[27] The administration of chondroitin sulfate-A to 60 patients with arteriosclerotic heart disease was associated with a single coronary event, while 13 clinical incidents occurred in a comparable control group.[28] Dextran lowered plasma lipid levels when given intravenously, but not orally.[29] The newest drug in this category is 3β, 5α, 6β-Cholestane Triol. This cholesterol analog was found to antagonize the hyperlipemic effects of atherogenic diets in several animal species[30] and to do so by inhibiting the intestinal absorption of cholesterol.[31] There have been no substantial clinical trials with this agent as yet. The attack on cholesterol in the intestine continues to be of great interest.

Endogenous cholesterol biosynthesis may be divided into three stages (Fig. 2). The first stage involves fatty acids and encompasses the conversion of acetate to mevalonate. The second stage is concerned with the decarboxylation of mevalonate and conversion to isoprenol pyrophosphates, the last of which is farnesyl pyrophosphate. The third stage

from Steinberg, D, Advances in Pharmacology, Vol. I, 1962

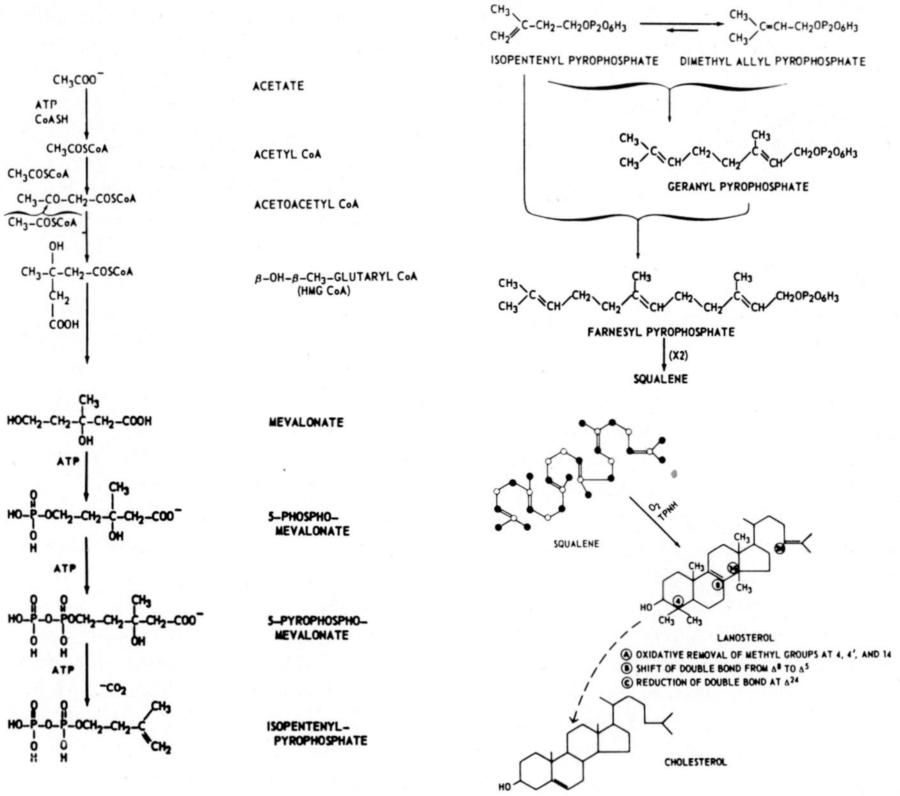

FIG. 2. The biosynthesis of cholesterol. The first stage involves fatty acids and encompasses the conversion from acetate to mevalonate. The second stage is concerned with the decarboxylation of mevalonate and conversion to isoprenol pyrophosphates, the last of which is farnesyl pyrophosphate. The third stage involves the production of squalene from farnesyl pyrophosphate, the cyclization of squalene to lanosterol, and the synthesis of cholesterol via various steroidal intermediates.

involves the production of squalene from farnesyl pyrophosphate, the cyclization of squalene to lanosterol, and the synthesis of cholesterol via various steroidal intermediates.

The first inhibitor of cholesterol biosynthesis to be thoroughly studied was benzmalacene, a uricosuric agent found to inhibit cholesterol biosynthesis from mevalonate, thus indicating a second or third stage inhibition[32] (Fig. 2). In clinical trials it did indeed lower blood cholesterol, but gastrointestinal and other side effects prohibited continued clinical use.[33] Curiously, cholesterol lowering was associated with a rise in triglyceride and phospholipids.[33]

The next cholesterol-biosynthesis inhibitor, triparanol or MER 29, acted at the third stage of the chain.[34] It inhibited the reduction of the $\triangle 24$ (side chain) double bond in steroid precursors of cholesterol.[35] As a result, biosynthesis progressed to desmosterol instead of cholesterol.[36] This caused an accumulation of desmosterol, a C-24 unsaturated steroid, in the tissues and experimental and pathological studies indicated desmosterol shared at least some of the atherogenic properties of cholesterol.[37] These observations, plus the occurrence of severe side effects—cataracts, hair loss, ichthyosis and others—necessitated its withdrawal from the market.

Clofibrate (ethyl-p-chlorophenoxyisobutyrate, CPIB, Atromid-S) (Fig. 3) is also considered to be an inhibitor of endogenous cholesterol biosynthesis, acting in the first phase, between acetate and mevalonate.[38] Since this activity was demonstrated in liver slices and intact animals but not in preparations of liver homogenate, the possibility of an indirect inhibition was raised.[38] The observations that clofibrate lowers plasma free fatty acid levels could provide the basis for such a mechanism.[39] Reduction in plasma free fatty acid levels has been observed in humans as well as in animals.[40] Since the acetate needed for the biosynthesis of cholesterol is par-

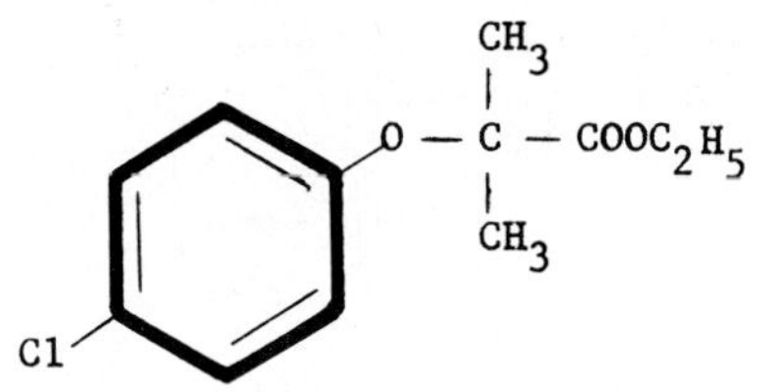

ETHYL p-CHLOROPHENOXYISOBUTYRATE

Fig. 3.   Structure of clofibrate (Atromid-S).

tially provided by the hydrolysis of fatty acids in the liver, the action of clofibrate in suppressing free fatty acid release from tissue depots could reduce the amount of acetate available for the synthesis of cholesterol. This action also reduces the supply of free fatty acid available for incorporation into triglycerides, and may explain the prominent effect of clofibrate on this lipid fraction. This may not, however, be the only mechanism by which clofibrate affects triglycerides since several investigators have reported a decreased production of triglycerides when radioactively labeled fatty acids were presented to the liver.[41-44] It has also been suggested that clofibrate accelerates triglyceride clearance.[45]

These experimental observations have been amply confirmed by clinical trials demonstrating favorable effects on cholesterol, free fatty acid, triglyceride and lipoprotein blood levels.[7,46-49] In concurrence with the experimental data, numerous reports have emphasized the greater effect on triglycerides than on cholesterol.[50-52] In terms of lipoproteins, the very low density triglyceride rich fraction (S.F. 20-400) is most affected, but the cholesterol rich, low density fraction (S.F. 0-20) is also reduced.[53] The net effect is an average reduction of plasma triglyceride levels of 30 to 40 per cent, and cholesterol levels of 15 to 25 per cent in 85 per cent of patients treated.[54] When subjects with hyperlipemia are phenotyped according to the classification of Fredrickson and Lees, clofibrate has been found to be most effective in Type III, modestly effective in Type II and ineffective in Type I.[55] Types IV and V patients may respond favorably to clofibrate, but dietary management is much more important in these groups of subjects.[55] Perhaps more important are the observations that clofibrate therapy may reduce tissue deposits as well. These involve the regression of xanthomatous lesions and clearing of diabetic retinopathy.[13,56]

An effect on thrombus formation was noted early in the clinical use of clofibrate. Oliver and associates[57] reported a potentiation of anticoagulants affecting the prothrombin time. The principal reason for this is that clofibrate displaces such anticoagulants bound to albumin from their binding sites making more pharmacologically active drug available.[58] However, several factors may be involved. Clofibrate has been reported to reduce blood fibrinogen levels,[59] reduce platelet stickiness[60] and prevent the accelerated clotting associated with postprandial hyperlipemia.[61] In view of the proposed role of thrombosis in the atherosclerotic process, these observations may be indicative of beneficial actions as well as of potential side effects. When patients on anticoagulants are given clofibrate, the dose of the anticoagulant should be reduced by a third to a half until a new maintenance requirement is established.

Clinical reports indicate clofibrate is quite safe. Oliver[56] reported patients treated for up to four years without significant side effects. Transient elevations in serum glutamic oxalacetic transaminase (SGOT) levels may occur early in treatment,[62] but this is not indicative of liver toxicity.[54] Minor gastrointestinal disturbances and one questionable instance of reversible agranulocytosis have, however, also been reported.[63] In subjects with hyperuricemia or hypertriglyceridemia, blood uric acid levels are lowered.[64]

Some recent reports suggest that the combination of clofibrate with dextrothyroxine[65] or thyroxine[66] may be more effective than the individual agents used alone. SaH-2348 [(bis-p-chlorophenoxy) acetic acid] 1-methyl-4-piperidyl ester is chemically similar to clofibrate, but is pharmacologically nine times more active.[67] It has been reported to lower cholesterol and triglyceride levels in humans, but further studies are needed to establish its safety and efficacy relative to existing agents.[67]

One approach to the inhibition of endogenous biosynthesis attempts to simulate the negative feedback effects of cholesterol itself on cholesterol biosynthesis. The physiologic control of cholesterol biosynthesis occurs in the first stage; i.e., the reduction of β-hydroxy-β-methylglutarate to mevalonate.[68] The site of this control mechanism is in the microsomal membrane fraction of the liver. To imitate cholesterol, Counsell and his associates[69,70] prepared a series of diaza and aza isomers; that is, compounds identical to cholesterol except that one or two nitrogens are substituted for carbons in the side chain. These agents lowered serum cholesterol and total body sterols in animals, and 20, 25 diazacholesterol was effective in man.[71] However, an accumulation of desmosterol indicated an effect on desmosterol reductase similar to that of triparanol, thus these drugs were in fact third-stage inhibitors.[72]

A compound reported to inhibit in the first stage

A.

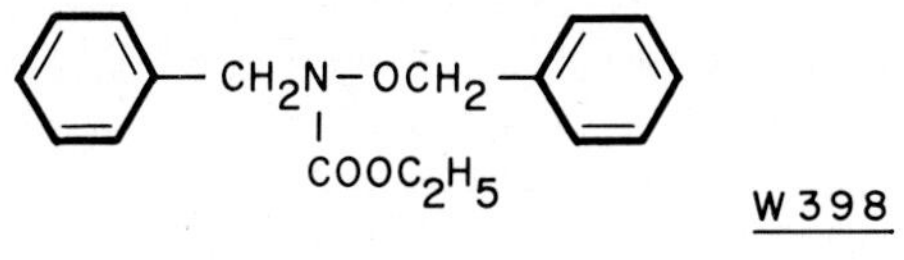

W 398

B.

AY 9944

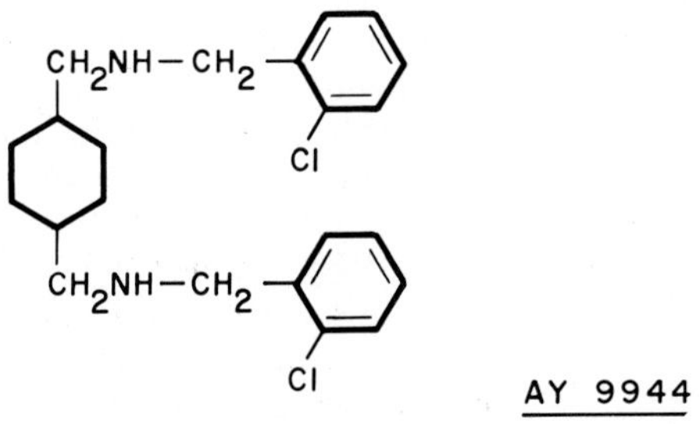

Fig. 4. *A,* Benzyl-N-benzyl carbethoxyhydroxamate (W-398). *B,* AY 9944.

is benzyl-N-benzyl carbethoxyhydroxamate (W-398)[73] (Fig. 4, A). This agent caused a disappearance of arterial lesions in cholesterol-fed rabbits and reduced serum cholesterol in rabbits and rats fed a hypercholesterolemic diet. In vitro studies indicated inhibition between acetate and mevalonate. Some recent evidence suggests it reduces the recirculation of cholesterol after its uptake by the liver from the systemic circulation.[74] On the negative side, Kritchevsky and Tepper[75] report an increase in the liver content of cholesterol when W-398 is administered to rats on a cholesterol-free diet. Clinical data have not yet been reported.

Although a number of isoprenol analogs have been prepared in attempts to inhibit cholesterol biosynthesis in the second stage, none have been successful to date. Third-stage inhibition, as mentioned above, tends to accumulate steroidal precursors of cholesterol and this was shown to be true for triparanol and the azacholesterols with the production of desmosterol. It has also been true for a new group of third-stage inhibitors, the best known of which is AY 9944[76] (Fig. 4, B). These substances, acting on the △7-reductase system, interfere with the conversion of 7-dehydrocholesterol to cholesterol. Thus, 7-dehydrocholesterol accumulates in the blood and tissues.[77]

As mentioned above, liver microsomal enzyme systems, which are important for the metabolism or detoxification of drugs, are also involved in cholesterol biosynthesis.[78] It was logical, therefore, to study agents which inhibit these enzyme systems for possible antilipemic effects and indeed two such agents, SKF 525-A[79] and phenyramidol,[80] have been shown to lower cholesterol levels in animals and man. Phenyramidol is currently employed as an analgesic. In spite of the many problems involved, the search for new inhibitors of endogenous cholesterol biosynthesis goes on.

Turning now to the possibility of increasing cholesterol excretion, two groups of substances come to mind, polyunsaturated fatty acids and the thyroxine derivatives. It has generally been held that the anticholesterolemic effect of polyunsaturated fatty acids increases with the degree of unsaturation.[81] On this basis we studied the effects of Eiocosa—5:8:11:14 tetraynoic acid, designated Ro 3-1428, a 20 carbon fatty acid with four triple bonds, synthesized by Dr. J. M. Osbond and associates at Roche Products Ltd. The administration of Ro 3-1428 to 19 subjects was associated with a modest reduction in the serum cholesterol levels which was, however, not dose related. Subsequently, Bender[82] treated 32 subjects for up to 48 weeks and confirmed the cholesterolpenic effects of this agent, but noted a significant incidence of minor gastrointestinal and dermatologic side effects. The search for a well tolerated, highly unsaturated synthetic fatty acid could lead to a useful product, but such agents are difficult to make, expensive, unstable and likely to require large doses. Furthermore, doubts exist about their mechanism of action. The ability of polyunsaturated fatty acids to increase bile acid excretion has been the subject of many reports over the last decade.[81] Ahrens,[83] however, has been unable to confirm this concept and has advanced the possibility that polyunsaturates lower plasma cholesterol by increasing tissue deposition.

As is well known, the cholesterol-lowering properties of thyroid hormone were exploited by the preparation of a number of thyroxine derivatives in which the effects on cholesterol were to some extent dissociated from the metabolic actions. The most intensively studied of these is dextrothyroxine, which has about one tenth the calorigenic action of levothyroxine, the natural substance.[84] In doses of 4 to 8 mg. per day, dextrothyroxine can be expected to produce a 20 to 25 per cent drop in serum cholesterol in 80 to 85 per cent of patients treated. The mechanism of the cholesterolpenic action has been assumed to be like that of thyroxine; namely an increase in cholesterol excretion as bile acids.[85] Studies by Hollander[63] suggest, however, that d-thyroxine may merely increase the turnover of cholesterol and perhaps alter its distribution, but may not decrease the body content of cholesterol. There is also some evidence that thyroid hormones inhibit the biosynthesis of cholesterol from acetate.[86] The major clinical problem with Choloxin concerns its propensity to increase angina and myocardial irritability in subjects with arteriosclerotic heart disease.[63,87] There is, however, a considerable difference of opinion regarding the frequency and significance of these actions.[85,88] In a recent review it was reported that first attacks of angina pectoris occurred in only five of about 2000 cardiac patients treated with dextrothyroxine.[89] There were also 36 myocardial infarctions and 17 cardiac arrhythmias. This incidence was not considered to be excessive. It was also noted that chest pain improved as often as it worsened in subjects with pre-existing angina pectoris. Nevertheless, dextrothyroxine is currently not recommended for use in subjects with organic heart disease. Other problems include production of congestive heart failure, aggravation of diabetes and potentiation of anticoagulants.

Progress in the use of thyroid substances for the treatment of hyperlipemia awaits clarification of the mechanism of action and agents with even less metabolic effects. To this end, Wechter and associates[90] have prepared a series of thyroalkanols, alcoholic analogs of thyroxine. Pharmacologic studies indicate a wider dissociation of the hypocholesterolemic and calorigenic effects than with the thyroalkanoic acids of which dextro- and levothyroxine are members.

The other hormonal substances of interest in the cholesterol problem are the estrogens. It has long been appreciated that premenopausal women have less coronary disease than do men, and this difference disappears later in life. Young women also have lower plasma concentrations of cholesterol and beta (low density) lipoproteins than do their male counterparts.[91] Furthermore, the administration of estrogens to subjects with coronary heart disease lowers plasma cholesterol and phospholipid concentrations, reduces beta (low density) lipoproteins and increases alpha (high density) lipoproteins.[92] The doses capable of producing such effects, however, also produce gynecomastia, loss of libido and impotence in males. The estrogenic oral contraceptives have the antilipemic properties of other estrogens.[93]

Long term mortality and morbidity studies have failed to establish the ability of estrogens to alter the natural history of coronary artery disease. On one hand Marmorston, *et al.*[94] found that "well tolerated" doses of conjugated estrogens markedly improved survival in a group of coronary patients.[94] This benefit could not be correlated with changes in serum lipids. On the other hand, Oliver and Boyd[95] found that 50 men given full doses of ethinyl estradiol had the same incidence of new coronary events as a matched control group. Stamler, *et al.*[96] observed 275 survivors of myocardial infarction for

over ten years. Treatment with conjugated estrogens in small initial doses, gradually increased, was associated with significantly better survival in "poor risk" patients (severe and/or multiple infarcts). Survival was also better in "good risk" patients (single mild infarcts), but statistical significance was not achieved.[96] Large doses given within three months of an infarction, however, was associated with an increased mortality.

Studies of the mechanism of action are also unclear. In tissues taken from estrogen treated rats, cholesterol biosynthesis was inhibited. In vivo, however, the antilipemic effects were associated with a shift in cholesterol from the blood into the liver.[97] The medicinal chemists remain busy trying to find substances which can exert antilipemic effects at doses free from hormonal actions and which act by favorable mechanisms.

The last group of cholesterol lowering agents to be considered are the compounds related to nicotinic acid. Since 1955, nicotinic acid[98,99] has been extensively used as an antilipemic agent and, more recently, nicotinyl alcohol tartrate.*[100,101] Zeller[100] found daily doses of 1—2 gm. of the latter as effective as the recommended 3-6 gm. of nicotinic acid in lowering serum cholesterol in normo- and hypercholesterolemic subjects.[100] Clinically, these agents may be expected to reduce cholesterol levels 20 to 30 per cent in 80 per cent of patients treated.[99] The changes are associated with falls in triglycerides, total lipids, free fatty acids and beta lipoprotein cholesterol.[99,102] Skin and tendon xanthomas tend to reduce in size and may disappear. Such effects would be of benefit to patients with Type II and possibly Type III lipoprotein abnormalities. Types IV and V might also respond, but as mentioned, these forms are best treated with weight reduction and diet.[55] Side effects consist of flushing, dry skin, pruritus, indigestion, reactivation of duodenal ulcer, disturbances in liver function, hyperuricemia and impairment of carbohydrate utilization.[99,101,103-105]

Such untoward effects are reversible on discontinuation of drug.

Studies at the Special Treatment Unit, Maryland Medical Center, corroborated the antilipemic effects of nicotinyl alcohol. Six hypercholesterolemic subjects, three of whom were mild diabetics, were started on a dose of 450 mg. twice daily for one week and then increased to 900 mg. twice daily for the remainder of the drug period. A one-month "stabilization" period was allowed prior to therapy. Three of the subjects were maintained on a diet consisting of 450 to 550 mg. of cholesterol, 60 to

* Roniacol Timespan

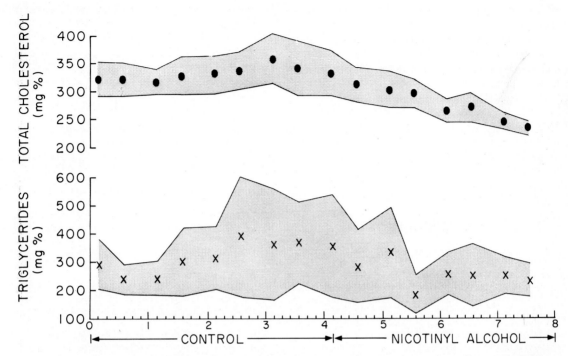

F<small>IG</small>. 5.   Serum cholesterol (•) and triglyceride (X) levels obtained twice weekly for four weeks before and four weeks during therapy with nicotinyl alcohol tartrate. The graphs show the mean values ± standard errors for the six subjects in the study. The dose of nicotinyl alcohol tartrate was 450 mg. twice daily for one week, then 900 mg. twice daily for three weeks. Analysis of variance comparing the values obtained during the third and fourth control weeks and the third and fourth treatment weeks indicated significant declines in these parameters.

70 gm. of protein, 70 to 80 gm. of fat (25% polyunsaturated), 225 to 250 gm. of carbohydrate, and 2000 to 2200 total calories per day. Serum concentration of cholesterol and triglycerides were measured twice weekly.

Figure 5 demonstrates the decline in serum cholesterol and triglycerides during treatment. Statistical analysis using weeks three and four of the control period versus weeks three and four while on drugs confirmed the significance of the declines.

The antilipemic mechanism of nicotinic acid and nicotinyl alcohol is unknown; however, a number of possibilities have been proposed and studied: (1) prevention of the release of free fatty acids;[106,107] (2) decreasing of the low-density and very-low-density lipoproteins;[98] (3) increasing cholesterol breakdown;[102,108–110] and (4) inhibition of cholesterol biosynthesis.[99]

Free fatty acids in the plasma that are released from adipose tissue are sequestered by the liver, synthesized into triglycerides, and released into the plasma as lipoproteins. Therefore, compounds that prevent the release of free fatty acids from adipose tissue might retard the formation of triglycerides. Nicotinic acid not only lowers plasma free fatty acids, but also inhibits their rise under norepinephrine provocation. It also reduces free fatty acid levels and liver glycogen content in mice and elevates fructose-1, 6-diphosphate, dihydroxyacetone-phosphate, and pyruvate in liver. These data are interpreted to show accelerated carbohydrate breakdown for energy production since free fatty acids are less available for this purpose. Therefore, the antilipemic effect of nicotinic acid and its aggravation of diabetes may be a consequence of the reduction of free fatty acid levels in serum. It is to be recalled that clofibrate may act by a similar mechanism.

Goldsmith, Miller and Hamilton[102,108,110] have obtained evidence that nicotinic acid does not act by competition for methyl groups or glycine nor by increasing the excretion of sterols and bile acids in the feces. The latter is indirect evidence that enhanced oxidation of cholesterol to bile acids by the liver is not responsible for the antilipemic effect of nicotinic acid.

Another possible mechanism is an effect on the biosynthesis of lipids, particularly cholesterol. Parsons' experiments,[99] using ^{14}C-acetate, imply that conversion into free and esterized serum cholesterol and erythrocyte cholesterol was much reduced during nicotinic acid administration. He also found that this compound influences lipid transport by lowering beta-lipoproteins and increasing alpha-lipoproteins in the serum which may account in part for its antilipemic activity.

In summary, cholesterol and other lipids involved in atherogenesis may be attacked at every site in their metabolic chains. Although it is possible to lower plasma cholesterol with currently available drugs and dietary measures, and even better agents are sure to follow, only time will tell if such therapy influences the natural course of atherosclerosis.

REFERENCES

1. Myant, N. B.: The regulation of cholesterol metabolism, Postgrad. M. J. *44*:86, 1968.
2. Hernandez, H. H., Peterson, D. W., Chaikoff, I. L., and Dauben, W. G.: Absorption of cholesterol-4-C[14] in rats fed mixed soybean sterols and beta-sitosterol, Proc. Soc. Exper. Biol. & Med. *83*:498, 1953.
3. Pollak, O.J.: Reduction of blood cholesterol in man, Circulation *7*:702, 1953.
4. Farquhar, J. W., Smith, R. E., and Dempsey, M. E: The effect of beta-sitosterol on the serum lipids of young men with arteriosclerotic heart disease. Circulation *14*:77, 1956.
5. Best, M. M., and Duncan, C. H.: Modification of abnormal serum lipid patterns in atherosclerosis by administration of sitosterol, Ann. Int. Med. *45*:614, 1956.
6. Hashim, S. A., and Van Itallie, T. B.: Cholestyramine resin therapy for hypercholesteremia, J. A. M. A. *192*:89, 1965.
7. Berkowitz, D.: Selective blood lipid reductions by newer pharmacologic agents, Am. J. Cardiol. *12*:834, 1963.
8. Howard, R. P., Brusco, O. J., and Furman, R. H.: Effect of cholestyramine administration on serum lipids and on nitrogen balance in familial hypercholesterolemia, J. Lab. & Clin. Med. *68*:12, 1966.
9. Tennent, D. M., Siegel, H., Zanetti, M. E., Kuron, G. W., Ott, W. H., and Wolf, F. J.: Plasma cholesterol lowering action of bile acid binding polymers in experimental animals, J. Lip. Res. *1*:469, 1960.
10. Schneider, D. L., Gallo, D. G., and Sarett, H. P.: Effect of cholestyramine on cholesterol metabolism in young adult swine, Proc. Soc. Exper. Biol. & Med. *121*:1244, 1966.
11. Fallon, H. J., and Woods, J. W.: Response of hyperlipoproteinemia to cholestyramine resin, J.A.M.A. *204*:1161, 1968.
12. Khachadurian, A. K.: Cholestyramine therapy in patients homozygous for familial hypercholesterolemia (familial hypercholesterolemic xanthomatosis), J. Atherosclerosis Res. *8*:177–188, 1968.
13. Roe, D. A.: Essential hyperlipemia with xanthomatosis. Effects of cholestyramine and clofibrate, Arch. Dermat. *97*:436, 1968.
14. Samuel, P., and Steiner, A.: Reduction of the level of serum cholesterol in man by neomycin, Circulation *18*:494, 1958.

15. Samuel, P., and Waithe, W. I.: Reduction of serum cholesterol concentrations by neomycin, para-aminosalicylic acid, and other antibacterial drugs in man, Circulation *24*:578, 1961.
16. Samuel, P., Holtzman, C. M., Meilman, E., and Shalchi, O. B.: Reduction of the rapidly miscible pool of cholesterol by neomycin in man, Circulation *32*:(II), 28, 1965.
17. Samuel, P., Holtzman, C. M., and Goldstein, J.: Longterm reduction of serum cholesterol levels of patients with atherosclerosis by small doses of neomycin, Circulation *35*:938, 1967.
18. Goldsmith, G. A., Hamilton, J. G., and Miller, O. N.: Mechanisms used by unsaturated fats, nicotinic acid and neomycin: Excretion of sterols and bile acids-lowering of serum lipid concentrations, Arch. Int. Med. *105*:512, 1960.
19. Van den Bosch, J. F., and Claes, P. J.: Correlation between the bile salt precipitating capacity of derivatives of basic antibiotics and plasma cholesterol-lowering effect in vivo, 2nd International Symposium on Drugs Affecting Lipid Metabolism, Milan, Italy, September, 1965.
20. Eyssen, H., Evrard, E., and Vanderhaeghe, H.: Cholesterol-lowering effects of N-methylated neomycin and basic antibiotics, J. Lab. & Clin. Med. *68*:753, 1966.
21. Fisher, H., Van der Noot, G. W., McGrath, W. S., and Griminger, P.: Dietary pectin and plasma cholesterol in swine, J. Atherosclerosis Res. *6*:190, 1966.
22. Leveille, G. A., and Sauberlich, H. E.: Mechanism of the cholesterol-depressing effect of pectin in the cholesterol-fed rat, J. Nutrition *88*:209, 1966.
23. Griminger, P., and Fisher, H.: Anti-hypercholesterolemic action of scleroglucan and pectin in chickens, Proc. Soc. Exper. Biol. & Med. *122*:551, 1966.
24. Riccardi, B.A., and Fahrenbach, M.J.: Effect of guar gum and pectin N. F., on serum and liver lipids of cholesterol fed rats, Proc. Soc. Exper. Biol. & Med. *124*:749, 1967.
25. Morrison, L. M., Murata, K., Quilligan, J. J., Jr., Schjeide, O. A., and Freeman, L: Prevention of atherosclerosis in sub-human primates by chondroitin sulfate A, Circulation Res. *19*:358, 1966.
26. Brahmankar, D. M., and Connor, W. E.: Effect of high molecular weight dextran on experimental hypercholesterolemia, Circulation Res. *21*:817, 1967.
27. Palmer, G. H., and Dixon, D. G.: Effect of pectin dose on serum cholesterol levels, Am. J. Clin. Nutrition *18*:437, 1966.
28. Morrison, L. M.: Treatment of coronary arteriosclerotic heart disease with chondroitin sulfate-A: Preliminary report, J. Am. Geriatrics Soc. *16*:779–785, 1968.
29. Blohme, G., Kerstell, J., and Svanborg, A.: The effect of dextran on plasma lipids. A study on patients with essential hypercholesterolemia or hyperlipemia, Acta med. scandinav. *183*:481, 1968.
30. Aramaki, Y., Kobayashi, T., Imai, Y., Kikuchi, S., Matsukawa, T., and Kanazawa, K.: Biological studies of cholestane-3β, 5α, 6β-triol and its derivatives. Part 1. Hypocholesterolemic effects in rabbits, chickens and rats on atherogenic diets, J. Atherosclerosis Res. *7*:653, 1967.
31. Imai, Y., Kikuchi, S., Matsuo, T., Suzuoki, Z., and Nishikawa, K.: Biological studies of cholestane-

3β, 5α, 6β-triol and its derivatives. Part 2. Effect of cholestane-3β, 5α, 6β-triol on the absorption, synthesis, excretion and tissue distribution of cholesterol in rats, J. Atherosclerosis Res. 7:671, 1967.

32. Cooper, E.: Inhibition of cholesterol biosynthesis in man, Circulation 20:681, 1959.

33. Sachs, B. A., Danielson, E., and Sperber, R.: Hypocholesterolemic effects of N-(1-methyl-2-3-di-p-chlorophenylpropyl)-maleamic acid in hyperlipemic and normolipemic man, Circulation 20:762, 1959.

34. Blohm, T. R., and MacKenzie, R. D.: Specific inhibition of cholesterol biosynthesis by a synthetic compound (MER-29), Arch. Biochem. 85:245, 1959.

35. Goodman, D. S., Avigan, J., and Steinberg, D.: Studies of cholesterol biosynthesis. V. The time course and pathway of the later stages of cholesterol biosynthesis in the livers of intact rats, J. Biol. Chem. 238:1287, 1963.

36. Avigan, J., Steinberg, D., Vroman, H. E., Thompson, M. J., and Mosettig, E.: Studies of cholesterol biosynthesis. I. The identification of desmosterol in serum and tissues of animals and man treated with MER-29, J. Biol. Chem. 235:3123, 1960.

37. Blankenhorn, D. H., Maronde, R. F., and Scholtz, J. R.: Occurrence and distribution of demosterol in human arteries following treatment with triparanol, Circulation 24:889, 1961.

38. Avoy, D. R., Swyryd, E. A., and Gould, R. G.: Effects of L-p-chlorophenoxyisobutyryl ethyl ester (CPIB) with and without androsterone on cholesterol biosynthesis in rat liver, J. Lip. Res. 6:369, 1965.

39. Barrett, A. M., and Thorp, J. M.: Studies on the mode of action of clofibrate; Effects on hormone-induced changes in plasma free fatty acids, cholesterol, phospholipids and total esterified fatty acids in rats and dogs, Brit. J. Pharmacol. 32:381, 1968.

40. Hunninghake, D. B., and Azarnoff, D. L.: Clofibrate effect on catecholamine-induced metabolic changes in humans, Metabolism 17:588, 1968.

41. Duncan, C. H., Best, M. M., and Despopoulos, A.: Inhibition of hepatic secretion of triglyceride by chlorophenoxyisobutyrate (CPIB), Circulation (Suppl. 3) 30:7, 1964.

42. Azarnoff, D. L., Tucker, D. R., and Barr, G. A.: Studies with ethyl chlorophenoxyisobutyrate (Clofibrate), Metabolism 14:959, 1965.

43. Feinberg, L. J., Sandbeerg, H., Van der Stichele, E., Warner, H., and Bellet, S.: Effects of hypocholesteremic drugs on the incorporation of C14-labeled tripalmitin into lipoproteins, Circulation 32:(II), 12, 1965.

44. Mishkel, M. A., and Webb, W. F.: The mechanisms underlying the hypolipidaemic effects of atromid S, nicotinic acid and benzmalecene—I. The metabolism of free fatty acid-albumin complex by the isolated perfused liver, Biochem. Pharmacol. 16:897, 1967.

45. Ryan, W. G., and Schwartz, T. B.: The dynamics of triglyceride turnover: effect of atromid-S, J. Lab. & Clin. Med. 64:1001, 1964.

46. Hellman, L., Zunoff, B., Kessler, G., Kara, E., Rubin, I. L., and Rosenfeld, R. S.: Reduction of cholesterol and lipids in man by ethyl p-chloro-phenoxyisobutyrate, Ann. Int. Med. 59:477, 1963.

47. Danowski, T. S., Novak, J. F., Saul, R. W., Vester, J. W., and Moses, C.: Hypolipidemic effect of chlorophenoxyisobutyrate in adult-onset diabetes mellitus, Clin. Pharmacol. Ther. 7:631, 1966.

48. Rifkind, B. M.: Effect of CPIB ester on plasma free fatty acid levels in man, Metabolism 15:673, 1966.

49. Orgain, E. S., Bogdonoff, M. D. and Cain, C.: Clofibrate and andosterone effect on serum lipids, Arch. Int. Med. 119:80, 1967.

50. Braunsteiner, H., Herbst, M., Sandhorfe, F., and Sailer, S.: Langzeitbehandlung von bisher therapierefraktaeren Faellen primaerer Hypertriglyceridaemie des Erwachsenen mit Aethyl-p-chlorophenoxyisobutyrat, Deutsche, med. Wchnschr. 92:2303, 1967.

51. Feinberg, L. J., Sandberg, H., Stichele, E. van der, Warner, H., and Bellet, S.: The effects of clofibrate on the metabolism of C14 labeled tripalmitin in the human subject, Metabolism 16:618, 1967.

52. Hagopian, M., and Robinson, R. W.: The effect of chlorophenoxyisobutyrate on plasma composition of cholesteryl esters and on levels of neutral lipids, J. Atherosclerosis Res. 8:21-27, 1968.

53. Strisower, E. H.: The response of hyperlipoproteinemias to atromid and ethyl chlorophenoxyisobutyrate, J. Atherosclerosis Res. 3:445, 1963.

54. Sachs, B. A.: Appraisal of clofibrate as a hypolipidemic agent, Am. Heart J. 5:707, 1968.

55. Levy, R. I., and Fredrickson, D. S.: Diagnosis and management of hyperlipoproteinemia. Am. J. Cardiol. 22:576, 1968.

56. Oliver, M. F.: The current status of Atromid-S and its use in the prevention of ischaemic heart disease. 2nd International Symposium on Drugs Affecting Lipid Metabolism, Milan, Italy, September 1965.

57. Oliver, M. F., Roberts, S. D., Hayes D., Pantridge, J. F., Suzman, M. M., and Bersohn, I.: Effect of atromid and ethyl chlorophenoxyisobutyrate on anticoagulant requirements, Lancet 1:143, 1963.

58. Solomon, H. M., and Schrogie, J. J.: The effect of various drugs on the binding of warfarin-14C to human albumin, Biochem. Pharmacol. 16:1219, 1967.

59. Cotton, R. C., Wade, E. G., and Spiller, G. W.: The effect of atromid on plasma fibrinogen and heparin resistance, J. Atherosclerosis Res. 3:648, 1963.

60. Carson, P., McDonald, L., Pickard, S., Pilkington, T., Davies, B., and Love, F.: Effect of atromid on platelet stickiness, J. Atherosclerosis Res. 3:619, 1963.

61. McAndrew, G. M., and Fullerton, H. W.: The effect of atromid on the recalcified plasma clotting time after high fat meals, Lancet 3:634, 1963.

62. Oliver, M. F.: Further observations on the effects of atromid and of ethyl chlorophenoxyisobutyrate on serum lipid levels, J. Atherosclerosis Res. 3:427, 1963.

63. Hollander, W.: The pharmacologic actions of anti-lipemic drugs, in Cardiovascular Drug Therapy, edited by A. N. Brest and J. H. Moyer, New York, Grune and Stratton, Inc. 1965. p. 339.

64. Berkowitz, D.: The effects of chlorophenoxyisobutyrate with and without androsterone on the serum lipids, fat tolerance and uric acid, Metabolism 14:966, 1965.

65. Best, M. M., and Duncan, C. H.: Effects of clofibrate

and dextrothyroxine singly and in combination on serum lipids, Arch. Int. Med. *118*:97, 1966.

66. Strisower, E. H.: The combined use of CPIB and thyroxine in treatment of hyperlipoproteinemias, Circulation *33*:291, 1966.

67. Berkowitz, D., De Felice, E., and Arcese, P.: The effect of SaH-2348 on the blood lipids (Abs.), Circulation *38*:(Suppl. VI) 41, 1968.

68. Siperstein, M. D., and Fagan, V. M.: Feedback control of mevalonate synthesis by dietary cholesterol, J. Biol. Chem. *241*:602, 1966.

69. Counsell, R. E., Klimstra, P. D., Nysted, L. N., and Ranney, R. E.: Hypocholesterolemic agents. V. Isomeric azacholesterols, J. M. Pharmacol. Chem. *8*:45, 1965.

70. Ranney, R. E., and Cook, D. L.: The hypocholesterolemic action of 20,25-diazacholesterol, Arch. Int. Pharmacodyn. *154*:51, 1965.

71. Sachs, B. A., and Wolfman, L.: 20–25-diazacholestenol dihydrochloride—inhibition of cholesterol biosynthesis in hyperlipemic subjects. Arch. Int. Med. *116*:366, 1965.

72. Dvornik, D., and Kraml, M.: Accumulation of 24-dehydrocholesterol in rats treated with 22, 25-diazacholestenol dihydrochloride: A new inhibitor of cholesterol biosynthesis, Proc. Soc. Exper. Biol. & Med. *112*:1012, 1963.

73. Berger, F. M., Douglas, J. F., Ludwig, B. J., and Margolin, S.: Effect of benzyl-N-benzyl carbethoxyhydroxamate (W-398) on experimental atherosclerosis and hypercholesteremia, Proc. Soc. Exper. Biol. & Med. *114*:337, 1963.

74. Douglas, J. F., Ludwig, B. J., Margolin, S., and Berger, F. M.: Studies on the mechanism of the hypocholesterolemic action of benzyl N-benzyl carbethoxy-hydroxamate. (W-398), J.Atherosclerosis Res. *5*:90, 1966.

75. Kritchevsky, D., and Tepper, S. A.: Effect of benzyl N-benzyl carbethoxyhydroxamate on cholesterol metabolism in the rat, Proc. Soc. Exper. Biol. & Med. *121*:1162, 1966.

76. Horlick, L.: Effect of new inhibitor of cholesterol biosynthesis (AY-9944) on serum and tissue sterols in the rat, J. Lipid Res. *7*:116, 1966.

77. Dvornik, D., and Hill, P.: Effect of long-term administration of AY-9944, an inhibitor of 7-dehydrocholesterol △ 7-reductase, on serum and tissue lipids in the rat, J. Lipid Res. *9*:587-595, 1968.

78. Popjak, G.: Biosynthesis of cholesterol and related substances, Ann. Rev. Biochem. *27*:533, 1958.

79. Dick, E. C., Greenberg, S. M., Herndon, J. F., Jones, M., and Van Loon, E. J.: Hypocholesterolemic effect of β-diethylaminoethyl diphenylpropylacetate hydrochloride (SKF 525-A) in the dog, Proc. Soc. Exper. Biol. & Med. *104*:523, 1960.

80. Schrogie, J. J., and Solomon, H. M.: The hypocholesterolemic effect of phenyramidol, Clin. Pharmacol. Ther. *7*:723, 1966.

81. Abrams, W. B.: The use of polyunsaturates as antilipemic agents, *in* Cardiovascular Drug Therapy, edited by A. N. Brest and J. H. Moyer, New York, Grune and Stratton, Inc., 1965, p. 364.

82. Bender, S.: Unpublished data.

83. Spritz, N., Ahrens, N., and Grundy, S.: Sterol balance in man as plasma cholesterol concentrations are altered by exchanges of dietary fats, J. Clin. Invest. *44*:1482, 1965.

84. Bender, S. R.: Thyroid analogs in the treatment of hyperlipidemia, *in* Cardiovascular Drug Therapy, edited by A. N. Brest and J. H. Moyer, New York, Grune and Stratton, Inc., 1965, p. 349.

85. Owen, W. R.: Efficacy of drugs in lowering blood cholesterol, M. Clin. North America *48*:347, 1964.

86. Eskelson, C. D.: The effects of some thyroid hormones on *in vitro* cholesterol biosynthesis, Life Sci. *7*(Part 2):467, 1968.

87. Taxay, E. P.: Clinical evaluation of a thyroid analog in patients with hypocholesterolemia, angina, claudication and diabetes, Am. J. M. Sc. *244*:191, 1962.

88. Moses, C., Jablonski, J. R., Sunder, J. H., and Katz, L. B.: The use of sodium dextro-thyroxin in patients with angina pectoris, Am. J. M. Sc. *244*:731, 1962.

89. Moyer, J. H.: A current appraisal of drug therapy of atherosclerosis, Arch. Environ. Health *14*:337-347, 1967.

90. Wechter, W. J., Phillips, W. A., and Kagan, F.: Hypocholesterolemic agents. Thyroalkanols, J. M. Chem. *8*:474, 1965.

91. Russ, E. M., Eder. H. A., and Barr, D. P.: Protein-lipid relationships in human plasma. I. In normal individuals, Am. J. Med. *11*:468, 1951.

92. Russ, E. M., Eder, H. A., and Barr, D. P.: Influence of gonadal hormones on protein-lipid relationships in human plasma, Am. J. Med. *19*:4, 1955.

93. Brody, S., Kerstell, J., Nilsson, L., and Svanborg, A.: The effect of some ovulation inhibitors on the different plasma lipid fractions. Acta med. scandinav. *183*:1, 1968.

94. Marmorston, J., Moore, F. J., Hopkins, C. E., Kuzma, O. T., and Weiner, J.: Estrogen therapy in men with myocardial infarction, Proc. Soc. Exper. Biol. & Med. *110*:400, 1962.

95. Oliver, M. F., and Boyd, G. S.: Influence of reduction of serum lipids on prognosis of coronary heart disease, a 5 year study using estrogen, Lancet *2*:499, 1961.

96. Stamler, J., Pick, R., Katz, L. N., Pick, A., Kaplan, B. M., Berkson, D. M., and Century, D.: Effectiveness of estrogens for therapy of myocardial infarction in middle-age men, J. A. M. A. *183*:106, 1963.

97. Merola, A. J., Dill, R. R., and Arnold, A.: Effects of estrogens on cholesterol biosynthesis and tissue distribution in rats, Arch. Biochem. Biophys. *123*:378, 1968.

98. Altschul, R., Hoffer, A., and Stephen, J. D.: Influence of necotinic acid on serum cholesterol in man, Arch. Biochem. Biophys. *54*:558 (1955).

99. Parsons, W. B., Jr.: Treatment of hypercholesterolemia by nicotinic acid, A. M. A. Arch. Int. Med. *107*:639 (1961).

100. Zeller, W.: Untersuchungen uber die Behandlung der hyperlipamischen Atherosklerose und der Leberepithelverfettung mit B-Pyridylcarbinol, Klin. Wchnschr. *44*:1022, (Number 17) 1966.

101. Gant, Z. N., and Taylor, W. J. B.: Effects of large doses of nicotinyl alcohol on serum lipid levels and carbohydrate tolerance, J. Clin. Pharmacol. and J. New Drugs *8*:370, Nov-Dec., 1968.

102. Miller, O. N., Hamilton, J. G., and Goldsmith, G. A.: Investigation of mechanism of action of nicotinic acid on serum lipid levels in man, Am. J.

Clin. Nutrition *8*:480 (1960).

103. Gurian, H., and Aldersberg, D.: The effect of large doses of nicotinic acid on circulating lipids and carbohydrate tolerance, Am. J. M. Sc. *237*:12 (1959).

104. Parsons, W. B.: Studies of nicotinic acid use in hypercholesterolemia, A. M. A. Arch. Int. Med. *107*:653, 1961.

105. Molnar, G. D., Gerge, K. G., Rosevear, J. W., McGuckin, W. F., and Achor, R. W. P.: The effect of nicotinic acid in diabetes mellitus, Metabolism *13*:181 (1964).

106. Carlson, L. A., and Oro, L.: The effect of nicotinic acid on the plasma free fatty acids, Acta. Med. scandinav. *172*:641, 1962.

107. Dalton, C., and Kowalski, C.: Cholesterol lowering mechanism of nicotinic acid and nicotinyl alcohol tartrate, Fed. Proc. *26*:806 (1967).

108. Goldsmith, G. A.: Mechanisms by which certain pharmacologic agents lower serum cholesterol, Fed. Proc. *21*:81, 1962.

109. Kritchevsky, D., Whitehouse, M. W., and Staple, E.: Oxidation of cholesterol-26-C^{14} by rat liver mitochondria. Effect of nicotinic acid, J. Lipid Res. *1*:154, 1960.

110. Miller, O. N., Hamilton, J. G., and Goldsmith, G.A.: Mechanism of action of nicotinic acid in lowering serum lipids, Am. J. Clin. Nutrition *10*: 285, 1962.

A Critical Appraisal of the Use of Anticoagulants

Irving S. Wright

Anticoagulant therapy has been subjected to most comprehensive investigation during the past 30 years. These drugs producing profound changes in the coagulation balance have been studied in terms of their basic chemistry, pharmacology, pathophysiologic actions, adverse effects and clinical values by experts of many disciplines. As might be expected when dealing with such complex syndromes in man and with drugs of such varying potency, there has not been complete unanimity in conclusions regarding their therapeutic use or efficacy.

They are not entirely successful in the prevention or dissolution of thrombi and they do not prevent the inexorable ravages of progressive atherothrombosis. Nevertheless they do frequently exert the effort of tilting the coagulation balance against the formation of thrombi and this has produced marked reduction in the incidence of thromboemboli in many conditions. Among the easiest conditions in which to demonstrate their value are venous thrombi with secondary pulmonary emboli. It was quickly found by Barker and Zilliacus and others that in these conditions both death and disability can be sharply reduced and this finding was widely accepted but, strangely, the full significance of venous thromboembolism has only recently been fully appreciated. In many hospitals today thrombophlebitis with pulmonary embolism has now been acknowledged as the number one cause of death from pulmonary disease when one includes both acute and recurrent embolization. It has been found to be the number one cause of pulmonary hypertension. It is the number one cause of death following fractures of the pelvis, hip or femur. It is the number one cause of death during labor and the post partum period. Evidence for these striking facts which we have been emphasizing for many years is now being accepted and in each instance the use of anticoagulant therapy has sharply reduced the morbidity and mortality statistics. Ten years ago it was difficult to find fracture surgeons or obstetricians who were willing to use these drugs. Today they are rapidly becoming standard therapy on these services. Fifteen years ago

the use of anticoagulants in the treatment of cerebral vascular disease was characterized as heresy and too dangerous. Today the indications for their use are clarified to a greater degree as indicated in Table 1. For further details the reader is referred to references 1 and 2.

TABLE 1
Cerebral Vascular Disease. An Evaluation of Anticoagulant Therapy

Condition	Evidence
Embolic strokes after first 3 days	Strong
Transient ischemic attacks	Strong
Progressive strokes	Good
Completed strokes (prevent T.E.C.)	Good
Effect on present stroke (local lesion)	Poor
Old strokes	Poor
Hemorrhagic strokes	Adverse
Senile dementia	Poor—new evidence to be evaluated

There has been greater difficulty in establishing their value in arterial than in venous thromboembolism but with continued investigation there has been some clarification of this problem. The fresh thrombi occurring in veins are more apt to be soft and sludge-like, especially those associated with dependency edema or enforced inactivity as after surgery or during a serious illness. Platelets and fibrin play a smaller role than with arterial thrombi during the early stages. It is easy, therefore, for them to become fragmented, detached in toto, or disintegrated by fibrinolysis. This condition may produce small and massive pulmonary emboli when not treated. There has consistently been a marked reduction in risk when anticoagulation permits the action of fibrinolysis to take place early. The older the thrombus the less likely the results are to be satisfactory. The typical arterial thrombus has several different characteristics. Among the most important is the fact that it is usually initiated and propagated in the setting of a more rapid flow. Platelets play a major part in the formation of the arterial thrombi. Probably softer components are swept away leaving only the tougher body remaining, and in the development of this fibrin plays a leading role. It has been found that coumarins and in-dandiones are relatively less effective against platelet fibrin agglomeration of the arterial thrombi than the softer venous thrombi where platelets play a less important early function. This helps to explain why their effects are more significant in venous than in arterial thromboembolism. There is nevertheless strong evidence that the use of anticoagulants in arterial disease is frequently effective. Adequate anticoagulation can reduce the incidence of arterial thrombosis in a wide variety of conditions as well as the propagation of already existing thrombi. However, of greater importance in this respect is the fact that in such cases venous thrombosis is frequently also present as a result of enforced inactivity, or injury, and with myocardial infarction fragile mural thrombi are extremely common in the chambers of the heart. They may also be attached to plaques on the walls of major atherosclerotic arteries. These represent major hazards and anti-coagulant therapy is relatively effective in con-trolling them. It has recently been demonstrated that aspirin (but not salicylic acid), phenylbutazone, guanidinosuccinic acid and persantin can exert an inhibiting effect on platelet agglomeration by action on platelet Factor 3 and other clotting factors. This may be of significance in man but at present must be considered as highly experimental in vitro and in vivo. Pending further study it is not to be recom-mended that these drugs be added to the oral anti-coagulants for clinical use. Their synergistic action may greatly enhance the anticoagulant activity and thereby increase the risk of hemorrhage.

Of the large number of studies of the effects of anticoagulant therapy in the treatment of myocardial infarction more than 90% have reported favorable results. The remainder have reported slight or no improvement. No series of significant size has shown a higher mortality rate in the treated group. If the favorable results had been based on chance alone a considerable number would have fallen on the negative side. It is true that the protocols of some reported series are not satisfactory by critical standards. They vary greatly in their protocols, yet the uniformity of results from many countries and from both sides of the iron curtain presents us with an extremely heavy weight of evidence in favor of the use of anticoagulants. Investigation into the reasons why a few seemingly well structured studies have failed to confirm the findings of the majority have led to the following deductions:

1. The protocols for the studies have varied wide-ly, from simple case reports to large and detailed but controlled experiences, and finally to well planned prospective double blind studies. In such studies the size is of great importance. Statistical studies based on projections from small series rather than adequate numbers of cases are not acceptable for this type of investigation. A double blind study is not necessarily satisfactory. Several reports have demonstrated that this does not insure adequate dosage levels.

2. The manner of laboratory control of the study has varied widely depending on the skill of the technician, the technic used and the thromboplastic material used; e.g., commercial thromboplastin, P & P (Owren), Thrombotest (Owren), or brain, or lung thromboplastin prepared locally. The curves used to determine satisfactory levels of activity of prothrombin, Factor VII, and other factors, vary widely. This variation can cause serious difficulties. For example, a large study was conducted using, as a therapeutic objective, a level of 15 per cent activi-ty as measured by the Thrombotest. It was apparent-ly assumed that this was therapeutically equal to 15-20 per cent by the one-stage Quick test. Actual-ly, using the Thrombotest we have found that for therapeutic purposes it is necessary to maintain the level at 7-10 per cent activity. It was not surprising, therefore, that the above study did not result in satisfactory therapeutic results.

3. The amount of anticoagulant used also is an important factor.

In our original reports of more than twenty years ago, we emphasized the need for adequate, but not excessive dosage of anticoagulant drugs. We recom-mended dosage levels of coumarin compounds which would prolong the prothrombin times to one and one half to two times the control. This averages to be 18-24 per cent activity (Quick). Heparin should be given in dosages adequate to insure maintenance of Lee-White clotting times of two times normal before the succeeding dose. The subcutaneous route of administration is generally satisfactory except for emergency or surgical pur-poses. The intervals between doses varies from 4–12 hours depending on the length of time necessary to return to the level of twice the normal time. For details regarding the practical managment of anticoagulants see Reference 3. However, some patients are even now receiving token therapy, such as 5000 units (50 mg.) of heparin a day or 10,000 units (100 mg.) twice a week. Others receiving oral anticoagulants have been kept at 40 per cent levels of prothrombin activity, or even higher levels. These are known to be ineffectual. In one long-term double blind study otherwise carefully planned, it was found that in only 70 per cent of the time was the prothrombin activity below 30 per cent. The optimal therapeutic level should be 20-25 per cent (Quick test). This meant that in roughly 100 days of each year the patients did not receive adequate therapy. Under such conditions satisfactory control of thromboembolism could hardly be expected and was not obtained. In another large study in which the P & P test was used, the activity level averaged about 40 per cent (Quick) apparently because of a miscalculation. The results were less than satisfactory as could have been predicted. In contrast the U. S. Veterans Administration study,[4] which resulted in statistically favorable results in the long-term treatment for myocardial infarction, was remarkable in that 89 per cent of the time the prothrombin activity was below 25 per cent. Loeliger and his co-workers have reemphasized this point in their recent report.[5]

These results confirm the conclusions drawn in 1954 (The Report of the American Heart Association Committee on Anticoagulants for Myocardial Infarction)[6] that the rate of clinical thromboembolic complications occurring at dosage levels producing prothrombin activity of 25 per cent or greater activity, was twice that occurring at levels less than 25 per cent activity (Quick one-stage test). No further gain was to be expected by higher dosage, and the risk of hemorrhage increases with markedly increased dosages. It is regrettable that more attention has not been paid to this conclusion in the development of some recent studies. It is equally applicable for studies of anticoagulant therapy for all types of thromboembolic conditions. Lack of adherence to it has led to confusion in the minds of many clinicians not expert in this field.

I have used the problems arising from studies dealing with myocardial infarction as examples of the effects of inadequate control of anticoagulant therapy. However, similar errors have been common with the use of these drugs in many other thromboembolic states. We have reviewed the evidence dealing with the use of these drugs as it has accumulated throughout these three decades. In Tables 1—5 we have listed the chief conditions for which anticoagulant therapy has been advocated and an evaluation of the evidence from the world literature. In most of the conditions mentioned the evaluation also reflects the experience on our services in which anticoagulants have been tested and used from their inception. Doubtless some will disagree with these ratings but most clinicians who thoroughly review the literature based on actual studies in this field should find them acceptable. In the future additional uses for these drugs may prove to be of value. In some of these the present evidence

must still be rated as only fair or poor—meaning inadequate as opposed to adverse.

TABLE 2
Conditions for Which Anticoagulant Therapy Should Be Considered. Thromboembolic States: Acute, Recurrent, Impending

Condition	Evidence
Acute thrombophlebitis	Strong
Acute pulmonary embolism	Very strong
Chronic thrombophlebitis (active)	Strong
Chronic venous insufficiency without active phlebitis	Poor
Recurrent thrombophlebitis (preventive)	Good
Thrombophlebitis in pregnancy or post-partum	Good

TABLE 3
Rheumatic Heart Disease. An Evaluation of Anticoagulation Therapy

Condition	Evidence
Valve damage—rhythm regular	Poor
Valve damage—rhythm regular with embolization	Good
Atrial fibrillation flutter without embolization	Good
Arrhythmia flutter fibrillation with embolization—pulmonary or peripheral	Strong
Before conversion	Good
Cardiac failure	Fair
With thromboembolism	Very strong

TABLE 4
Atherothrombotic Heart Disease. An Evaluation of Anticoagulant Therapy

Condition	Evidence
Acute myocardial infarction	Strong
Recurrent myocardial infarction	Strong
Prevention recurrence—to 2 years	Strong
Prevention recurrence—to 4 years	Good
Under 60 years of age	Strong
Over 60 years of age	Good
With arrhythmia	Very strong
With embolization	Very strong

TABLE 5
Conditions for Which Anticoagulant Therapy Should Be Considered

Condition	Evidence
After cardiac surgery valve replacement	Good
Commissurotomy	Good
Vineberg procedures	Poor
After arterial surgery	Good—Fair
Varicose vein surgery	Poor
Retinal vein thrombosis	Fair
Retinal artery thrombosis	Fair
After abdominal surgery (selective)	Fair—Good
After pelvic surgery	Good
Fractures—pelvis, hip, femur	Strong

TABLE 6

Anticoagulant Drugs for Oral Use, Suggested Dosage

	Loading Dose (mg.) First 24 to 48 Hours	Maintenance Dose (mg.)	Time to Produce Therapeutic Levels (Hours)
Coumarin Compounds			
Cyclocoumarol	125–200	12.5–50	36–72
Bishydroxycoumarin	200–300	25–150	36–72
Ethyl biscoumacetate	1800–2400	150–900	18–36
Nicoumalone	36–52	2–12	24–42
Phenprocoumon	18–30	0.75–6	30–48
Sodium warfarin	25–30	2.5–10	36–48
Indandione Compounds			
Anisindione	800–900	75–100	36–60
Diphenadione	30–45	3–5	48–60
Phenindione	200–300	25–200	36–48

CONCLUSIONS

It is a cardinal rule of therapeutics that adequate therapy is essential for satisfactory results. Table 6 indicates the average therapeutic dosage for the more commonly used anticoagulant drugs. The dosage must still be controlled by suitable prothrombin tests to maintain an activity of 18-23 per cent (2-2½ times the control time) for acute episodes and 20-25 per cent (1½-2 times the control level) for long-term therapy. (Quick one-stage test as the standard.) We are anticipating the use of new agents in the near future—including urokinase, and Malayan pit viper venom (Fraction 6) (Arvin) but these are both in the experimental stage at present. The clinical use of drugs including acetylsalicylic acid and phenylbutazone which may prove more active against platelet agglomeration is also being evaluated. The evidence does not yet justify their acceptance as effective therapeutic agents in the thromboembolic and atherothrombotic states.

REFERENCES

1. Wright, I. S.: Strokes—diagnosis and modern treatment (1), Mod. Concepts Cardiovas. Dis. *7*, 1965.
2. ———: Ibid, (2) *8*, 1965; (3) *8*, 1965.
3. Wright, I. S.: Anticoagulant therapy—practical management, Am. Heart J. in press.
4. U. S. Veterans Administration Study, Ebert, R. V., Chairman: Long term anticoagulant therapy after myocardial infarction, J. A. M. A. *193*:929, 1965.
5. Loeliger, E. A., Hensen, A., Kores, F., Van-Dijk, L. M., Fekkes, N., De Jonge, H., and Hemker, H. C.: A double blind trial of long-term anticoagulant treatment after myocardial infarction, Acta med. scandinav. *182*:549, 1967.
6. Wright, I. S., Marple, C., and Beck, D. F.: Myocardial Infarction. Report of the Anticoagulant Committee of the American Heart Association, New York, Grune and Stratton, Inc. 1954.
7. Wright, I. S.: A history of anticoagulants—a symposium, Circulation *29*:110, 1959.
8. Douglas, A S: Anticoagulant Therapy, Oxford, Blackwell Scientific Publications, 1962.
9. Friedberg, C.: Anticoagulant therapy, Heart Bulletin *17*:27, 33, 40, 1968.
10. Udden, P.: Treatment of angina pectoris with anticoagulant (Sintrome) until "bleeding close," Svenska Lakartidninger *60*:220, 1963.
11. Hartenauer, G., Dervers, R. L., and Krieger, E. M.: Acute myocardial infarction, Delaware M. J. *35*: 167, 1963.
12. Fischer, S.: Pathology of Coronary Occlusion With Special Reference to Anticoagulation Medication, Copenhagen, Store Nordiske Viderskabsboghandel, 1963.
13. British Medical Research Council: An assessment of long-term anticoagulant administration after cardiac infarction, Second Report, Brit. M. J. *2*:837, 1964.
14. Asperstrom, G., and Korsan-Bengtsen, K.: A double blind study of Dicumarol prophlaxis in coronary heart disease, Acta med. scandinav. *176*:563, 1964.
15. Wright, I. S.: A Critical Appraisal of Anticoagulant Presented before 46th South African Medical Congress, Durban, July 21, 1967, Accepted for publication in South African M. J.
16. Wright, I. S.: Answers to questions regarding the present day role of anticoagulants in clinical medicine, Hospital Medicine *3*:5, 1967.
17. Merskey, C., and Drapkin, A.: Anticoagulant Therapy, Blood *25*:567, 1965.
18. McDevitt, E., and McDowell, F.: Anticoagulant therapy of the completed stroke, Geriatrics *23*, 135, 1968.

New Dimension in Angina Pectoris Therapy: Propranolol-Nitrate Synergism*

Henry I. Russek

Although it is now almost two centuries since Heberden's classic description of angina pectoris,[1] few notable advances in the therapy of this distressing syndrome have been made. One hundred years ago, Brunton[2] reported on the use of amyl nitrite and a dozen years later Murrell[3] indicated that equally successful results could be achieved from the administration of nitroglycerin. Since those historic contributions, except for the introduction of certain longer acting nitrates, there has been virtually no progress in the medicinal therapy of angina pectoris. Moreover, this static state has persisted during the past many decades despite the introduction of countless new and allegedly effective drugs for this disorder.

It is only recently, with the introduction of propranolol, that a new dimension in antianginal, anti-ischemic therapy has been made available. By decreasing heart rate and ventricular systolic force, propranolol appears to reduce myocardial oxygen requirements to a level more readily satisfied by restricted coronary blood flow. Thus accumulating evidence clearly indicates that this beta adrenergic receptor blocking agent is frequently effective in alleviating angina pectoris which is refractory to conventional modes of therapy.[4-9] Our early experience indicated, however, that the benefits from propranolol in many patients were not appreciable and often hardly exceeded those observed from the use of long-acting nitrates. Moreover, the appearance of angina and ischemic electrocardiographic patterns at lower heart rates with propranolol strongly suggested that the drug may actually exert an adverse subsidiary effect on coronary-myocardial relationships and/or ventricular dynamics.

That propranolol reduces coronary blood flow either through vasoconstriction or through loss of vasodilation has been documented by both animal and human studies.[10-12] Elimination of this partially

*Portions of this article have appeared in geriatrics, *24:* 81, 1969.

negating influence, therefore, could conceivably enhance the action of the drug in angina pectoris. Inasmuch as the nitrates have been shown to increase regional blood flow to ischemic myocardium, their use in combination with propranolol appeared worthy of study. Moreover, since the oxygen-wasting tachycardia frequently attending nitrate administration might be blocked by the negative chronotropic action of propranolol, the possibility of a useful synergism could not be readily dismissed. Indeed, the present study clearly confirms the occurrence of this unusual therapeutic phenomenon.

MATERIALS AND METHODS

To date 115 patients have received propranolol-nitrate therapy. All of this series were markedly restricted by angina of effort and required the frequent use of nitroglycerin. The diagnosis of coronary disease was confirmed by a history and electrocardiographic evidence of previous myocardial infarction, a positive exercise-electrocardiographic response or angiographic evidence of significant coronary vessel involvement. In each instance symptoms had been present for one year or more and the disorder had remained static for several months prior to the trial. In 28 of this number, exercise tolerance and exercise-electrocardiographic tests were preformed to compare the responses to propranolol and isosorbide dinitrate administered singly or in combination. In these selected cases, there was not only a classic history of chest pain on exertion or excitement but also a reproducible ischemic S-T segment pattern following the onset of pain induced by standard exercise and limited or equivocal benefit from the use of long-acting nitrates. Fourteen of the 28 patients in this portion of the study had suffered previous myocardial infarction and 5 were on maintenance digitalis therapy as a result of antecedent congestive heart failure. Clinical features in these 28 cases are shown in Table 1. All patients were told that a new drug was under investigation and that a placebo would be employed in its evaluation. Tablets of propranolol and placebo were identical in appearance and as nearly identical as possible in taste.

Exercise-electrocardiographic tests were obtained by conventional means with the patient ascending and descending the Master two-step staircase at his customary rate under carefully standardized conditions. Only two exercise tests were obtained on any one day. All patients were accustomed to the routine of the test procedure, several control responses

having been recorded in each case prior to undertaking the study. Control electrocardiographic patterns after exercise were almost identical in the individual patient whether recorded on the same or consecutive days. All patients were ambulatory and resided at home in their accustomed environment. All tests were made by one observer, the author, employing the usual facilities of a private medical office.

The first 12 patients were studied in the following manner: After a light breakfast and at a variable interval following the administration of placebo, the

TABLE 1

Clinical Data on 28 Patients With Severe Angina of Effort

Case	Age Sex	Duration of Angina (years)	Previous Myocardial Infarction	Angina at Rest	Resting ECG	Remarks
1	65 M	3	—	None	Nonspecific ST-T abnormality	Secondary anemia and lead poisoning
2	78 M	2	—	None	Nonspecific ST-T abnormality	
3	60 M	2	2 yr. before	None	Normal	
4	78 F	8	5 yr. before	Moderate	Old posterior infarction	Previous CHF,* digitalized
5	60 M	2	—	None	Normal	
6	56 M	2	—	None	Normal	
7	58 F	4	—	None	Nonspecific ST-T abnormality	
8	54 F	3	2 yr. before	None	Nonspecific ST-T abnormality	
9	71 M	10	10 yr. before	Moderate	Old anterior infarction	Vineberg operation one year before
10	54 M	7	—	None	Nonspecific ST-T abnormality	Hypertension, "stroke," digitalized
11	52 M	3	—	None	Normal	
12	73 M	5	15 yr. before	None	Old anterior infarction	
13	63 M	15	15 yr. before	Occasional	Coronary insufficiency	Severe pain on sexual intercourse
14	52 M	1	—	None	Normal	Hypertension, diabetes mellitus
15	72 F	2	—	None	Nonspecific ST-T abnormality	Digitalized
16	68 F	1	—	None	Nonspecific ST-T abnormality	Previous CHF, digitalized
17	53 M	11	11 yr. before	Occassional	Coronary insufficiency	
18	60 M	2	—	None	Normal	
19	52 M	2	9 yr. before	None	Old anterior infarction	
20	29 M	1	1 yr. before	None	Normal	Cerebral palsy, gout
21	65 M	1	1 yr. before	Occasional	Old posterior infarction	
22	78 F	5	—	Occasional	Nonspecific ST-T abnormality	Previous CHF, digitalized
23	71 M	15	—	None	Nonspecific ST-T abnormality	
24	73 F	10	6 yr. before	None	Nonspecific ST-T abnormality	Diabetes mellitus
25	73 M	11	7 yr. before	Occasional	Coronary insufficiency	
26	40 M	1	1 yr. before	None	Old posterior infarction	
27	62 M	5	4 yr. before	None	Old posterior infarction	Diabetes mellitus
28	76 M	2	—	None	Normal	

*CHF=congestive failure

patient was exercised until he reported the onset of typical anginal pain. Exercise was then discontinued and, with the patient supine, the electrocardiogram was recorded immediately and at one minute intervals up to ten minutes. The number of trips to pain was then recorded, thus providing a standard for further testing. In this manner exercise stress was held constant for each patient. At the completion of the first test, a 30-minute interval was allowed to elapse before isosorbide dinitrate was given sublingually in a dosage of 5 mg. At a variable period thereafter (5 min. to 2 hr.) the exercise-electrocardiographic test was repeated in identical fashion. On the second day of study, the same procedure was followed, placebo being administered before the first test and propranolol before the second in a dosage of 40 to 80 mg. a half to two hours before stress. On the third day, the placebo test was again repeated, and this was followed by a final test in which both propranolol and isosorbide dinitrate had been administered as premedication. The dosage and time intervals before exercise with combined therapy were generally similar to those employed in the tests with the individual drugs. Upon completion of exercise-electrocardiographic testing, a new series of measurements was made to determine exercise tolerance to the end point of pain. The same sequence of drugs, dosage and time intervals before exercise was followed as in the first part of the study. For these tests, however, each patient was exercised to the point of pain without being restricted to control exercise levels, and the numbers of trips were carefully recorded and compared.

For the remaining 16 patients in the selected group, the protocol was intentionally altered by substituting random administration of the various test drugs for the set pattern of administration employed in the earlier evaluations. This change was deemed necessary to exclude possible variations in the results which may arise solely as a consequence of a fixed order of drug adiministration. In all other respects, however, the procedures throughout the study followed an identical pattern. Following this alteration in the technic of study, only one test was performed in a given patient on a single day.

In the final phase of the study each of the 115 patients was given propranolol, 40 to 80 mg. orally, four times daily before meals and at bedtime, and isosorbide dinitrate, 5 mg. sublingually, at least four times daily after meals and at bedtime on a continuing basis.

RESULTS

The data obtained from exercise testing are summarized in Table 2. The most striking findings pertain to alterations in anginal pain, heart rate, ischemic electrocardiographic patterns and exercise tolerance. Inasmuch as the observed trends in the data showed a striking uniformity throughout the series, it seemed evident that the fixed order of drug administration in the first 12 patients studied did not play a significant role in determining the results. Accordingly, data are presented for the individual cases as well as for the group as a whole.

Anginal Pain

In the standard exercise tests, isosorbide dinitrate completely prevented the onset of pain in 8 of the 28 patients and diminished its severity in 18. Propranolol prevented its onset in 8 and diminished its severity in 19. In sharp contrast, combined therapy

TABLE 2

Physiologic Data

Case	Medication	Dosage	Time interval before test (min.)	No. of trips	Heart rate Resting	Heart rate Maximal	Pain	Max. S-T seg. depr. (mm.)	Trips to pain
1	Placebo	...	60	26	75	125	++	3.5	26
	Isosorbide dinitrate (ISD)	5 mg.	60	26	86	125	+	3.0	32
	Propranolol	40 mg.	120	26	68	108	+	2.5	34
	ISD and prop.	Same	120	26	63	80	0	0	50*
2	Placebo	...	120	40	80	150	++	5.0	40
	ISD	5 mg.	15	40	107	150	+	3.0	44
	Propranolol	40 mg.	120	40	58	88	+	2.0	44
	ISD and prop.	Same	120	40	66	100	0	0.5	52
3	Placebo	...	120	30	84	125	++	4.0	30
	ISD	5 mg.	120	30	90	135	+	2.5	36
	Propranolol	40 mg.	120	30	59	100	+	2.0	34
	ISD and prop.	Same	120	30	78	95	0	0.5	54*

*No pain experienced at termination of test. Limit of tolerance greater than that recorded.

TABLE 2

Physiologic Data (continued)

Case	Medication	Dosage	Time interval before test (min.)	No. of trips	Heart rate Resting	Heart rate Maximal	Pain	Max. S-T seg. depr. (mm.)	Trips to pain
4	Placebo	...	120	8	76	110	++	4.0	8
	ISD	5 mg.	15	8	76	110	++	3.5	8
	Propranolol	40 mg.	120	8	53	75	+	1.0	10
	ISD and prop.	Same	120	8	53	70	0	0.5	16
5	Placebo	...	60	26	63	85	+++	2.0	26
	ISD	5 mg.	15	26	80	88	+	0.5	34
	Propranolol	40 mg.	60	26	55	78	+	1.0	33
	ISD and prop.	Same	60	26	58	76	0	0	52*
6	Placebo	Same	5	36	75	100	++	2.0	36
	ISD	5 mg.	5	36	80	96	0	0.5	44
	Propranolol	80 mg.	120	36	66	90	0	1.0	42
	ISD and prop.	Same	120	36	75	100	0	0	54*
7	Placebo	...	60	16	63	108	++	2.0	16
	ISD	5 mg.	10	16	74	110	+	0.5	22
	Propranolol	40 mg.	30	16	56	88	+	1.5	20
	ISD and prop.	Same	60	16	50	71	0	0.5	34
8	Placebo	...	60	22	75	100	++	2.0	22
	ISD	5 mg.	25	22	80	100	0	1.5	28
	Propranolol	40 mg.	60	22	58	83	0	0	32
	ISD and prop.	Same	60	22	60	85	0	0	44*
9	Placebo	...	60	26	65	105	+	2.0	26
	ISD	5 mg.	10	26	74	108	0	1.0	32
	Propranolol	40 mg.	60	26	60	88	0	1.0	32
	ISD and prop.	Same	60	26	63	87	0	0	44
10	Placebo	...	60	16	88	136	++	5.0	16
	ISD	5 mg.	30	16	94	138	+	4.0	20
	Propranolol	40 mg.	60	16	65	108	+	3.0	24
	ISD and prop.	Same	60	16	72	108	0	2.0	34
11	Placebo	...	60	34	94	138	++	4.0	34
	ISD	5 mg.	60	34	100	132	+	1.5	42
	Propranolol	40 mg.	120	34	74	110	+	3.0	40
	ISD and prop.	Same	120	34	70	106	0	0.5	48
12	Placebo	...	60	30	92	130	++	3.0	30
	ISD	5 mg.	60	30	104	128	0	1.0	38
	Propranolol	40 mg.	60	30	68	96	+	1.5	36
	ISD and prop.	Same	60	30	75	94	0	0	50*
13	Placebo	...	60	28	64	124	++	3.0	28
	ISD	5 mg.	60	28	74	130	0	1.5	34
	Propranolol	40 mg.	120	28	56	96	+	2.0	34
	ISD and prop.	Same	120	28	54	100	0	0	50
14	Placebo	...	60	18	100	160	++	2.5	18
	ISD	5 mg.	60	18	108	160	+	2.0	24
	Propranolol	80 mg.	120	18	68	120	+	2.0	22
	ISD and prop.	Same	120	18	66	120	0	0	40
15	Placebo	...	60	20	84	142	++	2.5	20
	ISD	5 mg.	60	20	94	144	+	2.0	24
	Propranolol	40 mg.	120	20	60	100	0	1.5	28
	ISD and prop.	Same	120	20	62	100	0	0	42*
16	Placebo	...	60	16	96	136	+++	2.0	16
	ISD	5 mg.	60	16	104	136	+	1.5	22
	Propranolol	40 mg.	120	16	60	96	0	1.0	26
	ISD and prop.	Same	120	16	52	94	0	0	44*
17	Placebo	...	60	16	80	166	++++	3.5	16
	ISD	5 mg.	60	16	80	136	++	3.0	20
	Propranolol	40 mg.	120	16	58	95	++	2.5	20
	ISD and prop.	Same	120	16	63	96	0	2.0	40

*No pain experienced at termination of test. Limit of tolerance greater than that recorded.

TABLE 2

Physiologic Data (concluded)

Case	Medication	Dosage	Time interval before test (min.)	No. of trips	Heart rate Rest-ing	Heart rate Maxi-mal	Pain	Max. S-T seg. depr. (mm.)	Trips to pain
18	Placebo	...	60	32	92	142	++	2.5	32
	ISD	5 mg.	60	32	96	140	0	1.0	38
	Propranolol	60 mg.	120	32	62	96	0	1.0	40
	ISD and prop.	Same	120	32	60	98	0	0	52*
19	Placebo	...	60	24	88	142	++	2.5	24
	ISD	5 mg.	60	24	96	140	+	2.0	28
	Propranolol	40 mg.	120	24	60	106	+	2.0	30
	ISD and prop.	Same	120	24	60	108	0	0.5	46
20	Placebo	...	60	16	84	148	++	1.5	16
	ISD	5 mg.	60	16	82	146	+	1.0	22
	Propranolol	60 mg.	120	16	66	110	+	1.0	24
	ISD and prop.	Same	120	16	65	112	0	0	36*
21	Placebo	...	60	34	72	136	++	2.0	34
	ISD	5 mg.	60	34	78	138	+	1.5	36
	Propranolol	80 mg.	120	34	64	104	0	1.0	38
	ISD and prop.	Same	120	34	64	100	0	0	48
22	Placebo	...	60	16	84	124	+	1.5	16
	ISD	5 mg.	60	16	96	128	+	1.0	18
	Propranolol	60 mg.	120	16	68	100	+	1.0	20
	ISD and prop.	Same	120	16	66	96	0	0.5	30
23	Placebo	...	60	28	60	136	++	2.0	28
	ISD	5 mg.	60	28	72	134	+	1.5	34
	Propranolol	40 mg.	120	28	44	100	+	1.5	34
	ISD and prop.	Same	120	28	46	96	0	0.5	46*
24	Placebo	...	60	20	72	140	++	2.5	29
	ISD	5 mg.	60	20	78	142	0	1.0	26
	Propranolol	40 mg.	120	20	56	106	+	1.5	26
	ISD and prop.	Same	120	20	56	104	0	0.5	38
25	Placebo	...	60	24	96	146	+++	2.5	24
	ISD	5 mg.	60	24	106	146	+	1.5	30
	Propranolol	40 mg.	120	24	60	102	+	1.5	30
	ISD and prop.	Same	120	24	60	100	0	0.5	50
26	Placebo	...	60	30	78	134	++	2.0	30
	ISD	5 mg.	60	30	88	136	+	1.5	36
	Propranolol	40 mg.	120	30	56	96	+	1.5	36
	ISD and prop.	Same	120	30	58	96	0	0.5	52*
27	Placebo	...	60	20	84	120	++	2.0	20
	ISD	5 mg.	60	20	88	120	+	1.5	24
	Propranolol	60 mg.	120	20	64	92	+	1.0	26
	ISD and prop.	Same	120	20	64	92	0	0.5	44
28	Placebo	...	60	24	72	124	+	2.0	24
	ISD	5 mg.	60	24	86	124	0	1.0	30
	Propranolol	40 mg.	120	24	54	96	0	1.0	30
	ISD and prop.	Same	120	24	56	94	0	0	48

*No pain experienced at termination of test. Limit of tolerance greater than that recorded.

protected all 28 patients from experiencing any discomfort as a result of exercise.

Heart Rate

Prior to exercise with the patients reclining, the heart rate after propranolol was an average of 24 per cent below that after placebo. The heart rate after isosorbide dinitrate averaged 11 per cent greater than that after placebo. Propranolol blocked the acceleration of the heart induced by isosorbide dinitrate. Following exercise, the maximal heart rates were only slightly greater after isosorbide dinitrate than after placebo. The reduction in maximal heart rate averaged 32 beats/min. following administration of propranolol, and this degree of cardiac slowing was achieved whether or not isosorbide dinitrate had been administered ($p < 0.001$) (Table 2).

ISCHEMIC ELECTROCARDIOGRAPHIC CHANGES

In all 28 patients, the greatest S-T segment depression was found in the tests following placebo, the least after the combination of propranolol and isosorbide dinitrate. Propranolol or isosorbide dinitrate alone were followed by intermediate degrees of S-T segment depression in exercise-electrocardiographic tests. Tables 3 and 4 show the remarkable influence of combined therapy on maximum S-T segment depression, but of even greater significance is the strong suggestion of synergism between the drugs in individual cases. Figures 1 to 4 illustrate this phenomenon in representative patients whose responses to the separate drugs were relatively slight or inconsequential. This is also dramatically demonstrated in the records of exercise tolerance tests (Table 2).

Exercise Tolerance

In individual cases there was a marked correlation between improvement in exercise-electrocardiographic patterns and increased ability to perform exercise. The average increase in exercise tolerance with propranolol or isosorbide dinitrate alone was approximately 22 and 25 per cent, respectively, whereas with combined therapy it averaged more than 83 per cent (p < 0.001) (Fig. 5). These differences are highly significant statistically, as shown in Table 4. Moreover, since 12 of the 28 subjects had encountered no pain, but only mild fatigue, at the termination of the tests in which propranolol and isosorbide dinitrate had been used simultaneously (even though it was the intent of the test to induce angina), it is evident that the capacity for exercise when both drugs were administered was even greater than that recorded for these patients.

Continuous Therapy

Of the 115 patients, 109 have been observed on combined treatment for periods ranging from 6 to 20 months with striking and persistent amelioration

Table 3
Average Maximal S-T Segment Depression After Exercise

Placebo	2.7 mm.
Isosorbide dinitrate (ISD)	1.7 mm.
Propranolol	1.5 mm.
Propranolol and ISD	0.4 mm.

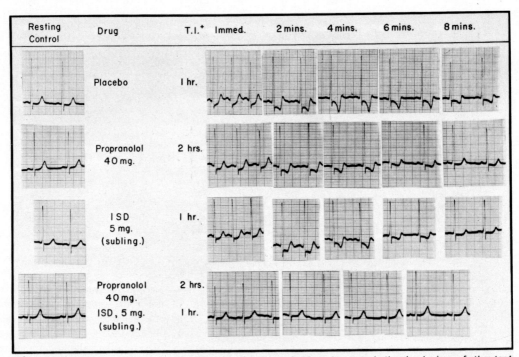

+ T.I. – *Time interval between the administration of the drug and the beginning of the test.*

FIG. 1.　Comparative ECG responses (lead V₅) to standard exercise (26 trips) following propranolol and/or isosorbide dinitrate. (R. D., 65-year-old male)

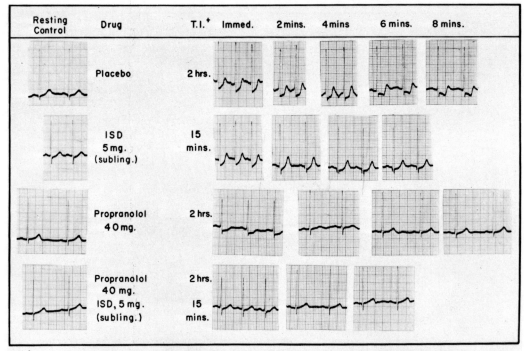

+ T.I. – *Time interval between the administration of the drug and the beginning of the test.*

FIG. 2. Comparative ECG responses (lead V₅) to standard exercise (40 trips) following propranolol and/or isosorbide dinitrate. (G. F., 78-year-old male)

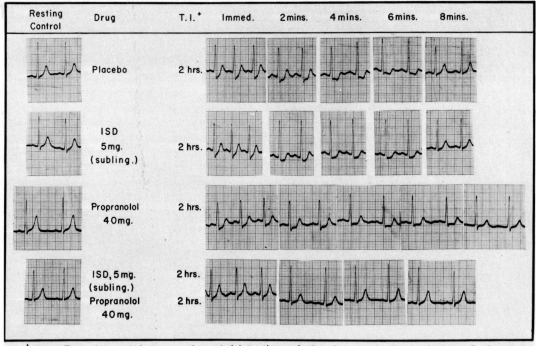

+ T.I. – *Time interval between the administration of the drug and the beginning of the test.*

FIG. 3. Comparative ECG responses (lead V₅) to standard exercise (30 trips) following propranolol and/or isosorbide dinitrate. (A. S., 60-year-old male)

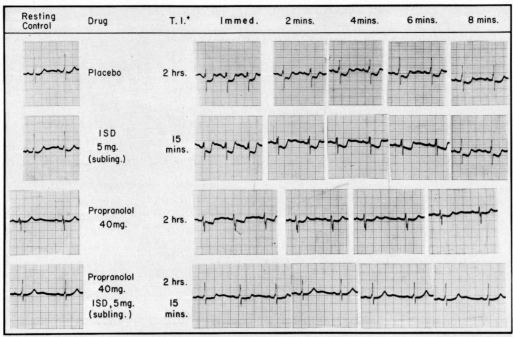

Resting Control	Drug	T. I.*	Immed.	2 mins.	4 mins.	6 mins.	8 mins.
	Placebo	2 hrs.					
	ISD 5 mg. (subling.)	15 mins.					
	Propranolol 40 mg.	2 hrs.					
	Propranolol 40 mg. ISD, 5 mg. (subling.)	2 hrs. 15 mins.					

*T.I. – *Time interval between the administration of the drug and the beginning of the test.*

FIG. 4.   Comparative ECG responses (lead V_5) to standard exercise (8 trips) following propranolol and/or isosorbide dinitrate. (H. F., 77 year-old female)

of symptoms (Table 5). Thus far, no instance of tolerance or "escape" from the favorable action of joint usage of the drugs has been encountered. Sudden return of symptoms of increased severity, however, heralded the onset of "acute coronary insufficiency" in two patients who subsequently recovered without discontinuance of therapy. Occasionally, minor adjustments in dosage and time of administration of the drugs have been necessary to achieve optimal response in individual cases. Two of the patients had been unrelieved by myocardial transplantation of the internal mammary and gastroepiploic arteries one year after surgery but became symptom-free upon administration of propranolol and isosorbide dinitrate. In only two patients of the total series was it found necessary to discontinue therapy because of the appearance of

dyspnea. To date four patients have succumbed from acute myocardial infarction after continuous therapy of 1, 4, 8, and 9 months respectively.

Dosage Range

Optimum results were obtained when propranolol was used in sufficient doses to slow the heart rate to approximately 60 beats per minute at rest. Of the 115 patients in the present series, 62 per cent required dosage levels of 40 mg. three or four times daily; 20 per cent required 60 mg. three or four times daily and 10 per cent required doses as high as 100 mg. t.i.d. or q.i.d. In 8 per cent of the patients only 20 mg. or less administered three times daily produced desired results.

TABLE 4
Statistical Analysis of Mean Difference in Maximal S-T Segment Depression and Trips to Pain in 28 Patients

	Placebo vs. ISD	Placebo vs. propranolol	Placebo vs. ISD and propranolol	ISD vs. propranolol	ISD vs. ISD and propranolol	Propranolol vs. ISD and propranolol
Maximal S-T depression	1.0 (p$<$0.001)	1.2 (p$<$0.001)	2.3 (p$<$0.001)	0.16 (Not sig.)	1.3 (p$<$0.001)	1.2 (p$<$0.001)
Trips to pain	5.4 (p$<$0.001)	6.0 (p$<$0.001)	20.1 (p$<$0.001)	0.7 (Not sig.)	14.7 (p$<$0.001)	14.0 (p$<$0.001)

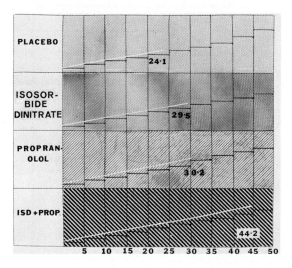

FIG. 5.   Average number of trips to pain in 28 patients.

arising from an underlying disproportion between myocardial oxygen demands and oxygen supply. Although this disparity may be altered either by agents which increase the coronary blood flow or by those which diminish the energy requirements of the heart, a dual approach toward correction, until now, has not been feasible. Consequently, the major objective of medicinal therapy has been improvement in perfusion of potentially ischemic myocardium by coronary vasodilator drugs. With the introduction of propranolol, however, a new dimension in anti-anginal, anti-ischemic therapy has been made available. Thus, it is now possible to decrease the oxygen needs of the heart muscle by blocking the cardiac inotropic and chronotropic effects of the catecholamines. By limiting cardiac responses to physical and emotional stresses, propranolol is proving distinctly useful in ameliorating symptoms and increasing exercise tolerance in anginal patients

TABLE 5

Response of 115 Patients with Angina Pectoris to Propranolol and Isosorbide Dinitrate

Type of angina	No. of patients	Symptom Response							Duration of therapy (months)
		Excellent			Fair	Poor	Myocardial infarction	Deaths	
		No angina	Occasional Angina	Total					
Moderate	48	43	4	47	0	1	1	1	
Severe	67	40	22	62	3	2	4	3	
Total	115	83	26	109	3	3	5	4	6–20

Side Effects

Two patients complained of dizziness following the administration of isosorbide dinitrate sublingually at a time when the propranolol effect was already in evidence. Moderate hypotension was associated with the symptoms in each case. Since both patients had previously exhibited a hypersensitivity to isosorbide dinitrate manifested by lightheadedness, only a half to two thirds of the sublingual tablet was used in subsequent tests without sacrifice of benefits and without recurrence of side effects. In one of these patients, moreover, the use of a weaker nitrate preparation, pentaerythritol tetranitrate, was also found effective (Fig. 6). Three patients experienced mild drowsiness while 4 reported a "very relaxed" feeling. In six there was transient mild diarrhea, in one slight nausea and in ten varying degrees of "heaviness" or weakness in the legs. Increasing dyspnea required discontinuation of therapy in two patients only one of whom suffered from significant diminution in myocardial reserve.

DISCUSSION

Angina pectoris is acknowledged as a syndrome

known to be refractory to conventional modes of therapy. Of even greater promise is the synergism which appears to exist between this agent and certain of the long-acting nitrates.

By administering propranolol in conjunction with isosorbide dinitrate or pentaerythritol tetranitrate, it appears possible to achieve remarkable results even in patients with relatively unsatisfactory response to each of these drugs alone (Figs. 1 and 6). Thus, careful analysis of the data in the 28 selected patients in the present study leads one to conclude that the combined actions of these agents may be not only additive and complementary but also synergistic. Each drug decreases the work of the heart, propranolol by reducing its force and rate and isosorbide dinitrate by diminishing peripheral resistance and venous return. Each agent tends to prevent myocardial ischemia, propranolol by blocking the oxygen-wasting influence of the catecholamines and isosorbide dinitrate by improving perfusion to hypoxic myocardium. Nevertheless, it is primarily through canceling out adverse subsidiary effects that the two drugs appear to achieve therapeutic synergism. Propranolol, in reducing the energy requirements for cardiac contraction. also reduces coronary blood flow either through vaso-

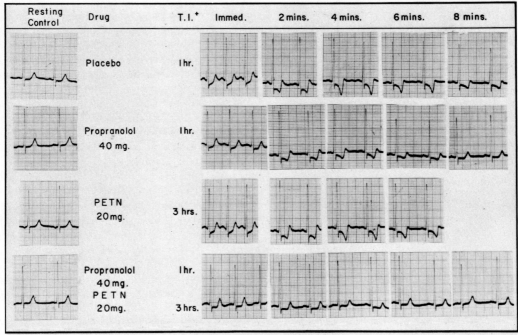

+ T.I. – *Time interval between the administration of the drug and the beginning of the test.*

FIG. 6. Comparative ECG responses (lead V_5) to standard exercise (26 trips) following propranolol and/or pentaerythritol tetranitrate. (R. D.)

contriction or loss of vasodilation.[10–12] This undesirable action, which may partially negate the benefits derived from the "suppression of unneeded and inappropriate cardiac overactivity," is effectively blocked by the simultaneous use of an active nitrate preparation. Contrariwise, propranolol prevents the oxygen-wasting tachycardia induced by isosorbide dinitrate and other related compounds. The total effect of the concurrent administration of both agents, therefore, should be expected to exceed appreciably the sum of the responses evoked when the two drugs are administered independently. This was actually the finding in the present study and is best revealed by the markedly augmented capacity for exercise without pain. Thus, while the average increase in exercise tolerance with propranolol or isosorbide dinitrate alone did not exceed 25 per cent, the increment with combined therapy was more than three times this value, averaging more than 83 per cent. Indeed, combination therapy frequently produced a "one plus one equals four effect" (Table 2).

With isosorbide dinitrate, 5 mg. sublingually, a potent effect is obtained which persists for two hours or more[13] but the drug is also effective by the oral route as shown in Figure 7. Nonetheless, isosorbide dinitrate by the sublingual route excels all other of its formulations in rapidity of action, potency, duration of effect, and dependability. Although

sustained-action preparations of isosorbide dinitrate and pentaerythritol tetranitrate have been found to be relatively weak and ineffectual when prescribed alone,[13] benefits from their use in conjunction with propranolol are often observed in subjects who are hypersensitive to the more potent nitrates. For most patients, however, these formulations fall far short of fulfilling necessary requirements for optimum response when used concurrently with propranolol.

The ability of propranolol to attenuate the resting heart rate and the tachycardia induced by exercise was found to be a prerequisite for its synergistic action with the nitrates. Since absorption appears to vary considerably among patients, individual dosage schedules must be established and periodically adjusted to maintain maximal response. In most of the patients in the present study, 160 mg. of propranolol in divided doses four times daily was effective in obtaining a resting pulse rate of 55 to 60 beats/min. At this dosage level the concomitant administration of isosorbide dinitrate was found to be singularly effective. Others,[9] however, have reported the need for considerably greater doses, as high as 400 mg. per day, when propranolol is administered alone for alleviation of symptoms. Only 10 per cent of our patients actually required such peak dosage levels for optimum response in combination therapy.

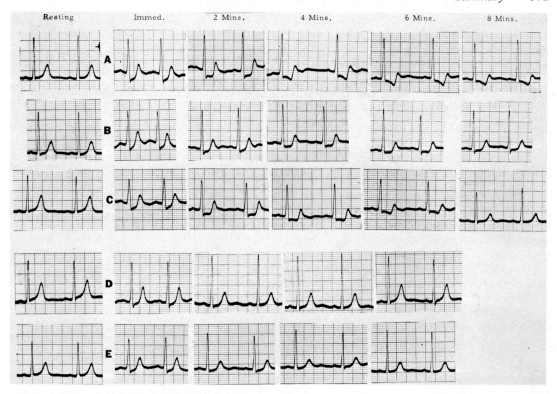

Fig. 7.   Electrocardiographic response (38 trips). *A,* Following placebo; *B,* Isosorbide dinitrate, 5 mg. sublingually, 15 minutes before test; *C,* Propranolol, 60 mg., 1 hour before test; *D,* Isosorbide dinitrate plus propranolol, 1 hour before test; *E,* Isosorbide dinitrate orally plus propranolol, 1 hour before test.

While our earlier studies have demonstrated the existence of a remarkable therapeutic phenomenon,[4,15] the present investigation has shown its applicability to clinical practice. Thus, continuous therapy in 115 patients has clearly established that long-term relief is now available for most patients suffering from severe and refractory forms of angina pectoris. Additional studies are indicated to determine whether propranolol-nitrate therapy is also capable of influencing the ultimate prognosis in such cases. Although pain has been the major focus of attention in treatment, patients who are completely free of symptoms not uncommonly reveal striking ischemic electrocardiographic alterations when monitored during the performance of daily routine activities or comparable stress tests in the laboratory. There is good evidence to believe that such ischemic changes with or without associated coronary artery spasm may progress to acute myocardial infarction or trigger fatal arrhythmias. Consequently, "silent" coronary insufficiency may often require the same degree of circumspection in therapy that now prevails for symptomatic cases.

Considerable emphasis has recently been placed upon the value of physical reconditioning in the rehabilitation of the coronary patient. It is apparent that beta adrenergic receptor blockade in conjunction with nitrate vasodilation may produce a number of desirable hemodynamic responses earnestly sought in organized programs of physical training. If such medicinal therapy does not eliminate the need for systematic physical activity, it may have adjuvant value and provide a greater margin of safety in such programs.

Forty-two of the 115 patients in the present study have already been on propranolol-nitrate therapy for more than one year. The striking results consistently observed open to question the justification for surgical revascularization of the myocardium in the anginal patient. From the data at hand, it appears highly unlikely that surgical intervention can match the results now available from medicinal therapy alone. An answer is being sought in comparative studies now in progress.

SUMMARY

A remarkable synergism has been found to exist between propranolol, a beta adrenergic receptor blocking agent, and isosorbide dinitrate. The phenomenon was demonstrated objectively in a series of 28 selected patients with severe and refractory forms of angina pectoris and was manifested by striking improvement in pain experience, ischemic electrocardiographic patterns, and capacity for exercise. That these results can be maintained on a long-term basis was clearly shown by the dramatic and persistent relief of symptoms in 109 of 115 patients on continuous therapy for periods now ranging from 6 to 20 months. Further studies are indicated to determine the range of applicability of propranolol-nitrate therapy in angina pectoris, in asymptomatic coronary insufficiency and in programs of physical reconditioning for coronary patients. Data are also necessary to determine the influence of this form of treatment on the ultimate prognosis in various types of coronary heart disease.

Propranolol-nitrate therapy appears to represent an important breakthrough in the treatment of refractory and hitherto intractable angina pectoris. In the light of these findings, justification for surgical revascularization procedures as a means of alleviating anginal symptoms must be reassessed.

REFERENCES

1. Heberden, W.: Some account of a disorder of the breast, M. Trans. R. C. P. (London) *2*:59, 1772.
2. Brunton, T. L.: On the use of nitrite in amyl in angina pectoris, Lancet *2*:97, 1867.
3. Murrell, W.: Nitroglycerine as a remedy for angina pectoris, Lancet *1*;80, 113, 151, 224, 1879.
4. Wolfson, S., Heinle, R. A., Herman, M. V., *et al.*: Propranolol and angina pectoris, Am. J. Cardiol. *18*:345, 1966.
5. Hamer, J., and Sowton, E.: Effects of propranolol on exercise tolerance in angina pectoris, Am. J. Cardiol. *18*:354, 1966.
6. Grant, R. H., Keelan, P., Kernohan, R. J., *et al.*: Multicenter trial of propranolol in angina pectoris, Am. J. Cardiol. *18*:361, 1966.
7. Gillam, P. M. S., and Prichard, B. N. C.: Propranolol in the therapy of angina pectoris, Am. J. Cardiol. *18*:366, 1966.
8. Rabkin, R., Stables, D. P., Levin, N. W., and Suzman, M. M.: The prophylactic value of propranolol in angina pectoris. Am. J. Cardiol. *18*:370, 1966.
9. Ginn, W. M., Jr., and Orgain, E. S.: Propranolol hydrochloride in the treatment of angina pectoris, J. A. M. A. *198*:1214, 1966.
10. McKenna, D. H., Collins, R. J., Sialer, S., Zarnstorff, W., Crumpton, C., and Rowe, G.: Effect of propranolol on systemic and coronary hemodynamics at rest and during simulated exercise, Circulation Res. *19*:520, 1966.
11. Chamberlain, D. A., Davis, W. G., and Mason, D. F.: Effects of beta-blockade on coronary flow, Lancet *2*:1257, 1967.
12. Reale, A., D'Intino, S., and Vestri, A.: Effects of beta-blockade on coronary flow, Lancet *1*:52, 1968.
13. Russek, H. I.: The therapeutic role of coronary vasodilators: glyceryl trinitrate, isosorbide dinitrate and pentaerythritol tetranitrate. Am. J. M. Sc. *252*:43, 1966.
14. ———: Propranolol and isosorbide dinitrate synergism in angina pectoris. Am. J. M. Sc. *254*:406, 1967.
15. ———: Propranolol and isosorbide dinitrate synergism in angina pectoris, Am. J. Cardiol. *21*:44, 1968.

Management of Refractory Angina Pectoris

Louis F. Bishop

DEFINITION

The term "refractory angina pectoris" is difficult to define. One dictionary definition of the word "refractory" is "resisting ordinary treatment." As far as angina is concerned, when unusual or severe pain occurs, various other terminologies are used; for example, "preinfarctional angina," "intermediate coronary syndrome" and "status anginosus." Sometimes the term "refractory" is not meant to imply that myocardial infarction will take place, but is concerned with the patient whose frequent attacks occur with minimal effort or emotion, at rest, at night, often without any precipitating factor. The pain is sometimes relieved by nitroglycerin, but in doses greater than usually required. These patients live in constant fear of attacks. They become complete invalids and even drug addicts. They frequently consult many physicians and clinics in the hope of relief. They may have minimal or marked coronary disease. Frequently in the syndrome of refractory angina, there is a superimposed anxiety state. This clinical description is probably more frequent than has been thought in the past, because the patients, failing to be helped by their own physicians, find their way to medical centers, where refractory patients are increasingly being reported.

A more precise method has been used to indicate the degree of angina pectoris and that is to assess the speed with which a patient is able to walk, not the distance. Four grades are as follows:

Grade I. Pain is only provoked by hurrying or walking up hills or several flights of stairs.

Grade II. Walking on the level at an average speed causes pain, usually within the first 300 yards.

Grade III. Pain occurs even when walking slowly.

Grade IV. There is pain at rest and total incapacity.

HISTORICAL

The term "refractory" does not usually occur in the description of angina by older authors, but Sir James Mackenzie, in his classical monograph *Angina Pectoris,* does state that there are patients in whom ordinary treatment is not effective. He wrote, "Unfortunately there are attacks which do not respond to nitroglycerin or nitrite of amyl where the pain is of that lingering kind coming in waves of intensity, and lasting, it may be, for many hours."[1]

In all probability he was describing the refractory type of pain, where there was impending or actual infarction.

As far as drug treatment was concerned, it is interesting to note that he used narcotics, and even chloroform.

MANAGEMENT OF REFRACTORY ANGINA

The management of a refractory case should always begin with a reassessment of the simple measures used in office practice. Has the patient been reassured and a proper explanation of the problem been given him? Has weight loss been accomplished? Weight loss is by no means easy. Has the life situation of the patient with regard to emotional problems been properly explored? This may take a great deal of time and involves a good doctor-patient relationship. Has the use of nitroglycerin been properly evaluated? Have the long-acting nitrates received a fair trial? Have tranquilizers had a proper trial? What is also most important is whether the patient is really controlling the use of tobacco, coffee and other drugs that may be contributing to the refractory angina.

Office re-evaluation may not be enough. It takes great wisdom to decide whether to hospitalize the patient when faced with refractory angina. If one knew that the angina was preinfarctional, there would be no question. Hospitalization is often the best course and in this respect it is not unlike the situation where congestive heart failure is refractory to ambulatory treatment.

The value of complete rest for a period of time in a hospital away from ordinary activities gives the physician a chance to study all of the "trigger mechanisms" that may be playing a role. Among the most important are (1) arthritis, (2) cervical or dorsal spondylitis, (3) peptic ulcer, (4) hiatal hernia, (5) chronic pancreatitis, (6) cholelithiasis, (7) prostatism, (8) bronchitis and emphysema, (9) severe anemia, (10) hyperthyroidism, (11) hypothyroidism, (12) left ventricular failure, (13) hypoglycemia, and (14) ectopic rhythms.[2]

It is obvious that a search for aggravating and precipitating factors that are amenable to treatment cannot be easily made without hospitalization.

In our experience, among the commonest trigger mechanisms, uncovered by a careful search, has been unrecognized mild congestive heart failure, treatment of which resulted in abrupt cessation of anginal episodes.

Coexistence of symptoms referrable to upper abdominal organs is very common. Hiatal hernia is perhaps the commonest, but not infrequently, peptic ulcer and gall bladder disease are discovered.

Associated musculoskeletal disorders of the chest wall may be a trigger mechanism.

Too much examination may be harmful to the patient with severe angina, and x-rays, for example, may have to be postponed.

Under close observation, there is the opportunity to re-evaluate the use of drugs. As in the refractory patient with congestive heart failure, where the use of digitalis must be carefully evaluated, the refractory patient with angina must have a restudy of his use of nitroglycerin. Has it been properly emphasized to the patient that nitroglycerin can be used prophylactically as well as symptomatically? In some patients, there is a definite fear of its use which has to be removed. Some patients are sensitive to nitrates and it is forgotten that the available doses range from 1/400 gr. (0.15 mg.) up to 1/100 gr. (0.6 mg.) The effective dose can be determined in the refractory case by progressive increments at hourly intervals until a slight headache is produced. In our experience 1/200 gr. (0.3 mg.) repeated in five minutes is usually effective.

The value of the long-acting vasodilator drugs has been firmly established and here the frequency and dosage have to be adjusted to the needs of each particular patient. The long-acting coronary dilator drugs certainly deserve a trial in the refractory patient. Unfortunately, we have had severe reactions,

such as fainting in elderly patients, which has made us cautious in their use.

In the same way that nitrates have to be re-evaluated in the refractory patient, the treatment of anxiety associated with angina by the use of central acting drugs may need reconsideration. The usual regime has been phenobarbital 30 mg. four times a day with a sedative at bedtime, but the refractory patient may do better with one of the tranquilizer drugs, such as meprobamate or diazepam. If there is an agitated depression, associated with severe angina, psychiatric consultation may be indicated.

The relatively new drug, propranolol, may have a very important role in the management of the refractory anginal case, particularly combined with the nitrates. It has now been widely used and a recent statement has been made that this is the first significant advance in the treatment of angina since the introduction of nitroglycerin 100 years ago.[3] It seems to be effective in patients where angina is due to coronary atherosclerosis. This was proved in a series of patients where cinearteriograms were done. Its effect is dependent on lowering the heart rate primarily, although other effects may play a role. A dose should be given that is adequate to lower the heart rate to between 56 and 60. The dosage appears to be varied and ranges between 40-480 mg. per day. At present it appears to be customary to begin with 40 mg. and then to increase. A testing dose of 20 mg. to note the effect on the heart rate can be given in the office. In the use of this drug for angina that is refractory to ordinary treatment, one must be alert for the patient who will develop cardiac failure. It is also contraindicated in an anginal patient subject to bronchial asthma.

The combination of propranolol and isosorbide dinitrate may be the most effective modern method in the treatment of refractory angina. There appears to be a synergistic action and recent hemodynamic studies have been done to help prove this.

The refractory anginal patient may be benefited by a carefully regulated exercise program in the form of frequent, brief, slow walks, but not after meals. This program may have great psychological as well as physical benefit.

The management of refractory angina must include methods that involve surgical procedures including carotid-sinus stimulation. Carotid-sinus stimulation depends on the fact that recent experimental studies have demonstrated that oxygen requirements of the heart are directly related to the heart rate, to the inotropic state of the myocardium and to the intraventricular pressure, which is a reflection of the intramyocardial wall tension. Carotid-sinus pressure will decrease arterial pressure, heart rate and myocardial contractility. As a result of these observations, one of the methods of relief of angina pectoris has been a mechanical method of electrical stimulation of the carotid-sinus nerves. The rationale of this method is that stimulation of these buffer nerves reduces sympathetic efferent traffic with consequent decrease in arterial pressure, heart rate and myocardial contractility.[4]

This appears to be a relatively simple procedure for a refractory patient, where medical management has failed. The number of patients in whom these radiofrequency carotid-sinus nerve stimulators have been implanted is relatively few (18) but improvement has been marked in most.

The value of revascularization operations in the treatment of refractory angina pectoris is far from a settled question at this time. Angina pectoris has been the graveyard of a number of once widely performed surgical procedures now completely discarded. They include cervical sympathectomy, dorsal rhizotomy, total thyroidectomy, ligation of the internal mammary artery, paravertebral alcohol block, procaine hydrochloride injection of the chest wall and many others.

There are now an imposing list of revascularizing operations and there is no question that some patients with refractory angina have been benefited.

It is difficult to set up controls such that the effect of medical management in a hospital over a suitable period of time could be compared with surgical results.

Just as many other early surgical procedures for angina are no longer being done, so it is with attempts to improve the coronary circulation.

Direct operations, such as thromboendarterectomy, are rarely, if ever, now attempted. The most commonly used are the various implant procedures. The latest one described is the anastomosis of the internal mammary with the coronary artery.[5]

If there is a place for this type of surgery in the management of refractory angina, the selection of a patient for it still remains a most difficult problem. Certainly the criteria should be strict. Young patients particularly might benefit from such a surgical procedure. There should be evidence by cineangiography of severe and focal disease. There should be severe and progressive angina pectoris. There must be acceptance of surgery by the patient.

CONCLUSIONS AND SUMMARY

In the management of refractory angina pectoris, we should re-evaluate all of the simple measures that are used in office practice. A decision must be made whether to hospitalize the patient, particularly if infarction is a possibility. Hospitalization will allow for a detailed study to be done.

The use of beta-adrenergic drugs in combination with the nitrates seems to influence the pathophysiology of even the most refractory patient with angina.

There may be a time in the future when structural pathology can be influenced by surgery.

Although refractory angina may be more frequent than is generally thought, a patient who cannot be helped is rare.

REFERENCES

1. Mackenzie, J.: Angina Pectoris, London, Oxford Medical Publications. 1923. p. 145.
2. Harrison, T. R., and Reeves, T. J.: Principles and Problems of Ischemic Heart Disease, Chicago, Year Book Medical Publishers, Inc. 1968, p. 262.
3. Russek, H. I.: Propranolol and isosorbide dinitrate synergism in angina pectoris, Am. J. Cardiol. *21*:44, 1968.
4. Braunwald, E., Epstein, S. E., Glick, G., Wechsler, A. S., and Braunwalk, N. S.: Relief of angina pectoris by electrical stimulation of the carotid-sinus nerves, New England J. Med. *277*:1278, 1967.
5. Bailey, C. P., and Hirose, T.: Successful internal mammary-coronary arterial anastomosis using a "minivascular" suturing technique, Int. J. Surg. *49*: 416, 1968.

Rationale for the Use of Beta Blockade as Therapy for Angina Pectoris

Steven Wolfson, Ezra A. Amsterdam, and Richard Gorlin

The myocardial circulation, like most systems in equilibrium, normally functions in balance between supply of, and demand for, substrates. The supply of oxygenated blood, if limited by the presence of atherosclerotic lesions, may be relatively fixed. Anterograde flow may vary only with changes in aortic perfusion pressures. Some potential for increasing collateral flow to ischemic zones does exist.

Myocardial O_2 demands, however, are quite variable as the oxygen uptake of the heart has been shown to correlate with changes in the force, velocity and duration of cardiac contraction, as well as the heart rate.[1-5] It is largely through changes in these variables that the stimulation of myocardial oxygen consumption produced by physical exercise and catecholamine infusion becomes manifest. Currently available evidence suggests that beta blockade functions in this setting by decreasing the mechanical demand upon the heart to a level within the capacity of the coronary circulation.[6,7]

MATERIAL AND METHODS

The data to follow are the results of investigations performed at the time of diagnostic cardiac catheterization in patients with angina pectoris. Measurements performed included arterial and left ventricular pressures, indocyanine green cardiac outputs, and arterial and coronary sinus manometric oxygen content and capacity. By methods previously described by this laboratory,[8] coronary flow was measured utilizing the gaseous radioisotope Krypton.[85] These data were recorded during a control rest state and 20 minutes after the intravenous infusion of 5 mg. of propranolol. The hemodynamic measurements were recorded in a total of 27 subjects; coronary flow and oxygen determinations in 20 subjects. In six patients, these data were also obtained during

Supported by USPHS Grants 5-R01-HE-8591, 5-T01-HE-05679 and 1-P01-HE-11306.

identical levels of supine leg exercise both before and after propranolol administration. In one study, the above measurements were made at rest, after propranolol and then 4 minutes after sublingual nitroglycerin (0.4 mg.). In three patients, heart rate was held constant by pacing with a Goodale-Lubin pacemaker catheter placed in the coronary sinus. The atria were also depolarized by this technic; an A wave was inscribed in the left ventricular pressure tracing prior to isometric contraction; the QRS complex was normal and neither systemic pressures nor cardiac output were altered. Thus, the effects of propranolol were determined exclusive of any alteration of heart rate.

RESULTS

Hemodynamics

At Rest. Propranolol reduced the average heart rate from a control of 79 to 74 beats per minute ($P < 0.001$). Pressure time per minute (the "tension-time index") fell from an average of 2780 to 2383 ($P < .001$). The average left ventricular end-diastolic pressure was lowered from 15 to 12 mm. Hg ($P < 0.01$). The cardiac index decreased from 2.5 to 2.1 L./min./M² ($P < .001$). No significant change ($p < .05$) was noted in stroke index. Brachial artery systolic mean pressure fell from 118 to 115 ($p < 0.05$) (Table 1).

During Exercise. Supine leg exercise was performed on a bicycle ergometer set at 874 foot-pounds per minute before and after the administration of propranolol, with resting measurements also recorded in each state. The mean heart rate, left ventricular external work, pressure time per minute, and cardiac index of the six patients studied, all rose to lower levels during exercise performed after the administration of propranolol (Fig. 1).

After Isoproterenol. In four patients, isoproterenol was infused at an average rate of 3 µg. per minute.

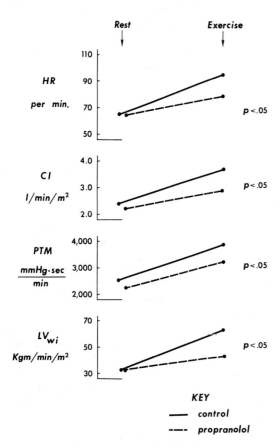

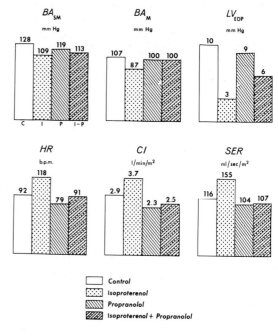

FIG. 2.   Blockade of hemodynamic response to isoproterenol. Less response is shown to a 3.5 ug./min. isoproterenol infusion after propranolol than to a 3 ug./min. infusion before propranolol. (Average for four patients.)

FIG. 1.   Attenuation of hemodynamic response to exercise. Heart rate (HR), Cardiac index (CI), Pressure-time per minute (PTM) and external left ventricular work index (LVwi) were lower (p < 0.05) during identical levels of supine leg exercise performed after propranolol.

This decreased brachial artery systolic mean pressure, brachial artery mean pressure and left ventricular end-diastolic pressure; and increased heart rate, cardiac index, and mean systolic ejection rate. Propranolol was then infused and the isoproterenol infusion was repeated with a mean dose of 3.5 μg. per minute. In the presence of beta blockade, isoproterenol produced no significant change in brachial artery systolic or mean pressure, or left ventricular end-diastolic pressure. Heart rate, reduced by propranolol from the resting state, was not brought back to the control level by isoproterenol challenge. No significant change in either cardiac index or mean systolic ejection rate was now produced (Fig. 2).

Myocardial Oxygen Consumption and Coronary Flow

At Rest. The average myocardial oxygen consump-

TABLE 1
Hemodynamic Effects of Propranolol (n=27)

	Control $\pm SE$	Propranolol $\pm SE$	"P"
Heart rate (beats/min.)	79$\pm$3.4	71$\pm$2.5	<0.001
Pressure-time/min. (systolic mean pressure $\times$SEP)	2780$\pm$93	2383$\pm$94	<0.001
Left ventricular EDP (mm.Hg)	15$\pm$1.5	12$\pm$1.6	<0.01
Cardiac index (liters/min./M²)	2.5$\pm$.08	2.1$\pm$.09	<0.001
Arterial systolic mean pressure (mm. Hg)	118$\pm$2.5	115$\pm$3.2	<0.05
Coronary Hemodynamic Effects of Propranolol (n=27)			
Coronary flow (ml./100 Gm. LV/min.)	98$\pm$5.2	80$\pm$4.1	<0.001
Myocardial oxygen consumption (ml./100 Gm. LV/min.)	11.4$\pm$0.71	9.1$\pm$.36	<0.001

tion for the 19 subjects tested fell from 11.4 to 9.1 ml. per 100 Gm. left ventricular mass per minute (p < .001) after propranolol. The average coronary flow declined from 98 to 80 ml. per 100 Gm. left ventricular mass per minute (p < 0.001) (Table 1).

During Exercise. An identical level of leg exercise

was performed before and after propranolol administration. Before propranolol, exercise increased the average myocardial oxygen consumption in the six patients to 17.4 ml. per 100 Gm. left ventricular mass per minute. After beta blockade oxygen consumption rose to only 14 ml. per 100 Gm. left ventricular mass

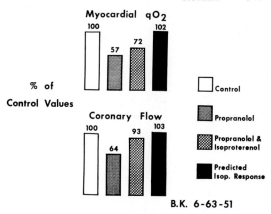

FIG. 4. Effect of propranolol on the coronary response to isoproterenol. Isoproterenol infused at 4 μg./min. failed to completely overcome the beta blockade. The resultant values fell short of control, prepropranolol levels of myocardial oxygen consumption (qO_2) and coronary flow. They also fall far short of the predicted response to this dose of isoproterenol.[9]

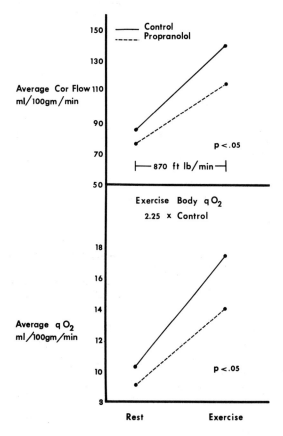

FIG. 3. Effects of propranolol upon oxygen requirements during exercise. During identical levels of supine leg exercise after propranolol, myocardial oxygen consumption (qO_2) and coronary flow (CF) were lower ($p < 0.05$) than before beta blockade.

per minute ($p < .025$, paired "t" test) (Fig. 3). As with myocardial oxygen consumption, beta adrenergic blockade also reduced the coronary flow required during supine leg exercise from 140 ml. per 100 Gm. left ventricular mass per minute before blockade to 115 ml. per 100 Gm. left ventricular mass per minute after propranolol ($p < 0.05$).

After Isoproterenol Infusion. In addition to the hemodynamic changes described above, myocardial oxygen consumption and coronary flow were measured in one subject at rest, after propranolol, and during an isoproterenol infusion in the presence of

beta blockade. As shown in Figure 4, isoproterenol infused at 4 μg. per minute failed to return either coronary flow or myocardial oxygen consumption to the control level recorded before propranolol administration.

Effects of Nitroglycerin in the Presence of Beta Adrenergic Blockade

When sublingual nitroglycerin was given after propranolol, the results were nearly identical to those previously reported for nitroglycerin in the absence of beta blockade.[10] The left ventricular end-diastolic pressure, already reduced from 10 to 4 mm. of mercury by propranolol, fell to 0. The cardiac index declined from 3.3 L./min./M² to 2.3 after blockade, and then dropped to 1.7 L/min./M² after nitroglycerin. Myocardial oxygen consumption decreased from 7.9 to 6.2 ml. per 100 Gm. left ventricular mass per minute after nitroglycerin, with coronary flow falling from 79 to 57 ml. per 100 Gm. left ventricular mass per minute. Nitroglycerin did decrease systemic pressure, brachial artery systolic mean pressure falling from 102 mm. Hg to 82 mm. Hg, but the reflex tachycardia usually associated with nitroglycerin administration was abolished by propranolol (Fig. 5). These results support the clinical impression that propranolol and nitroglycerin may have additive effects upon anginal symptoms.

Effects of Propranolol With Unchanged Heart Rate

Many of the effects of propranolol were un-

EFFECTS OF NITROGLYCERINE DURING BETA-BLOCKADE

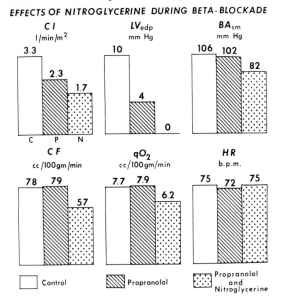

FIG. 5. Additive actions of nitroglycerin and propranolol in one patient. The response to nitroglycerin is identical to that seen under normal conditions but for the absence of a compensatory tachycardia. (See text)

TABLE 2
Controlled Heart Rate*

	Control	Propranolol
Heart rate (bpm)	85	85
Cardiac index (L./min./M²)	2.4	2.1
Stroke index (ml./bt/M²)	29	25
LV systolic mean pressure (mm. Hg)	125	119
Pressure-time per minute (mm. Hg. systolic sec.)	3120	2926
LV end diastolic pressure (mm. Hg)	16	17
LV end diastolic volume (ml./M²)	85	97
Force time /min. (dynes sec./min.)	4683	5267
Myocardial O₂ consumption (ml./100 Gm. LV/min.)	10.0	10.6
Coronary flow (ml./100 Gm. LV/min.)	88	93

*Average values for three patients.

altered by the prevention of reduction in heart rate (Table 2). However, only a minimal decrease in pressure time per minute was observed in these three patients. Average left ventricular end-diastolic volume, determined by cinearteriography,[11] actually increased. Force time per minute,[12] therefore, which varies with intracavitary volume as well as pressure, also increased. Presumably in response to these mechanical differences, propranolol administered during electrical pacing produced no change in either myocardial oxygen consumption or coronary flow. The key role played by changes in heart rate in the decrease in oxygen usage usually produced by propranolol is supported by experimental data.[13] In man, this finding is given added impact by the observation that angina occurs at a given product of systolic pressure and heart rate.[7]

Clinical Results

The ultimate rationale for the use of any clinical agent must be efficacy and safety. These have been evaluated in a controlled study in patients with angina pectoris over the last three years. Criteria for admission to this study were: angiographic diagnosis of the presence or absence of coronary artery disease; double blind trial including placebo; determination of optimal dosage of propranolol by carefully observed escalation; prolonged follow-up, averaging 18 months to this date. Results were judged to be significant if: 50-100 per cent reduction of the former anginal attack rate occurred; former nitroglycerin usage was reduced by 50-100 per cent; one or more of the multiple provoking factors of angina was lost.

Of 104 angina patients with documented coronary atherosclerosis, 90 (86 per cent) were significantly improved by the use of propranolol. Twenty-three patients with the anginal syndrome, but without coronary atherosclerosis, on coronary arteriography were also studied. Only four (17 per cent) had a significant decrease in their symptoms. Thus, it would appear that the effects of propranolol are specific for pain related to the atherosclerotic lesion.

At present, 143 patients have received propranolol for the treatment of either angina or chronic recurrent arrhythmias. The most frequent side-effect encountered was gastrointestinal distress, either mild nausea or diarrhea. This gave an incidence of 25 per cent. Of the 36 patients involved, however, it was necessary to discontinue propranolol in only three. Dizziness was reported in nine subjects, postural hypotension in three, excessive fatigue in 22 (15.3%). An increase in pre-existing bronchospasm was noted in two patients, and bradycardia (less than 50 beats per minute) in three subjects. Twelve patients (8.4%) reported either the appearance or exacerbation of peripheral edema or dyspnea. It was necessary to discontinue therapy in only two of these patients, adjustment of dosage or addition of either a diuretic or digitalis serving to ameliorate the cardiac decompensation in all other patients. Thus, of 143 subjects receiving the drug, propranolol caused side-effects serious enough to require discontinuation in only five.

Effects on Mortality

While control of anginal symptoms alone is certainly a sufficient goal for therapy, the ultimate end point for treatment must be its impact upon the mortality of the disease process. We have attempted to determine if treatment with propranolol alters survival rate of patients with angina pectoris.[14] Once it had been established that propranolol successfully treated anginal symptoms, it was felt ethically mandatory to continue patients on the drug. Therefore, controls for this study were difficult to obtain. Retrospectively, however, it was possible to compare patients treated with propranolol to other patients who had been seen prior to the introduction of this drug or who for a variety of nonmedical reasons either would not or could not be placed on the drug. Thus, the propranolol treated and controlled groups were neither randomly selected nor deliberately matched. The groups were, however, examined for the incidence of all factors which have been reported to affect the mortality of patients with coronary artery disease. Analyzed by Chi Square only two factors were found to be statistically different (p <.05). The propranolol treated group had a greater incidence than did the control group of coronary artery disease involving all three major coronary vessels (visualized by selective cineangiography). The control group, on the other hand, had a significantly greater number of patients with clinically overt or latent heart failure documented at the time of cardiac catheterization. On the possibility that these two differences offset each other, a life table analysis of survival[15] in the two groups was set up and the monthly survival rates compared by student's "t" test. Each patient's cardiac catheterization (for the controls) or onset of propranolol therapy was set as time zero. Significance was determined by p <.05.

As shown in Figure 6, the survival rate of the untreated patients fell below that of the propranolol series at four months, with a significant difference appearing at 6 months and continuing out to 24 months at this time.

It is recognized that the number of patients involved in this study is small, that adequate controls were precluded by the nature of the study and that 24 months is the minimal time period for an analysis to determine survival rates in chronic disease. We feel that it can at least be stated that these results strengthen the impression that propranolol is a safe drug for the treatment of patients with coronary artery disease. In addition, it is hoped that these data will provide the impetus for a more extensive controlled prospective study of the effects of propranolol on the mortality of coronary artery disease.

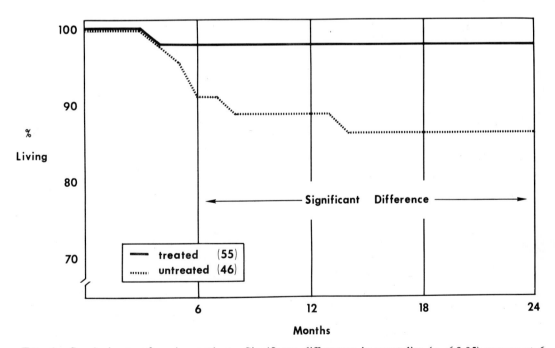

FIG. 6. Survival rate of angina patients. Significant differences in mortality (p < 0.05) appear at 6 months and persist till 24 months of observation.

SUMMARY

Propranolol, a beta adrenergic blocking agent, appears to decrease anginal symptoms by lowering the mechanical effort expended by the heart. The result is a decrease in myocardial oxygen consumption and coronary flow, presumably lowering both to within the limits set by atherosclerotic lesions. This drug is shown to be both safe and effective in treating angina pectoris. The suggestion is made that propranolol may improve survival rate in symptomatically improved patients.

REFERENCES

1. Sarnoff, S. J., Braunwald, E., Welsh, G. H., Jr., Case, R. B., Stainsby, W. N., and Macruz, R.: Hemodynamic determinants of oxygen consumption of the heart with special reference to the tension-time index, Am. J. Physiol. *192*:148, 1958.

2. Monroe, R. G., and French, G. N.: Left ventricular pressure-volume relationships and myocardial oxygen consumption in the isolated heart, Circulation Res. *9*:362, 1961.

3. Gorlin, R., Yurchak, P. M., Rolett, E. L., Elliott, W. C., and Cohen, L. S.: Inferential evidence for the Fenn effect in the human heart, J. Clin. Invest. *42*:939, 1963.

4. Sonnenblick, E. H., Ross, J., Jr., Covell, J. W., Kaiser, G. A., and Braunwald, E.: Velocity of contraction as a determinant of myocardial oxygen consumption, Am. J. Physiol. *209*:919, 1965.

5. Taylor, R. R., Cengolani, H. E., Graham, T. P., and Clancy, R.: Myocardial oxygen consumption, left ventricular fiber shortening and wall tension, Cardiovas. Res. *1*:219, 1967.

6. Wolfson, S., Heinle, R. A., Herman, M. V., Kemp, H. G., Sullivan, J. M., and Gorlin, R.: Propranolol and angina pectoris, Am. J. Cardiol. *18*:345, 1966.

7. Robinson, B. F.: Relation of heart rate and systolic blood pressure to the onset of pain in angina pectoris, Circulation *35*:1073, 1967.

8. Cohen, L. W., Elliott, W. C., and Gorlin, R.: Measurement of myocardial blood flow using Krypton[85], Am. J. Physiol. *206*:997, 1964.

9. Krasnow, H., Rolett, E. L., Yurchak, P. M., Hood, W. B., Jr., and Gorlin, R.: Isoproterenol and cardiovascular performance, Am. J. Med. *37*:514, 1964.

10. Brachfeld, N., Bozer, J., and Gorlin, R.: Action of nitroglycerin on the coronary circulation in normal and in mild cardiac subjects, Circulation *19*:697, 1959.

11. Klein, M. D., Herman, M. V., and Gorlin, R.: A hemodynamic study of left ventricular aneurysm, Circulation *35*:614, 1967.

12. Rolett, E. L., Yurchak, P. M., Cohen, L. S., Elliot, W. C., and Gorlin, R.: Relation between ventricular force and oxygen consumption, Fed. Proc. *22*: (Part I,) 345, 1963.

13. Whitsitt, L. S., and Lucchesi, B. R.: Effects of propranolol and its stereoisomers upon coronary vascular resistance, Circulation Res. *21*:305, 1967.

14. Wolfson, S., Amsterdam, E. A., and Gorlin, R.: Prognostic significance of angina therapy: Preliminary report, Circulation *36*:Supp.II, 274, 1967.

15. Cutler, S. J., and Ederer, F.: Maximum utilization of the life table method in analyzing survival, J. Chronic. Dis. *8*:699, 1958.

Rationale for Treating Coronary Patients With Psychotherapeutic Agents

J. Campbell Howard

Is there *raison d'etre* for psychotherapeutic agents in the "coronary patient"? This question can be approached in three ways: (1) by examining personality characteristics, (2) evaluating outside influences, and (3) pragmatically.

To identify some of the personality characteristics of individuals prone to coronary heart disease, Brozek[1] used the Minnesota Multiphasic Personality Inventory (MMPI) and Thurstone's Temperament Schedule in his prospective study. This was an extension of the studies initiated in 1948 by Keys to assess the potential factors and characteristics of the coronary prone subject.

A group of Minneapolis and St. Paul business and professional men, ages 45 to 55, who were clinically healthy at the time of the first examination were selected for this evaluation. Valid data had been obtained from 258 subjects at the time of the report, February 1966. Thirty-one had developed coronary heart disease, 24 infarction, and 7 classical angina and electrocardiographic evidence of ischemia. These could be compared with a control group of 138 subjects who remained clinically normal. There was a statistically significant difference from the control group in the MMPI, hypochondriasis, and the masculinity scales in the coronary disease group. Although the depression and hysteria scales were similar in direction, they did not reach statistical significance.

In the Thurstone Temperament Scale, the "A" or Active Scale was statistically significantly greater in the coronary group. According to Thurstone's criteria, this represents a subject likely to be on the go—one who speaks, walks, writes, works, and eats fast even though he does not have to do so.

In evaluating his results, Brozek wrote that "the potential candidates for ischemic heart disease were shown psychometrically to exhibit a higher 'concern for their bodily functions' which could be interpreted as a manifestation of anxiety and a higher 'activity drive.'" This description is not so detailed as that of the Friedman and Rosenman[2,3] coronary prone behavior pattern Type A patient (the individual with an excessive sense of time urgency, preoccupation with vocational deadlines, and enhanced competitive drive) but certainly would well fit the pattern.

Cady, et al.,[4] employed four factors from the Cattell 16 Personality Factor Questionnaire,[5] factors A, F, H, and L, including such items as blood lipids, blood pressure, etc., to assess a group of 35 patients with coronary disease and an equal number of controls. Using the Cattell Scale terminology, the study team suggested the following traits characterize coronary patients: (Cyclothymic, warm and sociable; Desurgency, a person who tends to inhibit any emotional expression—grim, sober, serious; and Relaxed Security, accepting and adaptable).

Shekelle and Ostfeld[6,7] used the MMPI and 16 Personality Factor Questionnaire in evaluating 1990 men, ages 40 to 55, at the Hawthorne works of the Western Electric Company. These men were free of clinical heart disease at the time of initial examination. The authors reported that 50 men developed angina pectoris without myocardial infarction, and 38 sustained an infarct in a period of four and one-half years. These data were sufficient to be broken into an angina and an infarction group.

In the Ostfeld study there were significant differences between those who had infarction and those who simply had angina. The hypochondriasis score was markedly higher in the angina subgroup (64) when compared to the noncoronary group (57.3). In contrast, the infarct group with a score of 55.1 was below the mean control.

A rigid comparison with the Brozek data cannot be made because he evaluated the coronary group as a whole (Table 1). Like the angina group in the Ostfeld study, the hypochondriasis score for the entire Brozek coronary group was higher (54.1) than the control mean (50.8). However, there were also differences in that there was a stronger masculinity (50.6) trait vs. control (54.9). which was not true in the Ostfeld data (54.5 vs. 55.5).

If we turn now to the Personality Factor Questionnaire, the Ostfeld group had a significantly higher "L" factor for the total coronary, that is, the angina and infarct patients, than the control group. The "L" factor, which is entitled "protension," had a high score suggesting a paranoid trend with suspiciousness, jealousy, self-sufficiency, and withdrawal. These data (Table 1) are in direct contrast to the Cady findings, wherein the "L" factor was low, indicating a tendency toward inner relaxation, trustfulness, understanding, composure, and social ease. The "C" factor, emotional stability, was much lower in the angina group than the coronary group. The only other correlative factor in the Ostfeld-Shekelle[8] data is the Q-2 factor, which was not evaluated in Cady's study.[9] This had a higher value than the noncoronary controls and indicates a self-sufficiency direction. This attribute of self-sufficiency,

occupation groups, reported a marked relationship to the emotional stressfulness of occupational activity. Although not substantiated by psychometric studies or detailed personality evaluations, the occupations associated with the higher incidence of coronary artery diseases would also seem to permit inclusion of these men in the same categories as the Friedman type A personality or the Brozek and Ostfeld "coronary prone patients."

What do these retrospective and prospective psychometric evaluation data mean in coronary heart disease? Two tentative conclusions can be drawn: (1) Before any over-all conclusions about personality factors and coronary proneness can be accepted or rejected, a much larger series must be collected. However, now with the aid of computers, adequate multifactorial analyses can be carried out; and we hope such will be done. (2) The second conclusion is that there are some core findings

TABLE   1
Psychometric Scales: Coronary Patient Group vs. Control

	Brozek	Cady	Shekelle—Ostfeld	
			Angina	Infarction
MMPI				
Hypochondriasis	↑●	—	↑	↓●
Masculinity	↑●	—	N.D.	↑
Depression	↑	—	↑	N.D.
Hysteria	↑	—	↑●	N.D.
Thurstone T.S.	↑●	—	—	—
Cattell 16 P.F.				
A	—	↑●	N.D.	N.D.
C	—	N.D.	↓●	N.D.
F	—	↓	N.D.	N.D.
L	—	↓●	↑●	↑●
Q-2	—	—	↑●	↑●

↑↓ = Greater tendency toward or away
● = Statistically significant <5%
= = No difference from control
— = No test

along with those included in the high "L" factor of the Ostfeld study, would likely be found in the Friedman Type A personality.[10] On the other hand, the apparent major psychologic variant ascertained from the MMPI analysis undertaken by Hellerstein, *et al.*,[11] in their evaluation of postcoronary patients was depression.

Russek,[12] in his survey of 12,000 men in 13

which do equate certain personality characteristics with an apparent coronary proneness. These strongly suggest a rationale for the use of psychotropic agents in the management of this group. But there are sufficient differences to indicate that psychotropic agents should not be stereotyped; i.e., not everyone should be given phenobarbital.

Aside from personality characteristics of the

patient with coronary artery disease, anxiety resulting from external causes also produces significant effects on the cardiovascular system. Through stimulation of the hypothalamus, a marked response of the sympathetic side of the autonomic nervous system is evoked. This stimulation triggers the anginal cycle, consisting of an increase in heart rate, an outpouring of cardiac and adrenal catecholamines, and thus an increase in the work of the heart, producing a myocardial oxygen deficit. This, in turn, results in pain, the pain causing more anxiety, and thus the cycle. (Fig. 1)

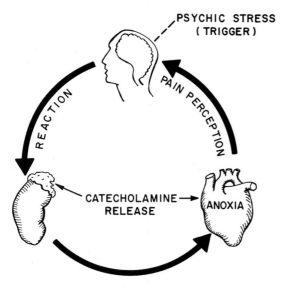

FIG. 1.   The psyche and the cycle of angina.

The cycle can be interrupted in a number of ways. In the management of the patient with angina pectoris per se, it is often useful to employ not one, but several of these methods. The use of psychotropic drugs may block the emotional trigger. The use of a "coronary vasodilator" may improve the myocardial oxygen relationship; i.e., block the effort trigger. As Russek[13] has recently advocated, the addition of propranolol* will aid by blocking the catecholamine effect and thus decreasing the demands put on the myocardium. (Fig. 2)

This still, however, omits the extracardiac effects of anxiety and its resultant effect on the sympathetic nervous system, such as blood pressure increase because of the vasoconstriction or its effect on cholesterol and free fatty acids. Further, in some series, 50 per cent or more of the patients had a substantiated history of emotional stress before the myocardia infarction.[14,15] These are potent reasons for considering the use of psychotherapeutic agents.

*Inderal (Ayerst)

Approaching the subject from a different aspect, or to be more pragmatic, as we just said, the need for a psychotherapeutic agent for the patient who has recently sustained myocardial infarction is obvious. Here the primary requirement for its administration is to calm and alleviate fear and anxiety. But, what of the patient well on the way to recovery, far along in the convalescent phase, or perhaps even starting back to work? Here the therapeutic reasoning may be similar or entirely different and dependent upon the individual himself—his background, his response to life situations, his family situation, his job security, and the like. There may be, as Hellerstein found, depression: "Most subjects with angina pectoris or myocardial infarction are initially quite depressed as shown by their personality inventory scores (MMPI)."[16] Not infrequently, the postcoronary patient is beset with both anxiety and depression. The patient might also be an aggressive individual who has made a good recovery and needs to be held down from overactivity.

Concerning the individual with angina pectoris, regardless of whether or not he may have also suffered a myocardial infarction, the indications for a psychotherapeutic agent apply in the same way as for the individual recovering from a myocardial infarction. In such a patient, the presence of both factors, anxiety and depression, might even be greater.

Finally, what about the individual without overt coronary artery disease—the individual who has all the factors which would indicate he might be the type to develop a myocardial infarction—the man who fits the Friedman-Rosenman Class A personality with the family history of hypertension, diabetes, etc.? Here the need for psychotropic agents may be even greater, but possibly difficult to administer.

In the latter type of patient, the potential subject for coronary artery disease, the minor tranquilizers such as oxazepam,† chlordiazepoxide,** or meprobamate†† are preferred to the more sedative, inactivating barbiturates. The term "minor tranquilizer" is used because these compounds are not antipsychotic, they produce a lesser degree of tranquilization and, unlike the phenothiazines, do not have autonomic side effects such as dry mouth, visual disturbances, and blood pressure or pulse changes. (Table 2)

Thus, the diazepine and meprobamate tranquilizers are preferable for this coronary prone patient who resists being slowed down, doesn't like the feeling of being sedated, and often compulsively

†Serax (Wyeth)
**Librium (Roche)
††Miltown (Wallace)

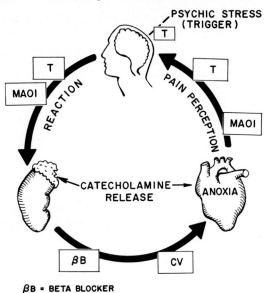

βB = BETA BLOCKER
T = TRANQUILIZER
CV = CORONARY VASODILATOR
MAOI = MONOAMINE OXIDASE INHIBITOR

FIG. 2.   The psyche and the cycle of angina, showing ways of interrupting the cycle.

refuses to take medication. Prognosis is usually bad in these cases because they are really denying that they are sick. When you prescribe for them, tell them it is to make them function better. Don't tell them it is to slow them down or because they are sick.

The presence of hypertension in the coronary prone patient may be an indication for reserpine* or a phenothiazine type tranquilizer with mild adrenergic blocking properties, such as acetophenazine.† These antipsychotropic agents are classed as major tranquilizers because they have been used to control psychotic patients and are potent. Actually, reserpine was initially evaluated because of its antihypertensive and bradycardic properties. The potential of this compound, however, to slow the patient down too much, and, in continuous use, to cause depression, must be taken into consideration. (Table 2)

The phenothiazine derivatives, although having some antihypertensive properties, also have side effects as indicated before, including tachycardia, dizziness, and others. The Parkinson-like side effects about which there may be concern are seen with the high doses of phenothiazines and reserpine but do not occur with the low doses given for these purposes.

The minor tranquilizer, the barbiturate type

*Naquival (Schering)
†Tindal (Schering)

sedative, or even the major phenothiazine type tranquilizer can be used in the patient who has recently had coronary thrombosis and myocardial infarction. In the acute stages of a myocardial infarction, because of the ability of phenothiazines such as perphenazine* to control nausea, they may be particularly valuable when administered in low dosage.[17] Where hypotension is a serious problem, care should be taken with phenothiazines because of their adrenergic blocking properties. (Table 2.)

As previously mentioned, the postcoronary patient during the recovery stage is often depressed, and depression is often missed or overlooked because it is masked or disguised as symptoms resembling those seen in cardiac patients. Such a patient is a suitable candidate for an MAO (monoamine oxidase) inhibitor or a tricyclic antidepressant.

On the basis of reports that they have some value in the relief of angina, some might prefer an MAO inhibitor such as isocarboxazid.** However, with the exception of ipmoniazide, the original MAO inhibitor/antidepressant, which was found to have antianginal properties, the others have not been as helpful. Because of their hypotensive action, the hypertensive crises following the ingestion of cheese, and the potential for serious liver damage, they are not very popular. The tricyclic antidepressants such as amitriptyline†† and imipramine,*** even with their tendency to lower blood pressure and their anticholinergic effects such as dry mouth and blurred vision, seem to be more acceptable. But when used in the coronary patient, care should be taken because they may prolong A-V conduction. (Table 2.)

In the postcoronary patient, where anxiety is a factor, the diazepine group or the meprobamate group are generally more suitable than the depressant sedative barbiturates. But, Dale Friend has commented, "Patients who seem to exhibit pure depression often have masked agitation, and once the depression is relieved the agitation becomes apparent, leading to new and sometimes frightening symptoms which may affect the entire program of therapy. The reverse is also commonly observed. When agitation is relieved, the masked depression then becomes a problem."[18] As Ayd said, "anxiety and depression scarcely ever exist alone."[19] Thus, a combination antidepressant and antianxiety medication, such as perphenazine and amitriptyline††† may be most valuable. (Table 2.)

In summary, it is apparent from the aspects of

**Trilafon (Schering)
††Marplan (Roche)
***Elavil (Merck)
**Tofranil (Geigy)
†††Etrafon (Schering)

TABLE 2
Types of Coronary Artery Disease and Appropriate Psychotropic Medication

CORONARY PRONE SUBJECT *Friedman-Rosenman Class A Personality*			
Minor tranquilizers		Librium	15–30 mg./day
		Serax	30–45 mg./day
		Valium	6–15 mg./day
	meprobamate	Equanil	1200–1600 mg./day
		Miltown	1200–1600 mg./day
Sedative	barbiturate	Luminal	45–90 mg./day
		Butisol, etc	45–90 mg./day
CORONARY PRONE WITH HYPERTENSION			
Rauwolfia	reserpine	Serpasil	0.1–0.5 mg./day
	alseroxylon	Rauwiloid	2–4 mg./day
	powdered root	Raudixin	50–300 mg./day
Phenothiazines	acetophenazine	Tindal	40–80 mg./day
	chlorpromazine	Thorazine	30–75 mg./day
	thioridazine	Mellaril	40–100 mg./day
RECENT CORONARY THROMBOSIS			
Minor tranquilizers & sedatives	As above		
Major tranquilizers with antiemetic Properties	perphenazine	Trilafon	6–8 mg./day
	prochlorperazine	Compazine	5–15 mg./day
POST-MYOCARDIAL INFARCTION *Late Recovery Phase*			
Antidepressants Monoamine oxidase inhibitor	isocarboxazid	Marplan	10–30 mg./day
	nialamide	Niamid	25–100 mg./day
	phenelzine	Nardil	15–45 mg./day
TRICYCLIC	desipramine	Pertofrane	75 mg./day
	imipramine	Tofranil	50–150 mg./day
	amitriptyline	Elavil	40–75 mg./day
	nortriptyline	Aventyl	20–100 mg./day
Tranquilizers & sedatives	As above		
Combinations	perphenazine & amitriptyline	Etrafon	2–10 to 2–25 mg. t.i.d.

psychometric evaluation, externally caused anxiety, as well as somatic symptomatology, there is a rationale for treating the coronary prone patient with psychotropic medications. However, based on the individual's psychiatric and somatic requirements, the use of psychotropic agents should not be stereotyped. They should be individualized according to the needs of the patient.

REFERENCES

1. Brozek, J., Keys, A., and Blackburn, H.: Personality differences between potential coronary and noncoronary subjects, Ann. New York Acad. Sc. *134*: 1057, 1966.
2. Friedman, M., and Rosenman, R. H.: Association of a specific overt behaviour pattern with increases in blood cholesterol, blood clotting time, incidence of arcus senilis and clinical coronary artery disease, J.A.M.A. *169*:1286, 1959.
3. Rosenman, R. H., and Friedman, M.: Association of a specific overt behaviour pattern in females with blood and cardiovascular findings, Circulation *24*: 1173, 1961.
4. Cady, L. D., Jr., Kirtler, M. M., and Woodbury, N. A.: Clues to the development of coronary heart disease, Geriatrics *16*:69, 1961.
5. Cattell, R. B., Saunders, D. R., and Stice, G.: Handbook for the Sixteen Personality Factor Questionnaire, Champaign, Illinois, The Institute for Personality and Ability Testing, 1957.
6. Ostfeld, A. M., Libowitz, B. Z., Shekelle, R. B., and Paul, O.: A prospective study on the relationship between personality and coronary heart disease, J. Chronic Dis. *17*:265, 1964.
7. Shekelle, R. B., and Ostfeld, A. M.: Psychometric evaluation in cardiovascular epidemiology, Ann. New York Acad. Sc. *126*:696, 1965.
8. *Ibid.*
9. Cady, L. D., Jr., Gertler, M. M., Gotsch, L. D., and Woodbury, M. A.: The factor structure concerned with coronary artery disease, Behavioral Sc. *6*:37, 1961.
10. Friedman, M., and Rosenman, R. H.: *op. cit.*
11. Hellerstein, H. K., *et al.*: The influence of active conditioning upon subjects with coronary artery

disease. Cardiac respiratory changes during training in 67 patients, Canad. M. A. J. *96*:758, 1967.

12. Russek, H. I.: Emotional stress and coronary heart disease in American physicians, dentists and lawyers, Am. J. M. Sc. *243*:716, 1962.

13. Russek, H. I.: Propranolol and isosorbide dinitrate synergism in angina pectoris, Am. J. Cardiol. *21*:44, 1968.

14. Dreyfuss, R.: Role of emotional stress preceding coronary occlusion, Am. J. Cardiol. *3*:590, 1959.

15. Weiss, E., Dolin, B., Rollin, H. R., Fischer, H. K., and Bepler, C. R.: Emotional factors in coronary occlusion. Arch. Int. Med. *99*:628, 1957.

16. Hellerstein, H. K., *et al.: op. cit.*

17. Bjerkelund, C., Nitter-Hauge, S., and Jakobsen, E.: Perphenazin (Trilafon) in the prophylaxis of nausea and vomiting following acute myocardial infarct. Acta med. scandinav. *177*:729, 1965.

18. Friend, D. G.: Treatment of psychological maladjustments in adults, Dis. Nerv. System *28*:7, 1967.

19. Ayd, F. J.: Perphenazine-amitriptyline combination. Int. Drug Therapy Newsletter *1*:4, 1966.

Emotional Rehabilitation of the Coronary Patient

John Francis Briggs

The rehabilitation of a patient with an acute myocardial infarction begins the moment the physician has made the diagnosis. The physician must approach the patient and relatives with confidence, assurance, and optimism. Unless the patient is desperately ill and in shock, the physician can assure the family and the patient that in all likelihood he is going to recover from his infarct and be able to return to the same work he was doing before the infarction occurred.

To do this the physician must analyze his own emotional reactions to the patient with a myocardial infarction. To many physicians this patient is a threat to his own security. As a result, he may develop empathy to the patient or, even worse, he may become so insecure in the management of the acute phase of the disease that the patient and his relatives sense his insecurity. This has an emotional impact on both the patient and his relatives so that they may question whether or not the physician is competent to handle the patient. Just as there are many surgeons whose emotional overreaction makes it advisable that they not operate, so there are many internists and cardiologists who are not emotionally equipped to handle the problems of the acutely ill heart patient (Fig. 1). Self-analysis will tell the physician whether or not the infarcted patient is a threat to himself. Should he feel this he should never take care of acutely infarcted patients.

A great many patients are now admitted to coronary care units. This can be a traumatic emotional experience for both the patient and his family. Often the patient has had a previous infarct, and being placed in a coronary care unit may make both him and his family suspicious that his condition is more grave. It must be emphasized to the patient and to his family that he is in the coronary care unit because recent progress has demonstrated how much this betters the care of the myocardial infarcted patient. It must be explained that life threatening disorders that might complicate an acute infarct can now be prevented by electrical monitoring. The patient is in the unit to *prevent* problems and not

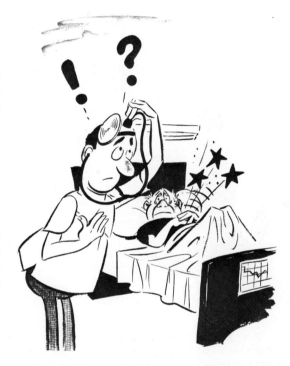

FIG. 1. Many physicians are not emotionally equipped to handle the problems of the acutely ill heart patient.

because he is critically ill. When there is no further need for the specialized care of the unit he will be removed from it. It is important to recognize the fact that the patient may become too dependent upon the protective atmosphere of the unit and thus should be removed as soon as it is safe to do so. This should be done for the patient and his family.

It is important to note whether the nurses are developing an abnormal empathy for the patient which may lead to his insecurity and may affect his care. There is no question that the coronary care unit has benefited the coronary patient, but it has also led to very many emotional problems when there is a feeling of insecurity in the nurses, the family and, even worse, in the attending physician, who may then be afraid to have the patient moved from the unit.

Once the diagnosis is established the physician must make a thorough physical examination of the patient. This helps to establish rapport with both patient and family. The physician should spend time with the patient and his family to explain exactly what has happened to the patient (Fig. 2). The

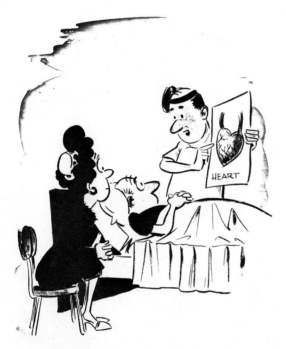

FIG. 2.   The physician should spend time with the patient and his family to explain exactly what has happened.

physician should give them a "lay course in myocardial infarction." He should tell them that a small portion of the heart muscle has died as a result of an insufficient supply of blood to that part of the myocardium. He also should emphasize that 75 or 80 per cent of the patients not only recover from the acute attack but return to a relatively normal life and are able to do their previous work. It is important to re-emphasize to the patient, and to the relatives, that at first there will certainly be restrictions placed upon him. These are the "don'ts" but as his progress continues satisfactorily the "don'ts" will be gradually removed and he will be told the "do's."

It is important that the physician, with the permission of the patient, contact the employer or the personnel director of the firm where the patient works. It is the physician's responsibility to tell the

employer the status of the patient and whether or not he will need to find a permanent replacement for his employee. Usually, the employer can be told that, in all likelihood, the individual will be able to return to work. It must be emphasized to the employer that in those areas where there is a secondary injury fund, the employee when he returns to work should be placed in the fund. The employer should receive frequent notices as to the employee's progress so that he knows when to anticipate his return to work, first on a part-time basis and finally full time.

It will help the attending physician greatly if he analyzes his patient from the emotional standpoint.

Some patients look upon the myocardial infarction as a punishment and suffering it as their penance. This individual (Fig. 3) points out that he doesn't

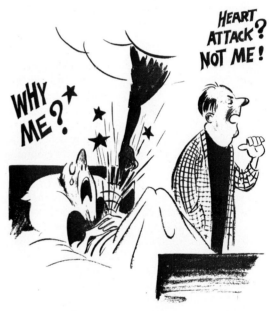

FIG. 3.   Some patients look upon infarction as a punishment, and suffering it as their penance. The patient at the left has a friend who carouses constantly and never had a heart attack. The patient at the right argues with his physician that this couldn't possibly be a heart attack because no one in his family ever had one.

drink, he doesn't smoke, he doesn't chase women and yet he has had an infarct. "Why has God done this to me?" He may point out a friend or relative who carouses constantly and never had a heart attack. This requires a sympathetic ear, reassurance and a reaffirmation that God is not punishing him.

A patient may be told he has had a myocardial infarction but he won't accept it (Fig. 3). He argues with the attending physician that this couldn't possibly be a myocardial infarction. No one in his family ever had a heart attack. This type of denial also requires reassurance to the patient that the electrocardiograms, the enzyme studies and the clinical course prove that he had a myocardial infarction despite the fact this has never occurred to any other members in his family.

The patient who refuses to accept the diagnoses, refuses to follow orders, insists on going to the bathroom, refuses his medications and signs out of the hospital against advice is indeed difficult. There is little any physician can do with such a patient. The physican must protect himself and the hospital by detailed notes as to his discussion with the patient and that despite this the patient left the hospital.

The physican will easily recognize the patient who actually enjoys his acute myocardial infarction (Fig. 4). This is the individual who has been faced with

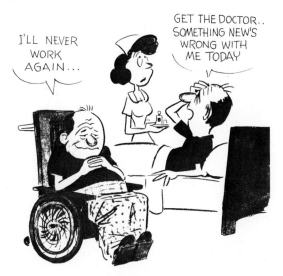

FIG. 4.   At the left, the patient has been under constant pressure and now the pressures are removed. The patient at the right has hypochondri-acal tendencies, belongs to the "Symptoms of the Day Club" and needs reassurance.

stresses and strains to which he could not adapt nor adjust. He had been under constant pressure and suddenly the myocardial infarction relieved him of the need to adapt and adjust and removed the pressures from him. He almost gladly retreats into his illness. The understanding of this patient's problem will be of help later in his rehabilitation. It may become a difficult task to return this person to his work.

The physician must recognize the patient who enjoys his myocardial infarction. He receives both

financial and emotional reward to such an extent that he refuses to be rehabilitated.

The physician can also recognize other personality problems in the patient. Does the patient have some organic or other form of psychosis that makes it difficult to treat him? The psychotic who suffers a myocardial infarction is most difficult to treat and the physician must have a psychiatrist in constant consultation in the treatment of this patient.

If the patient has a simple anxiety tension state in which he is worried about the present, feels guilty about the past and fears the future, he can be helped by constant reassurance.

If the patient has hypochondriacal tendencies, the physician may have much difficulty. These people belong to the "Symptoms of the Day Club." Each day they face the physician with a new set of complaints and new disorders for which no organic basis can be found (Fig. 4). Should one of these patients die suddenly, the relatives are disturbed because they know the patient rendered complaints on the day of sudden death. The physician can only reassure the patient that he does not have other organic disease and the symptoms of which he complains are not cardiac in origin.

Many patients with an acute myocardial infarction are severely depressed. This is an acute reactive depression which in some degree is normal. Reassurance and support of the patient soon result in the lessening of this reactive depression.

There are, however, some patients who are truly depressed individuals and whose depression antedated the myocardial infarction.

The true depressive who suffers a myocardial infarction needs psychiatric assistance. The physician must be particularly watchful for the smiling depressive. It is only through rapport with the patient that the physician will discover the patient is a depressive individual in need of psychiatric help.

The psychopathic person such as the alcoholic or the drug addict who has a myocardial infarction must have psychiatric help during the acute myocardial infarction and following it.

The individual with conversion problems also needs psychiatric care in conjunction with the care of the myocardial infarction.

The family physician and internist can handle the great number of patients who have neurotic disturbances during their myocardial infarction, but there are certain patients who must have psychiatric assistance when needed. The physician caring for the patient should not hesitate to ask for such assistance.

At the time of discharge from the hospital, the physician, the patient and his wife should have a confidential discussion in depth concerning the patient's problem. In lay terms it should be explained what has happened to the patient, what his future is and how he can be returned to gainful life.

It is most important that the problem of coitus be discussed (Fig. 5). The physician should tell the

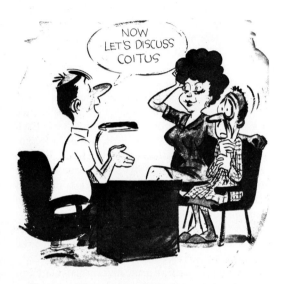

FIG. 5.   The physician should tell the husband and wife that they may continue to have a normal sexual life.

husband and wife that they may continue to have a normal sexual life. It should be explained that the victim of the infarct should be the less active participant in coitus, the healthy partner performing a greater part of the physical activities. If the husband has had the infarct, it may be well that his wife assume the superior position. This may also hold true if the wife had the infarct although usually the husband may be able to be more active in the superior position but should be especially considerate about supporting his weight on his knees and arms. Should the patient find himself having anginal pain with intercourse he should take nitroglycerin before performing the act and possibly also thereafter. Mutual understanding and consideration will lessen the likelihood of angina and there will be little problem concerning the coital act. Unless properly instructed, the man may develop psychic impotence because of fear of precipitating pain. This often leads to marital discord.

The successful rehabilitation of the patient suffering a myocardial infarction is dependent upon a well established rapport between the patient, the family, the employer and the physician. It depends also on constant reassurance and recognition of the various personality problems that arise. Returning these patients to normal life will result from proper treatment of the individual who has had the infarction and not the infarction that has had the individual.

Programs for the Rehabilitation of the Coronary Patient

Jerome S. Tobis

The field of physical medicine and rehabilitation (Rehabilitation Medicine) is concerned primarily with patients who have musculoskeletal or neuromuscular disabilities. However, the limitations of motor performance in the arthritic, the hemiplegic, the amputee or paraplegic at our hospital were often not due to the neuromusculoskeletal disability, but rather were the result of cardiovascular impairments. Thus our group of physiatrists has developed programs for cardiacs, particularly for the coronary patient who looks able-bodied but who may have a "hidden disability."

The coronary patient is often a chronically ill individual with psychological, social and vocational problems along with physical deconditioning resulting from the necessary acute treatment of the heart attack. The physiatrist has traditionally been interested in a comprehensive approach to the care of the chronically ill patient. He is familiar with exercise as a treatment method and has developed liaisons with helpful community agencies. Therefore, in the gray area between acute cardiology and the return of the patient to community living—at the interface—the physiatrist may join with the cardiologist in providing professional assistance to the cardiac patient. The material which follows will explain the rationale and results of our ongoing programs for these purposes at Montefiore Hospital in New York City.

Cardiac rehabilitation programs have been established elsewhere and have been concerned with improving the physical performance of the cardiac, such as Hellerstein's program in Cleveland,[1] evaluating the psychological performance of the cardiac —such as Gelfand's program in Philadelphia,[2] and assessing the vocational performance of the cardiac exemplified by some 50 work evaluation units throughout the country[3] among others. Methods vary. Exercise prescribed may be on a treadmill,[4] walking,[5] bicycling,[6] rope skipping,[7] jogging,[8] calisthenics,[9] or sports. Psychologic methods include psychometrics, attitude and personality testing, psychiatric stress interviews and counseling. Vocational methods include job evaluation, matching by energy cost, trial employment in sheltered shops, and retraining programs. Our programs are a synthesis of several of these methods. We have found it feasible, safe and appropriate to offer such programs out of a Rehabilitation Medicine Division.

For this presentation, four different clinical programs for the cardiac patient will be discussed. These include: (1) a program of exercise training for patients with angina pectoris, (2) a cardiac rehabilitation inpatient program, (3) an exercise program for postmyocardial infarction patients conducted at the 63rd Street YMCA in Manhattan and (4) an exercise and recreation program at the Mosholu-Montefiore Community Center, (on the property of the hospital) for recent postacute myocardial infarction patients.

ANGINA PECTORIS PROGRAM*[6]

The work tolerance of patients with angina pectoris is first evaluated at graded levels of bicycle exercise in the supine position, using measurements of energy cost, blood gases, lactic and pyruvic acids and electrocardiogram. The patients then train three times weekly for six weeks at exercise levels just below that which consistently produces angina. Subsequently, each patient undergoes a six-week "placebo" period. A double blind procedure is used. The "placebo" is compressed air administered as if it were oxygen, with interdiction of exercise during this period. Alternatively placebo and exercise periods are carried out in reverse order. Measurements are repeated after the six and twelve week intervals. The patients reported a decrease in the frequency of angina, a lessened need for nitroglycerin and increased work capacity consistently accompanied by a feeling of well-being. There was an increased ability to exercise to higher levels of performance in 6 of 18 patients. Electrocardio-

*Supported by Grant HD00599 from the National Institute of Child Health and Human Developnemt, USPHS.

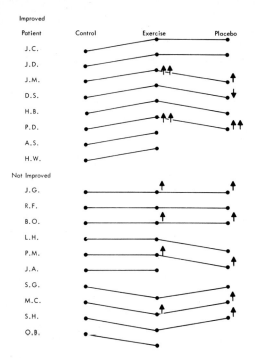

FIG. 1. Changes in the electrocardiographic findings in 18 patients with angina pectoris. Improvement (upward sloping lines), lack of change (horizontal line), or deterioration (downward sloping line), irrespective of the magnitude of the changes. Arrows upward indicate clinical improvement with the ability to exercise at one or more higher levels. Downward arrows indicate loss of clinical ability.

graphic changes indicated improvement in 8 patients (Fig. 1). A typical electrocardiographic change is seen in Figure 2. There was a tendency for oxygen debt to decrease and lactate/pyruvate ratios to increase when electrocardiographic improvement occurred. In the 8 patients in whom improvement was demonstrated by electrocardiography, no evidence was obtained to account for the change other than as a peripheral training effect. Subsequently, an additional 4 patients have confirmed the patterns described.

Briefly then, patients with angina can be improved considerably through a program of monitored, graded exercise, even within 6 weeks. Such programs can be provided through a rehabilitation service in a general hospital. Interestingly, the objective improvement does not strictly parallel the subjective.

CARDIAC REHABILITATION INPATIENT PROGRAM

The term "cardiac rehabilitation" refers to the restoration of the individual to that level of physical and mental activity compatible with the functional capacity of his heart.[11] To accomplish this goal in rehabilitation, comprehensive care of the cardiac patient should include graduated and monitored physical activity programs during convalescence, education of the patient concerning his current medical status and possible means of preventing future disability, vocational planning, and psychologic and social considerations. Since 1964 such an inpatient program has been provided on the Rehabilitation Medicine Service at Montefiore Hospital. Any cardiac patient was accepted provided he might derive benefit from a multidisciplinary approach to care, and that his cardiac status was stable. The chief prerequisite, however, was that the patient required the assistance of other professionals in addition to the cardiologist to achieve the best possible recovery. Patients have been accepted as early as a week after occurrence of the acute myocardial infarction, or at any point in the patient's hospital course. The experience of the first 18 months of this program has been reported.[10]

Two principles guided the program as follows: (a) the "equi-caloric" concept and, (b) radiomonitoring during activity. "Equi-caloric" expenditure is a term that we have devised for a method of prescribing physical and occupational therapy caloric levels by matching to those which are permitted the patient by his cardiologist for activities of daily living. For example, (Table 1), if the private physician permitted the patient to wash his hands and face, the patient was performing at an energy expenditure of approximately 2.5 calories per minute. It was permissible therefore, to allow the patients to carry out other activities at or below this level of energy expenditure, activities such as propelling a wheel chair (2.4 calories) or walking at a slow rate of 1 mile per hour (2.0 calories) or painting for recreation (2.0 calories). Since there was uncertainty regarding how many times per day such equi-caloric activity was permissible, and whether each subject was in actuality participating without undue stress in the prescribed activity, monitoring procedures were used. These consisted of telemetered electrocardiograms during activity and/or measurement of the energy cost of an activity as performed by a patient with his therapist.

The patient's activity was limited if the pulse rate exceeded 120 beats/min. during the activity, if there were significant changes in the ST or T waves, if chest, neck or abdominal discomfort resulted, or if numerous premature contractions occurred during activity. Although premature ventricular contractions at rest were not considered an indication for restriction of activity, if they increased in frequency with activity, the patient was restricted. In addition, when possible, an exercise test was monitored just prior to the time of discharge. It consisted in the rapid ascent of two flights of stairs. This "two flight test" has been equated, in terms of physical demand, to the energy expenditure during coitus.

TABLE 1
Equi-Caloric Prescription-Patient S.S.

Cardiologist permits	Rehabilitation staff matches
1.2 sitting	1.2 leather lacing
1.4 eating	1.5 passive ROM to uppers or lowers
1.4 conversation	1.7 active exercise to uppers
2.5 washing own hands and face	2.0 active exercise to lowers
3.6 walking 2.5 miles/hour	calisthenics progressing to 3.6

The entire therapy program for nursing, physical and occupational therapy, and prevocational evaluation was guided by these principles. Maximal caloric limits were prescribed, and the staff was taught not to exceed these prescribed levels and to approach them gradually.

To date, 43 patients have participated in the program since its inception in January 1965. In the original report for an 18-month period, there were 19 males and 9 females with an average age of 56 years. Fifteen of these patients were private and 13 were service cases. Seven patients returned to full time activity (6 to full time employment) within two months after the occurrence of the myocardial infarction. Fifteen other patients did return to work, but more than 2 months after the infarct. This contrasts with a report by Clark[12] on 60 employable patients with myocardial infarction. Of these, only two patients returned to work in less than two months. In the present series, service cases returned to work sooner than private cases. Patients less than 60 years old were better candidates for cardiac rehabilitation than those over 60 years. There were no untoward effects during the follow-up period resulting from early resumption of activities and employment.

At least 4 other inpatient programs for cardiac rehabilitation have been described in the literature. In 1952, Newman and associates reported on 527 patients with acute myocardial infarction who were managed on a medical service in a Veterans Administration Hospital.[13] A description of the program was included but no further data were provided. In 1957 a graded series of exercises and activities for the cardiac patient was outlined by Kornblueh and Michels.[14] Neither of these papers refers to the use of electrocardiographic monitoring of the patient.

Cain[15] studied 335 cardiac patients in a County Hospital. Electrocardiographic monitoring was performed on all their patients. A graded activity program was established in which patients moved through 10 levels of performance. Presumably each of these levels required higher energy expenditure and produced greater cardiovascular stress. However, no attempt to determine the energy requirements of these levels was described, although the report emphasizes the importance of the electrocardiographic monitoring.

In 1964, Torkelson in a Veterans Administration Hospital[16] outlined a regimen for comprehensive rehabilitation of patients with acute myocardial infarction. In that program, graded levels of exercise were established which were increased in severity week by week. Electrocardiographic monitoring was conducted during an exercise tolerance test. Fourteen patients were admitted to the study of whom ten were discharged at the time of the report. Another program is in progress in Atlanta employing progressive ambulation during the first 2 weeks following acute myocardial infarction.[17]

MONTEFIORE—Y.M.C.A. EXERCISE PROGRAM FOR THE POSTCORONARY PATIENT[18]

The most extensive organized program for reconditioning the coronary patient has been developed at the Y.M.C.A. and Jewish Community Center of Cleveland under the direction of Dr. Hellerstein.[19] His program involves restriction of diet, cessation of smoking, psychologic counseling and a program of exercises which are designed to promote cardiovascular fitness. He feels that by such a program the progression of coronary artery disease may be modified.

Based on this experience, a clinical program of exercise alone through the joint facilities of the Division of Rehabilitation Medicine at Montefiore and the West Side Y.M.C.A. on 63rd Street in Manhattan has been developed. An exercise prescription is determined at the hospital by having the patient actually perform the exercises he is to do at the "Y" with a physical educator during continuous EKG monitoring. The instructor then works with a class of postmyocardial infarction patients, each with his individual exercise prescription at the Y. To date, some 40 patients, mainly executives, have participated in this program, which has been in progress for the past 3 years. Patients

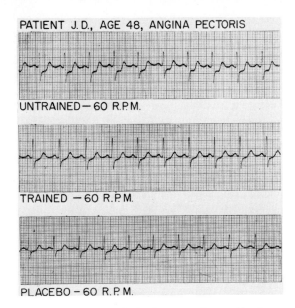

FIG. 2.   Patient had electrocardiographic improvement without improved tolerance to higher exercise levels.

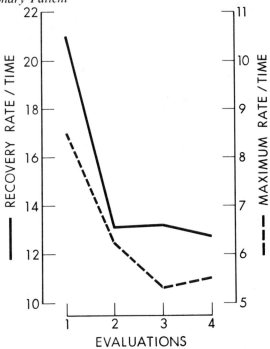

FIG. 3.   Effect of training program on maximum and recovery pulse rates.

are accepted to the program provided their infarction was sustained longer than 6 months previously. Evaluations are carried out on each member of this group at the hospital at approximately 4 month intervals in order to assess the progress during the previous period and to provide new exercise prescriptions for the ensuing 4 months.

The exercise starts with a warm-up consisting of brisk walking, jogging, arm pumping and walking on heels and toes with deep breathing. The remainder of the exercises consist of anterior, posterior, lateral and rotational trunk bends aimed at promoting flexibility, and thigh, leg and abdominal lifts prone and supine to promote strength. The progression is shown in Table 2. An attempt is made to avoid those exercises which require a Valsalva maneuver. The individual exercise prescription is tailored within safe limits by having the man rest during some of the calisthenics and join the group again for the final jogging. Competition between individuals is discouraged and improvement over one's own previous performance is stressed. Physicians are not present at the exercise sessions. Comparison of electrocardiographic monitoring done at the Y.M.C.A. and at the hospital showed fewer ST-T changes and slower heart rates at the Y.

The clinical results have been rewarding. All patients have felt considerably improved, reporting a carry-over into daily living in that physical activity is generally easier. Objective benefit is seen in the decreased resting, maximal and cumulative

recovery heart rates. The difficulty in comparing the pulse rate response to exercise periods of different duration is resolved here through ratios (Fig. 3). The average maximal heart rate is divided by the length of the exercise period, providing one ratio. The sum of heart rates during the first, second and third minutes following cessation of exercise divided by the total time exercised provides a second ratio. When viewed over time, these ratios show that most of the training effect occurred early. Subsequent evaluations have revealed that there has been a further dip during the second year for the majority of these patients. Electrocardiographic improvement is more difficult to assess since during the exercise re-evaluations the patients were not stopped at comparable exercise levels to permit technically adequate recordings (Fig. 4).

This program differs from existing programs for cardiacs in that it pretests the patient on exactly the exercises he will perform in the class rather than attempting to predict his performance ability from laboratory evaluation.

WORK EVALUATION UNIT IN CONJUNCTION WITH EXERCISE AND RECREATION PROGRAM AT MOSHOLU-MONTEFIORE COMMUNITY CENTER

This is the most recent of our programs for

TABLE 2
West Side Y.M.C.A. Exercise Pattern for Postcardiac Class

Level	Warm-up (laps)*		Calisthenics	Run-Walk	Calisthenics	Run-Walk
A Beginner 15 min.	Walk Jog Walk	3 4 2	1–4	Rest	5–11	Rest
B 4 mos. 20 min.	Walk Jog Walk	3–4 4–5 2	1–4	Rest	5–11	Walk 2 Jog 6 Walk 2
C 8 mos. 25 min.	Walk Jog Walk	4 5 2	1–4	Walk 2 Jog 6 Walk 2	5–11	Rest
D 12 mos. 30 min.	Walk Jog Walk	4 5 2	1–4	Walk 2 Jog 6 Walk 2	5–11	Walk 2 Jog 6 Walk 2

*1 lap walking=60 steps, 1 lap jogging=45 steps

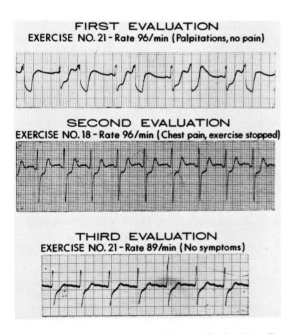

FIRST EVALUATION
EXERCISE NO. 21 - Rate 96/min (Palpitations, no pain)

SECOND EVALUATION
EXERCISE NO. 18 - Rate 96/min (Chest pain, exercise stopped)

THIRD EVALUATION
EXERCISE NO. 21 - Rate 89/min (No symptoms)

FIG. 4.   Exercise radiocardiograms (Patient No. 7).

cardiacs. It was organized approximately 2 years ago as a demonstration project with Federal Grant support.*

The program has the objective of rehabilitating the coronary patient for work, using the technics of a Work Assessment Unit and an Exercise—Recreation Program at the Community Center adjacent to the hospital. In addition, it includes a simulated work situation for the recent myocardial infarction patient at the hospital and on-the-job monitoring, utilizing telephone transmission technic (dataphone).

*Supported by Grant RD 1994-M from the Department of Health, Education and Welfare, Social and Rehabilitation Service.

Patients who are convalescing from myocardial infarctions sustained less than 2 months previously are evaluated by a team consisting of a physician, vocational counselor, social worker, psychologist and nurse. The physical and mental requirements of his job are determined and the patient is evaluated through performance tests and psychosocial interviews in regard to his ability to return to his job. The patient is placed in a simulated work situation in an office or shop in the hospital and is observed and monitored electrocardiographically while carrying out typical work assignments, including peak activities, for several hours. His electrocardiographic tracing (transmitted by dataphone) is observed continuously in our laboratory by a physician. If there are significant abnormalities in the tracing, such as the development of numerous or multifocal premature ventricular contractions, or a deep ST depression associated with chest pain, the patient is stopped from carrying out the task. Patients then are monitored in the actual job situation, using the same methods of telephone transmission of the electrocardiogram back to the hospital while the patients work. In this way the estimate of the patient's ability to return to work which was derived from the simulated job situation is rechecked in the real situation. During the assessment period and continuing three nights weekly thereafter, these patients are involved in a graduated reconditioning exercise program at the Mosholu-Montefiore Community Center which adjoins our hospital. In similar manner to the Y.M.C.A. program, the patient is pretested at a given level of exercise in the hospital setting. He is then permitted to participate in this group exercise program under the direction of a Physical Educator. The exercise pattern here, however, is less strenuous than at the Y.M.C.A. although the calisthenics used in both programs are patterned after Cureton. At the Community Center, five minute exercise periods are alternated with five minute rest periods, the exercise periods requiring approximately 3.0 calories per minute for calisthenics and walking sequences. As the patients develop tolerance to these exercises and no longer demonstrate substantial pulse increments (no greater than to 120) additional minutes of jogging are added in the rest periods, and monitored when the patient attempts to increase the amount of exercise he is doing for the first time. In addition, these patients participate in a group counseling session as well as other recreational, cultural and social activities which are conducted at the Community Center itself.

We believe that this type of program serves as a valuable transition for the patient with a recent myocardial infarction facilitating return to a wholesome community and family life and his earlier return to work.

The four programs described have been attempts to provide additional therapy beyond what is traditionally offered to patients with coronary heart disease by the cardiologist. The angina program of monitored exercise just below the point of pain results in significant clinical improvement with evidence of a peripheral training effect in all cases and electrocardiographic improvement in one third of the cases. The inpatient program permits rational prescription of activities during convalescence and smoothes the readjustment to community living and resumption of employment through psychologic, social and vocational guidance. The Y.M.C.A. exercise classes for active businessmen are an effort to prevent recurrence of myocardial infarction through exercise although it is realized at this time that there is no incontrovertible evidence that exercise prolongs life after a heart attack. The Work Assessment Program, which determines whether patients can work by on-line electrocardiographic observation during the real work situation, also supports a group reconditioning program. The latter takes place at a local Community Center and involves patients in recreational, social and group counseling programs which facilitate their cardiac rehabilitation.

These programs have been found to be feasible within an acute general hospital and permit the physiatrist to contribute in the care of the postacute cardiac patient by using a team approach and knowledge of exercise physiology. Such programs have been valuable teaching instruments for teaching of both house officers and medical students and have stimulated research into the pathophysiologic concomitants of exercise and the psychosocial problems which are deterrents to cardiac rehabilitation.

REFERENCES

1. Hellerstein, H. K., and Hornsten, T. R.: Assessing and preparing the patient for return to a meaningful and productive life, J. Rehab. *32*:48, 1966.
2. Gelfand, D.: Factors relating to unsuccessful vocational adjustment of cardiac patients, J. Occup. Med. *2*:62, 1960.
3. Whitehouse, F. A.: The Cardiac Work Evaluation Unit as a Specialized Team Approach, J. Rehab. *32*:66, 1966.
4. Naughton, J., Balke, B., and Nagle, F.: Refinements in method of evaluation and physical conditioning before and after myocardial infarction, Am. J. Cardiol. *14*:837, 1964.
5. Newman, L. B., Wasserman, R. R., Borden, C.: Productive living for those with heart disease: The Role of physical medicine and rehabilitation, Arch. Phys. Med. & Rehab. *37*:137, 1956.
6. Zohman, L. R., and Tobis, J. S.: The effect of exercise training on patients with angina pectoris, Arch. Phys. Med. & Rehab. *48*:527, 1967.
7. Rodahl, K.: Be Fit for Life, New York, Harper & Row, 1966.
8. Bowerman, W. J., and Harris, W. E.: Jogging, New York, Grosset & Dunlap, 1967.
9. Weiss, R. A., and Karpovich, P. V.: Energy cost of exercise for convalescents, Arch. Phys. Med. *28*:447, 1947.
10. Tobis, J. S., and Zohman, L. R.: A rehabilitation program for inpatients with recent myocardial infarction, Arch. Phys. Med. & Rehab. *49*:443, 1968.
11. de la Chapelle, C., as quoted *in* Cardiovascular Rehabilitation by White, P. D., Rusk, H. A., Williams B., and Lee, P. R., New York, McGraw-Hill Book Company. Inc. 1957, p. 55.
12. Clark, Richard J.: Experience of the Cardiac Work Classification Unit in Boston, Massachusetts, *in* Work and the Heart, New York, Paul B. Hoeber, Inc., 1959.
13. Newman, L. B., Andrews, M. F., Koblish, M. O., and Baker, L. A.: Physical medicine and rehabilitation in acute myocardial infarction, A. M. A. Arch. Int. Med. *89*:552, 1952.
14. Kornblueh, I. H., and Michels, E.: Outline of an exercise program for patients with myocardial infarction, Pennsylvania M. J. *60*:1575, 1957.
15. Cain, H. D., Frasher, W. G., and Stivelman, R.: Graded activity program for safe return to selfcare after myocardial infarction, J.A.M.A. *177*:111, 1961
16. Torkelson, L. O.: Rehabilitation of the patient with acute myocardial infarction, J. Chron. Dis. *17*:685, 1964.
17. Wenger, N., presentation at the Second National Meeting of Work Evaluation Unit Personnnel, 11/19/68, Bal Harbour, Florida.
18. Moreau, F. W., and Zohman, L. R.: A Postcoronary Exercise Program at the Y. M. C. A., presented at the New York Academy of Medicine, May 1967.
19. Hellerstein, H. K., Hornsten, T. R., Goldberg, A., Burlando, A. G., Friedman, E. H., and Hirsch, E. Z.: The influence of active conditioning upon subjects with coronary artery disease, Proc. Int. Symposium on Physical Activity and Cardiovascular Health, held in Toronto, Ontario, Oct. 11-13 1966.

New Methods of Work Prescription for the Coronary Patient

Lenore R. Zohman

The cardiologist or internist is generally the physician who must decide when it is medically permissible for a patient who has suffered a recent myocardial infarction to return to employment. The existing guidelines are meager. Reasonably, he awaits healing which, according to Mallory takes place within six to eight weeks in man. He interdicts work if there is any residual symptomatology and prescribes more rest and delayed resumption of employment if the infarction involved large areas of the myocardium according to the electrocardiogram, if the course was stormy, if the physical requirements of the job seem high, if the emotional pressures are great, if the patient is not motivated to return to work at the time, or if he is sympathetic to the patient's desires to make full use of his insurance benefits or disability funds. For a variety of reasons, therefore, patients may be unemployed for some three to twelve months or longer. This is not necessarily disadvantageous according to Bjork,[2] who feels that, since life span may be shortened by myocardial infarction, a man may well be entitled to a "terminal holiday" if he chooses to retire early. With due respect to the philosophies of both patient and physician, if the patient ultimately chooses to return to work, the physician is often asked to advise his patients as to whether their former jobs may be resumed safely.

CLINICAL METHODS

The usual procedure is to advise the patient who has been moderately active outside the hospital during convalescence to resume work on a part-time basis, two to four hours daily, avoiding, symptoms and fatigue as well as emotional tension. The patient is usually cautioned to avoid public transportation and rush hour traffic, as well as to limit his after-hours social functions. He may be asked to rest during the day if this is feasible. Empirically, he is guided back to full-time employment depending upon such qualitative factors as the patient's motivation, and the physician's past experience with similar cases. Some patients may be referred to the local Work Evaluation Unit for more detailed evaluation or vocational guidance.

WORK EVALUATION UNIT METHODS

There are approxiamtely 50 Work Evaluation Units throughout the country according to Whitehouse,[3] most of these supported by local Heart Associations. The major contribution of the Units has been in attempting to quantitate job requirements, providing information about the capacities of patients through performance testing, and recommending methods by which patient and the job may be matched safely and appropriately. By familiarizing physicians with the concept of caloric expenditure, or energy cost, Work Evaluation Units have given him the means to describe jobs semiquantitatively in terms of metabolic units (mets or M.U.) or multiples of the basal caloric expenditure. The basal energy cost is taken as 1.0 large calories per minute or approximately 200 cc. of oxygen consumed per minute. In actuality, basal oxygen consumption is usually more than 200 cc./min. and hence 1.0 basal = 1.39 calories for average size males. The physician, then, by history, using the caloric expenditure tables of Passmore and Durnin[4] or the simplified drawings of Gordon as shown in a pamphlet distributed by the Los Angeles Heart Association Work Evaluation Unit,[5] determines the approximate energy requirements of the job to which he would like to return his patient. He then carries out one of several types of performance tests — the single Master two-step test at 8.5 calories per minute or 3 to 4 times the basal energy cost, the double Master at 7-8 times the basal or the Bruce progressive treadmill test at 4 to 5 times the basal requirements (Fig. 1). If the patient can sustain this degree of activity without detriment, then he probably can carry out a job of equal caloric cost. While monitoring the patients, the following criteria may be used.

1. Using the electrocardiogram, the cardiac rate should probably not rise to more than 130 beats per

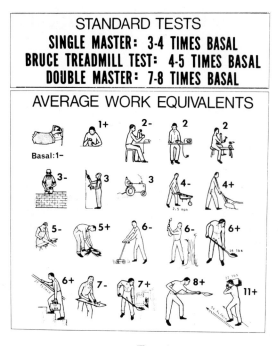

STANDARD TESTS
SINGLE MASTER: 3-4 TIMES BASAL
BRUCE TREADMILL TEST: 4-5 TIMES BASAL
DOUBLE MASTER: 7-8 TIMES BASAL

AVERAGE WORK EQUIVALENTS

FIG. 1.

minute during any peak effort, and there should be no significant alterations of the ST or T waves, nor should there be an increase in the number of premature contractions or the appearance of premature ventricular contractions if they were not present before the activity. The appearance of arrhythmias is also to be avoided.

2. The systolic blood pressure should rise from 10 to 40 mm. Hg mean pressure during heavy activity. The failure of the systolic blood pressure to rise, or a rise of the pulse rate to a level numerically greater than the systolic blood pressure during the activity is an indication of impaired exercise response with inadequate cardiac output[6] (Fig. 2). There should be a rapid return of pulse rate and blood pressure to the normal level. The sum of the pulse rates at one minute, two minutes, and three minutes, following cessation of activity, should be less than 350.[7]

3. All symptoms should be avoided including those which seem, on casual consideration, to be unrelated to the heart. It is of interest that Harrison reports eructation as a symptom accompanying ischemia in some patients, and in our own Unit we have found abdominal cramps, claudication, or

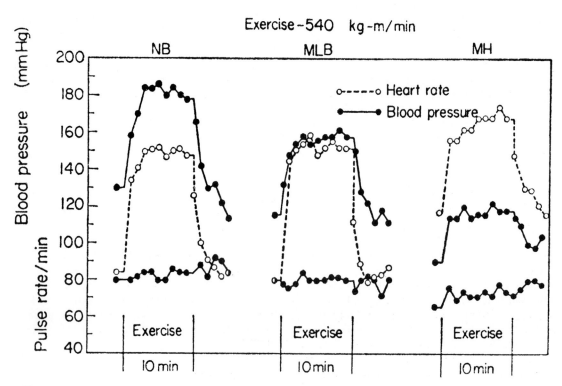

FIG. 2. Three kinds of numerical relationships between heart rate and systolic blood pressure values during muscular work.

dizziness sometimes to be concomitant with the appearance of ischemic electrocardiographic changes in the absence of symptoms referable to heart or lungs.

Using these methods, that is, matching the patient to the job in terms of the caloric expenditure required by the job and the ability of the patient to attain that caloric expenditure without symptoms, the patient may be returned to work according to seemingly objective criteria. However, the test procedure usually took less than one hour, and does not indicate for how many hours the patient may work. Brouha,[9] in studying heat stress, provides an example of the insidious effects of prolonged work, that is, over the entire workday, effects which would not be obvious within the first hour (Fig. 3). Only

minutes or longer.

The use of the New York Heart Association functional cardiac classification, has provided another possibly useful method of matching patient and job (Table 1). The normal individual is capable of carrying out work requiring more than 6.6 calories per minute. The Class I cardiac may work between 4.0 and 6.0, Class II between 2.7 and 4.0, and Class III between 1.5 and 2.7 calories per minute. Class IV cardiacs are obviously unable to do more than 1.5 calories per minute of work. In so doing, the oxygen debt of the Class I cardiac is insignificantly higher than that of a normal person, but the Class II and III cardiacs sustain twice and four times the debt respectively.[11] In using this information, the physician simply determines whether the job to

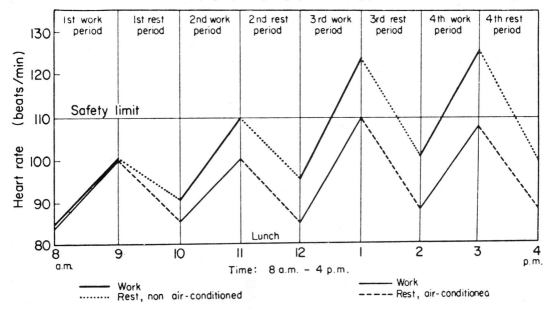

FIG. 3. Heart rates at the beginning and at the end of successive work and rest periods. One group was resting in a non-air-conditioned atmosphere, the other in an air-conditioned room.

in late afternoon did the cumulative effects of inadequate recovery of the pulse rate during rest periods become significant.

Further, since most industrial activities require between 2.0 and 4.0 calories per minute of sustained expenditure of energy,[10] it is only in the emergency situation that as much energy as that required by the Master test would be needed. It is conceivable therefore, that using performance tests in the office to predict job performance may err in both directions; namely, by proscribing work for the patient who does not pass the performance test, and by permitting work for many hours because a patient has been able to sustain a particular caloric expenditure for 3

which the patient returns is within the recommended caloric expenditure level according to the patient's functional cardiac classification. Alternatively, he may use the charts prepared by the State Division of Vocational Rehabilitation which list permissible jobs by name, within the functional cardiac classification framework (Fig. 4).

JOB MONITORING METHODS

With the advent of technical refinements in telemetry of the electrocardiogram, and the growing interest in cardiac rehabilitation, other methods of assessing whether patients can work have been

ILLUSTRATIVE TYPES OF ACTIVITY

Checkmarks indicate the classes for which the specified activities would be suitable — provided the therapeutic classification does not impose a greater restriction of physical activity than that indicated by functional capacity.

Occupation or Activity	I	II	III	IV
Farming—				
General (without excessive exertion)	x			
Light, using power equipment	x	x		
Poultry raising	x	x	x	
Supervision only, no exertion more than walking short distances	x	x	x	x
Millwork—				
Fast process, full day	x			
Slow process, part-time sitting	x	x		
Supervision only	x	x	x	
Store Clerk—				
Heavy merchandise, active	x			
Light merchandise, intermittent activity	x	x		
Small shop, intermittent activity	x	x	x	
Watchman-janitor—				
Firing boiler	x			
No stoking, walking, two floors	x	x		
Walking on level	x	x	x	
Sitting, no emergencies	x	x	x	x
Carpenter—				
Building construction	x			
Cabinetmaker, machine	x	x		
Benchwork, modelmaking, seated; no pressure for speed	x	x	x	
Handiwork—				
Sheltered industry, unhurried	x	x	x	x
Walking—moderate speed—				
On level, 3 miles	x			
1 mile	x	x		
½ mile	x	x	x	
Short distance	x	x	x	x
Stair climbing—unhurried—				
3 flights	x			
1 flight	x	x	x	

FIG. 4. From the Cardiac Disability Form of the Division of Vocational Rehabilitation, New York State Education Department.

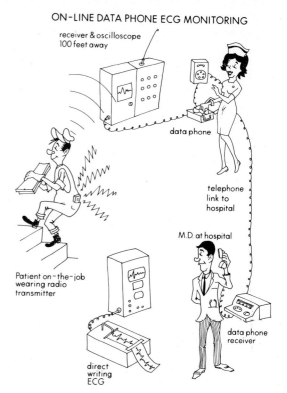

ON-LINE DATA PHONE ECG MONITORING

FIG. 5. On-the-job monitoring permits continuous observation of patient and ECG throughout the workday by telephone transmission of the ECG (dataphone) to the hospital.

developed. The ensuing paragraphs describe two such methods: (1) simulated job monitoring, a method borrowed from the rehabilitation of patients with neuromusculoskeletal diseases, and (2) on-the-job monitoring, an on-line method developed as an offshoot of the six to eight hour magnetic tape recordings used by Holter and others.[12]

Simulated job monitoring (SJM) duplicates the physical and sometimes the emotional requirements of a job on the hospital premises, permitting observation of the patient over gradually increasing periods of time. On-the-job monitoring (OJM)

permits continuous observation of the patient and electrocardiogram throughout the workday by telephone transmission of the electrocardiogram (dataphone) to the hospital (Figs. 5, 6). This differs from magnetic tape recording in that the tracing is observed continuously while the patient works so that he may be stopped from working immediately upon the appearance of detrimental alterations in the tracing, whereas the magnetic tape type of recording does not permit altering the patient's activity until much later, after the tape has been

TABLE 1

Relationship Between Functional Capacity (N.Y. Heart Association), Exercise Tolerance (Bruce Physical Fitness Index), Oxygen Debt, Estimated Work Capacity and Follow-up Mortality

Functional Classification	Normal	I	II	III	IV
Physical fitness index	17	17	15	9	2
Oxygen debt per cent	12	14	32	55	Not tested
Estimated work capacity (calories per minute)	More than 6.6	4.0–6.6	2.7–4.0	1.5–2.7	Less than 1.5
Per cent dead, 6-year average follow-up	4	25	31	53	60

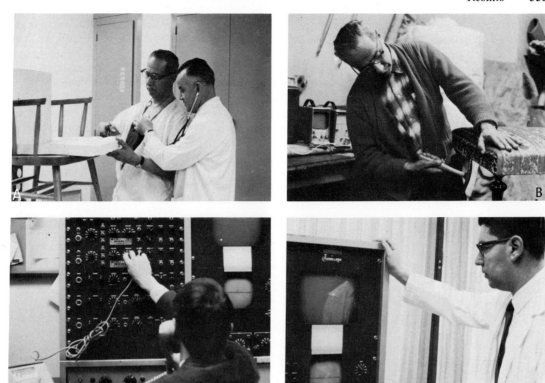

FIG. 6. *A*, Simulated job monitoring in the occupational Therapy Shop. The patient is an upholsterer and is being monitored while he upholsters a chair. *B,* On-the-job monitoring. At his own shop, the patient upholsters a chair. The radiotelemetry receiver and oscilloscope are seen in the background. *C,* At Montefiore Hospital, the electrocardiogram is received continuously via telephone (dataphone) during the work period. *D,* The cardiologist observes the tracing at the hospital, proscribing activities which are detrimental immediately by telephone.

reviewed.

In simulated job monitoring, Brozek[13] has described the use of miniature job samples, tasks of known physical and skill requirements which could be adjusted for studies of single psychophysiologic functions in a laboratory, or studies of output in job situations. The TOWER system (Testing Orientation and Work Evaluation in Rehabilitation) at the Institute for Crippled and Disabled in New York City, also presents a series of job sample tasks upon which the patients are graded.[14] These tasks are not exactly like what the individual did in his job, but quantitate his remaining skills and potential for a variety of different activities to see in what ways he may be helped by vocational rehabilitation. For the able-bodied cardiac, it is not often necessary to dissect the job into its component parts and have such a structured program of evaluation. In our hospital, after detailed description of the job by the patient, we have matched his job to those in our own hospital shops such as the laundry, engineering department, offices, etc. or have simulated the physical requirements of his job in the Occupational Therapy shop in Rehabilitation Medicine. Further, we have purposely imposed various psychologic stresses through the cooperation of heads of the shops, or a separate stress interview with a psychologist. A rotation of resident physicians, nurses and technicians with cardiologists constantly available provides for the monitoring by observation and on-line transmission of the electrocardiogram by telephone to an oscilloscope located elsewhere within the hospital.

RESULTS

Thirty-six patients with coronary heart disease, all of whom had sustained one or more myocardial infarctions have been involved in our program to date. Thirty-three patients were male and three were female. Three patients were less than 39 years of age and four were over 60. There were 15 patients between the ages of 40 and 49 and 14 patients between the ages of 50 and 59. Seventeen patients had simulated job monitoring and 7 patients had on-the-job monitoring. Twelve patients had both simulated and on-the-job monitoring. Twenty-two patients also had Master two-step tests. Patients were monitored using a true chest lead with the exploring electrode placed over the precordial lead showing residual changes of infarction or, if none remained, using the lead with the largest R wave. Gulton equipment with silver chloride electrodes was used, powered either by a 6 volt battery in an attaché case or via a car cigarette lighter connection to the battery or using alternating current. At times a converter was necessary for DC current in the business district. Patients studied at the beginning of the program were observed using the RKG 100 with the selector switch permitting observation of lead II and other related leads in patients who had posterior myocardial infarction. A nurse or trained technician accompanied the patient to the job simulation area of the hospital or to his job, set up the equipment and kept records of his performance throughout the workday.

Three important questions arise from these observations: (1) did job monitoring provide information not available through the usual clinical methods? (2) did job monitoring provide information not available from the Master two-step test? and (3) what are the relative advantages and disadvantages of simulated versus on-the-job monitoring.

Job Monitoring Compared to Traditional Clinical Methods

Monitoring of the patient at work, either in the simulated situation or on-the-job, provides useful information to the physician concerning the effects of this amount of activity on his patient, offers psychologic benefit to the patient since he once again sees himself as a useful member of the community, and provides information useful to employer as to what can be expected of the cardiac who has returned to work. It sometimes verifies, sometimes contradicts, clinical impressions but in all cases provides a rational adjunct to the clinical assessment. Ten examples are listed below:

Case 1. Mr. H. B., a 49-year-old male building superintendent sustained a posterior wall myocardial infarction on 4/26/66. The manager of the building in which he worked planned to hire the temporary superintendent on a permanent basis if the patient was not back at full-time work within one month. After 10 days of rest and chair treatment, he was progressively ambulated and put on an exercise reconditioning program followed by a simulated job activity designed to increase work tolerance. He

was monitored day after day for an increasing number of hours while waxing and mopping floors, and working in the plumbing shop of the hospital. He moved barrels of bricks (simulating emptying ashcans) outside on the roof of the hospital without detrimental ECG changes. He was instructed to request assistance in this activity, however, despite the negative findings. His physician permitted him to return to full-time work upon discharge from the hospital on 5/24/66. Follow-up studies revealed no deleterious effects of this early resumption of activities. Most physicians would be reluctant to permit this return to full activity after one month; yet job monitoring offered a rational approach to the dilemma of avoiding an economic and family crisis for the patient while protecting his myocardium.

Case 2. Mr. E. B., a 48-year-old truckman for an x-ray company, sustained an anterior wall myocardial infarction on 9/2/67. The company was reluctant to permit him to return to work because of the strenuous nature of his job, but the patient pleaded to be allowed to work because his former jobs as handyman were intermittent and provided only a meager wage. Job simulation involved moving 40 pound boxes of x-ray films using an interval pattern of work, that is, 30 seconds of lifting and 30 seconds of rest over a 15 minute period on 10/20/67. There was some exertional dyspnea and the pulse rate rose to 130 but there were no electrocardiographic changes. On 10/23/67 the patient worked again for 30 minutes, on 10/25/67 for several hours after which there was an inverted T III and AVF. The patient was not returned to work full time on the basis of these findings, but accepted this course with greater equanimity, feeling that every attempt had been made to return him to the preferred job.

Case 3. Mr. W. C., a 52-year-old gardener, sustained a posterior wall myocardial infarction on 5/31/66. He had a past history of chorea at the age of 6. His usual job entailed raking, shoveling, sawing wood, spraying and planting, the heaviest activity being the lifting of 80 pound bags of fertilizer. The job was simulated in one of the construction areas of the hospital while the patient raked leaves, pulled a cart, swept, sawed wood (Fig. 7) moved a wheelbarrow and an 80 pound waste can. He developed 2 mm. ST depressions and premature ventricular contractions with coupling at peak energy levels. Although the prematures disappeared within 3 minutes, the pulse rate returned to normal only after 15 minutes reaching a maximum of 120 beats per minute from a baseline of 91. On the basis of these findings, the private physician referred the

Resting

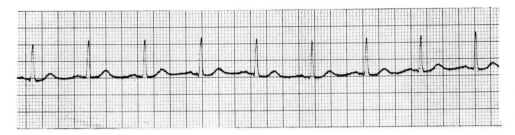

Sawing wood

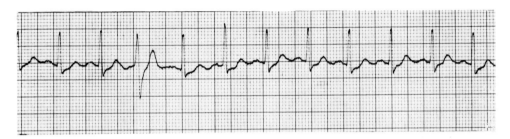

FIG. 7.   Electrocardiogram of patient W.C.

patient to the Division of Vocational Rehabilitation for retraining.

Case 4. Mr. J. S., a 48-year-old installer of thermostats, had his posterior wall myocardial infarction on 6/2/68. On August 12, 1968, he worked in the hospital machine shop straightening copper tubing by hammering and doing some light bench work. He developed premature ventricular beats and had to be stopped during the monitoring session to receive procaine amide. Subsequent monitoring in the hospital while carrying out the same activities on antiarrhythmic medication permitted him to work through most of the day. On the job, however, as he installed thermostat controls in a new building, when he was working at ceiling level and climbing up and down ladders, he developed numerous premature contractions and had to be stopped after 2 hours. Subsequently, treatment with propanolol enabled him to carry out heavy labor for the entire workday without ST-T changes or premature beats (Fig. 8). The use of appropriate medication in this case permitted a skilled worker to return to his former job. Although procaine amide was adequate during the simulated job situation in the hospital, it was not adequate as on-the-job treatment, whereas propanolol prevented the ECG alterations completely.

Case 5. Dr. E. K. a 55-year-old general practitioner who had been limiting his practice to office sessions, sustained a posterior wall myocardial infarction in 4/68. He was anxious to return to

practice as soon as possible and had his cardiologist's agreement. Stair climbing up one flight six weeks after infarct resulted in ST depression of 2 mm. across the precordial leads which subsided quickly. The subsequent on-the-job monitoring when the patient did go back to work in August 1968 was completely normal despite his very busy practice. In this situation simulated job monitoring showed that this physician did require a more prolonged convalescence than either he or his cardiologist anticipated.

Case 6. Mr. L. S. a 57-year-old man who sustained an anterolateral myocardial infarction on 11/17/67, described his job as the owner of a dry-goods store as very light work. After 3 months his physician felt that he could go back to work and wait on customers. Simulated job monitoring in the Occupational Therapy shop carrying 25 pounds of weight up and down stairs and moving objects from one place to another over a 4 hour period was normal. His heart rate rose from 70 to 120 beats per minute at the end of this session. However, on the job, when bending and lifting objects from the floor or climbing upstairs with boxes of curtains which had just been delivered, the patient developed bigeminy and ST elevations of 2 to 3 mm. He was stopped after 2 hours of work and quinidine was recommended. Subsequent monitoring when fully treated with quinidine showed only minimal T wave change (to biphasic) without the ST changes described previously. This man's job was seemingly light and

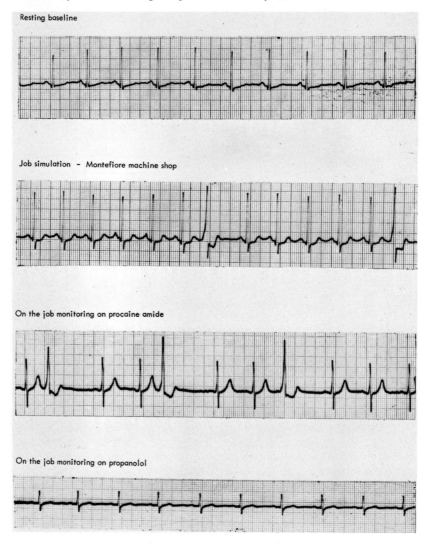

Resting baseline

Job simulation – Montefiore machine shop

On the job monitoring on procaine amide

On the job monitoring on propanolol

FIG. 8.   Electrocardiograms of patient J.S.

suitable for a cardiac except for the cardiac stress of peak loads, not suspected by the physician.

Case 7. Mr. S. C., age 48, had a posterolateral myocardial infarction on May 22, 1968. On 10/23/68, after monitoring, he was found to be able to resume his occupation as a house painter provided he did not lift the paint cans which weighed more than 60 pounds. In this case, the physician was able to individualize the safety requirements for this patient on the basis of job monitoring.

Case 8. Mr. B. A., a 45-year-old accountant who had a myocardial infarction on November 11, 1967, remained at home until March 1968 on the advice of his physician because of transient, sticking pains in his chest and shoulders. Both he and his wife were very worried about the persistence of symptoms.

On-the-job monitoring at the office, carried out from an adjacent room, without the knowledge of the clients, showed that this man had no electrocardiographic changes accompanying twinges of pain (finally determined to be musculoskeletal) and that he was quite capable of sustaining the desk work, interviewing and hectic pace of his office. The physician was then able to reassure the patient and his wife and return the man to work.

Case 9. Mr. R. H., a 44-year-old hat cutter, sustained a left hemiplegia and a myocardial infarction simultaneously in June 1967. The hemiplegia was transient, resulting in minimal weakness which in no way interfered with the patient's ability to carry out his job. On 7/27/67 he participated in job simulation in the hospital laundry for one hour and developed premature ventricular contractions on carrying, pushing or bending. Subsequent monitoring for 3 hours and 4 hours revealed the same arrhythmia. However, the arrhythmia appeared only during the first half hour of performance and the patient was seemingly able to participate in full activities for many hours after this with a normal tracing. He was therefore sent back to work. On 8/10/67 he was monitored in the hat factory from 9:15 A. M. to late afternoon while using an electric cutting machine, and lifting bolts of cloth. He developed occasional ventricular premature beats during the first 10 minutes of work which were not present at anytime thereafter. However, throughout the day, pulse rate continued to climb in the heat of the factory and because of the cumulative stress and pressures of the job as well as the fact that this man refused to take any rest periods throughout the day, his physician chose to retrain him for other employment of a more sedentary nature.

Case 10. Mr. A. R., a 53-year-old auto repairman (body and fender), had an anterior wall myocardial infarction on 5/2/68 and was thought ready to resume work on 6/20/68. Simulated job monitoring in the hospital engineering department while carrying out moderate work in the metal and carpenter shops for 6 hours revealed no ST-T changes or premature beats. However, after heavy work for 2 hours on 6/26/68, ST depression became evident persisting for 8 minutes after cessation of activity. On the job at an auto body establishment in the Bronx, several days later, the tracing remained negative while the patient sanded, polished and sprayed cars. Simulated job monitoring in this case conflicted with clinical judgment and on-the-job monitoring confirmed the correctness of the clinical impression. The job apparently entailed only moderate work which was well within the capacities of the patient (Fig. 9)

Thus, information is made available to the physician through job monitoring on which he

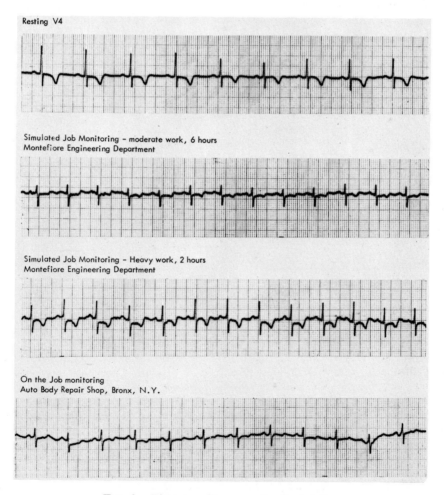

Resting V4

Simulated Job Monitoring – moderate work, 6 hours
Montefiore Engineering Department

Simulated Job Monitoring – Heavy work, 2 hours
Montefiore Engineering Department

On the Job monitoring
Auto Body Repair Shop, Bronx, N.Y.

FIG. 9. Electrocardiograms of patient A.R.

can base his decision as to whether a patient should or should not return to a job, for how many hours a day a patient may work, and whether there are any modifications of activity which should be made to permit the patient to carry on the same occupation as prior to his heart attack. The patient may psychologically adapt to work better than to several months of confinement at home and may even lose some of his symptoms, the psychosomatic nature of which becomes apparent only after on-the-job monitoring. Job monitoring also occasionally discloses the need for additional medication, the doses prescribed for the sedentary individual proving insufficient for the active patient.

Job Monitoring and the Master Two-Step Test

Does job monitoring offer any more information to the physician than does the Master test?

Twenty-two patients had the double Master two-step test, usually within 1 to 2 months of job monitoring. Of the 11 patients who had negative two-step tests, two patients subsequently showed premature ventricular and atrial contractions on simulated job monitoring. One of these had negative on-the-job monitoring 7 months later when he finally resumed work. The other patient had ven-

and supervision on the job. Of the 5 patients with positive Master two-step tests, the 3 who had simulated job monitoring showed no changes and 4 who had on-the-job monitoring similarly showed no changes.

Thus, if the Master test is negative, the patient probably will have negative job monitoring although there are exceptions depending on the peak stresses of the job. Of the 11 patients with borderline or even positive Master tests, detrimental electrocardiographic changes did not necessarily appear during job monitoring, that is, the presence of a positive Master test does not necessarily indicate that return to work will be accompanied by similar changes.

Further, in this series the anatomic location of the myocardial infarction was not related either to the presence of a positive Master test or to whether the job monitoring was normal or abnormal, with the distribution of positive Master tests and abnormal job findings, being approximately equal in the anterior and posterior wall groups.

Comparison of Simulated and On-the-Job Monitoring

Simulated job monitoring has both medical and technical concomitants. When a patient is observed for many hours in a hospital setting, the physician

TABLE 2
Double Two Step vs. Job Monitoring

| Double Two Step | | Job Monitoring | | |
No. Pts.	Results	No. Pts.	Results	Type
11	Negative	2	Atrial and vent. prematures	Simulated
		1	Vent. premature and high pulse rates	On-the-job
6	Borderline	1	ST-T changes	Simulated
		1	Occas. vent. premature	Simulated
		3	Vent. premat. on stress	On-the-job
5	Positive	3	no changes	Simulated
		4	no changes	On-the-job

tricular premature contractions and high pulse rates on the job so that in only two of the cases, the negative Master two-step test was not accompanied by negative job monitoring (Table 2).

Conversely, of the 6 patients with borderline double two-step tests, one showed significant ST-T changes in the simulated job situation and the other had occasional ventricular premature beats. On the job, the patient with ST-T changes had a normal tracing but the patient with the premature ventricular contractions had many more on lifting. There were two additional patients who developed premature ventricular contractions during the stress of heavy lifting or due to emotion related to personal contacts

has an opportunity to find an "indicator" by which the patient may gauge his own performance. Concomitant with detrimental configuration or rhythm changes on the electrocardiogram or alterations in blood pressure, the patient may experience some sensation which he may be taught to use as a warning to stop the activity being carried out or to limit it. As mentioned previously, the sensation need not necessarily be of cardiac origin. Often, casual office confrontation does not provide ample opportunity to seek out an indicator,

Simulated job monitoring also permits observation of the effects of work on the patient over a period of time (from hours to days) in graded doses permitting the patient to develop tolerance to resumption of activity. The physician may then proceed resumption of activity. The physician may then proceed more slowly and with more adequate information and need not make a decision which might unfairly limit or unwisely permit the patient to carry out activities.

Technically, not all activities can be simulated, particularly executive activities with their accompanying emotional tension. In the hospital setting, the activities of two accountants in the business environment could not be matched, nor could the operation of a mechanized bakery, the duties of a teacher, or the operation of a candy stand and stationery store which entailed both inside and outside work. The laundry could not be turned into an establishment which presses Dior gowns although it could be used to simulate a hat factory. The facilities of the Occupational Therapy area, hospital shops and offices and even the sheltered shop are inadequate for simulation of certain activities.

On-the-job activities could be monitored in 19 patients but not in the other 7 for the following reasons: portable equipment was not available at the time of monitoring of 5 patients. Six patients were unemployed. Either the patient or the physician refused monitoring in 3 cases since knowledge of the medical condition might interfere with the patient's being rehired. In one case it was unnecessary to monitor on the job because the job was duplicated precisely at the hospital. The remaining patients are not far enough from infarct for the physician to consider sending them back to work.

On the job, the psychosocial elements, as well as the physical stresses become important in the patient's over-all response to re-employment. He has a chance to react to his fellow employees and to his supervisors, to argue with clients or to feel reassured that he is getting back into life and that he will not be an invalid. The employer is made aware that the patient is capable of carrying out his job or is specifically advised as to limitations through the private physician. On-the-job monitoring is technically simple but poses many minor difficulties and is costly in terms of personnel and time. For example, although it is relatively easy to monitor heavy and moderately heavy labor even outdoors (with portable battery-powered equipment) large metal obstacles may obstruct radio-EKG transmission and the lack of power sources and telephone facilities in new buildings sometimes poses problems. Further, usually only one electrocardiographic lead is monitored since the patient is generally too involved in his job to permit changing to another lead. Further, it is difficult to take blood pressures on the job so that only the electrocardiogram is available to provide rate, rhythm and configuration changes. A technician or a nurse must remain at the job to describe the activities in which the patient is engaging during the monitoring and to be available in case of any emergency. It is possible to train a volunteer for such purposes, however, At the other end of the telephone line, constant observation of the oscilloscope screen is necessary. The audible tone of the monitor and a rotation of resident physicians makes continuous observation quite practical. Thus, the obstacles of time and cost are certainly not insurmountable.

SUMMARY

If the physician chooses to have the patient return to work, and if the patient is so motivated, new methods are available for monitoring the patient in either a simulated work situation or on his job. The simulated job situation may be set up in an acute general hospital using the shops and offices of the hospital. The monitoring on the job may be done by on-line telephone transmission of the electrocardiogram back to the hospital while the patient works at the actual job that he will resume. Using these methods to supplement clinical and office testing procedures, we have been able to provide useful information to the physician which assists him to make a more rational and objective decision about return to work after a coronary episode.

REFERENCES

1. Mallory, G. K., White, P. D., and Salcedo-Salgar, J.: Speed of healing of myocardial infarction: study of pathologic anatomy in 72 cases, Am. Heart J. *18*:647, 1939.
2. Bjorck, G.: The return to work of patients with myocardial infarction, Editorial, J. Chron. Dis. *17*:653, 1964.
3. Whitehouse, F. A.: The cardiac work evaluation unit as a specialized team approach, J. Rehab. *32*:66, 1966.
4. Passmore, R., and Durnin, J. V. G. A.: Human energy expenditure, Physiol, Rev. *35*:801, 1955.
5. Frasher, W., Stivelman, R., Horowitz, L.: Work prescription for heart patients, Work Classification Unit, Los Angeles County Heart Association.
6. Brouha, L.: Physiology in Industry, N.Y. Pergamon Press, 1960, p. 10.
7. Frasher, W., Stivelman, R., and Horowitz, L.: Office procedures as aids to work prescription for cardiac patients, Part II, Mod. Concepts Cardiovas. Dis. *32*:777, 1963.
8. Harrison, T. R., and Reeves, T. J.: Principles and Problems of Ischemic Heart Disease, Chicago, Year Book Medical Publishers, Inc., 1968, p. 209.
9. Brouha, L.: *Op. cit.,* p. 121.

10. Turrell, D. J., and Hellerstein, H. K.: Evaluation of cardiac function in relation to specific physical activities following recovery from acute myocardial infarction, Prog. Cardiovas. Dis. *1*:237, 1958.

11. *Ibid.* p. 241.

12. Holter, N. J.: New method for heart studies, Science *134*:1214, 1961.

13. Brozek, J., and Monke, J. V.: Miniature work situations as a research tool, Arch. Indus. Hygiene & Occup. Med. *2*:63, 1950.

14. Tower: Institute for the Crippled & Disabled, N. Y. 1967.

Laboratory and Clinical Experience in Orthotopic Cardiac Allotransplantation

Adrian Kantrowitz, Jordan D. Haller, Yasunori Koga, Eduard Sujansky, Hans E. Carstensen, Jose Caralps-Riera, Howard A. Joos, William Neches, William Pomerance, and Marcial M. Cerruti*

With the development of a feasible surgical technic by Lower and Shumway,[1] orthotopic cardiac allotransplantation has been on the threshold of clinical practicability for several years. We began a series of experimental studies of this procedure in 1963. Among the conditions appearing to warrant cardiac transplantation in infants, severe congenital malformations represent a major group. With this in mind, we gave major emphasis to studies on mongrel puppy allografts.

In mongrel puppies, as well as in infants, small size and homeostatic immaturity present special problems. Cardiopulmonary bypass is at best difficult and hazardous in infants. The alternative, circulatory arrest during profound hypothermia induced by external cooling, offered the advantages of a nearly bloodless surgical field and avoidance of the postoperative bleeding associated with the use of anticoagulants.

Studies of transplantations of adult canine hearts have been carried out in our program by methods similar to those reported by other investigators.[1-4] Since 1963, more than 250 puppy allografts have been transplanted. In this report, 166 cases will be analyzed, including 59 instances of delayed transplantation, or procedures in which the donor organ was excised and stored prior to implantation. Two clinical trials of the transplant procedure are also described.

SURGICAL TECHNIC

The surgical technic was that reported by Lower and Shumway[1] and modified in our laboratory by Y. Kondo.[5,6] Pairs of puppies were randomly selected on the basis of approximate match in weight. After premedication, the animals were

anesthetized with ether, intubated and ventilated.

Femoral arterial pressure and the ECG were continuously monitored, as was the temperature, measured intrarectally. A femoral vein was cannulated for continuous infusion and occasional CVP measurements.

After all preliminary preparations were completed, the recipient puppy was immersed in a bath containing ice cubes and water (Fig. 1). Anesthesia was discontinued when the temperature declined to 25°C.

A Schematic Drawing of Set-up for Puppy Heart Transplantation

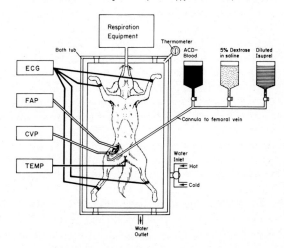

FIG. 1. Schematic drawing of set-up for puppy heart transplantation using external cooling for hypothermia.

The donor puppy was also anesthetized, similarly managed and subjected to moderate hypothermia (25 to 29°C.). Cooling was stopped when the recipient's temperature reached 20°C. and the donor's about 30°C. Ventricular fibrillation was never encountered during the cooling period (Fig. 2), and was seen infrequently during manipulation of the

*The authors are of the Department of Surgery, Maimonides Medical Center, Brooklyn, N.Y. Work supported by USPHS Grant HE-11173.

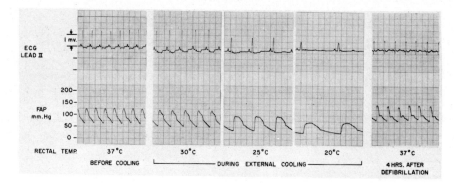

FIG. 2.   ECG tracings and femoral arterial pressures before transplantation, during cooling and 4 hours after defibrillation.

heart after thoractomy.

The surgery was performed by two teams. The first team prepared the recipient. The chest was opened bilaterally through the anterior fourth interocostal space and tourniquets were placed around the venae cavae and azygos vein. The pericardial sac was then opened widely and partly fixed to the chest wall. The aorta and pulmonary artery were cross-clamped through the transverse sinus and the vessels transected close to the valves. The atria were then cut close to the ventricles. Artificial respiration was stopped at this time.

While the recipient was being prepared, the second team opened the donor's chest cavity through the left fourth intercostal space, injected heparin (3 to 4 mg./Kg. body weight) into a pulmonary vein or the superior vena cava and excised the heart. Care was taken to include an undamaged sinus node in the excised specimen as well as to retain appropriately long segments of the aorta and pulmonary trunk. The graft was immediately placed in a cold isotonic solution (4 to 5°C.).

To implant the heart, stay sutures were placed at both ends of the atrial septal ridge (Fig. 3). The atrial walls, including the septum, were approximated with a continuous over-and-over suture. In the initial series we used 5-0 silk or Dacron. Subsequently, 5-0 chromic catgut was used beause the silk caused stricture of the suture line during the animal's subsequent maturation.[6,7] Finally, the aorta and then the pulmonary artery were anastomosed with 5-0 silk or Dacron. Initially, a continuous suture technic was employed, but thereafter, continuous suture for about two thirds of the circumference of each vessel and interrupted stitches for the remainder were used—again, to prevent stricture. The atria and the ventricles were flushed with cold saline before the last suture was placed, to expel air.

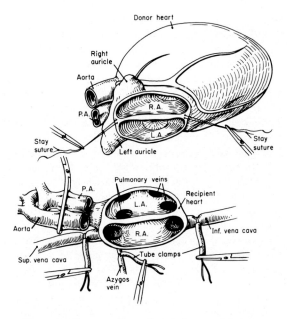

FIG. 3.   Preparation of recipient atrial stump and excised graft for orthotopic cardiac transplantation.

Cardiac massage, controlled respiration, blood transfusion and external and intrathoracic rewarming with warm saline solution with penicillin added were started simultaneously after removal of the clamp and tourniquets. The duration of circulatory arrest was 30 to 60 minutes in most experiments. Shortly after the start of cardiac massage, the heart began to fibrillate. Sodium bicarbonate was administered intravenously to correct metabolic acidosis. On a few occasions the heart began to beat spontaneously. In most instances, ventricular fibrillation was readily converted by countershock at 20 to 28°C. temperature.

Additional intermittent heart massage was sometimes required. A slow intravenous drip of *l*-norepinephrine or isoproterenol hydrochloride in 5 per cent dextrose during a brief interval was usually necessary to support the blood pressure and maintain the heart rate. In most cases, intraventricular or intravenous injection of calcium chloride was used for the same purpose immediately before and after defibrillation.

first 24 hours after operation.

Several factors accounted for these deaths (Table 1). Among 15 animals dying of early graft failure, in 5 the heart could not be resuscitated after implantation, either as a result of insufficient protection of the graft during the period between excision and implantation or as a result of technical errors (chiefly air embolism into the coronary arteries immediately after the start of cardiac massage).

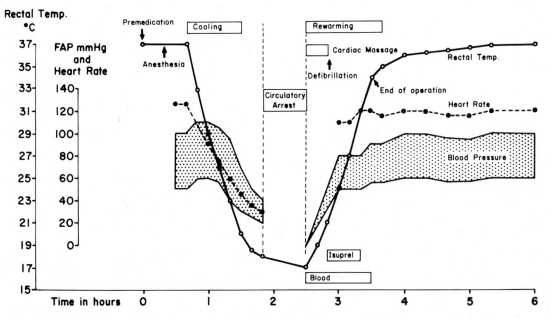

FIG. 4. Physiologic parameters and sequence of events during puppy heart transplantation.

Rewarming was continued until the temperature reached 36 to 37°C. The chest cavity was closed in three layers with a chest tube on each side for drainage. Blood (30 to 50 ml.) was transfused to replace the amount lost. Figure 4 shows hemodynamic parameters and the steps during an uneventful transplantation.

OBSERVATIONS ON DIRECT HEART TRANSPLANTS

Intraoperative and Immediate Postoperative Problems

Although the use of a technic involving complete circulatory arrest during hypothermia has advantages in infants when compared with methods requiring extracorporeal circulation, the method also has drawbacks, as may be shown by consideration of 107 direct orthotopic puppy heart allotransplantations. Of these animals, 40 died within the

TABLE 1
*Causes of Death in 40 Dogs
Dying Within 24 Hours After Transplantation*

Cause	No.		(%)
Early graft failure	15		(37.5)
Note resuscitatable		5	(12.5)
Resuscitatable but function inadequate		10	(25.0)
Brain damage	10		(25.0)
Respiratory failure	4		(10.0)
Hemorrhage	2		(5.0)
Others	9		(22.5)
Totals	40		(100.0)

In the other 10 animals in this group, the same factors led to early heart failure within 24 hours after operation.

10 of the 40 dogs died of brain damage which resulted from prolonged circulatory arrest or from insufficient circulation while rewarming was being carried out. In 4 instances, respiratory failure led to death. Two animals died of hemorrhage.

Of the remaining 9 dogs, 6 died as a result of technical errors in anesthesia administration (2 cases), surgical technic (3 cases) and postoperative care (1 case). In 3 dogs in which post-mortem studies disclosed no significant abnormalities, severe uncorrected metabolic acidosis was probably the cause of death.

In a study of 12 consecutive puppy heart transplants, arterial blood samples were taken during the procedures. Half of these animals were not treated, while half were given bicarbonate, 5 mEq./Kg. body weight, during rewarming. Figure 5 shows pH versus base excess before cooling, approximately 30 minutes after induction of anesthesia, and after rewarming, when the temperature had reached 36 to 37°C. All the animals were acidotic at the start of cooling. During cooling, decrease in pH continued—most markedly during the period of circulatory arrest. On rewarming, the decrease in pH and base excess was sustained in untreated animals to average pH values of 6.90 and base excess values of -25 mEq./L.

Although formidable, problems arising during the operation or during the first 24 postoperative hours can be prevented or minimized by careful, swift surgical technic, cautious administration of anesthesia, effective respiratory assistance and meticulous postoperative care; in short, the same requirements as for any other cardiac surgery on infants.

Late Postoperative Problems

The management of puppies surviving the hazards of the first 24 hours after transplantation involves two major problems—rejection and pulmonary infection. The latter is unquestionably the major factor accounting for nearly two-thirds of all deaths in transplantation.

Postoperatively, the puppies were treated according to three different regimens. One group received no immunosuppressive therapy. A second group received azathioprine, steroids and actinomycin-C on appearance of signs of rejection. In the third group, most puppies were treated from the third day with steroids and from the fifth day with azathioprine; three puppies in this group were given azathioprine, 4 mg./Kg. orally, for 3 to 8 days postoperatively. Azathioprine and methylprednisolone were given in doses of 5 or 10 mg./Kg., and during rejection crises, actinomycin-C in doses of 8 mg./Kg. was administered. Antibiotics were given to all the animals.

Table 2 shows the distribution of survival in the three groups. The findings are expressed as percentages of all puppies in the respective group. Although in individual instances it could be clearly seen (Fig. 6) that immunosuppressive treatment was effective in suppressing rejection of the graft, there was no difference in survival rate between the untreated and the treated groups.

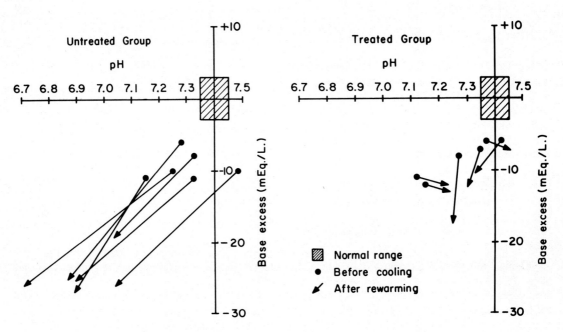

FIG. 5.   Base excess and pH before and after cardiac transplantation (at left) in untreated animals and (at right) in animals given bicarbonate, 5 mEq./kg. body weight, during rewarming.

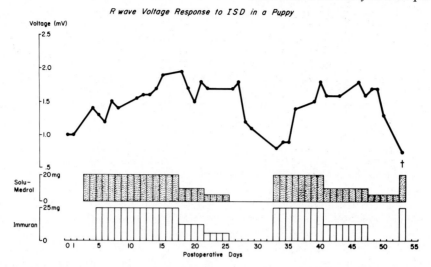

FIG. 6.   Postoperative course of R wave voltage (Lead II) and immunosuppressive therapy in puppy 6183. After withdrawal of azathioprine and methylprednisolone on the 26th day, a significant drop in R wave voltage and the development of heart failure indicated graft rejection. Repetition of immunosuppressive treatment restored R wave voltage and cardiac function. After a second withdrawal of treatment, the puppy died of acute rejection.

In all likelihood, the explanation for this derives from the difficulty of keeping the animals free of infection,[8] a problem enhanced during immunosuppressive treatment.

Table 3 shows the primary causes of death in the 67 puppies living for more than 1 day. The rate of

TABLE 2
Survival (%) According to Immunosuppressive Treatment Used

Alive More Than	No immuno- Suppression (37 Dogs)	Immuno- Suppression on Signs of Rejection (30 Dogs)	Immuno- Suppression Starting on Third day (40 Dogs)
1 day	75.0%	43.5%	65.0%
1 week	39.0%	33.3%	32.5%
2 weeks	29.7%	20.0%	27.5%
3 weeks	13.5%	10.0%	15.0%

TABLE 3
Causes of Death in 67 Dogs Living More Than 24 Hours After Transplantation*

Cause	No. of Animals	(%)
Pulmonary complications	42	(62.6)
Acute rejection	13	(19.4)
Brain damage	3	(4.5)
Stricture of suture line	2	(3.0)
Hemorrhage	1	(1.5)
Others	5	(7.5)
Totals	66	(98.5)

*One dog alive and well 28 months postoperatively.

pulmonary infection—whether associated with rejection or not—was higher in the treated groups (70 per cent versus 58 per cent), whereas the rate of death due to acute rejection crises was lower (15 per cent versus 25 per cent).

Currently available drugs are sufficiently potent to make management of many rejection crises possible. The solution to the problem of infection lies not in administration of antibiotics, but rather in prevention through isolation and observance of strict aseptic technics during the immediate postoperative period—a solution achieved only with difficulty in the animal laboratory.

OBSERVATIONS ON DELAYED TRANSPLANTS

An important aspect of heart transplantation is preservation of the graft. Since our study was initiated, we have implanted 59 hearts stored by various methods for as long as 24 hours. The methods fall into two groups—hypothermic storage (38 cases)[9] and normothermic storage (21 cases).[10,11]

Hypothermic Storage

Of the 38 hearts stored at 2 to 4°C., 32 were stored under O_2 pressures of 3 to 4 atmospheres. These hearts were all excised from living donors while beating. Several variations of the method were tried. The optimal technic appeared to be rapid cooling in Tyrode solution for 10 minutes and

TABLE   4

Results of Delayed Heart Transplantation Following
*Preservation by Hyperbaric Oxygenation During Hypothermia**

	No. of Exp.	Material	Preservation Time	Resuscitation Rate	Maximum Survival After Trans- plantation
Group I	7	Fresh heart	12 hours	100%	35 days
Group II	17	Fresh heart	24 hours	76%	5 days

*Oxygen pressure: 3 to 4 atm. absolute; temperature, 2 to 4°C.

subsequent dry storage in the refrigerated oxygen pressure tank. Table 4 shows the results in 24 hearts stored under hypothermic, hypobaric conditions. Thirteen of 17 hearts stored for 24 hours could be resuscitated and all of 7 hearts stored for 12 hours immediately resumed function. It was concluded that by this method fresh hearts can be safely stored for 12 hours.

Normothermic Resuscitation and Preservation

Although the duration of storage obtainable with hypothermic, hyperbaric preservation would seem sufficient to permit preparation of a recipient, there is need for preoperative evaluation of the functional capability of the heart. Normothermic preservation appeared to allow for the required observations.

Using normothermic coronary perfusion, the heart could be made to beat in vitro and its performance under these conditions evaluated.[11] This procedure, furthermore, allowed for resuscitation

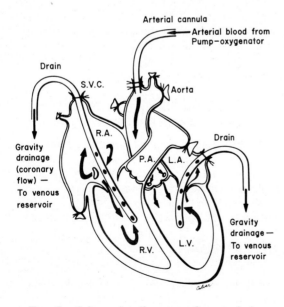

FIG. 7.   Schematic diagram of cannulations for isolated normothermic perfusion of the excised heart.

of hearts that had ceased beating for as long as 90 minutes.

The cannulations were performed as shown in Figure 7 and the hearts were connected to the perfusion circuit shown in Figure 8. From leads on the apex and the aorta, an ECG was recorded every 15 minutes and the flow from the coronary sinus measured. Sixty-four hearts were studied in this perfusion system. The initial experience comprises 30 hearts obtained from puppies sacrificed by an overdose of barbiturates. The hearts were left in the chest for 30 to 45 minutes before excision. These hearts were perfused at a variety of pressures—5 without and 25 with a pulsatile pressure generated by delivering an O_2-CO_2 gas mixture to the oxygenator from a respirator, with peak pressures ranging from 35 to 80 mm. Hg. No clear-cut difference was found in the use of pulsatile and nonpulsatile pressures. Although high pressures (> 40 mm. Hg.) caused a higher coronary flow, the myocardium did not tolerate these pressures well.

The use of hemodilution with 1 part low molecular weight dextran to 2 parts whole blood—employed in 9 instances—was found to increase the time for which normal electrocardiogram and function could be maintained to a maximum of $7\frac{1}{2}$ hours, as compared to $4\frac{1}{2}$ hours for hearts perfused with whole blood. In addition, 11 hearts were transplanted after perfusion. Of these, 8 hearts perfused with whole blood were in no instance—despite short durations of perfusion—able to keep the puppy alive for more than 8 hours. However, in three instances in which the hemodilution technic was used, the puppies survived for 17 hours and 5 and 17 days.

Table 5 presents our most recent experience,[11] using hearts taken 30 minutes after electrical asystole induced by asphyxiation.[8] In this series, a constant low pressure of 40 mm. Hg. was applied. As in the previous series, all hearts could be resuscitated, but hearts perfused with whole blood rapidly deteriorated. Hemodilution, which improves the flow, led to a longer duration of storage. An important observation was that the introduction of a microfilter greatly improved the flow. This was

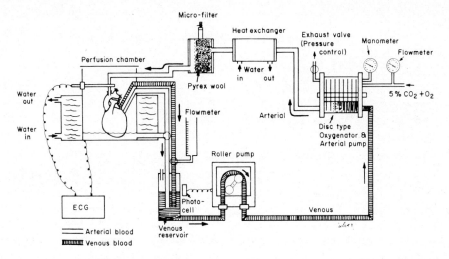

Schematic Drawing of Experimental Perfusion Circuit

FIG. 8.   Schematic diagram of circuit for isolated normothermic coronary perfusion. Flow is produced by delivery of an O_2-CO_2 mixture under pressure into the oxygenator.

TABLE 5
Resuscitation and Preservation of Canine Cadaver Hearts by Normothermic Coronary Perfusion in Vitro

		Resuscitation		
Anoxic Time After Cessation of ECG Activity	*No. of Exp.*	*Restoring of Sinus Rhythm*	*ECG Findings*	*Myocardial Contraction*
30 min.	23	+	normal	good
60 min.	2	+	normal	good
90 min.	1	+	low voltage	poor
		Preservation		
Perfusion Technique		*Number of Experiments*	*Preservation Time**	
Whole blood perfusion		4	mean 4.0 hrs. (3–5)	
Hemodilution		4	mean 5.8 hrs. (4-7)	
Hemodilution with micro-filter		5	mean 11.6 hrs. (10–15)	

*Time for which hearts studied during perfusion only retained sinus rhythm.

TABLE 6
Results of Cadaver Heart Transplants Following Normothermic Coronary Perfusion in Vitro

	Perfusion Time	*Immediate Cardiac performance*	*Survival Time*	*Cause of Death*
Whole blood perfusion	1 hr.	Poor with drug support	5 hrs.	Early graft failure
	2 hrs.	Poor with drug support	3 hrs.	Early graft failure
Hemodilution	1 hr.	Good	7 days	Late graft failure
	2 hrs.	Good with drug support	8 hrs.	Early graft failure
	3 hrs.	Good	1 hr.	Early graft failure
Hemodilution with Micro-Filter	2 hrs.	Good	2 hrs.	Respiratory failure
	4 hrs.	Good	7 days	Respiratory failure
	6 hrs.	Good	2 hrs.	Respiratory failure
	8 hrs.	Good	6 hrs.	Early graft failure
	10 hrs.	Good	24 hrs.	Early graft failure

clearly reflected in the length of preservation possible and in the ECG changes during perfusion (Table 5, Fig. 9). Microscopic examination of the perfused hearts gave evidence of the rationale for use of the microfilter. Histologic studies demonstrated numerous occlusions of arterioles by what

ECG Changes in Isolated Normothermic Heart Perfusion

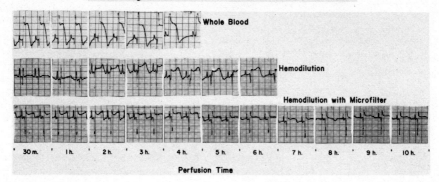

FIG. 9.   ECG tracings during isolated normothermic coronary perfusion with different perfusates.

appeared to be fibrin material.

Ten hearts in this series were transplanted (Table 6, Fig. 10). The hemodilution technic, with a filter in the arterial line, seemed superior to the previous methods. After 10 hours of perfusion, the heart could be made to maintain the circulation for 24 hours. Hearts perfused for 6 hours or less by this technic were comparable in all parameters to fresh hearts. The method is currently under further investigation.

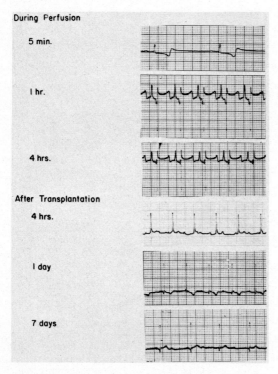

FIG. 10.   ECG tracings during isolated normothermic coronary perfusion and after transplantation of the graft into a puppy. Note the occurrence of two independent P waves.

In conclusion, the use of hyperbaric oxygen and cooling allows for up to 12 hours of safe storage of hearts but does not yield information on possible agonal damages to the myocardium. Normothermic perfusion using a hemodilution technic with microfiltration of the perfusate permits resuscitation of hearts up to 90 minutes after asystole. Observation of the graft's gross anatomy, ECG and performance allows for clarification of its functional capability—information that is essential before the irrevocable step of cardiectomy is performed in a recipient.

CLINICAL EXPERIENCE

The surgical technic of cardiac transplantation developed in our animal studies appeared satisfactory for clinical trial in July, 1966. At that time, an infant with a lethal cardiac lesion was under our care. We could not implement the decision to undertake transplantation in this case because a donor infant with a heart in good condition could not be found.

The next occasion on which we considered clinical implantation of a cardiac homograft was in November, 1967. A report of this experience, previously described elsewhere,[12] follows.

Case 1. A 2600 gm. Caucasian baby was born on Nov. 18, 1967, following a 40-week gestation. The mother was 37 years old and had previously delivered a living child. The antepartum course had been uneventful, but the intrapartum course was complicated by rupture of the membranes more than 48 hours before delivery. The baby's 1 minute Apgar score was 9/10, and the 5 minute Apgar score was 10/10.

At 16 hours of age, the patient was noted to be dusky in color, with circumoral cyanosis that became more marked with crying. The distal arterial pulses were equal and normal in amplitude. No

J. S. Diagnosis: Tricuspid Atresia 11/67

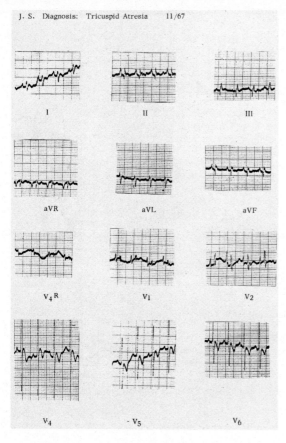

I   II   III

aVR   aVL   aVF

V₄R   V₁   V₂

V₄   V₅   V₆

FIG. 11. Preoperative ECG in Case 1.

cardiac murmur was heard. The second heart sound was single and decreased at the base. The liver edge was palpable approximately 5 cm. blow the right costal margin.

In the electrocardiogram taken at this time (Fig. 11), the P waves were tall and spiking. An rSR pattern was noted in the right precordial leads. Chest x-ray disclosed cardiac enlargement with decreased pulmonary vascular markings.

TABLE 7
Cardiac Catheterization Data in Case 1

Chamber	Pressure (mm. Hg.)	Oxygen Saturation (%)
Right atrium	mean 10	(35)
	A wave 10—13	
	V wave 7—9	
Pulmonary vein	mean 13	(—)
Left atrium	mean 12	(48)
Left ventricle	66—75	(48)
	5—15	
Heart rate: 130—140/min. and regular		

Cardiac catheterization was performed on Nov. 20 (Table 7). The catheter could not be passed into the right ventricle. Oxygen studies showed mixing of arterial and venous blood at the atrial level. Cineangiocardiography after injection of medium into the right atrium revealed opacification of a huge right atrial chamber with subsequent spill of dye into the left atrium, left ventricle and aorta. Visualization of the pulmonary vessels occurred only after opacification of the aorta. The conclusion was that the infant had a complete right-to-left shunt at the atrial level, most probably because of tricuspid atresia.

In view of the patient's difficulties, the severity of the underlying malformation and the poor prognosis, it was decided to attempt cardiac transplantation. A suitable donor was not available and a palliative procedure was therefore performed. On Nov. 20, when the patient was 63 hours of age, thoracotomy was undertaken and a 4 mm. intrapericardial anastomosis was constructed between the ascending aorta and the right pulmonary artery. Because of the patient's poor condition, exploration of the cardiac anatomy was not undertaken.

For the first three postoperative days, the patient remained critically ill with intermittent episodes of apnea and overt heart failure. After a few days the patient's condition improved slightly. The heart rate remained between 120 and 140/min. and the respiratory rate 40 to 60/min. with mild distress. The liver edge remained palpable 4 to 5 cm. below the right costal margin. Although the infant tolerated oral feedings, his weight remained at about 2500 gm. Serial chest x-rays disclosed progressive cardiac enlargement.

On December 4, an anencephalic infant became available. The infant required intubation with assisted ventilation to sustain its cardiac action. Evaluation by clinical examination, ECG and chest x-rays failed to demonstrate any cardiac abnormalities. The potential donor and the recipient were found to have the same major blood groups and a compatible cross match. Histocompatibility studies of lymphocytes also indicated a good match according to the irradiated hamster test.[13]

Following preoperative preparations, cooling of both recipient and donor was initiated at approximately 3:45 A.M. on Dec. 6. The donor was heparinized during cooling (Fig. 12). At 4:25 A.M., the donor infant's spontaneous cardiac activity ceased, his body temperature at that time being 27°C. The heart was immediately excised and immersed in normal saline solution cooled to 5°C. The donor heart manifested no gross abnormalities. A second surgical team began a thoracotomy at 4:25 A.M. on the recipient, when his body temperature had reached 19° C. The cooling proceeded without

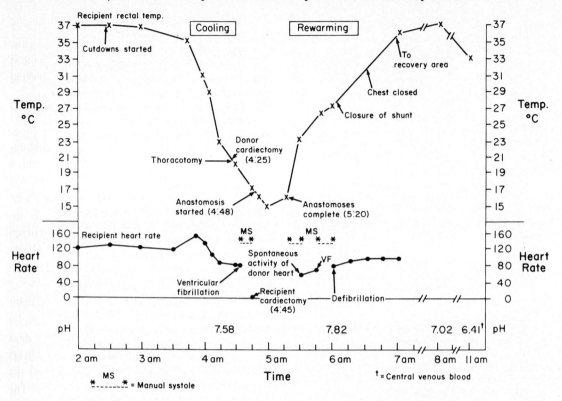

FIG. 12.   Sequence of events during cardiac transplantation in Case 1.

cardiac arrhythmias until 4:38 A.M., when manipulations induced ventricular fibrillation. Massage was given until cardiectomy at 4:45 A.M. The body temperature at this time was 17°C.

Implantation of the donor heart was begun at 4:48 A.M. The anastomoses were completed at 5:20 A.M. and cardiac massage was then instituted. The duration of circulatory arrest was approximately 40 minutes.

Rewarming was then carried out. At 5:30 A.M.,

with the body temperature at 23°C., spontaneous sinus rhythm was resumed. Cardiac massage was continued until the temperature had reached 26°C. At this time, strong ventricular fibrillation developed. Electrical defibrillation immediately restored regular ventricular contractions in sinus rhythm at a rate of 80 to 85 beats per minute. The aortic-right pulmonary artery anastomosis was then ligated. When the patient's body temperature had reached 32°C., the chest was closed. The patient was moved

TABLE 8
Blood Gas* and Electrolyte Data in Case 1

Date	Specimen	Temp. (O/C.)	Na (mEq./L.)	K (mEq./L.)	pH	PCO₂ (mm. Hg)	HCO₃ (mEq./L.)	Base excess (mEq./L.)	PO₂ (mm.Hg)	O₂ Sat. (%)
11/20	Before aortic-right pulm. art. anastomosis	36°	147	5.8	7.15	60	32	−6	35	(45)
11/24	After anastomosis	37°	135	5.3	7.32	44	25	+1	55	(80)
12/5	Transplant, preop.	37°	135	4.0	7.35	45	21	−1	50	(80)
12/6	Transplant, 4:15 A.M., before cardiectomy	23°	140	3.7	7.58	21	19	+1	28	(85)
12/6	Transplant, 6:00 A.M., postop.	27°	140	4.8	7.82	15	24	+6	51	(95)
12/6	Transplant, 8:00 A.M., postop.	35°	137	4.1	7.02	35	9	−23	66	(90)
12/6	Transplant, 11:00 A.M., postop.	33°	135	4.2	6.41†	122†	10†	>−25†	—	(—)

*Determinations made on capillary blood, except as noted.
†Central venous blood.

to an isolation area at 7:00 A.M., with a body temperature of 36°C. His vital signs were stable and the heart rate was 90 to 110 /min. (Figs. 12 and 13). Because of weak respiratory action, assisted ventilation was necessary. Spontaneous movement of the extremities was noted.

Postoperative:

Lead II - Continuous Rhythm Strip

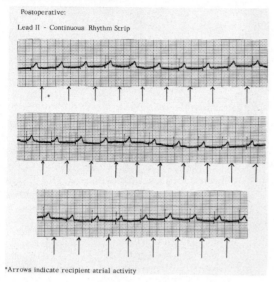

*Arrows indicate recipient atrial activity

FIG. 13. Postoperative ECG in Case 1.

During next few hours, the patient's temperature fell to 33°C. In addition, a profound metabolic and respiratory acidosis ensued (Table 8), despite corrective measures. At 12:10 P.M. bradycardia, with a rate of 60/min., suddenly developed. By 12:15 P. M., there was no cardiac rhythm and, despite attempts at resuscitation by both closed and open massage and direct electrical stimulation, there was no return of cardiac activity. The patient was pronounced dead at 1:00 P. M. on December 6.

Autopsy later that day disclosed diffuse areas of atelectasis in both lungs. The transplanted heart was normal in size and structure. Suture lines were intact. The aortic-pulmonary artery anastomosis had not been completely closed, as the shunt was patent.

In the recipient's excised heart, a severe Ebstein's malformation of the tricuspid valve and subvalvular, right ventricular outflow tract obstruction were found.

Case 2. A 57-year-old Caucasian male was admitted on December 10, 1967, for evaluation of chronic congestive heart failure.[12] In 1959, he had sustained an acute myocardial infarction for which he had been hospitalized for 2 months. In the following years, he was unable to return to work and was hospitalized on 14 occasions because of mani-

festations of progressive congestive heart failure. Mild diabetes was diagnosed in 1963.

At the time of admission, the patient was unable to walk more than 10 steps without experiencing angina and dyspnea and frequently had paroxysmal nocturnal dyspnea. His pharmacologic treatment included daily doses of digoxin, furosemide, hydrochlorothiazide, spironolactone, warfarin sodium and tolbutamide. His blood pressure ranged from 120/70 to 90/60 mm. Hg. The pulse was 70 beats per minute and regular. The neck veins were distended and filled from below with the patient at 30°C. There were mild atherosclerotic changes in the retinal vessels.

Examination of the heart disclosed a point of maximal impulse in the fifth intercostal space at the anterior axillary line, with systolic thrill and heave. $S_1M_1 > S_1M_2$; $S_2P_2 > S_2A_2$. S_2 was split paradoxically. A Grade II/VI pansystolic murmur was prominent at the apex and radiated into the axilla. The liver was blunt-edged and tender and could be palpated 4 cm. below the costal margin. No peripheral edema was present.

Laboratory findings were as follows: hematocrit, 37%; white blood cell count, 11,300/cu. mm.; urine reaction for protein, +1, for sugar and acetone, 0. The blood urea nitrogen level was 30 mg. %, the creatinine level, 1.5%. Serum electrolyte levels were as follows: Na, 139 mEq./L.; K, 4.5 mEq./L.; Cl, 81 mEq./L. The CO_2 combining power was 35.5 mEq./L. The fasting blood sugar was 122 mg.%. The prothrombin time was 27 seconds (control, 12 seconds). The blood type was AB, Rh positive.

Cardiac catheterization and angiocardiography were performed on December 18, 1967. The results are summarized in Table 9.

TABLE 9
Summary of Catheterization Data in Case 2

Chamber	Pressure (mm. Hg.)
Right atrium	2/2
Right ventricle	
inflow	22/2
outflow	47/3
Pulmonary artery truncus	47/18
Pulmonary capillary wedge	mean 19
Left atrium	5–3
Left ventricle	113/10–20*

Heart rate 72/min.
Cardiac index 3.1 ± 0.4 L./min./M.²
O_2 consumption (cc./min./M.²) 133 ± 14
Arterial O_2 % saturation 96.2 ± 1.4

*Left atrial "A" wave contribution to left ventricular end disastolic pressure.

The clinical diagnosis was atherosclerotic heart disease, severe left ventricular myocardial failure

TABLE 10
Isolated Heart Perfusion Through the Aortic Root in Case 2

Isolated heart perfusion	36 min.	
Implanted heart perfusion	2 hrs.14 min.	
Total duration	2 hrs.50 min.	
Isolated heart perfusion		
Temperature	Flow	Pressure
29.1 C. (av.)	42.9 cc./min. (av.)	48.7 mm. Hg.(av.)
(range 29°–30°C.)	(range 20–45 cc./min.)	(range 20–60 mm. Hg.)
Implanted heart perfusion (average)		
Temperature	Flow	Pressure
31.2°C. (av.)	54.9 cc./min. (av.)	54.0 mm. Hg.(av.)
(range 30°–34°C.)	(range 40–70 cc./min.)	(range 48–60 mm. Hg.)

and moderate pulmonary hypertension. Continued efforts to improve the patient's condition with medical therapy were unsuccessful, and no treatment appeared to offer any promise of reversing the course of this patient's progressive cardiac failure. The patient accepted the proposal that a heart transplant be attempted.

On January 9, 1968, a previously healthy 29-year-old, 90-pound woman was transferred to Maimonides Medical Center. The referring physicians stated that the patient had been comatose for 19 hours and that for the 9 hours preceding transfer she had required assisted ventilation. A cardiac arrest of indeterminate duration 9 hours prior to transfer had been managed by sternal compression.

On admission, both pupils were dilated and fixed bilaterally and she was completely areflexic and unresponsive to any stimuli. An electroencephalogram showed no cerebral cortical activity. The blood type was AB, Rh positive. A 12-lead ECG disclosed sinus tachycardia with nonspecific ST segment changes. The neurological diagnosis was massive intracranial hemorrhage, possibly secondary to a brain tumor with herniation through the foramen magnum.

Three hours after admission here, the patient's blood pressure began to fall, despite increasing doses of vasopressors, and she was moved to the operating room. At 1:00 P.M., effective cardiac action ceased and the patient was pronounced dead. At 1:10 P.M., cardiectomy was performed in the same manner as in the animal studies. At 1:16 P.M., the aorta of the donor heart was cannulated and the coronary arteries were perfused (Table 10) with a hemodilution technic at an average temperature, pressure and flow of 29.1°C., 48.7 mm. Hg. and 42.9 cc./min., respectively, for 36 minutes while the recipient was being prepared.

Continuous monitoring of the recipient's central venous pressure, radial artery pressure and ECG was instituted. Urine output, pH, pCO₂, pO₂, base excess and serum electrolytes were measured at frequent intervals. A median sternotomy and right femoral artery cutdown were performed simultaneously. The venae cavae were cannulated through a right atrial incision; the right femoral artery was also cannulated. Cardiopulmonary bypass (Table 11) was begun. Hypothermia averaging 31.9°C. and flow rates averaging 4206 cc./min. were established. Recipient cardiectomy leaving generous margins of the posterior atrial walls was performed, and the

TABLE 11
Extracorporeal Bypass in Case 2: Summary of Perfusion Data

Patient's weight: 63.18 kg.		
Body surface area: 1.72 M.²		
Calculated cardiac output:		4128 cc./min.
Pump rate:	High	5200 cc./min.
	Low	2400 cc./min.
	Average	4206 cc./min.
Patient's body		
temperature:	High	36.5°C.
	Low	30.5°C.
	Average	31.9°C.
Total perfusion time:		4 hrs. 41 min.
Operative perfusion time:		2 hrs. 29 min.
Support perfusion time:		2 hrs. 12 min.

donor heart was then implanted in a manner similar to that used in the animal studies.

Total cardiopulmonary bypass time was 4 hours and 41 minutes. Operative perfusion time was 2 hours and 29 minutes, with 2 hours and 12 minutes for support perfusion (Table 11).

At completion of the surgical procedure and discontinuation of support perfusion, the transplanted heart was beating spontaneously and was able to support the circulation of the recipient (Fig. 14). However, manifestations of progressive cardiac failure ensued. Phase-shift intra-aortic balloon pumping temporarily supported the left ventricle, but cardiac action ceased 10½ hours following surgery.

At post-mortem examination, the recipient's excised heart weighed 550 gm. The left ventricle was

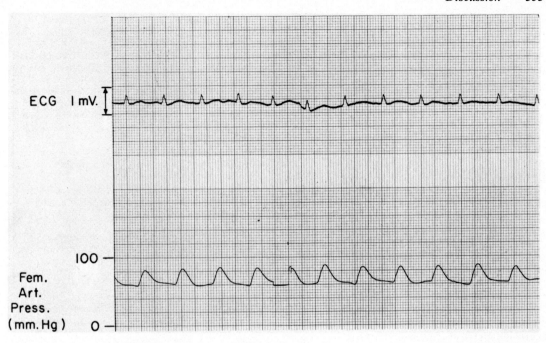

FIG. 14. ECG and femoral arterial pressure at conclusion of surgical procedure in Case 2.

a diffuse fibrotic sac. The left ventricular myocardium was thinned to approximately half the normal thickness and contained multiple areas of fibrous scarring. There was no valvular disease. There was diffuse coronary sclerosis with multiple areas of narrowing.

The donor heart weighed 250 gm. There were areas of subepicardial hematoma of recent onset. All suture lines were intact. Examination of the brain confirmed the clinical diagnosis of massive intracranial hemorrhage into a posterior fossa brain tumor, with herniation into the foramen magnum.

DISCUSSION

From our laboratory experience, we felt that enough evidence had been collected to warrant a clinical trial. The important points in this experience were as follows: (1) the surgery can be carried out with a reasonable risk for the recipient; (2) the excised donor heart can almost invariably be resuscitated; (3) graft-rejection reactions can be managed with present-day drugs; (4) a transplanted heart, although denervated, is able to maintain adequate circulation even under physical stress.[14,15] In addition, we found that both cooling in fluid media to 5 to 10°C. and isolated organ perfusion are adequate to protect the donor heart for 1 to 2 hours.

On the basis of this experience, we decided that heart transplants should be attempted in patients with potentially lethal cardiac conditions for which

there was no further surgical or medical treatment. This decision was reached in July, 1966, when an attempt to perform a heart transplant in an infant had to be given up because of lack of an adequate graft. The decision was finally implemented in December, 1967.

Both our patients died on the day of operation. In retrospect, the failure in Case 1 probably resulted from the combination of inability to maintain adequate respiration, inability to retain a normal body temperature and inability to correct severe metabolic and respiratory acidosis, despite vigorous treatment.

In Case 2, the reason for failure is not as clear. The poor performance of the heart was probably the result of damage sustained at the time of cardiorespiratory arrest, for which sternal compression and vasopressor treatment had been required. Additional damage from the hypothermia and isolated perfusion is less likely, but possible. The postoperative management of the low output syndrome was difficult, and the use of intra-aortic balloon pumping[16] did not rectify this condition.

In spite of our present clinical experience, it is our belief that human heart transplantation must be undertaken. This is an entirely reasonable possibility that must be explored to identify its ultimate place in the treatment of heart disease. In our laboratory, we are pursuing the development of mechanical cardiac-assist devices. We feel that these two methods eventually will prove to be complementary.

SUMMARY

We can now review our experience with orthotopic cardiac allotransplantation under profound hypothermia in mongrel puppies. In a series of 107 direct transplants, 40 died during the first 24 postoperative hours. Early graft failure (15 cases) and brain damage (10 cases) referable to errors in technic were the major causes of death. Among the 67 surviving more than 24 hours, pulmonary complications (42 cases) and rejection (13 cases) were the principal causes of mortality. One animal given a short course of immunosuppressive treatment postoperatively was well 28 months after the operation, and there was no evidence of rejection.

In 59 cases, delayed transplants were performed. Maximal survival of dogs receiving grafts after hypothermic and hyperbaric storage for 24 hours was 5 days, and after storage for 12 hours, 35 days. With normothermic coronary perfusion in vitro, hearts could be resuscitated up to 90 minutes after clinical death. Survival after perfusion using a hemodilution technic and microfiltration for 6 hours or less was comparable to that in direct transplants.

Two clinical trials of cardiac allotransplantation were attempted. In Case 1, a graft taken from an anencephalic infant was implanted under profound hypothermia in a 17-day-old boy suffering from an Ebstein's malformation of the tricuspid valve and subvalvular, membranous pulmonary artery stenosis. The recipient died 6 hours after operation of intractable metabolic and respiratory acidosis.

In Case 2, a graft taken from a 29-year-old woman, who died of an intracranial tumor in the posterior fossa with herniation into the foramen magnum, was implanted under extracorporeal circulation in a 57-year-old man with severe, progressive chronic congestive heart failure. The patient died approximately $10^1/_2$ hours postoperatively of a low cardiac output syndrome.

REFERENCES

1. Lower, R. R. and Shumway, N. E.: Studies on orthotopic homotransplantation of the canine heart. Surg. Forum, *11:*18, 1960.
2. Webb, W. R., Howard, H. S. and Neely, W. A.: Practical method of homologous transplantation. J. Thorac. Surg., *37:*361, 1959.
3. Cleveland, R. J. and Lower, R. R.: Transplantation of canine cadaver hearts after short-term preservation. Transplantation, *5:*904, 1967.
4. Hardy, J. D., Chavez, C. M., Erasalan, S., Adkins, J. R. and Williams, R. D.: Heart transplantation in dogs. Procedures, physiologic problems and results in 142 experiments. Surgery, *60:*361, 1966.
5. Kondo, Y., Grädel, F. and Kantrowitz, A.: Homotransplantation of the heart in puppies under profound hypothermia. (Abstract) Bull. New York Acad. Med., *40:*986, 1964.
6. Homotransplantation of the heart in puppies under profound hypothermia: Long survival without immunosuppressive treatment. Ann. Surg. *162:*837, 1965.
7. Heart homotransplantation in puppies: Long survival without immunosuppressive therapy. Suppl. I, Circulation, *31-32:*181, 1965.
8. Kondo, Y., Chaptal, P.-A., Grädel, F., Cottle, H.R. and Kantrowitz, A.: Fate of orthotopic canine heart transplants. J. Cardiov, Surg., *8:*155, 1967.
9. Immediate and delayed orthotopic homotransplantation of the heart. J. Thorac. Cardiov. Surg, *50:*781, 1965.
10. Dureau, G., Okura, T., Schilt, W. and Kantrowitz, A.: Transplantation orthotopique de coeur de cadavre chez le chien. Ann. Chir. Thor Car. C., *932:*1966.
11. Koga, Y., Carstensen, H. E., Sujansky, E. and Kantrowitz, A.: Resuscitation and preservation of canine cadaver hearts. Tr. Am. Soc. Art. Internal Organs, *14:*140, 1968.
12. Kantrowitz, A., Haller, J. D., Joos, H., Cerruti, M. M. Carstensen, H. E.: Transplantation of the heart in an infant and an adult. Am. J. Cardiol., *22:*782, 1968.
13. Cabasson, J., Joos, H., Dureau, G., Schilt, W., Samuels, S. and Kantrowitz, A.: Histo-compatibilité et transplantation cardiaque. Presse Méd., *55:*2825, 1967.
14. Dong, E., Hurley, E. J., Lower, R. R. and Shumway, N. E.: Performance of the heart two years after autotransplantation. Surgery, *56:*270, 1964.
15. Angell, W. W., Dong, E. and Shumway, N. E.: A humoral substitute for nervous control in the dog heart transplant. Surg. Forum, *18:*223, 1967.
16. Kantrowitz, A., Tjonneland, S., Krakauer, J., Butner, A. N., Phillips, S. J., Yahr, W. Z., Shapiro, M., Freed, P. S., Jaron, D. and Sherman, J. L., Jr.: Clinical experience with cardiac assistance by means of intrassortic phase-shift balloon pumping. Tr. Am Soc. Art. Internal Organs, *14:*344, 1968.

Acute Coronary Care Unit

Chairman

Eliot Corday, M.D.

Management of Acute Myocardial Infarction Without Complications

William J. Grace, M.D.

The Value of the Coronary Care Unit

Eduardo Rosselot, M.D.
Tzu-Wang Lang, M.D.
John K. Vyden
Eliot Corday, M.D.

Resuscitation for Cardiac Arrest Due to Myocardial Infarction

William J. Grace, M.D.
Richard J. Kennedy, M.D.

The Treatment of Shock Complicating Acute Myocardial Infarction

Max Harry Weil, M.D.
Herbert Shubin, M.D.

Problems in Myocardial Infarction

Thomas Killip, M.D.

Aggressive Management of Cardiac Arrhythmias

Leslie A. Kuhn, M.D.

Fluid and Electrolyte Problems of Patients on the Acute Coronary Care Unit

Raymond E. Weston, M.D.

Management of Heart Block Complicating Acute Myocardial Infarction

Simon Dack, M.D.
Ephraim Donoso, M.D.

Clinical Experience With Phase-Shift Pumping in Medically Refractory Cardiogenic Shock After Myocardial Infarction

Adrian Kantrowitz, M.D.
Joseph S. Krakauer, M.D.
Steinar Tjønneland, M.D.
Alfred N. Butner, M.D.

Management of Acute Myocardial Infarction Without Complications

William J. Grace

This discussion is based on the facts that arise from the natural history of acute myocardial infarction and is limited to the care of patients with acute transmural infarction, a type of infarct readily definable and described in adequate pathologic material.[1]

Why does at least one out of five patients suffering an infarct die before reaching the hospital? Recognizing an irreducible number of deaths it appears that of this 20 per cent, some could be saved by prompt treatment of arrhythmia during the earliest stage of the illness. This concept of on-the-site treatment has been put into practice by Pantridge and Geddes.[2] In October 1968 we inaugurated a mobile coronary care unit and have demonstrated that it is possible in the metropolitan center of New York to mobilize a coronary care team of physicians and nurses which proceeds to the location of a patient with an acute myocardial infarct. In actuality this consists in setting up in a restaurant, factory, subway station or the patient's home a temporary coronary care unit equipped with portable, battery operated equipment and the usual drugs necessary to cope with the arrhythmic complications of infarction.

Sufficient experience has not accumulated to demonstrate how many lives will be saved by such prompt treatment based on accurate diagnosis before the patient reaches the hospital.

THE RISK

What is the risk for a patient with acute myocardial infarction? To answer this question one must divide patients with infarction into three classes on the basis of clinical status and hemodynamic function.

Class I, No left ventricular dysfunction

Class II, Mild failure, dyspnea, orthopnea, diaphoresis, protracted severe chest pain

Class III, Acute pulmonary edema, shock

In each class the influence of age must be considered as an additional determining factor which affects mortality. In Table 1 mortality rates for the functional classes are shown and in Table 2 are shown mortality rates based on the age factor. In a smaller series, the combined influences of class and age are shown in Table 3. It is apparent that all patients are subject to a high mortality rate.

TABLE 1
Acute Myocardial Infarction: Mortality Rate*

Class I	17%	(10–22%)
Class II	38%	(33–55%)
Class III	72%	(–100%)

Based on 2174 patients in USPHS Study (1967)

TABLE 2
Acute Transmural Myocardial Infarction: Mortality Rate*

Age	Mortality	Range
55 or less	9%	(8—25%)
55 to 64	21%	(17—31%)
65 and over	37%	(30—47%)

Based on 2174 patients in USPHS study (1967)

TABLE 3
Mortality Rate, January 1965 to June 1966 Transmural Myocardial Infarction Only

	Years of Age			
	55 or Less	55 to 65	65 or Over	Total
CLASS I	9%	23%	50%	27%
CLASS II	33%	50%	42%	42%
CLASS III	66%	91%	90%	82%

St. Vincent's Hospital Series

In a group of 60 consecutive patients the incidence of cardiac arrest is shown in Table 4.

*Figures in Tables 1 and 2 in percentages indicate St. Vincent's Hospital series of patients. Figures in parentheses indicate the range of mortality reported by the various contributing hospitals.

TABLE 4
Sixty Consecutive Patients With Cardiac Arrest

18 were originally in Class III
27 were originally in Class II
15 were originally in Class I

It is worth noting that 25 per cent of patients with cardiac arrest were originally in Class I. Consequently we feel that all patients with acute myocardial infarction are at the risk of sudden and unexpected cardiac arrest.

The incidence of major life threatening arrhythmias in patients with acute myocardial infarction is shown in Table 5. These data indicate that all patients are subject to life threatening arrhythmias.

TABLE 5
One Hundred of Acute Myocardial Infarction

Class	Ventricular Fibrillation	Ventricular Tachycardia	CHB
No left ventricular dysfunction	4	0	2
Mild failure	7	8	2
Severe failure	9	4	10

A comparison of the incidence and survival rate of ventricular fibrillation which usually occurs on the first hospital day treated at two different sites is shown in Table 6. These data indicate that prompt monitoring for diagnosis and prompt treatment for control of ventricular fibrillation is very successful.

TABLE 6
Primary Ventricular Fibrillation (625) Patients

Patients with acute myocardial
infarction (Transmural) 625
Patients with primary ventricular
fibrillation............................ 85
  In Coronary Care Unit..............44
  In Emergency Room 32
                               76
  Over-All Survivors......................68%
    Survivors in Coronary Care Unit. ..41%
    Survivors in Emergency Room 75%

Department of Medicine, St. Vincent's Hospital, New York City

TABLE 7
Results of Resuscitation— Effect of Time Lag

Physician Immediately Available
  Permanent survivors   14 (22%)
  Fatalities   50
                                 64
Physician Not Immediately Available
  Permanent survivors   1 (2%)
  Fatalities   43
                                 44

Contrast this data to the data in Table 7. The influence of the immediate availability of trained personnel is apparent in Table 7.

IMPORTANCE OF OXYGEN

The successful electrical management of the major arrhythmias is well known and the modality is widely accepted. However, little attention has been paid to the relationship between hypoxia and the occurrence or persistence of arrhythmias. Our studies show that patients with acute infarction are hypoxic and alkalotic as demonstrated in Table 8 and Figure 1.

TABLE 8
Range and Average Values

		pH	pO$_2$	O$_2$SAT	pCO$_2$	HCO$_3$
10 Pts.	High	7.46	98.2	97.4	45.0	28.9
No MI	Low	7.40	75.0	94.0	30.2	20.8
	Mean	7.425	85.68	95.73	38.64	24.82
	S.D.	.019	8.28	1.08	4.86	3.02
35 Pts.	High	7.56	74.0	95.0	53.0	34.0
With MI	Low	7.24	37.0	70.2	28.4	19.0
	Mean	7.43	58.44	88.29	36.62	24.70
	S.D.	0.65	11.65	7.29	4.12	3.89

We feel that a major precipitating factor in arrhythmias is anoxia.[3] To deliver oxygen we use a "nasal cannula," rarely a face mask and occasionally positive pressure oxygen. In the event of mild failure or arrhythmic disorders the arterial blood pH, pO$_2$, pCO$_2$ and HCO$_3$ are determined. If pO$_2$ is low, positive pressure oxygen is given intermittently by face mask. In the event of respiratory alkalosis appropriate drugs are given to reduce the ventilation. Figure 2 shows atrial fibrillation unresponsive to repeated electrical cardioversion, digitalis and quinidine. The administration of oxygen by intermittent positive pressure was associated with a return to normal sinus rhythm.

NONSPECIFIC FACTORS IN TREATMENT

We start an infusion of glucose and water on all our patients. This is run continuously and slowly to "keep the vein open."

The patient with acute myocardial infarction should be on complete bed rest for 7 to 10 days and then modified bed rest for another 7 to 10 days. Moving about in the bed and the bedroom is generally permitted from the 10th to 14th day and, after the 21st day, unlimited mobility is encouraged. Discharge from the hospital is generally between the 21st and 25th hospital day.

Atrial Fibrillation with LBBB

Atrial Flutter with LBBB

Intermittent Atrial Flutter

Onset of Atrial Flutter and
development of LBBB

Sustained Sinus Rhythm

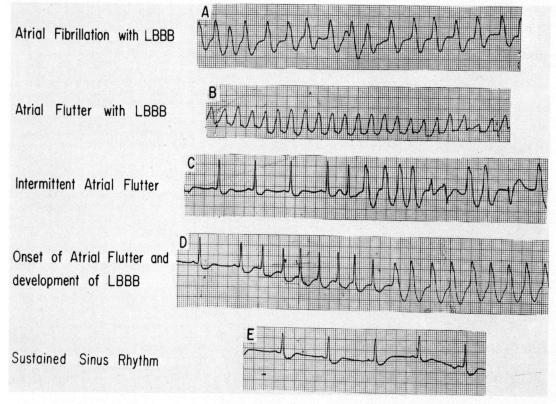

FIG. 1.   A series of arrhythmias in patient with acute myocardial infarction which were not responsive
to repeated cardioversion or drug therapy. After the patient was oxygenated via Bird respirator, sinus
rhythm was established.

There is no significant body of data pertaining to
the influence of the quantity of food intake of the
patient or the nature of the diet. Most physicians
prescribe a low caloric intake throughout the hospital course.

Anticoagulation using intravenous heparin is
carried out in all of our patients. After approximately the 7th day, the patient is shifted to an oral
tablet and all anticoagulation is discontinued on the
day of discharge.

Whether the patient is permitted to use the bedside
commode, or bathroom or whether he is forced to
use the bedpan is more a matter of individual
practice and feeling than it is of scientific information.

CORONARY CARE

The essence of the management of a patient with
acute myocardial infarction is coronary care. This
consists of:

1. Placing all the patients in the same area of the
   hospital
2. Continuous electronic monitoring of the EKG

3. Continuous observation of the monitored EKG
   by trained people
4. An especially trained staff eager to detect and
   treat the early warning signs of life threatening arrhythmias

The coronary care program should probably be
started by the mobile coronary care team at the
patient's home.

All patients should receive oxygen; all patients
should have a continuous intravenous infusion
running to keep a vein "open."

After 7 to 10 days of "coronary care" the patient
may be transferred to an intermediate unit or "step
down unit" where gradual mobilization is carried

TABLE 9
Acute Myocardial Infarction: Mortality Rate

	Alive	Dead	CCU Total	Hosp. Total	Hosp. Dead*
1964	119	56	N/A	175	32%
1965	100	34	134	190	26%
1966	132	50	182	227	27%
1967	142	31	173	208	17%

*Excludes death in Emergency Room.
All patients had transmural myocardial infarction.

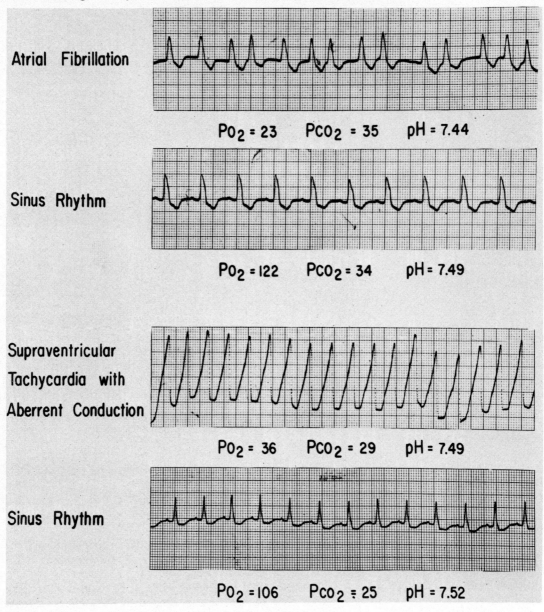

FIG. 2.   Two patients having atrial fibrillation and bundle branch block in the presence of severe anoxia. Correction of the blood gases by administration of oxygen resulted in the return of normal sinus rhythm.

out during further continuous or interrupted monitoring. Most patients are discharged from hospital between the 21st and 28th days.

Under such management the mortality rate in this hospital has declined as shown in Table 9.

REFERENCES

1. Grace, W. J.: Mortality rate from acute myocardial infarction—What are we talking about? Am. J. Cardiol. *20:* 301.
2. Pantridge, J. F., and Geddes, J. S.: A mobile intensive-care unit in the management of myocardial infarction, Lancet *271*, 1967.
3. Ayres, S. M., and Grace, W. J.: Inappropriate ventilation in the acutely ill, in press, Am. J. Med.

The Value of the Coronary Care Unit

Eduardo Rosselot, Tzu-Wang Lang, John K. Vyden and Eliot Corday

The concept of the coronary care unit (CCU) resulted from a dynamic coupling of advanced electronic technology with aggressive medical management. The basic foundation for the advance lay in experience gained in resuscitation,[1,2] electrical countershock treatment of arrhythmias,[3-6] and the increasing use of artificial pacemakers.[7,8] Segregation of patients to a specialized area equipped with sophisticated instruments and staffed with well trained personnel providing prompt diagnosis and treatment ensured speedy implementation of new coronary care concepts as they developed.

In the six years after the first CCU was opened,[12,13] considerable scientific data concerning their value was accumulated. Even though their efficacy was originally questioned,[14-16] enthusiasm for the CCU concept never diminished and continues to grow to this day.

This paper will discuss the clinical value, management, problems, and the impact upon the practice of medicine and community life of the CCU.

CLINICAL VALUE

The hospital mortality rate for cardiac infarction before the advent of intensive care was estimated at between 30–40 per cent.[17-21] The belief that this rate could be cut by one third by the aggressive management of life threatening arrhythmias and cardiac arrest is now confirmed.[22-26] Minor arrhythmias can trigger a deleterious hemodynamic disturbance in an infarcted heart[27,28] that may result in irreversible heart failure or cardiac arrest. It was shown in the CCU that early intervention and aggressive management of these minor problems prevent these serious complications from developing. When not accompanied by power failure of the heart, both ventricular fibrillation and standstill can usually be corrected promptly.[29,30] Their mortality rate was further reduced by delegating resuscitative procedures to expertly trained nurses because the nurse, unlike the physician, is in constant attendance, and if properly trained reacts with the split second precision needed

to overcome the emergency.[31]

CCUs offer invaluable scientific data providing detail of the natural history of cardiac infarction seldom available before their institution. This is particularly noticeable in providing more effective treatment for the complications of the infarction.

COMPLICATIONS OF CARDIAC INFARCTION

Electrical Dysfunction of the Heart

Major or minor arrhythmias are the most frequent complication of cardiac infarction, occurring in 60–90 per cent of patients. Eighty-five per cent of the arrhythmias occur during the first two days.[22,32-36]

Ventricular fibrillation is the most serious, occurring in about 8–10 per cent of patients. It[37] is often preceded by premonitory disturbances of the rhythm.[22,38] When ventricular fibrillation is not associated with heart failure or shock, about 75–80 per cent of instances are treated successfully. Later in the course of the infarction, it is generally secondary to severe hemodynamic or metabolic derangements, and then the possibility of successful resuscitation is generally only small.[37,39]

Ventricular premature contractions indicate ventricular irritability and frequently herald the appearance of cardiac arrest.[40-42] Hence when more than five occur per minute they are treated by an antiarrhythmic drug such as lidocaine, procainamide, or diphenylhydantoin.[28,43-45] Bursts of ventricular tachycardia, when persistent, are treated by cardioversion, even though the long-term evaluation of this procedure is unreliable because of the unpredictability of the arrhythmia. Many of these runs subside spontaneously and the patients are unaware of their existence.[46] Close monitoring is the only way to detect them. Nevertheless as ventricular fibrillation is a frequent terminal event of this rhythm, immediate treatment is essential with prophylactic antiarrhythmic drugs.[47]

Marked bradycardia is also a forerunner of escape

rhythms ending in ventricular fibrillation or heart block. In these circumstances, atropine, isoproterenol, and artificial pacing of the heart prevent more serious disturbances.[32,48]

Supraventricular arrhythmias, when unaccompanied by hypotension or decompensation, do not represent increased risk. They are usually successfully terminated by glycosides, quinidine, Tensilon, or lidocaine, and cardioversion is seldom needed.[34,46,49] There is, however, still some controversy on the significance of some supraventricular arrhythmias such as atrial fibrillation because some authors find them associated with a disproportionately high (74 per cent) mortality.[32]

Heart block complicates between 6–20 per cent of cases of cardiac infarction.[32,39,50] The higher the degree of block the worse the prognosis. First degree A-V block even though considered a premonitory event to higher degrees of conduction disturbance, is associated with a 25 per cent mortality rate.[32,39] The mortality rate in third degree A-V block is high[52,53] because a considerable percentage of these patients suffer extensive damage of the myocardium and usually die of shock or heart failure. Anterior wall infarcts with third degree A-V block have the worst prognosis with 100 per cent deaths in several reports.[39,53,54] Other ominous associations of A-V block are syncopal attacks, wide QRS complexes, especially in inferior infarction, electrocardiographic signs of previous infarction and mental confusion.[39,51,54]

Artificial pacing of the heart is widely used for the treatment of heart block complicating cardiac infarction, although its results are debatable.[39,51,53–55] It helps to restore to normal the depressed hemodynamics seen in slow rhythms. It is imperative for the treatment of ventricular standstill. However, in some patients with massive myocardial damage, no response to electrical stimulation is obtainable.[50,51] Most of these patients present a syndrome of downward displacement of the pacemaker with progressive widening of the QRS complexes or electromechanical dissociation refractory to artificial pacing.[33]

Power Failure of the Heart

Heart failure and cardiogenic shock remain a challenge for the skill of the coronary care staff. The mortality rates in patients suffering from these complications are not significantly different despite the new therapeutic setting.[30,46,47,56,57] However, hope lies in the prevention of their development by constant surveillance, and control of contributing disturbances such as arrhythmias.

Subtle signs of decompensation occur in about 80 per cent of patients suffering an acute cardiac infarction[58] with approximately 16 per cent developing pulmonary edema.[47] New, potent diuretics and the concept of subdigitalizing dosage to avoid glycoside toxicity are of significant benefit.[20]

Cardiogenic shock occurs in 13–20 per cent of patients.[48,56] Ventricular fibrillation and complete heart block are more frequent among patients with shock, and this partially accounts for the 60–80 per cent mortality rate reported for this type of patient.[37,47,48,51] Drugs do not influence survival significantly, but more promising results are expected from circulatory assist procedures.[20,59–62]

Metabolic Disturbances

Biochemical monitoring in the CCU allows recognition of early metabolic disturbances that further compromise the electrical and power function of the myocardium.[63–65] It is possible to correct acidosis and hypoxemia even though no effect on mortality is reported.[66] The finding of a high arterio/mixed venous oxygen content difference in patients following acute cardiac infarction, which tends toward normal during recovery, provides an index of circulatory competence of valuable prognostic value.[67]

Other Complications

Pulmonary or systemic thromboembolic phenomena, papillary muscle dysfunction or rupture, ventricular aneurysm, rupture of the heart, and hemopericardium or tamponade are dreaded complications of acute cardiac infarction. The coronary care setting allows early recognition of these events and not infrequently, radical therapeutic procedures are applied and prove lifesaving.

ASSESSMENT OF CLINICAL VALUE

Despite the considerable new knowledge, the promising therapeutic programs, and the technologic setting of the coronary care unit, assessment of its clinical value is difficult because no comparable groups are available to allow evaluation of its performance. However, one report by Marshall, Genton and Blount[68] who studied equivalent groups of patients with cardiac infarction arrived at the conclusion that the coronary care unit system successfully prevented ventricular fibrillation and treated cardiac arrest. Mortality was reduced to 19 per cent, compared to 33 per cent in comparable patients admitted to medical wards.

PROBLEMS IN MANAGEMENT

The six-year life period of the CCU was not devoid of problems. Retouches and improvements were accomplished in either structural design of units, equipment, attending staff, policies of admission and discharge, or therapeutic programs. Comment on these issues is relevant.

Where possible all coronary patients should have private or semi-private facilities for complete rest. However, those with complications such as arrhythmias, decompensation, and the shock syndrome need constant observation by the attending staff (direct vision or monitored). Instant availability at the bedside of resuscitative apparatus—i.e., defibrillator and closed chest resuscitation equipment—is another necessary addition to the monitoring devices. However, the physical design of the units is not perfect and regrettably there are all too many instances of patients undergoing the unnecessary psychologic stress attendant upon the witnessing of an emergency resuscitation on another patient in the same unit.[31,40] Whether this or just chance accounts for the multiple arrests at the same time in the same unit is undecided.

The most adequate number of beds for each coronary care area depends on the number of admissions, the availability of personnel and the financial support. The number of beds is no limitation. One bed is as satisfactory as a 16 bed unit provided the following fundamental requirements are met.[69] For the primary purpose of prevention and treatment of emergency situations, an electrocardiographic monitor system with oscilloscopic display, rate meter, alarm and recording device is essential. An external defibrillator, a pacemaker with transvenous catheter electrodes, emergency cart containing an intratracheal tube, resuscitator tray, intravenous fluids and other medications, completes the necessary instrumentation.

A venous line to measure central venous pressure and an arterial line for direct record of blood pressure is of great benefit when it is necessary to evaluate hemodynamics, as in the failing heart.

However, more sophisticated equipment offers great promise in disclosing possible underlying physiologic derangements that will help in assessing the circulatory and metabolic conditions of patients and provide a more pathophysiologic approach to treatment. Constant on-line systems for analysis of blood gases and pH are being used in several units, but only on a research basis.[70] Preliminary data obtained by following these parameters show the value of on-line analysis.[67,71] Such devices may lead to other refined technic that are badly needed to enhance the ability to follow myocardial performance, because it is likely that heart failure, hypotension, and shock in many patients are gradually occurring events rather than a sudden catastrophe.[48] If the early prodromes of heart failure and shock can be ascertained with more certainty, then preventive treatment could be utilized before their fatal evolution. Computerized methods of recognition of cardiac arrhythmias also promise to relieve the nurse of the difficult responsibility of providing pinpoint accuracy in the diagnosis of arrhythmias.[72,73]

The training of the personnel (software) is more important than the hardware in a coronary care unit.[74] Nurses must develop a proficiency in coronary care unit expertise before satisfactory results can be expected. In fact, the success in reducing mortality depends on their devotion and ability and a width of knowledge which allows them to function at all times with promptness and skill.[75,76] This allegiance is required of all the other members of the staff as well, including the unit director.[31] Continuous teaching programs and analytical meetings are suitable to maintain vivid motivation, knowledge that is honed razor sharp, and high morale.

One of the problems of evaluating results of the CCU depends on different admission and discharge policies of each unit. Preferences for the particular exclusion or inclusion of some types of severely ill patients, early discharges from the unit and the inclusion of the coronary suspect before a specific diagnosis can be confirmed make it difficult to compare the statistics of different CCUs.[14,16] Evolution of policies and criteria often make it impossible to compare results within the same unit year by year.

The optimal length of stay of a patient in CCU is uncertain. It is often dictated by administrative rather than pure medical reasoning. Three to four days seems to be the period during which most of the benefits of intensive care are obtained because most of the catastrophies that can be prevented or treated occur during this time.[33,37,51] However, several reports call for more prolonged observation of patients to avoid complications that develop past the first or second week.[42,69]

Drugs are often evaluated in the CCU setting. Close observation and monitoring provide a critical ground upon which to judge drug effects and side reactions. A word of warning has been given against indiscriminate use of opiates and other depressant drugs; i.e., analgesics and hypnotics that could further compromise cardiac function and enhance proneness to shock and myocardial failure.[65,71] Still unsettled is whether the best drug treatment for cardiogenic shock is vasoconstrictors or vasodilators.[60,77,78]

Complications arising from therapeutic procedures in the CCU have been described, but do not of themselves detract from the many benefits of the dynamic coronary care system. Ventricular fibrillation, secondary to artificial pacemaker activity[51] enhanced the search for better methods of artificial pacing. Perforation of the heart by the tip of the catheter electrode seems to cause no additional risk provided anticoagulant therapy is avoided.[51,54] Local infection in relation to venous lines or pacemakers sometimes occurs, but is controlled by adequate antibiotic therapy and replacement of the catheters. In a small number of post-mortem examinations clotting associated with the central venous catheter was found. Whether this represents a potential source for pulmonary emboli, representing an increased hazard to the patient, requires further study.

CONTRIBUTION TO SCIENTIFIC KNOWLEDGE

We need not emphasize further how a new understanding of the pathophysiologic changes associated with acute cardiac infarction resulted from the close monitoring of the electrocardiographic, hemodynamic and metabolic parameters in affiliated patients. Shillingford and his colleagues[42,67,71,80] pioneered the utilization of the coronary care area as a research unit where a considerable amount of new information is obtainable. Since knowledge of most of the factors that contribute to death in patients following acute cardiac infarction is fragmentary, this sophisticated approach is justified.

As a result, there is fuller understanding, regarding the following: (1) what the causes of death are following acute cardiac infarction; (2) the natural history of arrhythmias, their hemodynamic effects and possibilities of prevention and treatment; (3) the characteristics and incidence of heart failure and shock; (4) the respiratory alterations associated with cardiac infarction and its biochemical consequences, (5) the metabolic derangements that often seal a vicious cycle of irreversibility through arrhythmias; impaired myocardial function and peripheral vascular disturbances; (6) the neurohumoral reflex effects on the circulation among which catecholamine release is suspected to play a principal role,[71,80] and (7) the side-effects of drugs and other therapeutic measures that sometimes entangle treatment and impede survival.

Even though it is a very specialized area, the coronary care unit demonstrates that it provides excellent teaching for both the medical and paramedical professions. Nurses and physicians engaged in in-tensive coronary care can obtain wisdom and new insight into the interrelationship of difficult medical problems.

IMPACT ON COMMUNITY LIFE AND THE PRACTICE OF MEDICINE

The annual loss of life from coronary artery disease in the United States of America totals more than half a million.[19] Only 30–40 per cent of fatalities occur in the hospital,[81] and about one third of these will be prevented when coronary care units are established in hospitals throughout the country.[19] The experience with coronary care units clearly shows that cardiac catastrophies are responsive to treatment, and if more people could receive treatment, in time the mortality rate from cardiac infarction would be cut still further.

However, it seems necessary to take the coronary care service to the home and business surroundings where the cardiac attack takes place if the lives of many thousands each year are to be saved. The results expected from prototype flying squads[83-85] will give an answer about the possibility of such programs in conjunction with epidemiologic studies to assess the relevancy of this endeavor. However, training and educational programs should not just be confined to personnel in the coronary care area or mobile units. The spread of basic information from the CCU to the average man in the street is necessary concerning elementary measures for respiratory ventilation and external cardiac massage, and the need for convenient centers of coronary assistance.

In other respects, the coronary care unit represents a major therapeutic innovation,[47] and a new philosophy towards disease and treatment. The aphorism, "patients must die in peace and in dignity," is no longer tenable in view of the possibilities of long productive life after recuperation from cardiac arrest.[30] The influence of this attitude will not remain confined to only the treatment of the complications of coronary heart disease. Other fields of medicine also require an aggressive approach. Close monitoring, serial biochemical studies, detailed analysis of hemodynamics and neurologic function, together with bedside radiographic and scanning technics, will become accepted procedures to an adequate follow-up in the cerebral stroke, metabolic coma, and other life threatening diseases in which the actual medical attitude is no more than a contemplative passiveness.

If a change in attitude towards disease were the only contribution that the CCU concept made to curing the ills that afflict mankind, it would be welcome. However the exciting fact is that it offers much more.

REFERENCES

1. Kouwenhoven, W. B., Jude, J. R., and Knicker-bocker, G. G.: Closed chest cardiac massage, J.A.M.A, *173*:1064, 1960.
2. Johnson, J. D.: A plan of action in cardiac arrest, J. A. M. A., *186*:468, 1963.
3. Beck, C. S., Pritchard, W., H. and Feil. H. S.: Ventricular fibrillation abolished by electric shock, J. A. M. A., *135*:985, 1947.
4. Beck, C. S., Weckesser, E. C., and Barry, F. M.: Fatal heart attack and successful defibrillation. New concepts in coronary artery disease, J.A.M.A, *161*:434, 1956.
5. Zoll, P. M., Linenthal, A. J., Gibson, A. J., Paul, M. G., and Norman, L. R.: Termination of ventricular fibrillation in man by externally applied countershock, New England J. Med. *254*:727, 1956.
6. Lown, B., Amarasingham, R., and Newman, J.: New method for terminating cardiac arrhythmias. Use of synchronized capacitor discharge, J.A.M.A. *182*:548, 1962.
7. Zoll, P. M.: Resuscitation of the heart in ventricular standstill by external cardiac stimulation, New England J. Med. *247*:768, 1952.
8. Siddons, H., and Sowton, E.: Cardiac Pacemakers. Springfield, Ill., Charles C Thomas, 1967.
9. Julian, D. G.: Treatment of cardaic arrest in acute myocardial ischemia and infarction, Lancet, *2*:840, 1961.
10. Day, H. W.: A cardiac resuscitation program, Lancet, *82*:153, 1962.
11. Coburn, W. V.: Bedside monitors keep hearts beating, Mod. Hosp. *100*:79, 1963.
12. Day, H. W.: An intensive coronary care area, Dis. Chest, *44*:423, 1963.
13. Meltzer, L. E.: Concept and system for intensive coronary care, Acad. Med. New Jersey Bull. *10*:304, 1964.
14. Oliver, M. F., Julian, G. D., and Donald, K. W.: Problems in evaluating coronary care units. Their responsibilities and their relation to the community, Am. J. Cardiol, *20*:465, 1967.
15. Lown, B., and Shillingford, J. P.: Coronary care unit. Promise and challenge, Am. J. Cardiol. *20*:449, 1967.
16. Lown, B., and Selzer, A.: The coronary care unit, Am. J. Cardiol, *22*:597, 1968.
17. Honey, G. E., and Truelove, S. C.: Prognostic factors in myocardial infarction, Lancet *1*:1155, 1957.
18. Wahlberg, F.: A study of acute myocardial infarction at Seraphimer Hospital during 1950–1959, Am. Heart J. *65*:749, 1963.
19. Training technics for the coronary care unit. Second Bethesda Conference of the American College of Cardiology, Am. J. Cardiol. *17*:736, 1966.
20. Proceedings of the National Conference on Coronary Care Units. U. S. Dept. of Health, Education and Welfare. Public Health Service Publication No. 1764, March 1968.
21. Norris, R. M., Bensley, K. E., Caughey, D. E., and Scott, P. J.: Hospital mortality in acute myocardial infarction, Brit. M. J. *3*:144, 1968.
22. Julian, D. G., Valentine, P. A., and Miller, G. G.: Arrhythmias in myocardial infarction, Am. J. Med. *37*:915–927, 1964.
23. Annotations. Management of acute myocardial infarction, Lancet *2*:665, 1967.
24. Restieaux, N., Bray, C., Bullard, H., Murray, M., Robinson, J., Brigden, W., and MacDonald: 150 patients with cardiac infarction treated in a coronary unit, Lancet *1*:1285, 1967.
25. Lawrie, D. M., Greenwood, T. W., Goddard, M., Harvey, A. C., Donald, K. W., Julian, D. G., and Oliver, M. F.: A coronary care unit in the routine management of acute myocardial infarction, Lancet *2*:109, 1967.
26. Day, H. W.: Acute coronary care. A five year report, Am. J. Cardiol. *21*:252, 1968.
27. Corday, E., Gold, H., DeVera, L. B., Williams, J. H., and Fields, J.: Effects of cardiac arrhythmias on the coronary circulation, Ann. Int. Med. *50*:535, 1959.
28. Corday, E., Irwing, D.W., Gold, H., Bernstein, H., and Jaffe, H. L.: Recent advances in the treatment of arrhythmias and conduction defects, Am. Heart J. *64*:126–134, 1962.
29. Cohen, D. B., Doctor, L., and Pick, A.: The significance of atrioventricular block complicating acute myocardial infarct, Am. Heart J. *55*:215, 1958.
30. Geddes, J. S., Adgey, A. A. J., and Pantridge, J. F.: Prognosis after recovery from ventricular fibrillation complicating ischemic heart disease, Lancet *2*:273, 1967.
31. Corday, E., and Litauer, D.: Guidelines for the design and operation of a coronary care unit, Hospitals *40*:77, 1966.
32. Imperial, E. S., Carballo, R., and Zimmermann, H. A.: Disturbances of rate, rhythm and conduction in acute myocardial infarction, Am. J. Cardiol. *5*:24, 1960.
33. Spann, J. F., Moellering, R. C., Haber, E., and Wheeler, E. O.: Arrhythmias in acute myocardial infarction. A study utilizing an electrocardiographic monitor for automatic detection and recording of arrhythmias, New England J. Med. *221*:427, 1964.
34. Mounsey, P.: Intensive coronary care. Arrhythmias after acute myocardial infarction, Am. J. Cardiol, *20*:475, 1967.
35. Stock, E., Goble, A., and Sloman, G.: Assessment of arrhythmias in myocardial infarction, Brit. M. J. *2*:719–724, 1967.
36. Day, H. W., and Averril, K.: Recorded arrhythmias in an acute coronary area, Dis. Chest *49*:113, 1966.
37. Lawrie, D. M., Higgins, M. R., Godman, M. J., Oliver, M. F., Julian, D. G., and Donald, K. W.: Ventricular fibrillation complicating acute myocardial infarction, Lancet *2*:523, 1968.
38. Smirk, F. H., and Palmer, D. G.: A myocardial syndrome. With particular reference to the occurrence of sudden death and of premature systoles interrupting antecedent T waves, Am. J. Cardiol. *6*:620, 1960.
39. Symposium on cardiac pacing and cardioversion, The American College of Cardiology and Presbyterian University of Pennsylvania Medical Center, Philadelphia, The Charles Press, 1967.
40. Yu, P. N., Fox, S. M., Imboden, C A., and Killip, T.: Coronary care unit. A specialized care unit for acute myocardial infarction, Mod. Concepts

Cardiovas. Dis. *34*:23, 1965.

41. Nachlas, M. M., Miller, D. I., and Sieldband, M. P.: Continuous monitoring of patients with acute myocardial infarction, A 32 month experience, J. A. M. A. *119*:126, 1966.

42. Thomas, M., Jewitt, D. E., and Shillingdorf, M. P.: Analysis of 150 patients with acute myocardial infarction admitted to an intensive care and study unit, Brit. M. J. *1*:787, 1968.

43. Conn, P. C.: Diphenylhydantoin sodium in cardiac arrhythmias, New England J. Med. *272*:277, 1965.

44. Frieden, J.: Antiarrhythmic drugs. Part VII. Lidocaine as an antiarrhythmic agent, Am. Heart J. *70*:713, 1965.

45. Lown, B., Fakro, A. M., Wood, W. B., and Thorn, G. W.: The coronary care unit. New perspectives and directions, J. A. M. A. *199*:188, 1967.

46. MacMillan, R. L., Brown, K. W. G., Peckham, G. B., Kahn, O., Hutchison, D. B. and Paton, M.: Changing perspectives in coronary care. A five year study, Am. J. Cardiol. *20*:451, 1967.

47. Lown, B., Vassaux, C., Hood, W. B., Fakro. A. M., Kalplinsky, E., and Roberge, G.: Unresolved problems in coronary care, Am. J. Cardiol. *20*:494, 1967.

48. Killip, T., and Kimball, J. T.: Treatment of myocardial infarction in a coronary care unit, a two year experience with 250 patients, Am. J. Cardiol. *20*:457, 1967.

49. Lewitt, D. E., Balcon, R., Raftery, E. B., and Oram, S.: Incidence and management of supraventricular arrhythmias after acute myocardial infarction, Lancet *2*:734, 1967.

50. Corday, E., and Vyden, J. K.: Resuscitation after myocardial infarction. A clinical appraisal, J. A. M. A. *200*:781, 1967.

51. Lasser, B. W., and Julian, D. G.: Artificial pacing in management of complete heart block complicating acute myocardial infarction, Brit. M. J. *2*:142, 1968.

52. Paulk, E. A., and Hurst, J. W.: Complete heart block in acute myocardial infarction, Am. J. Cardiol. *17*:695, 1966.

53. Friedberg, C. K., Cohen, H., and Donoso, E.: Advanced heart block as a complication of acute myocardial infarction. Role of pacemaker therapy, Prog. Cardiovas. Dis. *10*:466, 1968.

54. Sutton, R., Chaterjee, K., and Leatham, A.: Heart block following acute myocardial infarction. Treatment with demand and fixed rate pacemakers, Lancet *2*:645, 1968.

55. Scott, M. E., Geddes, J. S., Patterson, G. C., Adgey, A. A. G., and Partridge, J. F.: Management of complete heart block complicating acute myocardial infarction, Lancet *2*:1382, 1967.

56. Bernstein, A., Rothfeld, E. L., Robins, B., Cohen, F., and Simon, F.: The treatment of shock accompanying myocardial infarction, Angiology *14*:560, 1963.

57. Symposium on the current status of intensive coronary care, The American College of Cardiology and Presbyterian University of Pennsylvania Medical Center, Philadelphia, The Charles Press, 1966.

58. Logue, R. B., Rogers, J. V., and Gay, B. B.: Subtle roentgenographic signs of left heart failure, Am. Heart J. *65*:464, 1963.

59. Goldman, A., Boszormenyi, F., Utzu, F., Swan, H. J. C., Enescu, V. and Corday, E.: Venoarterial pulsatile bypass for circulatory assist, Dis. Chest *50*:633, 1966.

60. Kuhn, L. A.: The treatment of cardiogenic shock, Am. Heart J. *74*:578 and 725, 1967.

61. Kantrowitz, A.: Initial clinical experience with intraaortic balloon pumping in cardiogenic shock, J.A.M.A. *203*:113, 1968.

62. Corday, E., Vyden, J. K., Rosselot, E., Carvalho, M., Lang, T. W., and Goldman, A.: Advances and controversy in the treatment of shock secondary to cardiac infarction, J.A.M.A. (in press).

63. MacKenzie, G. J., Taylor, S. H., Flenley, D. C., MacDonald, A. H., Stannton, H. P., and Donald, K. W.: Circulatory and respiratory studies in myocardial infarction and cardiogenic shock, Lancet *2*:825, 1964.

64. Neaverson, M. H.: Metabolic acidosis in acute myocardial infarction, Brit. M. J. *2*:383, 1966.

65. MacNicol, M. W.: Intensive care of patients with acute myocardial infarction, Postgrad. Med. *43*: 207-211, 1967.

66. Kirby, B. J., and MacNicol, M. W.: Acid base status in acute myocardial infarction, Lancet *2*:1054, 1966.

67. Valentine, P. H., Fluck, D. C., Mounsey, J. P. D., Reid, D., Shillingford, J. P., and Steiner, R. E.: Blood gases changes after acute myocardial infarction, Lancet *2*:837, 1966.

68. Marshall, R. M., Genton, E., and Blount, S. G.: Acute myocardial infarction. Influence of a coronary care unit, Arch. Int. Med. (to be published).

69. Smith, W. G.: A coronary care unit in a general medical ward, Lancet *1*:397, 1968.

70. Buzza, E. E., Leonard, T. E., Watanabe, H., and Carlsen, E. N.: A new electrode system for continuous measurement of pH, PCO_2, PO_2 and temperature on flowing blood, A.A.M.I. Meeting, Houston, Texas, July 18, 1968.

71. Shillingford, J. P., and Thomas, M.: Cardiovascular and pulmonary changes in patients with myocardial infarction treated in an intensive care and research unit, Am. J. Cardiol. *20*:484, 1967.

72. Pordy, L., Jaffe, H., Chesky, K., and Friedberg, C. K.: Computer analysis of the electrocardiogram; a joint project, J. Mt. Sinai Hosp. *34*:69, 1967.

73. Daly, J. M., and Johnson, G. G.: Automated method for monitoring ventricular ectopic beats, Lancet *2*: 813, 1968.

74. Corday, E.: The coronary care area. A tiger by the tail, Am. J. Cardiol. *16*:466, 1965.

75. Pinneo, R.: Nursing in a coronary care unit, Cardiovas. Nurs. *3*:1, 1967.

76. Symposium on aggressive nursing management of acute myocardial infarction. The Cedars Sinai Medical Center Department of Nursing, Philadelphia, The Charles Press, 1968.

77. Bradley, E. C., and Weil, M. H.: Vasopressor and vasodilator drugs in the treatment of shock, Mod. Treat. *4*:243, 1967.

78. Eichna, L. W.: The treatment of cardiogenic shock. Part III. The Use of isoproterenol in cardiogenic shock, Am. Heart J. *74*:848, 1967.

79. Beecher, H. K.: Ethical problems created by the hopelessly unconscious patient, New England. J. Med. *278*:1425, 1968.

80. Valori, C., Thomas, M., and Shillingford, J. P.: Urinary excretion of free noradrenaline and adrenaline following acute myocardial infarction, Lancet *1*:127, 1967.

81. MacNeilly, R. H., and Pemberton, J.: Duration of last attack in 988 fatal cases of coronary artery disease and its relation to possible cardiac resuscitation, Brit. M. J. *3*:139, 1968.

82. Beck, D. S., and Leighninger, D. S.: Hearts too good to die. Our problem, The Ohio State M. J. *56*:1221, 1960.

83. Pantridge, J. F., and Geddes, J. S.: Cardiac arrest after myocardial infarction, Lancet *1*:807, 1966.

84. Pantridge, J. F., and Geddes, J. S.: A mobile intensive care unit in the management of myocardial infarction, Lancet *2*:271, 1967.

85. Kernohan, R. J., and McGucken, R. B.: Mobile intensive care in myocardial infarction, Brit. M. J. *3*:178, 1968.

Resuscitation for Cardiac Arrest Due to Myocardial Infarction

William J. Grace and Richard J. Kennedy

At present the developing and major emphasis in coronary care is in the prevention of the life threatening arrhythmias and the management of congestive failure and shock.

In 1963 when our Coronary Care Unit was activated the main preoccupation was in the treatment of existing cardiac arrhythmias. The patient was monitored, the alarm set and one waited for a major arrhythmia or asystole to occur. With time it became apparent that the CCU should function as one of the first indicators of potentially fatal disturbances of cardiac rhythm so that treatment could be expectant. With this attitude attention was directed to prevention by the prompt recognition and early treatment of the premonitory signs of the major arrhythmias. Despite this anticipatory attitude cardiac arrest continues to occur, but with knowledge and experience considerable saving of life can be accomplished in these patients.

Ventricular Fibrillation

Here we are using the term "ventricular fibrillation" in the sense of a sudden onset of the arrhythmia in a patient who appeared to be doing well, who is not in shock or congestive failure. In our series of patients with acute cardiac arrest and myocardial infarction 75 per cent of arrests are due to ventricular fibrillation and 25 per cent to actual

TABLE 1
Primary Ventricular Fibrillation

Patients with Acute Myocardial Infarction (Transmural)...............	625
Patients with Primary Ventricular Fibrillation..........................	85
In CCU..............44	
In ER...............32	
76	
Overall Survivors.........................68%	
% Survivors in CCU....41%	
% Survivors in ER.... 75%	

Department of Medicine
St. Vincent's Hospital, New York City

cardiac standstill manifested by a straight-line ECG. Almost half of sudden, unexpected, ventricular fibrillation occurs within the first few hours of myocardial infarction, or during the first hospital day. Actually half of the episodes occur in such patients in the Emergency Room or in the ambulance.

Table 1 indicates our experience[1] with primary ventricular fibrillation during the past 4 years.

If one is not seeing ventricular fibrillation in the course of hospitalization, the probability is that the patients are not being seen early in the course and if the salvage rate of all patients with myocardial infarction is to be improved, a mobile coronary care unit must be instituted.

HISTORY OF RESUSCITATION IN CARDIAC ARREST

In reference to cardiac resuscitation, it is startling to read the following quotation from a surgical text written by Allan Burns[2] of Glasgow in 1809. "Where, however, the cessation of a vital action is very complete and continues wrong, we ought to inflate the lung, and pass electric shocks through the chest; the practitioner ought never, if the death has been sudden and the person not very far advanced in life, to despair of success, until he has unequivocal signs of real death."

Though it is not quite clear what was meant by electric shock, this has a strikingly modern ring, though written almost 120 years ago—a long interval before the suggestion was applied to everyday clinical emergencies by Zoll[3] who, in 1956, almost 100 years after Burns, terminated ventricular fibrillation in man by externally applied countershock.

In 1960, Kouwenhoven[4] demonstrated the efficacy of external cardiac massage in controlling the circulatory effects of ventricular fibrillation until external countershock could be applied.

In our experience from 1947 to 1960, nine patients with ventricular fibrillation survived. This figure means little, for the total patients with this arrhythmia are not known. Yet from 1960 to 1963, after the availability of the electrical defibrillator, we have records of 9 survivors in one quarter of the time delineated in the predefibrillator era. Since the institution of coronary care units in 1963 and orientation of the hospital staff to immediate defibrillation, we now count 15 to 20 successful resuscitations from ventricular fibrillation and cardiac arrest each year.[1] The high success rate is the result of intensive training of the staff in the technics of cardiac resuscitation.

CARDIAC RESUSCITATION

Three procedures constitute the essentials of successful resuscitation in cardiac arrest.

1. Electrical control of the cardiac arrhythmia.
2. Closed chest cardiac massage to provide adequate circulation.
3. Ventilation of the patient, first by mouth-to-mouth respiration and then by endotracheal intubation and a mechanical respirator to provide oxygenation.

These three essentials are considered out of their temporal sequence, for closed chest cardiac massage and mouth-to-mouth respiration ordinarily precede electrical defibrillation. In recent years, however, our instructions to the staff are as follows. "A patient with acute myocardial infarction who becomes pulseless should be defibrillated immediately without taking the time to record the EKG."

Electrical Control of Cardiac Arrhythmia

The control of ventricular fibrillation is determined for practical purposes by the prompt and efficient use of the electrical defibrillator. It is likely that if electrical defibrillation could be accomplished within 15–20 seconds after the onset of fibrillation, the other technic of cardiac resuscitation would not be necessary. To accomplish prompt defibrillation requires repeated in-service educational programs to familiarize personnel with equipment and to train them in efficient team cooperation.

At St. Vincent's Hospital weekly seminars of continuing education are conducted on the use of electrical defibrillation. All house officers on both the intern and resident levels are periodically rotated through this teaching program. Also, all nurses in the Intensive Care Unit, the Intermediate Coronary Care Unit and the Emergency Room participate on a regular basis in the program. The uses and hazards of the defibrillator are first explained. The staff then goes, step by step, through a mock procedure under supervision, using a mongrel dog who is under pentothal anesthesia and in normal sinus rhythm. As the staff becomes more familiar with the use of the defibrillator they are encouraged to increase the tempo of their activity which is timed by a stopwatch. When they reach the point where they can perform the mock procedure in 30 seconds or less, they are tested against "booby-trapped" equipment; electrodes are disconnected, electrode wires are snarled and tangled; the cap on the tube of electrode jelly is so firmly fixed that it requires pliers for removal. The first time the staff are confronted with these obstacles, more than 60 seconds pass before mock defibrillation is completed. With repeated exposure to these handicaps, the most experienced members of the staff can go through the defibrillation procedure in less than 30 seconds.

When the mock training period is completed, the dog is made to fibrillate by passing through its chest an ordinary 60-cycle household current by means of a special but simple piece of equipment. The fibrillating rhythm is recorded on an oscilloscope. When the animal's pulse disappears, defibrillation is initiated. Finally, fibrillation is initiated, the monitor is switched off and the individual student has to decide whether fibrillation is present on the basis of the presence or absence of the animal's peripheral pulses and to use the defibrillator if indicated.

As the program has been continued, great improvement in skill and increased confidence in electrical defibrillation have developed in those who have participated. Also, successes in the management of ventricular fibrillation have increased manyfold.

Failure of a patient to respond to electrical therapy for ventricular fibrillation or intractable ventricular fibrillation raises many questions. How often should a patient be defibrillated? In acute myocardial infarction, repeated ventricular fibrillation is not uncommon and each episode of the arrhythmia must be treated. We have seen complete recovery of a patient after 25 electric shocks in the course of a single hour. Another patient was treated for the arrhythmia by closed chest massage and defibrillation 29 times in a period of 30 days, to subsequently leave the hospital alive and relatively well. In short, as long as electrical activity is recorded by the ECG, one should tenaciously persist in attempts to resuscitate.

Closed Chest Cardiac Massage

Closed chest cardiac massage in temporal sequence is the first procedure employed in patients with cardiac arrest. This, described in 1961 by

Kouwenhoven, Jude, and Knickerbocker,[4] is really the basis of successful resuscitation. Essentially, it consists in exerting enough intermittent pressure on the patient's sternum to produce a femoral pulse by cardiac compression. While pressure is exerted, another person must continuously monitor femoral pulse. At this hospital, we use a manually operated mechanical device, the Rentsch cardiac press, for closed chest massage. We have found it effective and easily operated, even by a person of small stature. Other mechanical systems, electrically or gas-driven, are available.

Ventilation of the Patient

It is important to realize that persistent arrhythmias and underoxygenation are intimately related. Oxygen should be administered to all patients being resuscitated, immediately, by using the Ambu bag and a mouth airway and, as soon as possible, switching to endotracheal intubation and ventilation with either a pressure—or a volume-scaled respirator. Considerable education and experience are necessary for proper endotracheal intubation. The proper tube must be selected and the operator must be familiar with the various fittings and adaptors.

Endotracheal intubation should be done immediately in the unconscious patient undergoing resuscitation. One must be careful that the tube is not placed so far down, that is beyond the carina, so that only one major bronchus is ventilated. This can only be determined by stethoscopic examination of the chest which should immediately follow intubation. One other complication should be kept in mind; namely, the possibility of dislodging dentures into the larynx during intubation.

Another cause of defibrillation failure is severe metabolic acidosis. We assume that any patient without circulation has developed a severe degree of acidosis which must be corrected by the administration of 50 mEq. of sodium bicarbonate every 15 minutes during attempted resuscitation. As soon as possible arterial blood pH is determined and further doses of bicarbonate are determined by the degree of acidosis.

CONCLUSION

Since the institution of the CCU and repeated inservice educational programs it is apparant that resuscitation from cardiac arrest is successful. The success or failure of this program of cardiac resuscitation in patients with ventricular fibrillation is closely related to the skill and experience of the group. It is emphasized that repeated educational programs are of paramount importance in success.

REFERENCES

1. Grace, W. J., and Minogue, W. F.: Resuscitation for cardiac arrest due to myocardial infarction, Dis. Chest 50:173, 1968
2. Burns, A.: Observations on Some of the Most Frequent and Important Diseases of the Heart, London, Hafner Publishing Company, 1964. (Originally published 1809, Edinburgh)
3. Zoll, P. M., Linenthal, A. J., Gibson, W., Paul, M. H., and Norman, L. R.: Termination of ventricular fibrillation in man by externally applied counter-shock, New England. J. Med., 254:727, 1956.
4. Kouwenhoven, W. G., Jude, J. R., and Knicker-bocker, G. G.: Closed chest cardiac massage, J.A. M.A. 173:1064, 1960.

The Treatment of Shock Complicating Acute Myocardial Infarction*

Max Harry Weil and Herbert Shubin

INTRODUCTION

After acute myocardial infarction, the clinical course of approximately 12 per cent of patients is complicated by manifestations of circulatory shock.[1-4] Even with supportive treatment, including analgesic drugs and breathing oxygen, fewer than 1 out of 5 patients survive.[5] The initial enthusiasm for "vasopressor" drugs, introduced 15 years ago, has been sustained by reports that the survival rate doubled after introduction of these drugs.[6] Yet, others find no definitive evidence that these drugs have improved survival.[2,7,8]

Since our understanding of both mechanisms and treatment of acute myocardial infarction and its complications is still very meager, convention rather than proven efficacy guides much current practice in this field. After greater understanding of mechanisms is achieved, the rational basis for treatment will undoubtedly be greatly improved. Even modest improvement would profoundly alter the dismal outlook. A decrease in mortality of but 15 per cent would essentially double the number of survivors.

The conscientious clinician, however, is alerted not only to the potential benefits of newer drugs and other innovations of management but is properly suspicious that innovations are likely to entail greater risks before their ultimate value is established. With these considerations in mind, we reviewed experimental and clinical data on the treatment of shock complicating myocardial infarction, aided by the results of our own investigations in the University of Southern California Shock Research Unit at the Los Angeles County/USC Medical Center.[9] This contribution is intended as a guide or, preferably, as a resource to aid in the planning of bedside treatment. With the specialized staffs and facilities of coronary care units, superior monitoring and technically more demanding technics of therapy have been feasible.

CENTRAL VENOUS CATHETERIZATION

An objective inventory of the status of the patient in shock and a quantitative evaluation of his response to treatment are now provided by the use of a central venous catheter.[10] Such a catheter, which is advanced into the superior vena cava or the right atrium with minimal difficulty and risk, is unquestionably one of the most helpful initial maneuvers available for the routine management of the patient with myocardial shock. The central venous catheter serves seven purposes:

(1) *Measurement of central venous pressure.* Central venous pressure indicates the relationship between blood volume and cardiac competence. As such, it is a helpful guide for early recognition of congestive heart failure, particularly during infusion of fluids. A rise in ventricular diastolic pressure and, in turn, atrial and caval pressures precedes the onset of overt heart failure.

(2) *Phlebotomy.* Withdrawal of 250 to 750 ml. of blood is facilitated by the central venous catheter. A standard blood donor collection bottle (Vacutainer, Travenol) is kept in readiness at the bedside for this purpose. Phlebotomy is immediately effective in the treatment of congestive heart failure and its use is advocated when pulmonary edema threatens immediate survival.

(3) *Route for infusion and injection.* The central venous catheter provides direct access to the central circuit for administration of medication. This is particularly useful during cardiac arrest when epinephrine, alkali and calcium solutions

*This investigation was supported by the John A. Hartford Foundation, Inc., New York, and by United States Public Health Service Research Grants HE-05570 and HE-07811 from the National Heart Institute.

Portions of this text were previously published in Progress in Cardiovascular Diseases, *10* (no. 1): July 1967, and are herein reproduced with the generous permission of Grune and Stratton, Inc.

are administered through the central venous catheter without the added trauma of multiple cardiac punctures.

(4) *Source of blood for repetitive laboratory measurements.* The catheter provides ready access to the central venous reservoir and serves as an atraumatic source of blood samples for laboratory analysis, thus obviating the anxiety and discomfort provoked by repeated venous puncture. Moreover, pH and PCO_2 are reliably measured on central venous blood during shock.[11] The trauma of arterial puncture may be avoided.

(5) *Route for insertion of intracardiac pacing electrode.* A suitable wire for intracardiac pacing may be guided directly into the heart through the lumen of the catheter with optimal speed and reliability.

(6) *Indirect measurement of cardiac output.* An increase in central venous oxygen content, oxygen saturation or oxygen tension (PO_2) when oxygen content of inspired air is held constant usually reflects an increase in cardiac output; a decline usually indicates a fall in cardiac output. These measurements lose reliability when diffusion of oxygen into the alveolar capillaries is impaired because of major pulmonary or cardiac complications.

(7) *Respiratory measurements.* Changes in intrathoracic pressure imposed by respiratory efforts are readily observed and provide a more reliable indication of ventilatory stress than measurements of respiratory rate alone.[12]

ARTERIAL CATHETERIZATION

The practice of inserting a small catheter into the femoral or brachial artery is becoming routine for managing patients in shock centers. The sphygmomanometer does not function as a consistently reliable indicator of arterial pressure during shock, particularly in the case of patients who are being treated with arterial constrictor drugs. The intra-arterial catheter also serves as a source of blood samples for determination of arterial oxygen saturation or for measurement of cardiac output and velocity of blood flow (circulation time) by the indicator-dilution technic.[8,13-22]

VASOACTIVE DRUGS

Beginning in 1950 and continuing until about a year ago, the severity of myocardial shock was gauged by the level of the blood pressure and the effectiveness of treatment was judged by the extent to which blood pressure was restored. So-called vasopressor drugs came into wide use, particularly levarterenol (Levophed) and metaraminol (Aramine).[1,5-7,23-29]This approach was based on the dual assumption that the increase in arterial pressure reflected an increase in effective systemic blood flow and that the vasoconstriction induced by these drugs improved coronary flow by augmenting coronary perfusion pressure[30] without disproportionately increasing the heart's work load. Yet, in previous studies on hemorrhagic and traumatic shock, elevation of blood pressure did not necessarily improve the outcome. To the contrary, transection of the spinal cord,[31] ganglionic blockage,[32] or adrenolytic dibenamine[33]—all of which produced "vasodilation" and lowered arterial pressure— nevertheless improved survival. In the past 5 years, vasodilator agents have been more extensively tested in the treatment of patients with hemorrhagic, bacterial and even cardiogenic shock, especially after open-heart surgery, and beneficial responses were observed.[34-36] This promoted a rigorous reexamination of the relative merits of vasopressor and vasodilator drugs, including their established use for treatment of myocardial shock.

Pharmacodynamics.

The apparent differences between those who favored vasopressor and those who favored vasodilator drugs for treatment of myocardial shock were largely resolved by the realization that these terms actually describe the cardiovascular actions of individual drugs very poorly. Drugs that are clinically used to increase blood pressure are called vasopressor drugs. However, these agents do not increase arterial pressure by a single mechanism. The pressor action may be due to arterial vasoconstriction without a change in flow, to an increase in blood flow without arterial or arteriolar vasoconstriction, or to alterations both in arterial caliber and blood flow. Corresponding considerations apply to so-called vasodilator drugs. They may decrease blood pressure by dilating arteries or arterioles, by decreasing blood flow or by a combination of these effects. The imprecision of these terms necessitates examining the role of vasoactive drugs in a broader physiological spectrum. Moreover, not only the effects on the arteries, but also the effects on the volume of blood normally stored in the capacitance bed and on the contractility of the myocardial "pump" must be taken into account.

For the practical purpose of relating pharmacological characteristics to clinical usefulness, only the major hemodynamic actions of these drugs are considered in the present discussion. Actions of drugs on the heart are described in terms of their effects on rate, rhythm and myocardial contractility. The arteries and arterioles, which constitute the resistance blood vessels, react by vasoconstriction or vasodilation. The venules and veins that make up the capacitance blood vessels store blood, and the drugs may either enlarge the venous pools and decrease venous return or mobilize blood from the storage sites and increase the venous return (and hence the cardiac output).

The terminology we use in our clinical unit to describe these hemodynamic actions adopts, in part, the alpha and beta adrenergic concepts originally proposed by Ahlquist.[38] Although the intravascular receptors postulated by Ahlquist have not been anatomically demonstrated, drugs that act as if they block actions at these sites are described as either alpha or beta adrenergic receptor blocking agents.[39] We prefer a more general concept which describes modes of action rather than effects on specific receptor sites. This translates Ahlquist's concept into a practical outline useful for predicting the hemodynamic responses of patients to vasoactive drugs. We refer to alphamimetic and betamimetic vasoactive drugs. The drugs which oppose these adrenergic hemodynamic actions are referred to as alphalytic and betalytic agents, respectively.

Alphamimetic Drugs. Agents such as methoxamine (Vasoxyl) and phenylephrine (Neo-Synephrine) constrict arteries and arterioles, thereby increasing arterial resistance and, in turn, arterial pressure. The work load on the heart is increased because more force is needed to eject blood against greater arterial resistance. This group of drugs also constricts venous sphincters and consequently traps blood in capacitance vessels proximal to the constricted veins. Venous return and hence cardiac output may be reduced.[40] These drugs have no inotropic or chronotropic effects on the heart, except that their pressor action reduces heart rate through reflexes mediated by carotid and aortic baroreceptors. Slowing of the heart rate, which is mediated through the vagus nerve, is effectively blocked by vagotomy or atropine.

The alphamimetic drugs also increase hydrostatic pressure in the capillaries proximal to constricted veins, accounting for escape of fluid from the intravascular compartment into the extravascular space. For this reason, prolonged administration of alphamimetic drugs not uncommonly reduces plasma volume[41] and is clinically confirmed by a progressive rise in hematocrit. Protracted hypotension with apparent decrease in responsiveness to the pressor amine[42-44] is primarily due to hypovolemia, a complication of treatment with alphamimetic

agents. In most cases the patient is readily "weaned" by restitution of volume, guided by measurement of central venous pressure.

The relatively pure alphamimetic drugs, such as methoxamine and phenylephrine, do not by themselves improve myocardial contractility and are of no present benefit in the treatment of shock due to myocardial infarction.[45-47] Angiotension II (Hypertension) resembles alphamimetic drugs in its pressor actions, but unlike them is not blocked by alphalytic drugs. Judged by its ability to raise arterial pressure,[48,49] its effectiveness has been equated with that of levarterenol. However, angiotensin, unlike levarterenol, does not increase myocardial contractility and cardiac output, and angiotensin provides no apparent advantage in the treatment of myocardial shock.[50,51]

Betamimetic Drugs. Isoproterenol (Isuprel) and mephentermine (Wyamine) are primarily beta adrenergic or betamimetic drugs. They consistently increase cardiac output and heart rate but, during shock, their effects on blood pressure are variable.[52-57] A profound fall in arterial pressure is avoided by assuring adequacy of intravascular volume, guided by measurement of central venous pressure. Since these drugs, particularly isoproterenol, reduce arterial tonus, they lower arterial pressure unless the cardiac output is disproportionately increased. However, the betamimetic agents also reduce venous pooling, and increase venous return and cardiac output. Since the strength and rate of cardiac contraction are also increased, there is additional basis for augmentation of cardiac output.

Betamimetic agents tend to decrease arterial resistance and thus counteract the intense vasoconstriction now implicated as a cause of progressive perfusion failure. Isoproterenol and, to a lesser degree, mephentermine, precipitate ventricular arrhythmias, but this is largely dependent on dosage. Clinical trials with these betamimetic drugs, particularly isoproterenol, indicate their potential usefulness.[57] Isoproterenol has been administered in amounts of 3 to 10 micrograms per minute by intravenous infusion.

Though myocardial function and cardiac output are substantially augmented during treatment with isoproterenol, these beneficial hemodynamic effects have not consistently reversed the metabolic changes during shock. Isoproterenol increases metabolic rate and myocardial oxygen demand. However, the greater oxygen needs may not be met by a sufficiently large increase in coronary and systemic blood flow.[58] Gunnar and his associates specifically caution against the use of isoproterenol for treatment of shock due to myocardial infarction.[59] Clearly, the ultimate benefits and risks associated with the use of betamimetic drugs are not as yet established.

Alpha-betamimetic drugs. Levarterenol and metaraminol have both alpha and betamimetic actions.[28,60,61] In moderate doses, they increase both cardiac output and arterial pressure. In small doses, metaraminol and levarterenol increase cardiac output with minimal vasoconstriction. A paradoxical decline in arterial resistance resembling that of betamimetic drugs may be observed.[20] With large doses, vascular resistance is markedly increased and, as in the case of alphamimetic drugs, cardiac output may decline. In a previously normotensive patient, cardiac output is usually increased when systolic pressure is raised to approximately 100 mg. Hg. Further increases in arterial pressure fail to improve and sometimes even lower the cardiac output.[20]

The great differences in the hemodynamic and renal effects described by various investigators are largely explained by differences related to the amounts of the drug administered. Metaraminol, in an amount of 200 mg., or levarterenol in an amount of 16 ml. (4 ampules) of a 0.2 per cent solution, diluted in 1 liter of 5 per cent glucose in water, is administered at a rate sufficient to maintain arterial pressure at a level of 20 to 30 mm. Hg. below the "normal" level. This method maximizes effects on cardiac output and minimizes increases in arterial resistance and the work load on the heart.

After treatment with reserpine or guanethidine (Ismelin), catecholamine stores are characteristically depleted, accounting for selective refractoriness to metaraminol, since this pressor agent acts primarily by releasing norepinephrine from tissue stores.[62] This effect is of practical significance in patients with hypertension using these drugs at the time of myocardial infarction. Under other conditions, there is no apparent advantage to the use of levarterenol over metaraminol, even though levarterenol appears to be the same as endogenous norepinephrine. To the contrary, metaraminol is administered with little risk of ischemic injury and slough, which results from extravasation of levarterenol. The risk of such local injury may be greatly decreased by the addition of 5 to 10 mg. of phentolamine to each liter of the levarterenol infusion.

During perfusion failure, anoxic metabolism with accumulation of lactic acid and other acid metabolites progresses to advanced metabolic acidosis. Responsiveness to the alphamimetic action of vasoactive drugs is reduced.[63,64] Infusion of sodium bicarbonate restores this pressor response, but ultimate benefit is doubtful in the advanced states of perfusion failure.

Nervous System Blockade. The role of the autonomic system in the progression of cardiogenic shock is imperfectly understood. Some investigators, notably Agress and Binder,[65] postulate that an inhibitory reflex arising in the injured myocardium accounts for peripheral circulatory failure. In dogs, in whom shock was produced by embolization of the coronary arteries with small glass spheres, arterial pressure was improved after afferent cardiac sympathetic fibers were blocked by thoracic epidural analgesia. Application of this technic of neural block to management of patients has been too limited for adequate evaluation.[6] However, no consistent improvement has been demonstrated following transsection, cooling of the cervical vagi or vagal blockage with atropine.[65-67]

It has long been recognized that drugs or procedures which block transmission of sympathetic impulses through autonomic ganglia improve the survival rate in some types of experimental shock. In 1938, Freeman and his associates[68] demonstrated the beneficial effects of sympathectomy. A decade later, Glasser and Page[32] found similar improvement following autonomic blockage in experiments on shock caused by hemorrhage. Autonomic blockade, widely applied to the treatment of systemic hypertension, probably has some merit for controlling massive blood loss and, consequently, hypovolemic shock during surgery. Phenothiazine drugs, especially chlorpromazine (Thorazine), that also manifest ganglionic blocking effects, have also been tested.[69,70] The relative unpredictability of the acute actions of these drugs have discouraged their general use for treatment of shock.[71] With the availability of more specific adrenolytic drugs, interest in ganglionic blockade has largely disappeared.

Alphalytic agents. Phenoxybenzamine (Dibenzyline), which has not yet been released for clinical use, and phentolamine (Regitine) are the principal alphalytic agents currently available.[37,72,73] The primary action of these drugs is to counteract the arterial and venous constriction provoked by alphamimetic stimulus of endogenous or exogenous cause. Since the effect of alphalytic drugs is to leave beta adrenergic actions unopposed, their net effect closely resembles that of betamimetic agents.[37]

Phenoxybenzamine improves pulmonary perfusion and decreases pulmonary edema during myocardial shock in patients and under experimental conditions of the laboratory.[74] Increases in vascular (primarily venous) capacitance of 25 per cent or more demonstrate the effects of this alphalytic drug. At the same time, this increase in vascular capacitance is also the principal hazard accompanying the use of phenoxybenzamine. When intravascular volume is even moderately decreased, expansion of the intravascular capacity induced by the alphalytic drug may result in profound hypotension and accentuation of shock. Phenoxybenzamine and phentolamine, like isoproterenol and mephentermine, are safely used only after volume has been repleted. In phentolamine studies on a small group of patients in cardiogenic shock, Bradley[76] has observed a consistent increase in cardiac output even though blood pressure was reduced. Improvement in systemic blood flow was manifested by a decrease in the mean circulation time of dye injected into the right atrium, an increase in peripheral skin temperature and an increase in urine flow. Phentolamine may be administered by intravenous infusion in amounts of 0.5 to 1 mg. per minute. It is of greater usefulness than phenoxybenzamine because phentolamine is a short-acting drug and its effects are controlled with relative ease, whereas effects of phenoxybenzamine are protracted and persist for 24 hours or more. Further investigation of the hemodynamic and metabolic effects of the alphalytic drugs during treatment of shock following acute myocardial infarction must of necessity precede their introduction into clinical practice.

When an alpha-betamimetic pressor agent like levarterenol or metaraminol is combined with an alphalytic drug, like phentolamine, the betamimetic action becomes dominant. These features have been clearly delineated both experimentally in our laboratory[40] and, more recently, in clinical studies reported by Bradley.[76] Phentolamine is a short-acting drug. The action of phenoxybenzamine is slower in onset and its pharmacologic effects persist for 24 hours and longer. Since the effects of the combination depend on the dose of the component drugs, adjustment is simplified by use of the short-acting preparation. The addition of phentolamine to levarterenol prevents skin necrosis on extravasation and therefore cancels a major advantage of metaraminol over levarterenol.

The relative amounts of levarterenol or metaraminol and phentolamine may be tailored to achieve maximum cardiac output (betamimetic action) while maintaining a favorable perfusion pressure and heart rate (alphamimetic action). These are clinically judged on the basis of improvements in alertness, urine flow, peripheral skin temperature and lesser electrocardiographic manifestations of ischemia.

Results with the combination of levarterenol and phentolamine must be more carefully evaluated before their routine use can be recommended. However, in patients in whom metaraminol, used in amounts of up to 20 mg. per hour to increase arterial pressure to approximately 30 mm. below "normal"

levels, fails to indicate improvement of circulation, a trial with levarterenol, in amounts ranging from 3 to 30 micrograms per minute, or metaraminol, 0.1 to 2 mg. per minute, combined with phentolamine in amounts ranging from 0.1 to 1.0 mg. per minute is, in our opinion, justified. Treatment is simplified by maintaining separate solutions, but joining the intravenous tubing in "piggy-back" fashion.

Betalytic Agents. After Ahlquist published his theory, a specific search was conducted to identify effective beta receptor blocking (betalytic) drugs. Dichloroisoproterenol (D.C.I.)[77,78] and, subsequently, pronethalol (Nethalide)[79,80] and propranolol hydrochloride (Inderal)[81] have been introduced. Most recently, MJ 1998 and MJ 1999[82] have been made available for laboratory study. D.C.I. had limited practical value because it had both betalytic and betamimetic actions. Pronethalol was abandoned because it was regarded as potentially carcinogenic in the light of animal experiments,[83] and experience with patients indicated that nausea, vomiting and paresthesia were significant side effects.[84] However, propranolol is now marketed in the United States, but its use for therapy of shock, per se, is still regarded as experimental.[85-88]

Betalytic drugs, like alphamimetic drugs, tend to increase blood pressure,[89] reduce cardiac output and increase arterial resistance.[90] Betamimetic stimuli, which account for episodes of cardiac arrhythmia, are blocked by these drugs. Unfortunately, they also tend to block inotropic effects. If the stimulating action on the myocardium is blocked by betalytic drugs at a time when cardiac competence is limited, the threat of congestive heart failure is greatly increased. In patients with obstructive airway disease, bronchospasm may be increased by blocking the beta adrenergic effect on the bronchioles.[91] For these reasons, betalytic drugs are not of proven value for treatment of patients in shock after myocardial infarction, and their present use should be reserved for the treatment of serious and otherwise uncontrolled arrhythmias.

NARCOTIC, SEDATIVE AND ANTIEMETIC DRUGS

An impressive number of synthetic narcotic drugs have been introduced in recent years, but claims of decisive advantages of one drug over another in terms of potency, rapidity of onset, duration of action, freedom from side effects and margin of safety are largely unsupported. Morphine is still the least expensive narcotic drug and we find no reason to abandon it in favor of newer agents for the relief of the severe pain of acute myocardial infarction.

Morphine in amounts of 10 mg. usually provides effective analgesia. Although it is frequently prescribed as "morphine, grain 1/4th," this amount (equivalent to 16 mg.) is generally an excessive dose.[92] Some persons manifest idiosyncrasy or specific unfavorable side effects, and in these cases another narcotic may be selected. As an alternative to morphine, there is meperidine (Demerol), 75 mg. of which is equivalent to approximately 10 mg. of morphine. Two mg. of dihydromorphinone (Dilaudid) or 7 mg. of methadone (Dolophine) may be selected as other alternatives to the comparable 10 mg. of morphine.

When circulatory shock is profound, the customary subcutaneous (hypodermic) route of administration is disadvised, since the narcotic may be poorly absorbed when perfusion of the injection site is decreased.[93] Under such circumstances, half the usual dose, or 5 mg. of morphine, is injected intravenously over a period of 2 minutes. After a delay of an additional 10 minutes, and if respiratory depression is not manifest, a second dose, also of 5 mg. may be conveniently injected through the intravenous tubing. The injection of morphine may be followed by an increase in blood pressure if pain is relieved. However, a further decrease in pressure is frequently observed.[94] More recently, pentozocine (Talwin) has been favored as a non-narcotic analgesic. In amounts of 30 mg. injected intravenously, this drug has analgesic potency comparable to that of 10 mg. of morphine. No distinct advantage over morphine has been demonstrated with respect to incidence of circulatory depression, respiratory depression or nausea and vomiting.

It is relatively uncommon for a patient in profound shock to require an analgesic drug and even less common for him to require narcotics. Patients are much more likely to manifest anxiety rather than pain. To control anxiety, hydroxyzine (Atarax, Vistaril) by slow intravenous injection in amounts ranging from 75 to 150 mg. is recommended. This non-narcotic, sedative agent usually produces the desired calming effect without any significant respiratory or circulatory depression.[95] As an alternative to hydroxyzine, promethazine (Phenergan) may be employed in amounts of 25 to 50 mg. Diazepam (Valium) injected slowly by intravenous route in total amounts of 5 to 20 mg. is likely to relieve severe anxiety and agitation, particularly in patients requiring ventilatory assistance. It may be repeated at intervals of 2 to 4 hours.

A drug related to narcotics but actually a narcotic antagonist with analgesic properties is a helpful adjunct under circumstances in which the narcotic has produced respiratory depression. Hypoventila-tion with anoxemia and respiratory acidosis are particularly hazardous since they greatly increase the risk of ventricular arrhythmias. The narcotic antagonist, nalorphine (Nalline), is administered intravenously in amounts of 2.5 to 5 mg. and, if necessary, repeated at intervals of 2 hours.

A disconcerting side effect of narcotic drugs is nausea and vomiting. The concomitant administration of dimenhydrinate (Dramamine) in amounts of 50 mg. with the narcotic drug appears to decrease the incidence of vomiting.

Oxygen. The administration of 100 per cent oxygen by nasal catheter or tight-fitting mask, at a flow of 6 to 8 liters per minute, is widely practiced. MacKenzie and associates[96] have recently reemphasized that partial pressure of oxygen (PO_2) in arterial blood may be markedly reduced during shock. Physical signs of hypoxemia are usually lacking. In fact, the oxygen saturation is only minimally lowered. The decline in oxygen tension is actually due to arteriovenous shunt of blood through underventilated portions of the lung. The administration of as little as 40 per cent oxygen by face mask more than doubles the oxygen tension in arterial blood. Consequently, the amount of oxygen delivered to ischemic but viable areas of the myocardium at the periphery of infarction is significantly increased.[97] Our group has modified a loose fitting Ventimask to deliver inspired oxygen concentrations to levels exceeding 50 per cent.

Oxygen constricts arterial segments[98] and systemically increases arterial pressure. However, the benefit (or detriment) of this effect with reference to the treatment of shock due to myocardial infarction is not established, particularly since the blood pressure and cardiac output do not consistently change in the same direction.

Hyperbaric Oxygen. Hyperbaric oxygenation has been proposed as a potentially promising means of reversing tissue hypoxia during shock.[99] When a human patient is placed in a hyperbaric chamber in which the pressure of oxygen is increased to two atmospheres (1520 mm. at sea level), the amount of oxygen in the arterial blood is increased by more than 3 volumes per cent, but this is actually only about 15 per cent more than is normally present.[100] Yet, the oxygen tension (PO_2) of arterial blood increases more than tenfold and provides a greater pressure head for the diffusion of oxygen.

In the absence of capillary flow, the increase in oxygen tension of blood is of no importance.[101] Since oxygen diffuses for only short distances after it leaves the capillary, effective transfer of oxygen still is fully dependent on adequacy of blood flow, even if PO_2 is increased more than tenfold. Yet, the fundamental defect following coronary occlusion and, in fact, in shock itself, is the critical curtailment of effective flow. Hence, the initial enthusiasm for hyperbaric oxygen for treatment of myocardial shock is tempered even on theoretical grounds.

Beneficial effects have nevertheless been demonstrated. The mortality rate in dogs after coronary artery occlusion was decreased when they were maintained in a hyperbaric oxygen tank at two atmospheres pressure.[102,103] A reduction in the size of the infarct has been reported by Trapp and Creighton,[104] but studies by Kuhn and associates[102] failed to bear this out. The data based on clinical trials with hyperbaric oxygen is not yet adequate for objective evaluation.[105,107] Toxic effects, including pulmonary atelectasis, associated with its prolonged usage indicate the need for special caution.[108,109]

Pulmonary Complications. Mixtures of helium and oxygen are sometimes employed since these are lighter than air and presumably facilitate ventilation and the work of breathing. Clinical proof of their actual value is, however, lacking. While a mixture of 20 per cent oxygen and 80 per cent helium is only one-third as dense as air, it is considerably more viscous and its flow through bronchioles is actually hampered rather than facilitated.[110]

When heart failure, pneumonia and other parenchymal diseases of the lung complicate the clinical course, as they often do, the pulmonary compliance (i.e., the expansibility of the lung) may be markedly reduced. In these cases, pressure-controlled ventilators, especially intermittent positive pressure units, may not have enough pressure flow reserve (work capability) to overcome the excessive airway resistance. Volume-controlled ventilators, such as the Engström respirator, are then needed. Yet, their effective use requires that the patient's own respiratory efforts do not counter the control established by the mechanical ventilator. This may be achieved by neuromuscular paralysis with tubocurarine chloride (Tubarine) or succinylcholine (Anectine). More than 60 per cent of patients managed in the Shock Research Unit at the Los Angeles County/USC Medical Center required mechanical support of ventilation to reverse respiratory acidosis and anoxemia.

CARDIAC GLYCOSIDES FOR HEART FAILURE

The increased hazard of serious cardiac arrhythmias and the failure to demonstrate consistent improvement in circulation following the administration of digitalis have prompted some clinicians to caution against the use of digitalis for the treatment

of myocardial shock.[111] Opposed to this view are Gilchrist[112] and Dack,[113] who suggest that the increase in myocardial contractility and the consequent increase in cardiac output are significant advantages. Experimental observations in dogs, in whom shock was produced by embolization of the coronary arteries with microspheres, lend support to the later view.[114,115] Both cardiac output and arterial pressure were increased after ouabain. In recent studies, the demonstration that digitalis is capable of stimulating myocardial contractility even in the nonfailing human heart[116] has further reawakened a latent controversy with regard to its routine use following myocardial infarction.[117] However, population type data currently available on the use of digitalis glycosides in patients with myocardial infarction complicated by shock are not adequate to settle this point. Neither the evidence of efficacy nor the danger of arrhythmias is sufficiently well documented to justify a firm position for or against its routine use.

However, there is no reason for equivocation in the use of digitalis for emergency treatment of congestive heart failure or potentially serious supraventricular arrhythmias. Digoxin (Lanoxin) administered by intravenous injection in the initial amount of 0.75 mg. is the drug of our choice in our unit. Its greatest advantage is the ease with which the subsequent administration of digitalis may be regulated, either by parenteral injection or oral medication. The principal disadvantage, though not often of practical moment, is the 20-minute delay before the pharmacological action of digoxin ordinarily becomes fully manifest. However, we would consider phlebotomy as the most expedient maneuver in such cases in which cardiac failure threatens immediate survival. Ouabain has also been widely used in critical circumstances, since its effect becomes manifest within 5 minutes. An initial dose of 0.5 mg. is administered as a single intravenous injection. This may be followed by amounts of 0.1 mg. every hour for 2 or 3 additional doses. In patients in whom the possibility of prior digitalization cannot be excluded, the digitalizing dose should be diluted in 20 ml. and injected at a rate of 1 ml. per minute. Deslanoside (Cedilanid), though widely used for rapid digitalization, has no advantage over digoxin in onset of action. It may have a minor advantage in that it is excreted slightly more rapidly than digoxin, a consideration in patients in whom digitalis intoxication might be precipitated. Reductions in hepatic blood flow and renal clearance account for the protracted action of digitalis glycosides. In addition, the increased tolerance to digitalis drugs during hyperkalemia and the high incidence of digitalis intoxication in patients with hypokalemia require special precaution in the presence of shock.

AGENTS FOR THE CONTROL OF CARDIAC ARRHYTHMIAS

Cardiac arrhythmias may themselves be the cause of shock following myocardial infarction or may contribute significantly to the hemodynamic defect. When the cardiac rate is so rapid that diastolic filling is compromised, cardiac output is markedly decreased, accounting for the manifestations of circulatory shock. Conversely, pathologically-slow heart rates of less than 50 per minute may also result in profoundly reduced cardiac output.

In patients in shock, regardless of cause, respiratory failure is a common complication and probably accounts for as many acute deaths as circulatory failure. With restoration of more adequate ventilation, often requiring the use of respirator assistance, hypercapnia, hypoxemia and cardiac arrhythmias may be reversed.

Digitalis. Digitalization has been firmly established for many years as the ultimate treatment for atrial fibrillation or for atrial tachycardia or atrial flutter. The occurrence of these arrhythmias during myocardial shock, when cardiac output and coronary flow are already markedly reduced, is of ominous significance. Further reduction in coronary flow is poorly tolerated and the supraventricular arrhythmias are soon followed by onset of ventricular arrhythmias. In cases of supraventricular tachycardia, digitalization may still be the treatment of choice. However, termination of these arrhythmias by electrical means[118,119] merits special consideration.

Diphenylhydantoin (Dilantin). This drug, widely used for the treatment of cerebral dysrhythmias, is *occasionally* effective in reversing supraventricular arrhythmias other than atrial fibrillation. It has also been used successfully in the treatment of some ventricular arrhythmias, particularly those due to digitalis intoxication.[120-122] Direct myocardial depressant and peripheral vasodilating effects have been noted.[123] Diphenylhydantoin is administered by intravenous infusion in amounts of 50 mg. per minute, up to a total of 300 mg.

Atropine. Sinus bradycardia with heart rates of less than 50 beats per minute is usually due to excessive vagotonic activity. This arrhythmia is often reversed by 1 mg. of atropine sulfate injected intravenously.[65,124] The drying action of atropine on the tracheobronchial mucosa, particularly when used for protracted periods, probably has an undesirable side effect. It increases the likelihood of inspissation of tracheobronchial secretions and further accentuates respiratory complications.

Potassium. A solution containing 50 mEq. of potassium chloride and 20 units of insulin per liter of 10 per cent glucose in water, the so-called polarizing solution, has been recommended by Ponce de Leon[125] for treatment of patients with acute myocardial infarction. Day and Averill[126] suggest that the polarizing solution is, in fact, effective in preventing ventricular arrhythmias. Objective confirmation is still needed.

Potassium chloride is useful for control of digitalis intoxication manifested by potentially serious cardiac arrhythmias. It is administered in amounts 40 to 100 mEq. diluted in 5 per cent glucose solution. In patients in shock, however, renal failure may preclude the use of this agent unless serum potassium is clearly reduced.

Glucocorticoids. The acute onset of atrioventricular block is sometimes reversed by the administration of glucocorticoid hormones in pharmacological amount.[127-129] Cortisol (Hydrocortisone) is administered in amounts of 200 to 500 mg. and equivalent doses are readministered at intervals of 4 to 12 hours. When atrioventricular block is due to inflammation at the periphery of an acute myocardial infarct, it is potentially reversible. Corticosteroid treatment may be continued for a period of up to 5 days without commitment to prolonged steroid treatment.

Pacemakers. The most specific treatment for atrioventricular block is electrical pacing.[130-133] In this technic, an electrode catheter may be inserted through a jugular vein, a peripheral arm vein or through the lumen of the venous catheter and advanced to the apex of the right ventricle. Rates of 60 to 80 beats per minute are usually within the optimal range.

Procainamide and lidocaine. For the acute treatment of ventricular tachycardia, procainamide (Pronestyl) is administered by intravenous injection in amounts of 50 to 100 mg. per minute, to a total amount of 1 to 2 grams. Alternatively, lidocaine (Xylocaine)[134-136] may be given at a rate of 25 mg. per minute, to a total amount of 300 mg., and repeated at 20-minute intervals. The action of lidocaine is more transient than that of procainamide. Lidocaine has an order of effectiveness at least comparable to that of procainamide, but has a lesser hypotensive action and is therefore generally preferred.[113] When these agents are used for treatment of cardiac arrhythmias, continuous monitoring of the electrocardiogram is mandatory.

Quinidine. Parenteral quinidine is not widely employed because of the relatively high risk of untoward reaction. The delayed onset of action of quinidine when administered by the oral route limits its effectiveness in cases of ventricular tachycardia in which immediate reversal is mandatory to obviate onset of ventricular fibrillation. Direct countershock is highly effective for reversing ventricular arrhythmias. This reversal tends to be short-lived unless maintained with the aid of anti-arrhythmic drugs. Present experience suggests that electroconversion is probably safer and more predictable, [118,138,139] and that the important role of anti-arrhythmic drugs is to maintain normal rhythm after electrical conversion.

Drugs for treatment of ventricular fibrillation and arrest. In cases of ventricular fibrillation effective circulation is initially restored by cardiac massage. [140-142] Respiration is renewed by mouth-to-mouth breathing or endotracheal intubation, followed by mechanical ventilation. On occasion, ventricular fibrillation terminates spontaneously during cardiac massage. However, electroshock and, preferably, direct current countershock[143] reverse ventricular fibrillation if treatment is immediately instituted. If ventricular fibrillation persists, approximately 90 mEq. sodium bicarbonate is injected intravenously and preferably into a central venous catheter. Direct current countershock is then repeated.

If these measures fail, either isoproterenol or procainamide may be administered with a view to modifying myocardial activity during ventricular fibrillation. When ventricular fibrillatory waves are of *low* amplitude, a single intravenous injection of 20 to 50 µg. isoproterenol is advised. After the amplitude of fibrillatory waves is augmented, the D. C. shock is repeated. When the ventricular complexes are initially of *high* amplitude, procainamide or lidocaine are administered in amounts comparable to those used for treatment of ventricular tachycardia. After the amplitude of the fibrillation waves is reduced, the electrical shock is repeated.[144]

After ventricular arrest, closed chest cardiac massage precedes other treatment.[140-142] Occasionally a sharp "blow" over the precordium restores the heart beat.

Betamimetic adrenergic drugs restore an effective heart beat because of their inotropic (myocardial stimulant) and chronotropic (cardiac accelerator) actions. Epinephrine, in addition, increases peripheral resistance by its alphamimetic vasoconstrictor action, and thereby also increases coronary perfusion pressure. Since epinephrine and related sympathomimetic drugs are ineffective in an acidotic medium, [63,54] approximately 90 mEq. of sodium bicarbonate is injected intravenously, preferably through a central venous catheter. Subsequently, 3 ml. of a

1:10,000 solution of epinephrine hydrochloride is injected through the central venous catheter without interruption of cardiac massage. If asystole persists after an additional 1 to 2 minutes of massage, 20 µg of isoproterenol is injected. This is followed by 5 ml. of a 10 per cent solution of calcium chloride, or 10 ml. of a 10 per cent solution of calcium gluconate, to supplement the inotropic action. If an effective cardiac beat is still not restored, isoproterenol is infused at a rate of 3 to 10 µg per minute. Additional bicarbonate is advised if acidosis persists. Even in the absence of shock, ventricular fibrillation is successfully reversed in only approximately one-half of patients, and fewer than 25 per cent of patients recover spontaneous rhythm after cardiac asystole.[144,145] In the presence of shock or congestive heart failure, the outlook is very poor.

Alphamimetic Agents. Occasional cases of supraventricular tachycardia are reversed by the administration of alphamimetic vasoconstrictor drugs such as methoxamine in amounts of 3 to 5 mg., or phenylephrine in amounts of 0.5 to 2 mg., by slow intravenous injection.[45,146,147] The acute elevation in arterial pressure excites reflex vagotonia and depresses sinus activity and atrioventricular conduction through action mediated by the carotid sinus baroreceptors.

Conversely, sinus bradycardia may of itself complicate the use of vasoactive drugs with alpha or alpha-beta adrenergic activity, including methoxamine, phenylephrine, levarterenol and metaraminol. Isoproterenol and other epinephrine-like drugs with a primary betamimetic action may precipitate supraventricular or ventricular tachycardia. Reduction of the dosage of these drugs may terminate the arrhythmia.

Betamimetic Agents. Since shock may follow critical reductions in ventricular rate, epinephrine-like drugs with chronotropic action, such as ephedrine, have been widely used for the treatment of atrioventricular block. In recent years, the introduction of relatively pure betamimetic isoproterenol has greatly improved the success with which patients with complete heart block are managed. This drug is infused intravenously in amounts of 2 to 10 µg per minute. The ventricular rate is usually increased in direct relationship to the amount administered. Large doses of isoproterenol may precipitate hypotension because of the drug's vasodilator action on the peripheral arterial bed. Isoproterenol is unstable in saline, so it is preferable to add the drug to a 5 per cent glucose solution. Each solution should be freshly prepared at intervals of 8 hours. The electrode catheter inserted into the right ventricle for pacing is a preferred alternative to pharmacological treatment of heart block.[130-133]

Betalytic Drugs. Beta adrenergic blocking drugs are now regarded as potentially valuable for the treatment of both supraventricular and ventricular arrhythmias.[91,145,148-150] The betalytic drugs specifically block the chronotropic and inotropic actions (more specifically, the betamimetic actions) of adrenergic drugs. Since the betamimetic action of adrenergic agents or autonomic stimuli excites premature ventricular contractions and ventricular tachycardia, prevention of such effects by treatment with betalytic drugs has been regarded as potentially useful and clinical benefits have been reported.[39,151,152] Some of the betalytic agents like propranolol, but not MJ 1999, also exhibit a direct depressant effect on the heart, independent of their betalytic actions.

OTHER AGENTS AND PROCEDURES

Diuretics. Diuretic agents are ineffective during shock when renal perfusion is critically reduced. We regard the intravenous administration of aminophylline during shock as particularly hazardous.[153] A selectively high incidence of cardiac arrest has been observed immediately after its slow injection.[154] Osmolar diuretics, including mannitol and urea, are used for prevention of renal failure. However, their use also includes hazard since the increase in osmolar load and consequently in intravascular volume may precipitate acute congestive heart failure.

Corticosteroid and hormones. There is no evidence that adrenal insufficiency is a factor in the development of shock after acute myocardial infarction. To the contrary, plasma cortisol levels during shock are 3 to 17 times greater than normal values at rest.[155] Moreover, glucocorticoids in themselves do not potentiate the pressor effect of vasoactive drugs.[156]

Glucocorticoids reportedly decreased both the mortality and the area of residual fibrosis in experimental myocardial infarction.[157] Other studies have failed to confirm this.[158] Aldosterone is reported to have beneficial effects in experimental endotoxic shock,[159] but there have been no comparable observations in shock due to myocardial infarction. With the exception of heart block, and then only in a minority of instances, glucocorticoids are not of proven value for the management of either acute myocardial infarction or myocardial shock.[160]

In patients who have prior Addison's disease of unrelated cause or who have adrenocortical suppression due to prolonged treatment with corticosteroid hormones, requirements for maintenance doses of corticosteroid are tripled during the acute period after myocardial infarction. However, the same applies to all major physical stresses in the case of patients with adrenocortical insufficiency and is not a selective circumstance related to myocardial infarction or myocardial shock.

Heparin. Thrombotic occlusion of small blood vessels or increased coagulability and "sludging" is regarded by some workers as a potentially important factor accounting for progression of shock.[161 164] The routine use of heparin, advised for prevention of macrothromboembolic complications in patients with acute myocardial infarction,[165] is also defended on this basis.

Fibrinolysin. The rationale for administration of fibrinolysin is (1) dissolution of thrombotic or embolic obstruction of the coronary circuit and (2) prevention of extension of the infarct, securing maximal perfusion and viability of adjacent ischemic myocardium.[166,167] Intravenous infusion of fibrinolysin (Thrombolysin, Actase) reportedly does lyse recently formed thrombi in coronary arteries and reduces peripheral microthrombi related to shock. However, fibrinolysin has not clearly altered the mortality rate of acute myocardial infarction, whether or not complicated by shock.[168] In fact, its administration was followed by a decrease in myocardial contractility and a fall in arterial pressure.[169] When large amounts of fibrinolysin were administered, prothrombin and fibrinogen concentrations were critically reduced and hemorrhage complicated the subsequent course.[167] In 116 patients with myocardial infarction, Richter[170] was unable to demonstrate that fibrinolysin had any advantage when compared to treatment with anticoagulants. For these reasons, its use cannot be recommended at present.

Dextran. Low viscous or low molecular weight dextran (Rheomacrodex) has a molecular weight of approximately 40,000. It is not a plasma expander, since the small molecules diffuse relatively rapidly out of the vascular compartment. However, this solution promotes blood flow by decreasing viscosity and sludging.[171,172] Its specific value as an adjunct for treatment of myocardial shock is not established. Low molecular weight dextran is still an experimental drug in the United States and is only available for investigation.

Buffers. There is no convincing evidence that treatment of acidosis by infusion of alkaline solutions alters the underlying defect or improves the outcome of the patient in shock.[173] To the contrary, experiments by several investigators indicate a higher mortality when this type of acidosis is reversed, and blood pH is restored to within normal ranges by infusion of buffer solutions.[174]

THAM (Tris-hydroxyaminomethane), an organic buffer, enjoyed brief popularity.[175] Unlike sodium lactate or sodium bicarbonate, this buffer is distributed throughout the body, including the intracellular compartment. Its diuretic activity offers a minor advantage. Although this organic buffer, like sodium bicarbonate, reverses acidosis, it also fails to repair the fundamental metabolic defects that underlie perfusion failure. It has toxic effects, including respiratory depression, and has not been approved for routine clinical use in the United States.

Mechanical support of the circulation. Augmentation of cardiac output and/or blood pressure to decrease the work load on the heart is being seriously investigated. Mechanical measures which would supply the pumping action to assure adequate systemic and coronary artery flow would be desirable for sustaining these patients during the most critical period following onset of shock. Veno-arterial bypass[176-180] and synchronized arterial counterpulsation[181,182] have been examined. However, additional investigation and controlled trials are needed before the feasibility, hazards and value of such mechanical supports are established. None are developed to the point where clinical use in other than an investigative environment would be feasible.

CONCLUSION

After myocardial infarction, shock threatens immediate survival. Even under optimal conditions in coronary care units, myocardial shock is fatal in two-thirds of all cases. Heroic maneuvers of unproven value are often undertaken that particularly outside of an investigative environment, are likely to entail greater risks than gains.

Vasopressor drugs to increase arterial pressure are now less commonly used and drugs which act primarily to improve blood flow are receiving greater attention. The conventional alphamimetic vasopressor drugs, including methoxamine and phenylephrine, tend to increase arterial pressure by increasing arterial resistance without corresponding increase in effective blood flow. However, betamimetic agents such as isoproterenol and alphalytic drugs such as phentolamine effectively increase blood flow under some circumstances, even though they may lower arterial pressure. The combination of an alpha-beta adrenergic agent, either levarterenol or metaraminol, and alphalytic phentolamine is probably the best compromise for optimal pressor-perfusion actions. Digitalis glycosides remain the

TABLE 1
Management of Shock Due to Myocardial Infarction

Condition	Treatment	Guides
Pain	Morphine sulfate, 10 mg. i.v.	Symptomatic relief
Nausea	Dimehydrinate (Dramamine), 50 mg. i.v.	Symptomatic relief
Hypoxia	Oxygen, 100% by pressure tight face mask, flow 6–8 L. /min.	Arterial O_2 saturation or PO_2, PCO_2, pH
Hypotension	Metaraminol (Aramine), 0.05 to 1.50 mg./min. in 5% G/W i.v. to maintain systolic pressure 30 mm. Hg. below "normal" level; levophed (Levarterenol) 3 to 30 μg and phentolamine (Regitine) 0.1 to 1 mg./min.	Arterial pressure Urine flow Peripheral pulses Skin temperature
Congestive heart failure	Digoxin (Lanoxin), 0.75 mg. i.v. followed by 1 to 3 subsequent injections of 0.25 mg. at 1/2 to 3 hr. intervals; lanatoside C (Cedilanid) if previously digitalized 0.2 to 0.4 mg. i.v. at 1 hr. intervals for total of 0.4 to 1.2 mg.	Central venous pressure; circulation time (cardiac output)
Arrhythmia		
Atrial tachycardia, flutter, fibrillation	Digoxin; methoxamine (Vasoxyl), 3 to 5 mg. i. v.; phenylephrine (Neo-Synephrine) 0.5 to 2 mg. i. v.; diphenylhydantoin (Dilantin) 250 mg. i.v. followed by 100 to 200 mg. i. v. at 4 to 6 hr. intervals	Electrocardiogram
Ventricular tachycardia	Lidocaine (Xylocaine), 25 mg./min. until arrhythmia terminated, or up to a maximum of 300 mg. i. v.; diphenylhydantoin	Electrocardiogram
Ventricular fibrillation	Resuscitation; D. C. countershock	Electrocardiogram
Sinus bradycardia	Atropine sulfate, 1 mg. i. v.	Electrocardiogram
Atrioventricular block	Isoproterenol (Isuprel), 5 mg./L. of 5% G/W i. v. infusion rate to increase ventricular rate to between 60 and 80 beats/min.	Electrocardiogram
Digitalis toxicity	Potassium chloride, 40 to 100 mEq. in 500 to 1000 ml. 5% G/W or 85% saline i. v.; diphenylhydantoin	Electrocardiogram Serum potassium
Thromboembolism	Heparin, 5000 to 7500 units i. v. q 4 hr.	Coagulation time

mainstay for treatment of congestive heart failure.

Ventilatory failure and acute hypoxia are now recognized as immediate causes of fatal arrhythmias. Close attention to the effectiveness of ventilation and gas exchange by measurement of pH, PCO_2 or arterial oxygen saturation is especially desirable. Mechanical ventilation and, in selected cases, endotracheal intubation and neuromuscular paralysis may be required to restore adequate gas exchange.

Improved methods of controlling arrhythmias by both pharmacological and electrical means are also likely to improve the outcome.

Based on the experimental and clinical data included in this review, a program for management of shock due to myocardial infarction is outlined in Table 1. The effective use of this guide makes it possible to improve objective diagnosis and allows for continuing assessment of the response to treatment. Routine employment of a central venous catheter is advised. The ultimate value of a well-ordered approach based on objective measurements of clinical and hemodynamic status is firmly established.

REFERENCES

1. Binder, M. J., Ryan, J. A., Marcus, S., Mugler, F., Strange, D., and Agress, C. M.: (Review) Evaluation of therapy in shock following acute myocardial infarction. Amer. J. Med., *18:*622, 1955.
2. Malach, M., and Rosenberg, B. A.: Acute myocardial infarction in a city hospital. III. Experiences with shock. Amer. J. Cardiol., *5:*487, 1960.
3. Wahlberg, F.: A study of myocardial infarction at the Seraphimer Hospital during 1950–1959. Amer. Heart J., *65:*749, 1963.
4. Day, H. W.: Effectiveness of an intensive coronary care area. Amer. J. Cardiol., *15:*51, 1965.
5. Griffith, G. C., Wallace, W. B., Cochran, B., Nierlick, W. E., and Frasher, W. G.: The treatment of shock associated with myocardial infarction. Circulation, *9:*527, 1954.
6. Agress, C. M.: Therapy of cardiogenic shock. Prog. Cardiovasc. Dis., *6:*236, 1963.
7. Littler, T. R., and McKendrick, C. S.: L-noradrenalin in myocardial infarction. Lancet, *2:*825, 1957.
8. Binder, M. J.: Effect of vasopressor drugs on circulatory dynamics in shock following myocardial infarction. Amer. J. Cardiol., *16:*834, 1965.
9. Weil, M. H., and Shubin, H. (eds.): Diagnosis and treatment of shock. Williams & Wilkins, 1967.
10. Weil, M. H., Shubin, H., and Rosoff, L.: Fluid repletion in circulatory shock: Central venous pressure and other practical guides. J.A.M.A., *192:*668, 1965.
11. Zahn, R. L., and Weil, M. H.: Central veonus blood for monitoring pH and PCO_2 in the critically ill patient. J. Thoracic and Cardiovasc. Surg., *52:*105, 1966.
12. Meagher, P. F., Jensen, R. E., Weil, M. H., and Shubin, H.: Measurement of respiration rate from central venous pressure in the critically ill patient. IEEE Transactions on Biomed. Engineering, *13:*54, 1966.
13. Freis, E. D., Schnaper, H. W., Johnson, R. L., and Schreiner, G. E.: Hemodynamic alterations in acute myocardial infarction. I. Cardiac output, mean arterial pressure, total peripheral resistance, "central" and total blood volume, venous pressure and average circulation time. J. Clin. Invest., *31:*131, 1952.
14. Smith, W. W., Wikler, N. S., and Fox, A. C.: Hemodynamic studies of patients with myocardial infarction. Circulation, *9:*352, 1954.
15. Gilbert, R. P., Goldberg, M., and Griffin, J.: Circulatory changes in acute myocardial infarction. Circulation, *9:*847, 1954.
16. Gammil, J. F., Applegarth, J. J., Reed, C. E., Fernald, J. D., and Antenucci, A. J.: Hemodynamic changes following acute myocardial infarction using the dye injection. Method for cardiac output determination. Ann. Int. Med., *43:*100, 1955.
17. Lee, G. de J.: Total and peripheral blood flow in acute myocardial infarction. Brit. Heart J., *19:*116, 1957.
18. Broch, O. J., Humerfeld, S., Haarstad, J., and Myhre, J. R.: Hemodynamic studies in acute myocardial infarction. Amer. Heart J., *57:*522, 1959.
19. Malmcrona, R., Schröder, G., and Werkö, L.: Hemodynamic effects of metaraminol. II: Patients with acute myocardial infarction. Amer. J. Cardiol., *13:*15, 1964.
20. Shubin, H., and Weil, M. H.: Hemodynamic alterations in patients after myocardial infarction. *In* Shock and Hypotension, ed. by Mills, L. C. and Moyer, J. H. New York, Grune and Stratton, 1965, p. 499.
21. Thomas, M., Malmcrona, R., and Shillingford, J.: Circulatory changes associated with systemic hypotension in patients with acute myocardial infarction. Brit. Heart J., *28:*108, 1966.
22. Gunnar, R. M., Cruz, A., Boswell, J., Co, B. S., Pietras, R. J., and Tobin, J. R.: Myocardial infarction with shock. Hemodynamic studies and results of therapy. Circulation, *33:*753, 1966.
23. Kaindl, F., and Lindner, A.: Zur pharmakalogic und Klinischen Anwendung des nor-adrenalins. Wein Ztschr. im Med., *31:*377, 1950.
24. Liljedahl, S. O., and Norlander, O.: Noradrenalin vid behandling av operativ circulationskoppaps. Svenska lak., *48:*2762, 1951.
25. Miller, A. J., and Baker, L. A.: L-arterenol (Levophed) in treatment of shock due to myocardial infarction. A.M.A. Arch. Int. Med., *89:*591, 1952.
26. Kurland, G. S., and Malach, M.: Clinical use of norepinephrine in the treatment of shock accompanying myocardial infarction and other conditions. New Eng. J. Med., *247:*383, 1952.
27. Calenda, D. G., Uricchio, J. F., and Friedman, L. M.: Management of shock in myocardial infarction with *l*-norepinephrine. Amer. J. Med. Sci., *226:*399, 1953.
28. Weil, M. H.: Clinical studies on a vasopressor agent: Metaraminol (Aramine). II. Observations on its use in the management of shock. Amer. J. Med. Sci., *230:*357, 1955.
29. Gorlin, R.: Modern treatment of coronary occlusion

and insufficiency. Med. Clin. N. Am., *46:*1243, 1962.

30. Corday, E., and Williams, J. H., Jr.: Effect of shock and of vasopressor drugs on the regional circulation of the brain, kidney and liver. Amer. J. Med., *29:* 228, 1960.

31. Swingle, W. W., Kleinberg, W., Remington, S. W., Eversde, J. W., and Overman, R. R.: Experimental analysis of the nervous factor in shock induced by muscle trauma in dogs. Amer. J. Physiol., *141:*54, 1944.

32. Glasser, O., and Page, I. H.: Hemorrhagic shock-production and treatment. Amer. J. Physiol., *154:* 297, 1948.

33. Wiggers, H. C., Roemhild, F., Goldberg, H., and Ingrahma, R. C.: Dibenamine in hemorrhagic shock. Fed. Proc., *6:*226, 1947.

34. Nickerson, M.: Sympathetic blockade in the therapy of shock. Amer. J. Cardiol., *12:*619, 1963.

35. Lillehei, R. C., Lillehei, C. W., Grishmer, J. T., and Levy, M. J.: Plasma catecholamines in open-heart surgery; prevention of their pernicious effects by pretreatment with Dibenzyline. Surg. Forum, *14:* 269, 1963.

36. Indeglia, R. A., Levy, M. J., Lillehei, R. C., Todd, D. B., and Lillehei, C. W. (U.): Correlation of plasma catecholamines, renal function, and the effects of Dibenzyline on cardiac patients undergoing corrective surgery. J. Thoracic and Cardiovasc. Surg., *51:*244, 1966.

37. Weil, M. H. (ed.): Circulatory shock: A symposium on advances in our understanding of mechanisms and treatment. Calif. Med., *103:*310, 1965.

38. Ahlquist, R. P.: A study of the adrenotropic receptors. Amer. J. Physiol., *153:*586, 1948.

39. Moran, N. C.: Adrenergic receptors, drugs and the cardiovascular system I and II. Mod. Conc. Cardiovasc. Dis., *35:*93, 1966.

40. Weil, M. H., Lewis, C. M., Allen, K. S., and Silver, A.: Venoconstriction, a pharmacologic effect of unrecognized importance in selection of vasopressor agents. Fed. Proc., *22:*101, 1963.

41. Freeman, N. E.: Decrease in blood volume after prolonged hyperactivity of the sympathetic nervous system. Amer. J. Physiol., *103:*185, 1933.

42. Schmutzer, K. L., Raschke, E., and Maloney, J. V., Jr.: Intravenous *l*-norepinephrine as a cause of reduced plasma volume. Surgery, *50:*452, 1961.

43. Guss, J. H.: Chronic shock after myocardial infarction, its mechanisms and management. Ann. Int. Med., *58:*333, 1963.

44. Spoerel, W. E., Seleny, F. L., and Williamson, R. D.: Shock caused by continuous infusion of metaraminol bitartrate (Aramine). Canad. Med. Assoc. J., *90:* 349, 1964.

45. Gootnick, A., and Knox, F. H.: Management of shock in acute myocardial infarction. Circulation, *7:*511, 1953.

46. Gazes, P. C., Goldberg, L. I., and Darby, T. D.: Heart force effects of sympathomimetic amine as basis for their use in shock accompanying myocardial infarction. Circulation, *8:*883, 1953.

47. West, J. W., Faulk, A. T., and Guzman, S. V.: Comparative study of effects of levarterenol and methoxamine in shock associated with acute myocardial ischemias in dogs. Circ. Res., *10:*712, 1962.

48. del Greco, F., and Johnson, D. C.: Clinical experience with angiotensin II in the treatment of shock. J.A.M.A., *178:*994, 1961.

49. Derrick, J. R., Anderson, J. R., and Ronald, B. J.: Adjunctive use of biological pressor agent, angiotensin, in management of shock. Circulation, *25:* 263, 1962.

50. Udhoji, V. N., and Weil, M. H.: Circulatory effects of angiotensin levaraterenol and metaraminol in the treatment of shock. New Eng. J. Med., *270:*501, 1964.

51. Beanlands, D. S., and Gunton, R. W.: Angiotensin II in the treatment of shock following myocardial infarction. Amer. J. Cardiol., *14:*370, 1964.

52. Hellerstein, H. K., Brofman, B. L., and Caskey, W. H.: Shock accompanying myocardial infarction. Treatment with pressor amines. Amer. Heart J., *44:*407, 1952.

53. Li, T. H., Shimosato, S., and Etsten, B.: Hemodynamics of mephentermine in man, New Eng. J. Med., *267:*180, 1962.

54. Bernstein, A., Simon, F., Rothfelf, E. J., Robins, B., Cohen, F. B., and Kaufman, J. G.: Treatment of shock in myocardial infarction. Amer. J. Cardiol., *9:*74, 1962.

55. Udhoji, V. N., and Weil, M. H.: Vasodilator action of a "pressor amine, " mephentermine (Wyamine), in circulatory shock. Amer. J. Cardiol., *16:*841, 1965.

56. MacLean, L. D., Duff, J. H., Scott, H. M., and Peretz, D. I.: Treatment of shock in man based on hemodynamic diagnosis. Surg. Gynec. Obstet., *120:*1, 1965.

57. Bradley, E. C., and Weil, M. H.: Treatment of circulatory shock with a betamimetic agent. Abst. Circulation, *32:*57, 1965.

58. Weil, M. H., and Shubin, H.: Editorial. Isoproterenol for the treatment of circulatory shock. Ann. Int. Med., *70:*638, 1969.

59. Gunnar, R. M., Loch, H. S., Pietras, R. J., and Tobin, J. R.: Ineffectiveness of isoproterenol in shock due to acute myocardial infarction. J.A.M.A., *202:*1124, 1967.

60. Von Euler, V. S.: Some aspects of the role of noradrenaline and adrenaline in circulation. Amer. Heart J., *56:*469, 1968.

61. Sarnoff, S. J., Case, R. B., Berglund, E., and Sarnoff, L. C.: Ventricular function. V. The circulatory effects of Aramine. Mechanism of action of "vasopressor" drugs in cardiogenic shock. Circulation, *10:*84, 1954.

62. Harrison, D. C., Chidsey, C. A., and Braunwald, E.: Studies on the mechanism of action of metaraminol (Aramine). Ann. Int. Med, *59:*297, 1963.

63. Burget, G. E., and Visscher, M. B.: Variations of the pH of the blood and the response of the vascular system to adrenalin. Amer. J. Physiol., *81:*113, 1927.

64. Houle, D. B., Weil, M. H., Brown, E. B., and Campbell, G. S.: Influence of respiratory acidosis on ECG and pressor responses to epinephrine, norepinephrine and metaraminol. Proc. Soc. Exp. Biol. Med., *94:*561, 1957.

65. Agress, C. M., and Binder, M. J.: Cardiogenic shock. Amer. Heart J., *54:*458, 1957.

66. Constantin, L.: Extracardiac factors contributing to hypotension during coronary occlusion. Amer. J. Cardiol., *11:*205, 1963.

67. Guzman, S. T., Swenson, E., and Mitchell, R.: Mechanism of cardiogenic shock. Circ. Res., *10:*

746, 1962.

68. Freeman, N. E., Schaeffer, S. A., Schecter, A. E., and Holling, H. E.: The effect of total sympathectomy on the occurrence of shock after hemorrhage. J. Clin. Invest., 17:359, 1938.

69. Collins, V. J., Jaffe, R. J. and Zahony, I.: Newer attitudes in management of hemorrhagic shock. The use of chlorpromazine as an adjunct. Surg. Clin. N. Am., 44, 1:173, 1964.

70. Weil, M. H., and Allen, K. S.: Comparison of sympathetic blocking drugs in prevention of lethal effects of endotoxin. Proc. Soc. Exp. Biol. Med., 115:627, 1964.

71. Aviado, D. M.: Hemodynamic effects of ganglionic blocking drugs. Circ. Res., 8:304, 1962.

72. Nickerson, M., and Gourzis, J. T.: Blockade of sympathetic vasoconstriction in the treatment of shock. J. Trauma, 2:399, 1962.

73. Lillehei, R. C., Longerbeam, J. K., Bloch, J. H., and Manax, W. G., The modern treatment of shock based on physiologic principles. Clin. Pharmacol. Therap., 5:63, 1964.

74. Sukhnandan, R., and Thal, A. P.: The effect of endotoxin and vasoactive agents on Dibenzyline-pretreated lungs. Surgery, 58:185, 1965.

75. Bloch, J. H., Pierce, C. H., and Lillehei, R. C.: Reduction of external cardiac work in the treatment of cardiogenic shock. Circulation, 32:Suppl. II. 52, 1965.

76. Bradley, E. C.: Results with phentolamine (Regitine) in the treatment of selected patients with shock. In Circulatory Shock, A symposium on advances in our understanding of mechanisms and treatment. Ed. by Weil, M. H. Calif. Med, 103:314, 1965.

77. Powell, C. E., and Slater, I. H.: Blocking of inhibitory adrenergic receptors by a dichloro analogue of isoproterenol. J. Pharmacol. Exptl. Therap., 122: 480, 1958.

78. Moran, N. C., and Perkins, M. E.: Adrenergic blockade of the mammalian heart by a dichloro analogue of isoproterenol. J. Pharmacol. Exptl. Therap., 124:223, 1958.

79. Black, J. W., and Stephenson, J. S.: Pharmacology of a new adrenergic-beta-receptor-blocking compound (Nethalide). Lancet, 2:311, 1962.

80. Dornhorst, A. C., and Robinson, B. F.: Clinical pharmacology of a beta-adrenergic-blocking agent (Nethalide). Lancet, 2:314, 1962.

81. Black, J. W., Crowther, A. F., Shanks, R. G., Smith, L. H., and Dornhorst, A. C.: New adrenergic beta-receptor antagonist. Lancet, 1:1080, 1964.

82. Lish, P.: Personal communication.

83. Paget, G. E.: Carcinogenic action of pronethalol. Brit. Med. J., 2:1266, 1963.

84. Schroder, G., and Werkö, L.: Hemodynamic studies and clinical experience with nethalide, a beta-adrenergic blocking agent. Amer. J. Cardiol., 15: 58, 1965.

85. Gillam, P. M. S., and Prichard, B. N. C.: Use of propanolol in angina pectoris. Brit. Med. J., 2:337, 1965.

86. Hamer, J., Grandjean, T., Melendez, L., and Sowton, G. E.: Effect of propanolol (Inderal) on exercise tolerance in angina pectoris. Brit. Heart J., 28:414, 1966.

87. Harrison, D. C., Braunwald, E., Glick, G., Mason, D. T., Chidsey, C. A., and Ross, J., Jr.: Effects of beta adrenergic blockade on the circulation with particular reference to observations in patients with hypertropic subaortic stenosis. Circulation, 29:84, 1964.

88. Epstein, S. E., Robinson, B. F., Kahler, R. L., and Braunwald, E.: Effects of beta-adrenergic blockade on the cardiac response to maximal and submaximal exercise in man. J. Clin. Invest., 44:1745, 1965.

89. Lowria, M. H., Miller, A. J., and Kaplan, B. M.: Successful therapy of prolonged hypotension with an adrenergic beta-receptor blocking agent. Circulation, 29:Suppl.: 494, 1964.

90. Harris, W. S., Schoenfeld, C. D., Brooks, R. H., and Weissler, A. M.: Effect of beta adrenergic blockade on the hemodynamic responses to epinephrine in man. Amer. J. Cardiol., 17:484, 1966.

91. Rowlands, D. J., Howitt, G. and Markman, P.: Propanolol (Inderal) in disturbance of cardiac rhythm. Brit. Med. J., 1:891, 1965.

92. Morphine and demerol. The Medical Letter, No.4: 13, 1962.

93. Bauer, F.: Some observations on the peripheral circulation in patients with myocardial infarction. Angiology, 6:6, 1955.

94. Altschule, M. D.: Hazards in the treatment of cardiac decompensation. New Eng. J. Med., 248: 493, 1953.

95. Weil, M. H., and Sudrann, R. B.: Cardiovascular effects of hydroxyzine. Amer. J. Cardiol., 6:1085, 1960.

96. MacKenzie, G. J., Taylor, S. H., McDonald, A. H., and Donald, K. W.: Hemodynamic effects of external cardiac compression. Lancet, 1:1342, 1964.

97. Sayen, J. J., Katcher, A. H., Sheldon, W. F., and Gilbert, C. M., Jr.: The effect of levarterenol on polargographic myocardial oxygen, the epicardial electrocardiogram and contraction in non-ischemic hearts and experimental acute regional ischemia. Cir. Res., 8:109, 1960.

98. Carrier, O., Walker, J. R., and Guyton, A. C.: The role of oxygen in autoregulation of blood flow in isolated vessels. Amer J. Physiol., 206:951, 1964.

99. Smith, G., and Lawson, D. A.: Experimental coronary arterial occlusion: Effects of the administration of oxygen under pressure. Scot. Med. J., 3:346, 1958.

100. Illingworth, Sir C.: Treatment of arterial occlusion under oxygen at two atmospheres pressure. Brit. Med. J., 2:1271, 1962.

101. Burnett, W., Clark, R. G., Duthie, H. L., and Smith, A. N.: The treatment of shock by oxygen under pressure. Scot. Med. J., 4:535, 1959.

102. Kuhn, L. A., Kline, H. J., Wang, M., Yamaki, T., and Jacobson, J. H.: Hemodynamic effects of hyperbaric oxygen in experimental acute myocardial infarction. Circul. Res., 16:499, 1965.

103. Jacobson, J. H., Wang, M. C. H., Yamaki, T., Kline, H. J., Kark, A. E., and Kuhn, L. A.: Hyperbaric oxygenation—diffuse myocardial infarction. Arch. Surg., 89:905, 1964.

104. Trapp, W. G., and Creighton, R.: Experimental studies of increased atmospheric pressure on myocardial ischemia after coronary ligation. J. Thoracic Cardiovasc. Surg., 47:687, 1964.

105. Moon, A. J., Williams, K. G., and Hopkinson, W. I.: A patient with coronary thrombosis treated with

hyperbaric oxygen. Lancet, *1:*18, 1964.

106. Smith, G., and Lawson, D. D.: The protective effect of inhalation of oxygen at two atmospheres absolute pressure. Surg. Gynec. and Obst., *114:*320, 1962.

107. Cameron, A. J. V., Gibb, B. H., Ledingham, I. McA., and McGuinness, J. B.: Controlled clinical trial of hyperbaric oxygen in the treatment of acute myocardial infarction. *In* Hyperbaric Oxygenation, Proceedings of the Second International Congress, Glasgow, Sept. 1964. Ed. by Ledingham, I. McA. Edinburgh, E. & S. Levingston, 1965, p. 277.

108. Saltzman, H. A.: Use of hyperbaric oxygenation in cardiovascular disease. Modern Concepts of Cardiovascular Disease, *35:*87, May 1966.

109. McDowall, D. G.: Hyperbaric oxygen in relation to circulatory and respiratory emergencies. Brit. J. Anaesth., *36:*563, 1964.

110. Comroe, J. H., Dripps, R. D., Dumke, P. R., and Deming, M.: Oxygen toxicity. J.A.M.A. *128:*710 1945.

111. Master, A. M., Weiser, F. M., and Rabin, R.: The emergency treatment of the complications of acute coronary artery occlusion. Dis. of the Chest, *42:*457, 1962.

112. Gilchrist, A. R.: Problems in management of acute myocardial infarction. Brit. Med. J., *1:*215, 1960.

113. Dack, S.: Postoperative myocardial infarction. Amer. J. Cardiol., *12:*423, 1963.

114. Cronin, R. E. P., and Zsoter, T.: Hemodynamic effects of rapid digitalization in experimental cardiogenic shock. Amer. Heart J., *69:*233, 1965.

115. Marano, A. J., Kline, H. J., Cestero, J., and Kuhn, L. A.: Hemodynamic effects on ouabain in experimental acute myocardial infarction with shock. Amer. J. Cardiol., *17:*327, 1966.

116. Braunwald, E., Bloodwell, R. O., Goldberg, L. I., and Morrow, A. G.: Studies on digitalis. IV. Observations in man on the effect of digitalis preparation on the contractility of the non-failing heart and on the total vascular resistance. J. Clin. Invest., *40:*52, 1964.

117. Selzer, A., and Kelly, J. J., Jr.: Action of digitalis upon the nonfailing heart:A critical review. Progr. Cardiovasc. Dis., *7:*273, 1964.

118. Lown, B., Amarasingham, R. and Neuman, J.: New method for terminating cardiac arrhythmias: Use of synchronized capacitor discharge. J.A.M.A., *182:* 548, 1962.

119. Killip, T.: Synchronized DC precordial shock for arrhythmias: Safe new technique to establish normal rhythm may be utilized on an elective or an emergency basis. J.A.M.A., *186:*1, 1963.

120. Harris, S. A., and Kokernot, R. H.: Effects of diphenylhydantoin sodium (Dilantin sodium) and phenobarbital sodium upon ectopic ventricular tachycardia in acute myocardial infarction. Amer. J. Physiol., *163:*505, 1950.

121. Mosey, L. and Tyler, M. D.: The effect of diphenylhydantoin sodium (Dilantin), procaine hydrochloride, procaine amide hydrochloride and quinidine hydrochloride upon ouabain-induced ventricular tachycardia in unanesthetized dogs. Circulation *10:*65, 1954.,

122. Conn, R. D.: Diphenylhydantoin sodium in cardiac arrhythmias. New Eng. J. Med., *272:*277, 1965.

123. Mixter, C. G., Moran, J. M., and Austen, W. G.: Cardiac and peripheral vascular effects of diphenyl-hydantoin sodium. Amer. J. Cardiol., *17:*332, 1966.

124. Thomas, M., and Woodgate, D.: Effect of atropine on bradycardia and hypotension in acute myocardial infarction. Brit. Heart J., *28:*409, 1966.

125. Ponce de Leon, J. J., Oriol-Palon, A., and Sodi-Pallares, D.: Evolucion clinica en el infarcto agudo del miocardiotratado con la solucion polarizante de glucosa, insulina y potasio. Memorias del IV Congreso Mundial de Cardiologia. Mexico., *4B:* 209, 1962.

126. Day, H. W., and Averill, K.: Recorded arrhythmias in an acute coronary care area. Dis. Chest, *49:* 113, 1966.

127. Dall, J. L. G., and Buchanan, J.: Steroid therapy in heart block following myocardial infarction. Lancet, *2:*8, 1962.

128. Phelps, M. D., Jr., and Lindsay, J. D., Jr.: Cortisone in Stokes-Adams disease secondary to myocardial infarction. New Eng. J. Med., *256:*204, 1957.

129. Prinzmetal, M., and Kennamer, R.: Emergency treatment of cardiac arrhythmias. J.A.M.A., *154:* 1049, 1954.

130. DeSanctis, R. W.: Short-term use of intravenous electrode in heart block. J. A. M. A., *184:*544, 1963.

131. Levy, L., and Albert, H. M.: Therapy of complete heart block complicating recent myocardial infarction. J. A. M. A., *187:*617, 1964.

132. Samet, P., Jacobs, W., and Bernstein, W. H.: Electrode catheter pacemaker in treatment of complete heart block in presence of acute myocardial infarction. Amer. J. Cardiol., *11:*379, 1963.

133. Yuceoglu, Y. Z., Lunger, M., and Dresdale, D. T.: Transvenous electrical pacing of the heart. Amer. Heart J., *71:*5, 1966.

134. Kimmey, J. R., and Steinhaus, J. E.: Cardiovascular effects of procaine and lidocaine (Xylocaine) during general anesthesia. Acta. Anaesth. Scadinav., *3:*9, 1959.

135. Weiss, M. A.: Intravenous use of lidocaine for ventricular arrhythmias. Anesth. & Analg., *39:*369 1960.

136. Harrison, D. C., Sprouse, J. H., and Morrow, A. G.: The anti-arrhythmic properties of lidocaine and procaine amide. Clinical and physiologic studies of their cardiovascular effects in man. Circulation, *28:* 486, 1963.

137. Austen, W. G., and Moran, J. M.: Cardiac and peripheral vascular effects of lidocaine and procaine amide. Amer. J. Cardiol., *16:*701, 1965.

138. Alexander, S., Kleiger, R., and Lown, B.: Use of external electric countershock in the treatment of ventricular tachycardia. J.A.M.A., *177:*916, 1961.

139. Robinson, J. S., Sloman, G., Hjorth, R., and Goble, A. J.: Direct current countershock in cardiac arrhythmias. Med. J. of Australia, *1:*289, 1965.

140. Kouwenhoven, W. B., Judge, J.R., and Knickerbocker G. G.: Closed chest cardiac massage. J.A.M.A., *173:*1064, 1960.

141. Jude, J. R., Kouwenhoven, W. B. and Knickerbocker, G. G.: Cardiac arrest: Report of application of external cardiac massage in 118 patients. J.A.M.A., *178:*1063, 1961.

142. Minogue, W. F., Smessart, A. A., and Grace, W. J.: External cardiac massage for cardiac arrest due to myocardial infarction. Amer. J. Cardiol., *13:*25, 1964.

143. Lown, B., Neuman, J., Amarasingham, R., and Berkovits, B. V.: Comparison of alternatiing current with direct current electroshock across the closed chest. Amer. J. Cardiol., *10:*223, 1962.

144. Robinson, J. S., Sloman, G., Mathew, T. H., and Goble, A. J.: Survival after resuscitation from cardiac arrest in acute myocardial infarction. Amer. Heart J., *69:*740, 1965.

145. Stock, E.: Assessment of management of cardiac resuscitation. Med. J. of Australia, *1:*565, 1966.

146. Corday, E., and Irving, D. W.: Disturbances of heart rate, rhythm and conduction. Philadelphia, W. B. Saunders, 1961, pp. 207-224, 300-311.

147. Youmans, W. B., Goodman, M. J., and Gould, J.: Neo-synephrine in treatment of paroxysmal supraventricular tachycardia. Amer. Heart J., *37:*359, 1949.

148. Stock, J. P. P., and Dale, N.: Beta-adrenergic receptor blockade in cardiac arrhythmias. Brit. Med. J., *11:*1230, 1963.

149. Taylor, R. R., Johnston, C. I., and Jose, A. D.: Reversal of digitalis intoxication by beta-adrenergic blockade with pronethalol. New Eng. J. Med., *271:*877, 1964.

150. Sloman, G., Robinson, J. S., and McLean, K.: Propanolol (Inderal) in persistent ventricular fibrillation. Brit. Med. J., *1:*895, 1965.

151. Taylor, R. R., and Halliday, E. J.: Beta-adrenergic blockade in the treatment of exercise induced paroxysmal ventricular tachycardia. Circulation, *32:*778, 1965.

152. Erlij, D., and Mendez, R.: The modification of digitalis intoxication by excluding adrenergic influences on the heart. J. Pharmacol. and Exper. Therap., *144:*97, 1964.

153. Merrill, G. A.: Aminophylline deaths. J.A.M.A., *123:*1115, 1943.

154. Camarata, S. J., Bradley, E. C., and Weil, M. H.: A study of 150 cardiac arrests with implications for treatment. Unpublished data.

155. Klein, A. J., and Palmer, L. A.: Plasma cortisol in myocardial infarction. Amer. J. Cardiol., *11:*332, 1963.

156. Shubin, H., and Weil, M. H.: Failure of corticosteroid to potentiate sympathomimetic pressor response during shock. J.A.M.A., *197:*808, 1966.

157. Johnson, A. S., Scheinberg, S. R., Gerish, R. A., and Saltzstein, H. C.: Effect of cortisone on the size of experimentally produced myocardial infarcts. Circulation, *7:*224, 1953.

158. Hepper, N. G., Pruitt, R. D., Donald, D. D., and Edwards, J. E.: The effect of cortisone on experimentally produced myocardial infarcts. Circulation, *11:*742, 1955.

159. Bein, H. J.: Aldosterone and alterations in circulatory reactivity following endotoxins. *In* Shock-Pathogenesis and Therapy. Ed. by Bock, K. D. Heidelberg, Springer-Verlag Berlin Göttingen, 1962, p. 162.

160. Weil, M. H.: The cardiovascular effects of corticosteroids. Circulation, *25:*718, 1962.

161. Knisely, M. H., Eliot, T. S., and Block, E. H.: Sludged blood in traumatic shock. Arch. Surg., *51:*220, 1945.

162. Crowell, J. W., and Read, W. L.: In vivo coagulation—a probable cause of irreversible shock. Amer. J. Physiol., *183:*565, 1955.

163. Hardaway, R. M.: The role of intravascular clotting in the etiology of shock. Ann. Surg., *155:*3, 1963.

164. Zweifach, B. W.: Tissue mediators in the genesis of experimental shock. J.A.M.A., *81:*866, 1962.

165. Glueck, H. I., Ryder, H. W., and Wasserman, P.: The prevention of thromboembolic complications in myocardial infarction by anticoagulant therapy. Circulation, *13:*884, 1956.

166. Nydick, I., Ruegsegger, P., Bouvier, C., Hutter, R. V., Abarquez, R., Clifton, E. E., and LaDue, J. S.: Salvage of heart muscle by fibrinolytic therapy after experimental coronary occlusion. Amer. Heart J., *61:*93, 1961.

167. Hardaway, R. M., and Johnson, D. G.: Influence of fibrinolysin on shock. J.A.M.A., *183:*177, 1963.

168. Clifton, E. E.: Fibrinolysin and its relation to the management of coronary thrombosis. Prog. Cardiovasc. Dis., *6:*255, 1963.

169. Boucek, R. J., and Murphy, W. P., Jr.: Segmental perfusion of the coronary arteries with fibrinolysin in man following a myocardial infarction. Amer. J. Cardiol., *6:*525, 1960.

170. Richter, I. H., Cliffton, E. E., Epstein, S., Musacchio, F., Nassar, A., Favazza, A. G., and Katabi, G.: Thrombolysin therapy in myocardial infarction. Amer. J. Cardiol., *9:*82, 1962.

171. Gelin, L. E.: Studies in anemia of injury. Acta. Chir. Scand., *201:* (Suppl.) 1, 1956.

172. Bernstein, E. F., Emmings, E. F., Evans, R. L., Castaneda, A., and Varco, R. L.: Effect of low molecular weight dextran on red blood cell charge during clinical extracorporeal circulation. Circulation, *27:*816, 1963.

173. Anderson, M. N., and Mouritzen, C.: Effect of acute respiratory and metabolic acidosis on cardiac output and peripheral resistance. Ann. Surg., *163:*161, 1966.

174. Selmonosky, C. A., Goetz, R. H., and State, D.: The role of acidosis in the irreversibility of experimental hemorrhagic shock. Surg. Res., *3:*491, 1963.

175. Nelson, R. M., Poulson, A. W., Lyman, J. H., and Henry, J. W.: Evaluation of tris (hydroxymethyl) aminomethane (THAM) in experimental hemorrhagic shock. Surgery, *54:*86, 1963.

176. Helmsworth, J. A., Clark, L. C., Kaplan, S., and Sherman, R. T.: Clinical use of extracorporeal oxygenation with oxygenator pump. J.A.M.A., *150:*451, 1952.

177. Stuckey, J. H., Newman, M. M., Dennis, C., Berg, E. H., Goodman, S. E., Fries, C. C., Karlson, K. E., Blumenfeld, M., Weitzner, S. W., Binder, L. S., and Winston, A.: The use of the heart lung machine in selected cases of acute myocardial infarction. Surg. Forum, *8:*342, 1957.

178. Bacaner, M.: Human heart failure and shock treated by means of a mechanical veno-arterial by-pass without oxygenation. Ann. Int. Med., *55:*837, 1961.

179. Bor, N. M., and Rieben, A. P.: Partial extracorporeal circulation in acute heart failure. Amer. J. Cardiol., *8:*41, 1961.

180. Wyman, M. G., Weil, M. H., and Blankenhorn, D. H.: Reduction of cardiac work during venous blood perfusion of lower body. J. Appl. Physiol., *17:*54, 1962.

181. Clauss, R. H., Birtwell, W. C., Albertal, G., Lunzer, S., Taylor, W. J., Fosberg, A. M., and Harken, D. E.: Assisted circulation. I. J. Thoracic Cardiovasc.

Surg., *41:*447, 1961.
182. Jacobey, J. A., Taylor, W. J., Smith, G. T., Golin, R., and Harken, D. E.: A new therapeutic approach to acute coronary occlusion. II. Opening dormant coronary collateral channels by counter-pulsation. Amer. J. Cardiol., *11:*218, 1963.

Problems in Myocardial Infarction*

Thomas Killip, M.D.

Neither coronary artery disease nor its prime complication, acute myocardial infarction, are static processes. The natural history of myocardial infarction may conveniently be divided into three phases: Phase I, the precoronary state; Phase II, the occurrence of the infarction; Phase III, the events following loss of viable myocardium.

Although it is not the intention of this paper to discuss the precoronary state, it is worth pointing out, on the basis of data obtained by our own group, that the majority of patients who eventually suffer from acute infarction have clear-cut prodromata or warning. These prodromata, usually ischemic pains, wax and wane and represent the clinical and presumably metabolic expression of a dynamic interplay between cardiac work, coronary blood flow and the oxygen delivery capacity of the coronary system.

Once infarction has occurred, there are multiple clinical pathways which a given patient may follow. The factors which control the sequence or chain of events leading to recovery or serious complications and possible death are poorly understood. It is now recognized that a significant group of patients suffer from primary ventricular fibrillation shortly after the onset of infarction. This complication may occur in as many as 20 or 30 per cent of those patients who suffer from myocardial infarction.

Primary fibrillation has its highest incidence in the first 6 to 10 hours after an acute infarction (Fig. 1). The arrhythmia apparently does not relate to the size of the damaged area. Indeed, there is some evidence to suggest that it occasionally may occur during an ischemic attack which does not cause muscle necrosis. The threat of its occurrence is the prime motivation for close scrutiny of our techniques of delivering care to the patient within the first few hours after the clinical onset of cardiac infarction. Data from workers in Belfast, Ireland and Edinburgh, Scotland indicate that 50 per cent of all deaths from myocardial infarction occur within

two hours and 15 minutes after the onset of the acute attack. Risk of death from infarction is maximal early after occurrence and declines exponentially thereafter. It may be argued that the patient with myocardial infarction should receive an effective anti-arrhythmic agent when first seen by a medical person, whether the patient be in the home, in the office, on the job or in the hospital. In view of the high initial risk, it is certainly appropriate to carefully evaluate a variety of schemes for delivering high quality care soon after infarction.

According to our experience, about 20 per cent of hospitalized patients have no significant complications following myocardial infarction. At the present time, unfortunately, we are unable to isolate these patients from the larger group who develop significant and treatable complications. Were we able to select these patients properly they might very well be candidates for home treatment.

The majority of hospitalized patients develop complications of varying severity and complexity after cardiac infarction. The most important complications relate to changes in cardiac contractility or rhythm. Either a "pump" problem or a rhythm problem may be the primary complication and each can influence the other. What starts as a primary arrhythmia may rapidly lead to progressive heart failure, hypotension, or cardiogenic shock. On the other hand, a patient with progressive left ventricular failure may become hypoxic and acidotic; this, in turn, may lead to serious or possibly fatal dysrhythmia.

The incidence and number of rhythm abnormalities can be related to the clinical severity of the infarction as judged by a bedside evaluation of the state of left ventricular compensation. A most dramatic presentation can be made by relating arrhythmia to the presence or absence of shock. Our own data show, for example, that slow heart rates are much more common in patients with shock— largely due to a striking incidence of heart block. The slowing of the heart may be related to the size and location of the infarction, to a decline in

*Supported in part by U.S.P.H.S. Myocardial Infarction Research Unit Contract No. PH 43–67–1439.

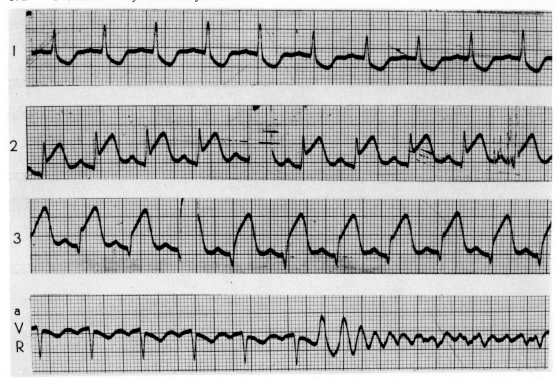

FIG. 1.   Primary ventricular fibrillation in acute myocardial infarction. This 44-year-old man was seen in the emergency room 20 minutes after onset of severe precordial pain. There was no evidence of ventricular failure or shock. Electrocardiogram, diagnostic of acute diaphragmatic (inferior) transmural infarction, shows onset of primary ventricular fibrillation. No ectopic beats preceded terminal dysrhythmia.

coronary perfusion pressure, or to a combination of factors. Death due to hypotension is commonly manifested by gradual slowing of the heart rate and descent of the pacemaker to lower centers, not infrequently culminating in asystole. The mechanism is almost certainly fundamentally metabolic in origin. Asystole is extraordinarily uncommon in the absence of cardiogenic shock.

Crude accumulations of statistics on arrhythmia or mortality are not very meaningful. Some time ago we began to evaluate each patient daily according to a simple clinical classification designed to give a crude estimation of left ventricular function. Many similar functional systems have been used by others, and we have found our method quite satisfactory. The patients are classified as follows:

Class   I   No evidence of heart failure
Class II   Evidence of mild heart failure with rales, change in heart sound, development of gallops
Class III   Pulmonary edema
Class IV   Cardiogenic shock manifested by systolic pressure less than 90, signs of peripheral vasoconstriction, reduced urine output

It is of interest that every aspect of myocardial infarction that we have studied can be correlated with one of the classifications described above. Thus, the incidence of arrhythmias, the degree of pulmonary congestion on x-ray, the blood lactate level, the arterial oxygen tension, the response to inhalation of oxygen and mortality are directly related to the severity of the infarction as determined by the above-mentioned classifications.

Utilizing the classification presented, mortality in myocardial infarction at The New York Hospital from 1965 through 1969 was as follows:

Class   I   5%
Class II   12%
Class III   37%
Class IV   85%

It is of interest that the mortality in Class I patients may be related to two prime factors. About half of the deaths were due to cardiac rupture; the other half were due to therapeutic misadventure. This latter category includes improper dosage or wrong choice of drug. It is not often that we have a chance to critically look at the delivery of medical care in the hospital setting. But if one assumes that Class I patients should survive, then one can carefully evaluate the quality of care received and determine the cause of death.

Let us now turn to certain objective measurements and their correlation with the functional severity of myocardial infarction. There has been a great deal of emphasis recently on the use of portable chest films in the evaluation of patients with myocardial infarction. We had an independent observer rate each daily film on our patients under study. The patients were classified daily as mentioned previously. The x-rays were rated on a scale of one to four, indicating increasing pulmonary congestion culminating in the pattern of pulmonary edema with effusion. There is a reasonable correlation between the clinical state and the x-ray pattern, but there is considerable overlap among the groups. (Fig. 2). We are not yet certain how much of this is

may be diffusion abnormalities. Respiratory depression due to overenthusiastic administration of narcotic drugs may also occur. Our own studies show a good correlation between the degree of arterial hypoxemia and the functional severity of the infarction (as determined by our classification) (Fig. 3). The important point is that there is a reasonable correlation between the bedside estimation of left ventricular function and an exact arterial measurement that reflects a functional cardiopulmonary derangement. Thus the use of a laboratory tool has sharpened our clinical skills.

CLINICAL and X-RAY CLASSIFICATION

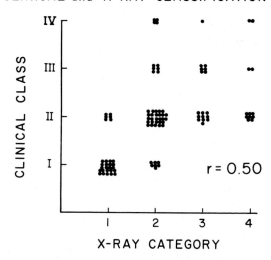

FIG. 2. Studies in myocardial infarction. Correlation between functional severity of infarction, clinical class as judged by bedside evaluation, and evidence of pulmonary congestion on portable chest film. See text for details.

CLINICAL CLASSIFICATION and $P_a O_2$

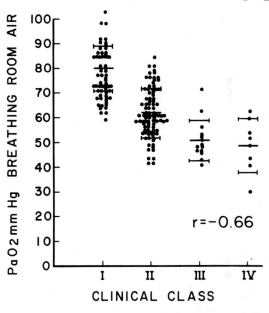

FIG. 3. Studies in myocardial infarction. Relationship between arterial oxygen tension while the patient is breathing room air and functional severity of infarction (clinical class). Arterial hypoxia becomes more severe with greater degrees of left ventricular failure.

related to the variable x-ray technic, since of necessity all of these films were obtained with a portable instrument, and how much is due to other causes. It is well known that patients may have high pulmonary venous pressure, heavy and wet lungs, but few clinical findings of congestion.

It is now recognized that some patients with myocardial infarction become markedly hypoxic. The mechanism of the reduced arterial oxygen tension has not been well explained. In some patients there is shunting of venous blood through poorly ventilated areas of lung. In other patients there

We have also evaluated the effect of oxygen inhalation in patients with myocardial infarction. The effectiveness of oxygen therapy relates directly to the functional severity of the infarction. In Class I patients, increasing the percent of oxygen in the expired air mixture by a variety of technics produce a satisfactory increment in arterial PO_2. As evidence of heart failure develops, however, and the patients become more anoxic, standard forms of oxygen therapy become progressively less satisfactory. Thus, while the patient with pulmonary edema or cardiogenic shock is breathing room air, arterial PO_2 may be only 40 to 50 mm. Hg. Breathing 28 per cent oxygen, which normally would produce an increment of 30 mm. Hg in arterial PO_2 may raise the oxygen tension only 5 to 10 mm. Hg, leaving the patient still severely hypoxic. The patient with progressive left ventricular failure and hypoxia develops acidosis and a rise in arterial lactate. These factors, in turn, may very well adversely influence cardiovascular function. One can easily see how a vicious cycle of positive feedback leading to progressive deterioration and finally death may develop. Our own experience with acutely ill patients in the cardiac unit indicates the value of frequent arterial blood gas measurements. A drop in arterial oxygen tension or a fall in pH may be the first sign of progressive deterioration. Vigorous treatment may forestall a fatality.

The coronary care unit concept has been flourishing for less than a decade. Prior to the introduction of coronary care units, mortality in myocardial infarction in large city hospitals frequently approached 40 per cent. Monitoring of the patient in specialized units that delegate authority and responsiblity to a properly trained nursing staff able to recognize arrhythmias and treat them promptly has reduced mortality in most institutions down to only 15 to 20 per cent. This salvage has been entirely due to aggressive treatment in prevention of serious arrhythmia. It should also be pointed out that the salvage has occurred entirely in hospitalized patients. As was mentioned earlier, in view of the hazard of primary fibrillation and the high early death rate in myocardial infarction, it is clear that the patient who reaches the hospital has already survived major hazards of his illness.

Many areas of treatment of myocardial infarction still require significant improvement. New forms of therapy and experiments in the improved delivery of medical care must be applied to the immediate pre- and post infarction period. Mortality in cardiac care units is largely related to problems of pump failure. Physiologic studies of the sort that have been outlined above indicate that much remains to be learned about the complications and the forms of treatment of myocardial infarction. The clinical therapist is becoming progressively more bold. Catheters are now being floated into the pulmonary artery and even into the left ventricle for precise measurement of cardiac function in the acutely ill patient. When cautiously applied and properly interpreted, such measurements should provide important information in evaluating our current therapy and should lead to significant improvement in morbidity and mortality.

Aggressive Management of Cardiac Arrhythmias in Acute Myocardial Infarction

Leslie A. Kuhn

Coronary care units have had their greatest impact in aiding the recognition and prompt treatment of significant arrhythmias and their precursors. Indeed, it is almost exclusively due to this ability that the mortality from acute myocardial infarction in hospital patients in the United States is generally reported to have declined from about 30 to about 17–18 per cent.

There is no doubt that monitoring has changed drastically our understanding of the frequency of various arrhythmias. Table 1 indicates the reported incidence of various arrhythmias in four large series of patients with acute myocardial infarction reported prior to the era of constant monitoring. There is a low incidence of all arrhythmias, 17–20 per cent, a very low incidence of the important ventricular tachycardia (1–4%), and no reported instance of ventricular fibrillation, undoubtedly because of inability to record the arrhythmias before rapid demise. The full significance of prognostically important ventricular premature beats was largely ignored. In contrast, in monitored patients with acute myocardial infarctions (Table 2), (six large series of 100–300 patients each), there is a much

TABLE 1
Arrhythmias in 927 Cases of Acute Myocardial Infarction Collected from the Literature*

	Series 1: 208 Patients (Per cent)	Series 2: 187 Patients (Per cent)	Series 3: 342 Patients (Per cent)	Series 4: 190 Patients (Per cent)
Arrhythmia				
Ventricular tachycardia	3	1	2	4
Atrial fibrillation	12	9	11	7
Atrial flutter	2	1	2	0
Atrial tachycardia	0	0	0	0
Nodal tachycardia	0	1	0	0
Atrioventricular block (all types)	3	6	4	6
Totals	20	18	19	17

*From Spann, J. F., Jr., *et al.*: Arrhythmias in acute myocardial infarction, New England J. Med. *271*:427, 1964.

TABLE 2
Incidence of Major Dysrhythmias in Continuously Monitored Patients with Myocardial Infarction

	Incidence (%)
Ventricular ectopic	
Premature beats	40–80
Tachycardia	6–28
Fibrillation	1–10
Supraventricular ectopic	
Premature beats	25–27
Tachycardia	4–19
Atrial fibrillation	7–16
Atrial flutter	1– 5
Bradycardias and blocks	
Sinus bradycardia	11–26
A-V nodal rhythm (with or without A-V dissociation)	3–10
A-V block: first degree	4–13
second degree	3–10
complete	2– 8

Collected by Marriott, Geriatrics, 23: Sept. and Oct. 1968.

higher incidence of all types of arrhythmias, particularly ventricular premature beats, ventricular tachycardia and ventricular fibrillation.

Increased mortality in acute myocardial infarction has been associated with the presence of arrhythmias, as seen in Table 3, which comprises patients cared for in general medical facilities. Note that the mortality associated with frequent ventricular ectopic beats was 41 per cent and that associated with ventricular tachycardia was 67 per cent. Of course, significant arrhythmias not only may be responsible for sudden death in hearts that are functioning well but may also cause further deteriorations of cardiac output and coronary flow in acutely ischemic hearts that are functioning poorly.

That this mortality may be diminished substantially as a result of careful monitoring and prompt treatment, was pointed out relatively soon after the establishment of coronary care units. In a study by Day of 126 patients (Table 4), there were 16 with 20

TABLE 3
*Patients With Acute Myocardial Infarction
Studied Before Monitoring: Higher
Mortality in Those With Arrhythmias**

Subjects	Incidence (Number)	Mortality (Per Cent)
All patients	100	31
Sinus tachycardia	43	44
Sinus bradycardia	14	21
Supraventricular ectopic beats	25	24
Ventricular ectopic beats (less than 1 in 10)	35	23
Ventricular ectopic beats (more than 1 in 10)	32	41
Ventricular ectopic beats (total)	67	31
Paroxysmal atrial tachycardia	4	50
Atrial flutter	2	**
Atrial fibrillation	16	31
Nodal rhythm	8	25
Ventricular tachycardia	6	67
Ventricular fibrillation	10	90
First degree heart-block	13	46
Second degree heart-block	10	30
Complete heart-block	8	37
Bundle-branch block	13	62
Paroxysmal sinus arrest	1	**

*Julian, D. G., *et al.*: Disturbances of rate, rhythm and conduction in acute myocardial infarction, Am. J. Med. *37*:915, 1964.
**Numbers too small to be analyzed.

TABLE 4
*Monitoring Hours and Clinical Course**

Total cases		126
Total hours on scope pacemakers		29,982
Deceased patient hours		1,099
Expected deaths (no resuscitation)		13
Number of patients with unexpected cardiac arrest		16
Number of patients alive and well		9
Unexpected episodes of cardiac arrest		20
Ventricular standstill	12	
Ventricular fibrillation	8	
Noncoronary monitoring hours		14,764

*From Day, H. W.: Effectiveness of an intensive coronary care unit, Am. J. Cardiol. *15*:51, 1965.

episodes of unexpected cardiac arrest and nine of these were apparently saved by prompt therapy. Similar results have been reported by many other groups.

TREATMENT OF SPECIFIC ARRHYTHMIAS

In general, with the exception of premature ventricular beats, sinus bradycardia and minor degrees of atrioventricular block, the treatment of specific arrhythmias is the same as that employed when infarction is not present, but since arrhythmias may be of more critical importance in the acutely ischemic ventricle, usually they must be treated more promptly and more decisively in the presence of acute infarction. In acute myocardial infarction, careful attention must also be given to alterations of arterial oxygen and pH.

Atrial Premature Beats, Sinus Bradycardia, Atrial Flutter, Atrial Fibrillation, and Supraventricular Tachycardia

Atrial arrhythmias are often, but not always, associated with rather severe cardiac functional impairment, sometimes with coexistent atrial infarction. Usually, possibly because of left hypertension, they are a result, rather than a cause of the functional impairment. Nevertheless, the associated rapid ventricular rates and, in the case of atrial flutter or fibrillation, the lack of effective atrial contractions, may be important in critically reducing an already low cardiac output.

Atrial premature beats are usually not treated unless they occur very frequently or produce significantly bothersome symptoms. Quinidine is the drug of choice for their suppression.

The treatment of atrial flutter or fibrillation is outlined in Table 5. If the ventricular rate is satisfactory and the patient is comfortable and manifests hemodynamic stability, no treatment need be given as these arrhythmias are usually transient and will subside spontaneously. If the ventricular rate is rapid, if the arrhythmia causes bothersome symptoms or if there are hemodynamic disturbances attributable to it, the ventricular rate should be slowed by digitalis, usually small doses intravenously; for atrial flutter, however, small energies of DC shock are almost invariably effective and this is probably the initial therapeutic method of choice for this arrhythmia. It is also of use in instances of atrial fibrillation in which the ventricular rate cannot be slowed appropriately. A preventive regimen with quinidine orally for several days is indicated after conversion to sinus rhythm.

In some instances, rapid atrial fibrillation may alternate with periods of sinus arrest. In such a patient, control of the rhythm and prevention of sinus arrest was accomplished with the insertion of a pacemaker. Pacemaker insertion is also advocated in the presence of sinus bradycardia alone, below 50/min., which does not respond to atropine or isoproterenol.

TABLE 5
Treatment of Atrial Flutter or Fibrillation

1. Digitalis to slow ventricular rate
2. No need to convert to NSR if rate satisfactory
3. If cannot control rate, DC countershock
4. If DC countershock not available, quinidine
5. Quinidine maintenance

Supraventricular tachycardia may be treated as outlined in Table 6. Digitalis is often effective because the arrhythmias generally occur as a manifestation of severe myocardial functional impairment.

Ventricular Premature Contractions

One of the significant advances made possible by coronary care units has been the prevention as well as the prompt treatment of ventricular fibrillation. This has been attributed by many authors to vigorous therapy of ventricular premature beats. As shown in Table 7, those ventricular premature beats which are multifocal, frequent or occur in the vulnerable phase of the cardiac cycle are generally considered to be precursors of ventricular tachycardia or fibrillation. Prompt administration of a bolus of lidocaine (50 or 100 mg. intravenously) is the method of choice, to be followed by continuous intravenous administration of 1–4 mg./min. Generally this is a well tolerated regimen, particularly since lidocaine is less apt to suppress arterial pressure and diminish cardiac output than are therapeutic doses of intravenous procainamide. The treatment is summarized in Table 8. Side effects, mainly muscle twitching, somnolence or convulsions may occur, however; these usually respond promptly to withdrawal of the medication. In some patients, lidocaine is ineffective for prophylactic purposes. Procainamide, 500 mg. every six hours intramuscularly or orally, or quinidine orally may then be used. Sometimes this must be supplemented by propranolol. Occasionally, multiple ventricular premature contractions may be associated with relatively slow ventricular rates and may fail to respond to suppressive agents or become more frequent with their use. This is probably because the slow heart rate produces inadequate cardiac output and coronary flow, rendering the ischemic ventricle more irritable. As seen in Figure 1, acceleration of the heart rate by isoproterenol, as in this patient, or by electrical pacing may then abolish the ectopic rhythms.

Ventricular Tachycardia

Ventricular tachycardia requires prompt attention because it may produce adverse hemodynamic effects and also may predispose to the development of ventricular fibrillation. Generally accepted treatment is outlined in Table 9. Before the institution of suppression therapy, it is important to maintain adequate arterial pressure with the use of vasopressor agents, preferably levarterenol. In some instances, this alone will be sufficient to revert the rhythm to normal, probably because of increase of coronary flow associated with the increase of coronary perfusion pressure. For short bursts of ventricular tachycardia, intravenous lidocaine administer-

TABLE 6
Treatment of Atrial Tachycardia

1. Vagal stimulation
2. Sedation
3. Digitalis
4. If persists, vasopressors
5. If persists, and vasopressors are poorly tolerated, DC shock

TABLE 7
Ventricular Premature Beats Requiring Prompt Treatment in Acute Myocardial Infarction

1. Frequency greater than 5/min.
2. Multifocal
3. Salvos of two or more
4. Occurrence in cycle interrupting T-wave (vulnerable period)

TABLE 8
Treatment of Ventricular Premature Beats in Acute Myocardial Infarction

1. IV lidocaine, 50 mg. bolus
2. If no response, 100 mg. bolus
3. When rhythm stabilized, IV lidocaine drip, 1-4 mg. per min.
4. If rhythm not stable, procainamide, 50-100 mg. per min.
5. Monitor arterial BP and have norepinephrine available
6. When rhythm stable, procainamide, 500 mg. every 6 hours IM or orally or quinidine, 0.4 Gm. q 6 h orally
7. Occasionally, propranolol or pacemaker may be necessary

TABLE 9
Treatment of Ventricular Tachycardia in Acute Myocardial Infarction

1. Maintain adequate arterial pressure with norepinephrine if necessary
2. Lidocaine IV, if unsuccessful, procainamide IV
3. With hypotension, congestive heart failure or syncope, or if above unsuccessful, DC shock. Follow with prophylactic lidocaine, procainamide or quinidine
4. Recurrent ventricular tachycardia
   a. Add propranolol orally (40–100 mg. daily) or IV-1-3 mg.
   b. If ineffective, atropine 1 mg. IV or isoproterenol, 1–4 mg. in 250 cc 5% glucose in water
   c. Pacemaker

ed in the manner previously outlined is the drug of choice. Procainamide administered intravenously (50 mg/min.) is an acceptable alternative. If there is circulatory deterioration or if there is sustained ventricular tachycardia, prompt DC countershock is

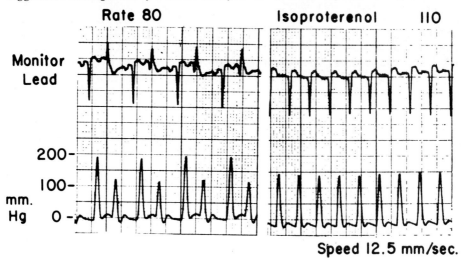

FIG.1.   Bigeminal rhythm present at ventricular rate of 80. Recurrent episodes of ventricular fibrillation were noted after administration of the suppressive agents, lidocaine and procainamide. When the ventricular rate was increased to 110 by isoproterenol infusion, ectopic beats were abolished. (From Lown *et al.*: Am. J. Cardiology *20:*500, 1967.)

usually effective. Ventricular tachycardia may be set off by a premature beat occurring on the T-wave of the preceding beat, during the "vulnerable" phase of the cardiac cycle.

A frequent therapeutic problem is that of recurrent ventricular tachycardia with its attendant risk of late ventricular fibrillation. Often, high doses of lidocaine, procainamide, orally or intramuscularly (2–4 gm. daily), or quinidine orally, are necessary prophylactically and, in some instances, this must be supplemented with propranolol (40–200 mg. daily orally), for full prophylactic effect. Such a regimen may be effective, but should be used with caution because of the negative inotropic effects of these agents. I have seen instances of ventricular tachycardia and fibrillation occurring several days after discharge from the Coronary Care Unit. Fortunately, prompt treatment allowed resuscitation, but such cases indicate the desirability of some monitoring facilities to cover a two- to three-week period after discharge from the Coronary Care Unit.

The cause of recurrent ventricular tachycardia or fibrillation in a period somewhat remote from the original myocardial infarction in an individual without evident hemodynamic impairment or new infarction is not clear, but it must be assumed that the acutely ischemic ventricle may retain its hyperirritability at least for a few weeks after the onset of acute myocardial infarction. In one patient, his emotional state appeared to have some importance in the precipitation of episodes of ventricular tachycardia. Here, ventricular tachycardia occurred

repeatedly upon notification of the patient that he would be discharged from the Unit. Although the precise role of the emotional state of the patient, with its attendant catecholamine release, in precipitating specific arrhythmias, is not clear, in some patients, as in this one, heavier than usual sedation may be a helpful adjuvant measure in preventing undesirable arrhythmias. Occasionally, hyperbaric oxygenation has been effective in the prevention of frequently recurring ventricular tachycardia in acute myocardial infarction.

Another technic for managing recurrent ventricular tachycardia which has been used relatively recently is that of increasing the intrinsic rate of the ventricle by drug administration (atropine or isoproterenol) or by electrical pacing. There have been reports of success with electrical pacing in preventing ventricular tachycardia, recurrence of the arrhythmias being noted when the rate slows. The rationale for this methodology rests on the assumption that above a critical rate, the ventricle may be "captured" by the pacemaker or drug induced impulse and therefore will not "escape" into ventricular tachycardia. Although this method may be effective, at times the rate required may be so high that the patient cannot tolerate it without the development of ischemic pain or other undesirable symptoms.

There is another type of ventricular tachycardia which occurs relatively frequently in patients with acute myocardial infarction (Fig. 2). This has been given a variety of designations, including "idioventricular rhythm," "slow ventricular tachycardia,"

CONTINUOUS ECG

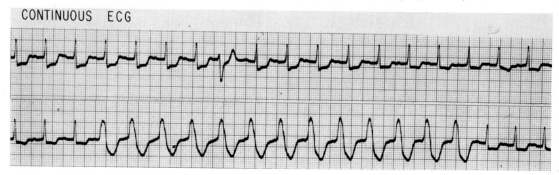

FIG. 2. Illustration of "slow ventricular tachycardia" or "idioventricular rhythm" in a patient with acute myocardial infarction. Note the nature and relatively slow rate of this arrhythmia.

"nonparoxysmal ventricular tachycardia," "accelerated intraventricular rhythm," and "atrioventricular dissociation with intraventricular rhythm." It is transient, recurrent and often associated with a slow sinus mechanism; hence it may be initiated by an "escape" or fusion beat. Its clinical features and comparison with the more serious "paroxysmal ventricular tachycardia" are indicated in Table 10.

TABLE 10
Comparison of Features of Idioventricular Rhythm and Usual Variety of Paroxysmal Ventricular Tachycardia

	IVER	PVT
Prevalence in this series	36%	8%
Site of infarction in myocardium	Inferior in 22 of 36	None specific
Rate per minute	60 to 100	>100
Onset	Idioventricular escape or ventricular fusion beat	Abrupt with R on T
Termination	Gradual slowing	Abrupt with compensatory pause
Fusion beats	Very common	Rare
Duration	Brief; 4 to 30 beats	Often sustained
Vital signs	Unchanged	Tachycardia; hypotension
SGOT	Same as in patients without ventricular arrhythmias	Significantly higher than in patients without ventricular arrhythmias
Prognosis	Favorable; spontaneous disappearance	Grave; 50% fatal

From Rothfeld *et al.,* Circulation *37*:206, 1968. By permission of Am. Heart Association, Inc.

Usually, it is of brief duration, disappears spontaneously and requires little therapy. If there is considerable sinus bradycardia, atropine or isopro-terenol may be indicated.

Perhaps the principal therapeutic advance attributable to coronary care units is the prompt, and often successful, treatment of ventricular fibrillation. The application of DC shock by nurses who are specially trained and constantly in attendance undoubtedly has resulted in increased numbers of survivors from what would otherwise have been a fatal arrhythmia. A few times, we have seen a patient with acute myocardial infarction who entered the Coronary Care Unit with premature ventricular beats and rapidly developed ventricular fibrillation while being put to bed before being seen by the physician of the Unit. Prompt defibrillation by the nurse in attendance resulted in cure of the arrhythmia and ultimate survival. Attention to the patient's airway and correction of acidosis or hypoxemia are important adjuvants to therapy in instances of more prolonged cardiac arrest.

As we look to future developments in coronary care units it is important to realize that, spectacular as the advances have been in prophylaxis and therapy of arrhythmias a major problem exists because of the large number of deaths (probably greater than 60% of all "coronary" deaths) occurring between the onset of symptoms and admission to the hospital. Table 11 illustrates the much higher incidence of ventricular fibrillation in patients admitted within four hours of the onset of symptoms as compared with those admitted later. The development of mobile coronary care units and accelerated admission procedures may help to reduce this incidence in the future. It should also be realized from these statistics that correct interpretation of the prophylaxis and therapy of ventricular fibrillation in a given coronary care unit must depend upon careful review of its admission policies and possible delays in entry to the unit, which, of itself, will result in a lower incidence of ventricular fibrillation within the unit. It should also be noted, as shown in Table 12, that success rate of defibrillation and survival is related generally to the age of the patient, with older patients faring more poorly than younger individuals. Some units have based admission policies on this trend, giving priority to younger individuals (below 70) in whom the probability of successful defibrillation is greater.

Although there is much that has been learned

TABLE 11
Incidence of Primary Ventricular Fibrillation Related to Time of Admission After Onset of Symptoms of Acute Myocardial Infarction

Patients	Number	Number Developing Primary Ventricular Fibrillation
Admitted within 4 hrs. of onset of symptoms	348	18 (5.5%)
Admitted more than 4 hrs. after onset of symptoms	252	2 (0.4%)

From Julian, Ann. Int. Med. *69*:610, 1968.

TABLE 12
Influence of Age of Patient on Survival after Ventricular Defibrillation in Acute Myocardial Infarction

Age yr	Number of Patients	Number of Deaths	Survivors from Ventricular Fibrillation	Survivors as Percent of Total Patients
30–39	16	1 (6%)	—	—
40–49	100	12 (12%)	9	9
50–59	236	24 (10%)	10	4
60–69	248	64 (26%)	6	2

From Julian, Ann. Int. Med. *69*:610, 1968.

about the management of arrhythmias in coronary care units, if we are to reduce mortality further, many more beds are needed, the patients should be observed for longer intervals than is currently allowed by the availability of beds in many institutions and patients must be monitored and treated much sooner after the onset of symptoms than is the current practice.

Fluid and Electrolyte Problems of Patients on the Acute Coronary Care Unit*

Raymond E. Weston

The fluid and electrolyte problems of patients in the acute coronary care unit reflect the hemodynamic, respiratory and metabolic consequences of acute circulatory insufficiency, often superimposed on the pathophysiological abnormalities of chronic cardiac disease and frequently modified by the effects of various immediate or more long-term therapeutic procedures. These phenomena are manifestations of congestive heart failure, which develops only when the cardiac output becomes inadequate for the body's metabolic needs (Fig. 1). Therefore, they are absent in the patient with minimal hemodynamic changes following a mild coronary occlusion and, when present in the sicker patient, may be completely reversed if normal tissue perfusion can be restored by the administration of inotropic agents like digitalis, isoproterenol or glucagon, or by application of one of the mechanical circulatory assist systems which are now being developed.

Thus, maintenance of an adequate cardiac output is the keystone of prophylactic or active treatment of these problems.[1] If this cannot be achieved, the various mechanisms which promote salt and water retention in congestive heart failure (Fig. 1) are successively activated more and more intensely as further hemodynamic deterioration occurs. Ultimately, unless the sequence is interrupted, the stage of intractable congestive failure is reached and little or no therapeutic response to any single drug or combination of pharmacological agents is possible.[2] Fortunately, new modes of therapy are now available, which permit correction of the severest fluid and electrolyte problems, even at this stage, thereby prolonging life and providing the time needed for the acutely damaged heart to heal.

In Figure 1, the interrelationships of the mechanisms that contribute to salt and water retention whenever cardiac output is inadequate for the

*Supported in part by grants-in-aid from the Western Foundation for Medical Research and Education, Beverly Hills, California, and from Mr. Ike West, Jr., Mrs. Nellie B. West, Mr. Sol West, III, Mr. and Mrs. Paul Van Cleef, Mr. George Elber, and the Mayer Family Foundation.

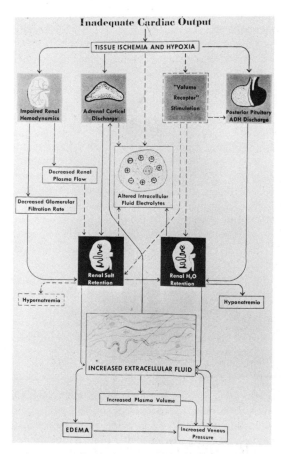

FIG. 1. Mechanisms affecting fluid and electrolyte excretion in congestive heart failure, when cardiac output becomes inadequate relative to body's metabolic needs.

body's metabolic needs are pictured. One manifestation of the generalized tissue ischemia is *impaired renal hemodynamics.* The well-documented decrease in glomerular filtration rate and the relatively greater reduction in renal blood flow lead to glomerulo-tubular imbalance, which promotes decreased sodium excretion. In addition, as Barger[3] suggested on the basis of studies in dogs with severe experimental congestive failure, there may be a disproportionately greater outer renal cortical ischemia that may reduce sodium excretion by decreasing particularly the perfusion of shorter, normally salt-losing nephrons.

In very severe congestive failure, *increased adrenal cortical production* of glucocorticoids occurs at times in response to stress, aldosterone or other stimuli. These steroids not only promote active tubular reabsorption of sodium and associated anions, but also stimulate the distal tubular base-conserving mechanisms that exchange ammonium, hydrogen and especially potassium ions for sodium in the distal tubular lumen of the salt-retaining patient.

Furthermore, the cardiovascular-renal hemodynamic impairment may upset the *volume-circulatory regulating system,* which normally protects the cardiac output, or effectively circulating blood volume, by increasing or decreasing the excretion of sodium and/or water whenever circumstances prevail. This suggests an increase or decrease, respectively, in extracellular fluid volume. Some as yet undefined stimulus, then, activates a receptor, probably somewhere in the cephalad portion of the circulation. As a result, depending upon the intensity of the stimulus, there may be changes in the renal hemodynamics and possibly in the distribution of blood flow between renal cortex and medulla. Changes may also occur in the aldosterone secretion,[4] and possibly in the release of both posterior pituitary antidiuretic hormones[1] and the so-called third factor, a natriuretic hormone postulated, on the basis of certain disputed experimental observations, to affect sodium excretion.[5]

In addition, *sustained production of antidiuretic hormone* may be maintained by severe stress or by some other extra-osmoreceptor system,[6] possibly an aberration in volume-circulatory regulation. The resulting retention of water, per se, may lead to the increasing edema and dilutional hyponatremia that we demonstrated[6] could develop during acute exacerbations of severe congestive failure in patients on low sodium intakes, unless fluid intake is vigorously restricted. Finally, *abnormalities in intracellular fluid and electrolytes* of patients in severe congestive failure may result from all these influences plus the effects of severe tissue ischemia and hypoxia, which produce lactic acid acidosis and other manifestations of impaired cellular metabolism. These intracellular changes not only may have effects on salt and water excretion but may contribute to both the morbidity and the mortality of cardiac failure when the more general intracellular potassium depletion affects the myocardium *(vide infra)*.

POTASSIUM DEPLETION

The intracellular potassium depletion in patients with congestive failure (Figure 2) reflects, in part, inadequate intake due to anorexia as well as losses via the gastrointestinal tract, at times resulting from ingested medications or visceral congestion. Of greater significance are the losses from cells, caused by metabolic acidosis, alkalosis, the catabolic effects of glucocorticoids, or the inability of metabolically impaired, anoxic "sick" cells to maintain the normally high intracellular-extracellular potassium concentration gradient. Finally, activation of the distal tubular ion exchange mechanism, discussed above, leads to continued losses of potassium in the urine, particularly if systemic acidosis or alkalosis develops.

Such urinary potassium losses are particularly great, as we reported some time ago,[2] when salt-retaining subjects are given any diuretic that increases the load of sodium delivered to the distal base-conserving mechanism. Under these circumstances, there is prompt increase in excretion of potassium ion, hydrogen ion and ammonia, if the diuretic does not also inhibit carbonic anhydrase. Consequently, during the ensuing diuresis, more chloride than sodium is excreted. Therefore, during the course of mercurial diuresis, in the normal fasting subject, potassium excretion continues to fall, whereas in the salt-retaining patient, it continues to increase steadily during and following maximal diuresis. A similar increase in potassium

ETIOLOGY OF POTASSIUM DEPLETION

1. ANOREXIA

2. G.I. LOSSES   (Vomiting, Diarrhea, Drainage)

3. INTRACELLULAR LOSSES

    a. Catabolic (Stress) Reaction

    b. Acidosis or Alkalosis

    c. "Sick Cell" Syndrome

4. URINARY LOSSES   due to:

    a. Distal Tubular Base Conservation

    b. Stress Reaction

    c. Acidosis or Alkalosis

    d. Diuretics

FIG. 2. Factors contributing to potassium depletion in cardiac failure.

excretion may be produced during such diuresis in the normal individual, if distal sodium conservation is activated by administering adrenal cortical steroids or by restricting sodium intake for a few days. Thus, continued administration of mercurials, thiazides, or the newer diuretics like ethacrynic acid and furosemide leads to substantial losses of potassium and consequent intracellular potassium depletion unless potassium intake is supplemented sufficiently.

Severe intracellular potassium depletion may contribute greatly to morbidity and particularly to the weakness of the cardiac patient. In addition, it may complicate other therapy and increase mortality by producing a dangerously increased incidence of arrhythmias, especially in digitalized patients, as illustrated by the data presented in Figure 3.

he excreted 800 ml. of urine in three hours, containing 74 mEq. of chloride, 45 mEq. of sodium and 19 mEq. of potassium, again without change in cardiac rhythm. The next day, when his cardiovascular status was somewhat improved after the previous two bouts of diuresis and a restricted fluid intake, he was given a third intravenous injection of the same potent diuretic. During the following four hours, he excreted 1930 ml. of urine, containing 221 mEq. of chloride, 130 mEq. of sodium and 131 mEq. of potassium. As a result, the serum potassium in this already potassium-depleted patient dropped from 4.4 to 3 mEq./1. and he developed paroxysmal atrial tachycardia with block and multiple ventricular contractions. As anticipated, there was a prompt reversion to normal sinus rhythm when he was given potassium chloride

POTASSIUM LOSS AND CARDIAC ARRHYTHMIA FOLLOWING DIURESIS

DATE	DURAT.	URINARY EXCRETION				ARRHY.
		K	H$_2$O	Na	Cl	
	(hrs.)	(mEq)	(ml)	(mEq)	(mEq)	
1/3/65	2	23	435	22	40	0
	3	19	808	45	74	0
1/4/65	4	28	1930	134	221	P.A.T. P.V.C.'S

FIG. 3. Urinary electrolyte excretion in digitalized, edematous patient who developed cardiac arrhythmia due to cumulative potassium losses following successive injections of a potent diuretic.

This particular patient, a massively edematous young man with severe cor pulmonale appeared to be terminally ill on admission to the hospital. In two hours, following the first intravenous injection of the potent diuretic, ethacrynic acid, he excreted 435 ml. of urine, containing 40 mEq. chloride, 22 mEq. of sodium and 23 mEq. of potassium, without change in his cardiac rhythm. Eight hours later, after receiving a second injection of the diuretic, intravenously.

Such arrhythmias due to myocardial potassium depletion induced by diuretics in digitalized patients generally are more easily prevented than treated. Therefore, whenever a digitalized cardiac patient is given potent diuretics, once diuresis has been achieved, potassium salts should be given orally or added in a concentration of 40 to 60 mEq./1. to any intravenous fluids being administered, in order to replace losses promptly.

Although this patient's serum potassium was initially low and dropped to subnormal levels simultaneously with the development of the arrhythmia, it should be emphasized that patients with severe intracellular and myocardial potassium depletion may have normal or even elevated serum potassium concentrations. This seemingly anomalous circumstance is not difficult to understand. First, the severe tissue ischemia and hypoxia that interfere with cellular metabolic function, leading to loss of the potassium from the intracellular fluid, make it difficult for cells to take up potassium unless the thermodynamic work required is reduced. Thus, by decreasing the concentration gradient, the rise in extracellular potassium may be compensatory, facilitating intracellular potassium uptake, Second, the metabolic acidosis of severe congestive failure leads to further intracellular potassium losses and increased serum potassium concentrations. As Scribner and his colleagues[7] demonstrated in men and animals, a tenth of a unit fall or rise in serum pH may lead to an inverse 1 to 1.25 mEq./l. rise or fall in serum potassium concentration. Third, the distal tubular ion exchange of potassium for sodium, which normally prevents increased serum potassium levels, may be impaired because metabolically-impaired cells are unable to take up needed potassium or because virtually no sodium reaches the distal tubular lumen for exchange, leading to hyperkalemia even in the face of potassium depletion.

Therefore, the serum potassium concentration is usually not reduced in the potassium-depleted cardiac patient. However, almost pathognomonic of intracellular potassium depletion is the metabolic alkalosis, with low serum chloride and elevated serum bicarbonate concentrations, that results from intracellular potassium losses. This serum anion pattern must be distinguished from respiratory acidosis by blood pH studies. Unfortunately, sometimes an underlying metabolic alkalosis may be masked by a superimposed metabolic acidosis that, because of the increase in organic acids, may lower the bicarbonate and the pH.

Such metabolic alkalosis and chloride depletion may interfere with the treatment or the prevention of potassium depletion, as emphasized by Schwartz and his colleagues.[8] They demonstrated that severe potassium depletion in the patient on a low sodium chloride intake with elevated serum bicarbonate and low serum chloride levels cannot be corrected by the administration of potassium bicarbonate, the ultimate metabolic equivalent of the commercially available oral potassium solutions, Kayon and

Potassium Triplex (Figure 4). However, when equivalent quntities of potassium chloride are given orally, retention of both potassium and chloride quickly corrects both the alkalosis and the potassium depletion and restores serum bicarbonate, chloride and pH levels to normal. Therefore, to prevent or to treat potassium depletion during diuretic therapy in patients on a low intake of chloride associated with the usual low sodium diet, chloride as well as potassium must be administered.

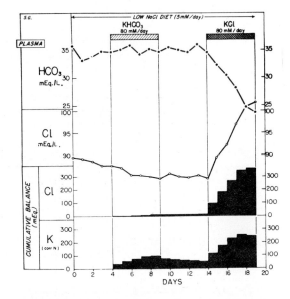

Fig. 4. Demonstration of successful correction of potassium depletion and metabolic alkalosis by oral administration of potassium chloride in contrast to potassium bicarbonate which was ineffective (From Kassiner, J.P. *et al.*: Amer. J. Med. *38*:172, 1965)

For a long time, enteric-coated potassium chloride tablets were widely prescribed to treat potassium depletion. However, the demonstration of ileal ulcers,[9] first in patients and later in experimental animals who were given enteric-coated tablets containing a combination of both potassium chloride and a thiazide diuretic, has led many to abandon the use of the enteric-coated potassium chloride tablets as well. However, four to twelve of the one gram potassium chloride Enseals have been taken daily by many of our edematous cardiac and cirrhotic patients for many years, without any signs of ileal lesions. Therefore, I continue to prescribe potassium chloride Enseals, particularly for use away from home. However, a variety of palatable 10 per cent potassium chloride syrups are now available, appropriately flavored, which are well tolerated in water or juices and apparently do not produce ileal ulcers.

In patients taking smaller or less frequent doses of the usual oral diuretics, potassium depletion generally may be prevented by concurrent administration of drugs like spironolactone[10] or triamterin,[11] which tend to inhibit the distal tubular mechanism exchanging potassium for sodium. However, these agents do not completely block distal tubular ion exchange. Therefore, patients taking higher doses of the more potent diuretics for long periods of time may require supplemental potassium administration. Under these circumstances, potassium must be given with considerable care, lest serious hyperkalemia result.

HYPERKALEMIA IN SEVERE CONGESTIVE FAILURE

The patient in severe congestive heart failure is particularly vulnerable not only to the development but also to the dangerous cardiac consequences of hyperkalemia. First, metabolic[7] and/or respiratory acidosis[12] lead not only to continued outpouring of potassium from the cells but also to intensification of the deleterious effects of the resulting hyperkalemia on cardiac irritability and conductivity.[13]

Second, the cellular metabolic effects of the reduced tissue perfusion that contribute to the intracellular potassium depletion also impair the capacity of even potassium-depleted cells to transfer potassium from the extracellular fluid, despite significant increases in serum potassium. Third, the capacity of the renal potassium secretory mechanism to prevent pathological increases in serum potassium levels is restricted by the virtual absence of sodium in the distal tubular urine, due to the intense reabsorption more proximally, as described above.

Therefore, it is not surprising that not infrequently an often unsuspected hyperkalemia may be present in very sick patients in the coronary care unit, even when only modest oral doses of potassium salts are being given several times daily to prevent or to treat potassium depletion. If metabolic or respiratory acidosis should insidiously increase, and particularly if potent diuretics that can increase the sodium load to the distal tubular potassium exchange mechanism are not given at least twice daily, dangerous hyperkalemia may result. We have seen serious arrhythmias develop under these circumstances, which were unsuccessfully treated as ventricular tachycardias until the correct etiologic diagnosis was made. Then, emergency treatment of hyperkalemia

rhythm.

The toxic effects of hyperkalemia, it should be emphasized, are not a function of serum potassium level alone. In the presence of hyponatremia, acidosis, hypocalcemia or myocardial damage, relatively small increases in serum potassium levels may produce electrocardiographic changes and even fatal arrhythmias that do not respond to standard treatment with electric countershock or pharmacologic agents such as lidocaine, quinidine, etc.

The emergency treatment of hyperkalemia, even before the development of serious electrocardiographic changes, is to discontinue parenteral or oral potassium therapy immediately. Then, to lower the serum potassium level, an infusion of 500 ml. of 50 per cent dextrose in water with 30 units of regular insulin should be started, 50 ml. being given rapidly to produce initial hyperglycemia. If these measures are not successful, a suspension in sorbitol of Kayexelate, a resin that exchanges sodium for potassium, may be given orally or by rectum. Finally, as discussed below, extracellular potassium can be definitively and rapidly removed from the body by peritoneal dialysis, if indicated.

Significant electrocardiographic changes, if present, can often be quickly reversed in patients who are not on digitalis glycosides by rapid intravenous injection of 10 ml. of a 10 per cent calcium gluconate solution. In digitalized patients in whom calcium injections are contraindicated, this can be accomplished by the rapid intravenous injection of 30 ml. of a 3 mEq. per ml. solution of sodium lactate or sodium acetate, if available*, or 50 ml. of a 7.5 per cent (0.88 mEq. per ml.) solution of sodium bicarbonate. Generally, due to the rapid increase in serum sodium concentration, the relative fall in potassium concentration and the partial correction of the acidosis, by the end of the injection of the concentrated sodium lactate, which takes only a minute or two, the hyperkalemic arrhythmia is abolished and cardiovascular improvement is marked.

---

*The 3 mEq./l. solutions of sodium lactate and acetate are about 3.5 times as concentrated as the 7.5 per cent sodium bicarbonate. Therefore, 30 ml. provides 90 mEq. of concentrated sodium, producing a more rapid and greater effect on serum electrolytes than the 44 mEq. in the 50 ml. of the most concentrated bicarbonate solution. It has been reported that concentrated sodium lactate is more effective in reversing hyperkalemic ECG changes than is either concentrated calcium gluconate or sodium bicarbonate when injected in dogs with experimental hyperkalemia. In recent years, particularly in patients with impaired lactate metabolism or lactic acid acidosis, we have used the 3 mEq. sodium acetate solution to provide the concentrated sodium in a small volume with a more rapidly

DIURETIC RESISTANCE

Failure to respond to conventional diuretics is another problem encountered in severely ill patients on the acute coronary care unit. As we demonstrated some years ago[2] with mercurial diuretics, this reflects not drug resistance but intensification of the factors promoting sodium and water retention in severe congestive failure due to the increasingly severe disproportion between cardiac output and the body's metabolic demands. Under these conditions, as a result of the greatly reduced filtration rate and increased proximal tubular reabsorption, the load of sodium is insufficient to exceed the reabsorptive or ionic exchange capacity of the more distal tubular segments, even after administering a diuretic, and little or no sodium and water diuresis results. At that time, we showed that increasing the filtration rate by intravenous injection of 0.25 to 0.5 grams of aminophyllin 2 hours after administering a mercurial diuretic, when there presumably is maximal mercurial depression of tubular sodium reabsorption, potentiates the diuretic response in patients previously resistant to mercurial diuretics. In patients in congestive failure, in contrast to normal subjects, the intravenous injection of aminophyllin increases cardiac output and renal blood flow for as long as 45 minutes, as well as produces a much more prolonged augmentation of glomerular filtration. However, the potentiation of mercurial diuresis following aimnophyllin injection may persist even after renal hemodynamic functions have declined to control levels. It is interesting to speculate whether the short period of increased cardiac output, relative to the body metabolic needs, produced by the aminophyllin injection may also have diminished the activation of other mechanisms that had been inhibiting diuresis by promoting intense renal salt and water retention.

Today, with the newer diuretics like ethacrinic acid[14] and furosemide,[15] which act in the ascending

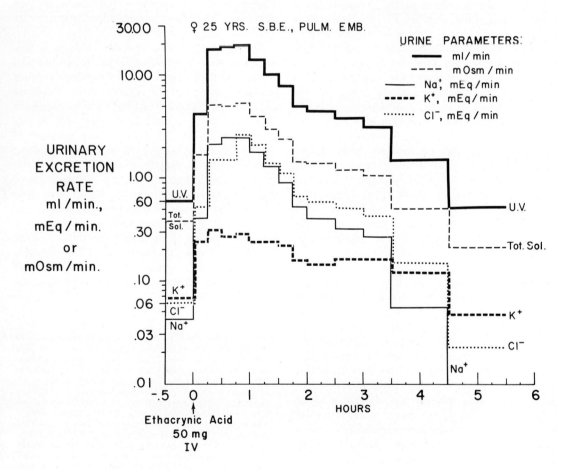

loop of the limb of Henle, remarkable diuretic responses can be achieved in the face of thiazide or mercurial resistance, as illustrated in Figure 5. This patient, who had pulmonary edema due to recurring pulmonary emboli, previously had given no diuretic response to mercurial or to thiazide diuretics. Nevertheless, after an intravenous injection of 50 mgm. of ethacrynic acid, urine output quickly increased to 25 ml. per minute and sodium excretion to 3.2 mEq. per minute. In a relatively short time, she excreted over 1,500 ml. of urine, promptly clearing her pulmonary congestion. Concurrently, her peak urinary potassium excretion, though less than 10 per cent of the tremendous sodium excretion in the first hour, was 18 mEq. per hour. As a result, she soon developed ventricular premature contractions, which subsided when she was slowly given potassium chloride intravenously.

However, the severity of the congestive failure and the state of the renal circulation may influence the diuretic response to even these newer, more potent drugs. Thus, as illustrated in Figure 6, a patient with congestive failure and renal impairment due to diabetic intercapillary glomerulosclerosis, when given an injection of ethacrynic acid, exhibited only a moderate diuresis that fell off after 75 minutes, in contrast to the usual 4 to 6 hour ethacrynic acid response, At that time, just as it would following a mercurial diuretic, intravenous administration of 250 mgm. of aminophyllin produced significant immediate augmentation of the diuretic response, which lasted for an additional 2 hours.

The dependence of diuretic response to ethacrynic acid on cardiovascular and renal hemodynamics is further illustrated by the data presented in Figure 7. During a hypotensive period following a myocardial infarction, this previously hypertensive patient in pulmonary edema, exhibited virtually no diuresis, despite receiving first ethacrynic acid and then an intravenous injection of aminophyllin. However, when his blood pressure was restored to

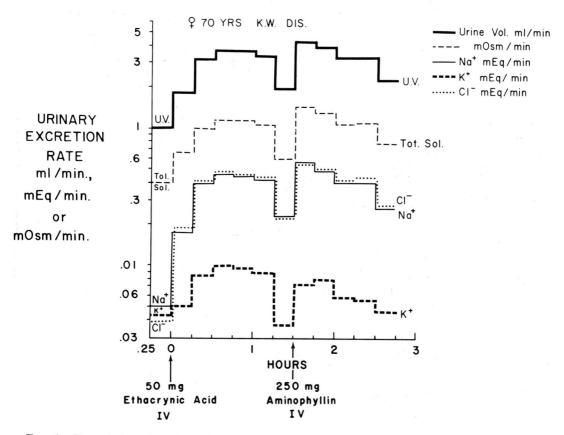

FIG. 6. Potentiation of waning ethacrynic acid diuresis following intravenous injection of 250 mgm. of aminophyllin in edematous patient with arteriosclerotic heart disease and Kimmelstiehl-Wilson's disease.

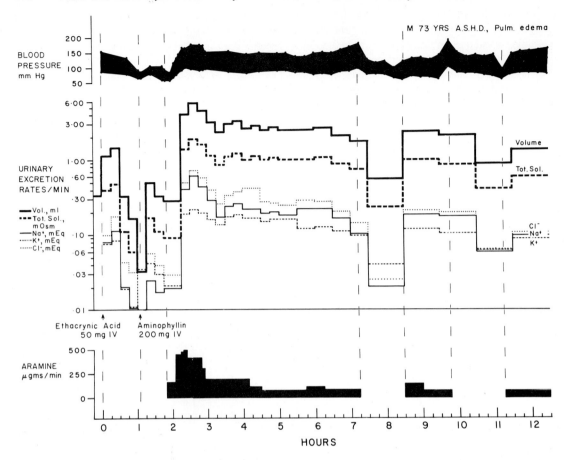

FIG. 7. Relationship between cardiovascular-renal hemodynamic status and diuretic response to ethacrynic acid in hypertensive patient in pulmonary edema, who became relatively hypotensive after
suffering acute myocardial infarction. Note failure to have significant diuresis after receiving intravenous
injection of ethacrynic acid, followed by aminophyllin one hour later, until blood pressure was maintained
at previously hypertensive levels by continuous infusion of vasopressor.

hypertensive levels by continuous infusion of
metaraminal, urine volume and excretion of sodium
and chloride increased promptly. Subsequently, the
typical ethacrynic acid diuresis was maintained as
long as the blood pressure and renal perfusion were
sustained by infusion of the vasopressor.

Finally, the data in Figure 8 illustrate a very limited
response to an initial injection of 50 mgm. of
ethacrynic acid given to an 88-year-old man with a
recent acute myocardial infarction. However, later,
when he was first given a priming dose of 250 cc.
of 20 per cent Mannitol and a sustaining infusion of
10 per cent Mannitol, an injection of only 25 mgm.
of ethacrynic acid produced a much greater and
more sustained output of urine and electrolytes.

The potency of the diuresis produced by the
administration of ethacrynic acid intravenously
makes such injections the treatment of choice for
pulmonary edema. In most patients, the almost

instant diuresis produces contraction of the extracellular fluid and blood volumes, with rapid
clearing of the pulmonary congestion. However,
as indicated above, in a very sick patient with a
markedly reduced cardiac output, no diuretic response may be achieved, even by an intravenous
injection of ethacrynic acid followed by aminophyllin. Moreover, if diuresis is achieved in well-
digitalized potassium-depleted subjects, severe
arrhythmias may result due to acute potassium loss
as indicated above in Figures 3 and 5.

Fortunately, an effective procedure is available
for correcting fluid and electrolyte abnormalities,
that is independent of cardiac or renal function;
namely, peritoneal dialysis. This technic, which
utilizes the peritoneal membrane as a means of
removing waste products and excess fluid from the
body has been well standardized for the treatment
of both acute and chronic renal failure.[16]

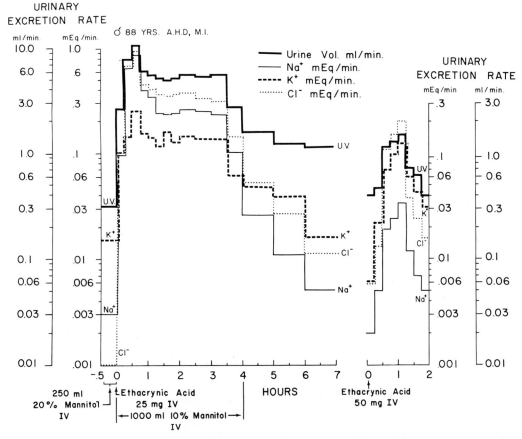

FIG. 8. Demonstration of mannitol infusion potentiating previously inadequate ethacrynic acid diuresis in a hyponatremic man in severe, acute congestive heart failure following recent myocardial infarction.

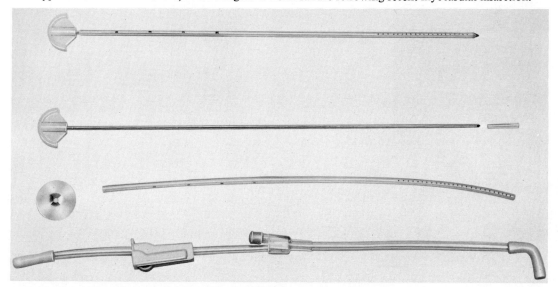

FIG. 9. Trocath stylet-catheter for peritoneal dialysis. From bottom up are illustrated the following: plastic set which connects dialysis catheter to fluid administration tubing during dialysis; peritoneal dialysis catheter with aluminum disc facilitating taping to skin; stainless steel stylet with triangular cutting tip; assembled trocath with stylet cutting tip protruding from catheter.

PERITONEAL DIALYSIS

The original method of peritoneal dialysis involved abdominal puncture with a No. 17 straight trochar to permit the insertion of a special nylon catheter into the peritoneal cavity. Inasmuch as an abdominal skin incision was required and bleeding sometimes resulted from passage of the rather large trochar, peritoneal dialysis was used with reluctance on sick cardiac patients, particularly those who were anticoagulated. More recently, Dr. Martin Roberts and I[17] developed the "trocath" stylet-catheter, which greatly simplifies the procedure. The solid tip of the regular peritoneal dialysis catheter was replaced with an open end, tapered to fit the protruding triangular trochar tip of a slightly longer, solid stainless steel stylet (Fig. 9). The trocath can be easily inserted into the peritoneal cavity in the avascular linea alba, without need for incision or abdominal trochar.

To distend the peritoneum in patients without ascites, 2 liters of peritoneal dialysis solution generally are introduced into the abdomen via a large spinal needle, prior to inserting the trocath.

In patients with ascites, a skin puncture wound is made, under local anesthesia, in the midline below the umbilicus, one-third of the distance to the pubis, either with a large spinal needle or by firmly pressing the protruding cutting tip of the trocath into the skin. Then, with a small mosquito hemostat, the cutaneous hole is dilated enough to permit the trocath to be passed into the peritoneal cavity by firm pressure with a twisting motion that utilizes the cutting effect of the stylet tip. Entrance into the peritoneal cavity is indicated by the sudden decrease in resistance and the rise of peritoneal fluid into the catheter. Once the catheter tip is in the peritoneal cavity, the stylus is withdrawn slightly so that the metal tip no longer protrudes into the peritoneal cavity and the tip of the catheter is passed into the right or left pelvic gutter. The stylet is removed and after the catheter is advanced maximally, a small metal disc is slipped over the catheter tip to facilitate taping to the skin. Finally, the connecting set is attached to the catheter and to the peritoneal dialysis fluid administration set and dialysis is begun (Fig. 10).

Table 1 presents the composition of the standard dialysis solution that we now use. In contrast to the

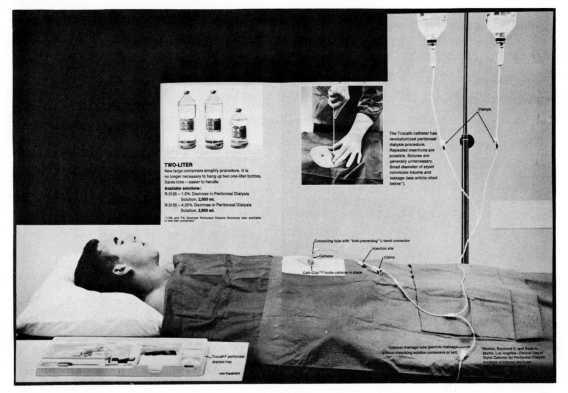

FIG. 10. Typical peritoneal dialysis set-up, illustrating technic of inserting trocath (right upper insert) and use of cath-clip for taping catheter to abdomen before connecting to peritoneal dialysis solution administration set.

TABLE 1
Composition of Peritoneal Dialysis Fluid

	mEq./liter	Gms./liter
Sodium	140.0	—
Chloride	101.0	—
Calcium	4.0	—
Magnesium	1.5	—
Acetate	45.0	—
Dextrose	—	1.5

*Potassium chloride or acetate, depending upon whether patient is alkaotic or acidoiic, respectively, is added in relation to patients serum potassium concentration (see text).

other commercially available solutions, the bicarbonate precursor in this product is acetate, not lactate. The change was instituted because of the possibly impaired lactate metabolism in patients with Laennec's or cardiac cirrhosis and/or with lactic acid acidosis such as that in severe congestive failure. To facilitate the rapid removal of potassium in uremic patients who are usually hyperkalemic before dialysis, standard peritoneal dialysis solutions are potassium free. In most cardiac patients, the serum potassium level is not too high and, from the start, potassium is added to the peritoneal dialysis solution. Particularly if the patient is digitalized, 8 to 10 mEq. of potassium should be added to each 2 liters of solution to prevent a fall in the serum potassium level with consequent rapid shifts of potassium from the myocardium. This averts the development of increased myocardial sensitivity to digitalis and consequent dangerous arrhythmias. The other electrolytes are present in dialysis solutions in concentrations equivalent to those of extracellular fluids.

To promote the transfer of fluid into the peritoneal cavity, the tonicity of the dialysis solution is augmented by increasing the concentration of dextrose to 1.5 per cent. However, when fluid must be removed more rapidly from the edematous patients, the tonicity of the dialysis solution is increased by raising the concentration of dextrose. As graphically presented in Figure 11, the volume of excess fluid removed in each 2-liter peritoneal dialysis exchange is roughly proportional to the concentration of dextrose in the dialysis solution. Originally, 1 liter of a peritoneal dialysis solution with 7 per cent dextrose was run in simultaneously with 1 liter of the standard peritoneal dialysis solution with 1.5 per cent dextrose, via a Y-tube set to produce 2 liters of peritoneal dialysis solution with a concentration of 4.25 per cent dextrose. Now, 2-liter containers are available of peritoneal dialysis solution with 4.25 or 1.5 per cent dextrose.

More recently, we have further modified the peritoneal dialysis solution by replacing the dextrose with sorbitol, a 6 carbon alcohol that has several advantages. First, it is much more slowly metabolized than is dextrose and then only after conversion to fructose, so that a concentrated solution produces less hyperglycemia in diabetic or uremic patients. Second, unlike dextrose, which carmelizes when heated unless the pH is acid, sorbitol is heat-stable when autoclaved. Therefore, the pH of sorbitol dialysis solution during and after sterilization can be maintained at almost neutral, thereby decreasing the potential peritoneal irritation and pain noted by some patients during rapid infusion of the more acid dextrose solutions.

Our standard technic is to infuse 2 liters of the 1.5 per cent dextrose or sorbitol peritoneal dialysis solution and leave it in the peritoneal cavity for 30 minutes before draining. Drainage of the 2 liters from the peritoneal cavity takes 10 to 20 minutes. To remove excess fluid more rapidly, for example, from a patient with pulmonary or peripheral edema, the 4.25 per cent solution is introduced into the peritoneal cavity and drained after only 10 minutes. By repeated exchanges with the 4.25 per cent dialysis solution, generally alternating with 1.5 per cent solution, as much as 500 to 1,000 cc. of excess fluid may be removed per hour, even from hypotensive, edematous patients, totally resistant to any type of diuretic therapy. With peritoneal dialysis, fluid is removed in diuretically-resistant patients and simultaneously, any or all electrolyte and/or acid-base abnormalities such as hyponatremia, hypochloremia, hyperkalemia or hypokalemia and even

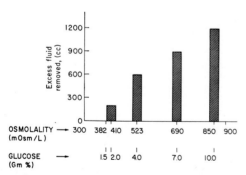

Relation of osmolality of dialysis solution to negative water balance. Height of bars represents excess fluid removed 60 minutes after insertion of 2 L containing indicated amounts of glucose. Figures are average values from 22 experiments.

FIG. 11. Relationship between increasing concentrations of dextrose in peritoneal dialysis solutions and the volume of excess fluid removed with each 2 liter exchange. (Maxwell, M. and Kleeman, C.R.: Clinical Disorders of Fluid and Electrolyte Metabolism, McGraw-Hill, New York, 1962)

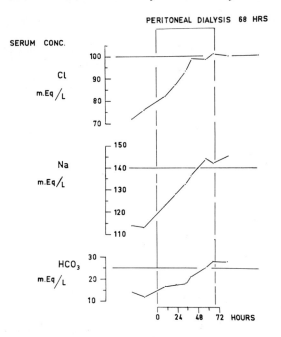

FIG. 12. Correction of hyponatremia, hypochloremia, and acidosis by peritoneal dialysis.

severe acidosis are corrected (Fig. 12). This is in striking contrast to the dangerously increased electrolyte abnormalities, particularly the rapid losses of potassium, resulting from mobilization of edema fluid by use of the potent diuretics.

These therapeutic effects are illustrated(Fig. 13) by the results of peritoneal dialysis in the patient with severe cor pulmonale in refractory congestive failure, discussed above, who had developed cardiac arrhythmias due to potassium losses during diuretic therapy (Fig. 4). Before peritoneal dialysis, this patient was hyponatremic, hypochloremic and azotemic and had an uncompensated severe metabolic alkalosis despite his severe respiratory insufficiency. Following peritoneal dialysis, during which he lost 11 kgms. of edema without developing any cardiac arrhythmias, his serum sodium and potassium were normal, his serum chloride increased and his serum pH became somewhat acidotic, reflecting the severe respiratory acidosis resulting from his pulmonary dysfunction. Moreover, he became increasingly responsive to ethacrynic acid and diuresed, losing an additional 7 kgm. during the next 6 days. At that time, his improved cardiovascular-renal status, following reduction in pulmonary and peripheral congestion, was reflected by the further decrease in his BUN and the return of his serum creatinine and electrolyte levels towards normal.

Recently, it has been emphasized by others[18] that peritoneal dialysis not only mobilizes edema fluid in patients unresponsive to diuretic therapy but, at

THERAPEUTIC EFFECTS OF PERITONEAL DIALYSIS IN REFRACTORY CONGESTIVE FAILURE

| TIME | Wt. | SERUM ELECTROLYTES | | | | ARTERIAL | | B.U.N. | CREAT. |
		Na	K	CO_2	Cl	pH	pCO_2		
	(kg)	(mEq/L)	(mEq/L)	(mEq/L)	(mEq/L)		(mm Hg)	(mgm%)	(mgm%)
Pre—P. D.	75	128	4.6	34	72	7.50	45	117	—
Post — P. D.	65	140	4.5	34	86	7.33	73	90	2.3
6 DAYS Post — P. D.	61	146	5.0	32	98	7.41	72	43	1.1

FIG. 13.   Correction of serum electrolyte abnormalities and metabolic alkalosis during mobilization of 10 liters of edema fluid by peritoneal dialysis in patient in previously intractable congestive failure. Note continued improvement and increased diuretic responsiveness (see text) over subsequent 6 days.

the same time, corrects serum electrolyte and acid base abnormalities. Table 2 summarizes the indications for peritoneal dialysis in acute or chronic failure. These are as follows: 1) intractable edema, either pulmonary or peripheral; 2) electrolyte abnormalities with or without edema, including hyponatremia, hypochloremic alkalosis, hyperkalemia or hypokalemia, and hypercalcemia or hypocalcemia; and 3) lactic acid acidosis. In lactic acid acidosis, peritoneal dialysis with solutions containing acetate as the bicarbonate precursor not only permits removal of accumulated organic acids but also permits rapid and repeated injections of as much concentrated sodium acetate or sodium bicarbonate as needed to correct the severe acidosis, without fear of intensifying the pulmonary and/or peripheral edema of the oliguric, diuretically-resistant patient in severe cardiac failure. Peritoneal dialysis also 4) corrects the hyperuricemia frequently present after long-term treatment with thiazide, furosemide or ethacrynic acid. Finally, peritoneal dialysis also 5)

corrects the prerenal azotemia of severe congestive failure.

The major precaution to be observed during peritoneal dialysis is to avoid too rapid or excessive removal of edema, which may produce transient hypovolemia and, later, excessive contraction of extracellular fluid volume in some edematous patients. The possibility of overly dehydrating

TABLE 2
Indications for Peritoneal Dialysis in Congestive Failure

Intractable Edema
  Pulmonary Edema
  Peripheral Edema
Electrolyte Abnormalities
  Hyponatremia
  Hypochloremia Alkalosis.
  Hyperkalemia or Hypokalemia
  Hypocalcemia
Lactic Acid Acidusis
Hyperuricemia
Azotemia

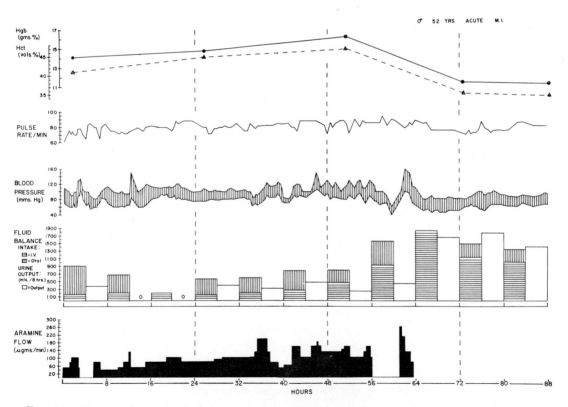

FIG. 14. Hypotension, tachycardia, and oliguria caused by dehydration in patient following myocardial infarction required aramine infusion to maintain blood pressure until rehydration was achieved by infusing 5% dextrose in water solution intravenously. Note initially increasing hemoglobin and hematocrit, reflecting decreased plasma volume and producing hypovolemia and reduced central venous pressure. After hemoconcentration and reduced plasma volume are corrected, urine output increases and blood pressure is maintained without vasopressor infusion.

patients in intractable congestive failure may appear paradoxical. However, recently there has been increasing recognition that, frequently, patients with a primary decrease in cardiac output after myocardial infarction may also have circulatory consequences secondary to a relative reduction in blood volume that generally is reflected by a decline in central venous pressure.[19] The decreased venous return ultimately leads to the renal and hemodynamic consequences of a falling cardiac output.

This sequence is illustrated by the data in Figure 14. In the course of his myocardial infarction, this patient, who was never subjected to peritoneal dialysis, developed oliguria, tachycardia and hypotension. His blood pressure was initially raised by infusing metaraminol for a number of hours. Nevertheless, his oliguria persisted until it was recognized that he had become dehydrated, possibly from his continual diaphoresis. A central venous catheter, inserted percutaneously, revealed a low pressure and his rising hematocrit gave further indication of a decreasing plasma volume. Therefore, he was rehydrated by rapidly infusing 5 per cent dextrose in water, intravenously.

When his total body water and plasma volume were re-expanded, as indicated by the decrease in hemoglobin and hematocrit, not only was his blood pressure sustained without administration of metaraminol but his urine output was promptly increased. Subsequently, he was maintained on an increased oral fluid intake without incident and required no more vaso-constrictor drugs.

Such excessive contraction of the extracellular fluid has a number of deleterious effects, as shown in Figure 15. The renal ischemia and impairment in electrolyte and water excretion following reduction in extracellular fluid volume and the ultimate cardiovascular hemodynamic consequences of hemoconcentration and uncorrected hypovolemia are well known. Another less appreciated effect influencing morbidity is the thickening of respiratory secretions, tending to promote the development of pulmonary complications and inducing atelectasis. It has been recently emphasized that relative hypovolemia and/or excessive extracellular fluid reduction may be produced in cardiac patients by improper evaluation of "normal" central venous pressure readings.[20] In patients in congestive failure, such normal values may actually be dangerous, reflecting insufficient venous return. Modern tendency to restrict fluid intake in congestive failure may lead to subtle development of occult dehydration due to insensible

SEQUELLAE OF EXTRACELLULAR FLUID CONTRACTION

1. RENAL ISCHEMIA
    a. Oliguria
    b. Impaired Electrolyte and Acid-Base Regulation
    c. Azotemia

2. HEMOCONCENTRATION AND HYPOVOLEMIA
    a. Vasoconstriction ⟶ tissue ischemia and anoxia
        1) General ⟶ lactic acid acidosis
        2) Specific
            a) Splanchnic
                1. Gastrointestinal ⟶ atony ⟶ ileus
                2. Hepatic ⟶ metabolic problems
            b) Myocardial
            c) Cerebral
    b. Decreased Cardiac Output
    c. Hypotension
    d. Shock

3. THICKENED RESPIRATORY SECRETIONS

FIG. 15.   Deleterious effects of excessive extracellular fluid contraction.

losses, particularly when these are exaggerated by fever or dyspnea. As illustrated, change in hemoglobin concentration and hematocrit may detect contraction of the plasma volume early. Then, testing the renal and cardiovascular effects of a rapid infusion of 5 per cent dextrose in water solution, as indicated above, may quickly determine if relative hypovolemia or dehydration are present.

Significant contraction of the extracellular fluid during peritoneal dialysis is generally easy to avoid in the average patient on an acute coronary care unit where important physiological parameters are continually monitored. As discussed, excessive fall in central venous pressure, decrease in blood pressure and unexplained tachycardia may indicate too rapid removal of extracellular fluid with consequent hypovolemia, generally reflected by a rising hemoglobin and hematocrit. In the very edematous patient, plasma volume may be sustained by applying elastic bandages to the legs to promote more rapid reabsorption of peripheral edema as fluid is being removed during dialysis. If hypovolemia develops in the absence of such a convenient source of fluid, infusion of 5 per cent dextrose in water or some other isotonic fluid may suffice until reequillibration between extracellular fluid and plasma volume can occur.

With these precautions, peritoneal dialysis is a most important therapeutic aid in the management of the seemingly terminal coronary patient. It permits removal of excess fluid and correction of severe electrolyte abnormalities, including acidosis, without over-burdening the circulation, thereby prolonging life and permitting the damaged myocardium to heal.

ABNORMALITIES IN ACID-BASE BALANCE

On the acute coronary care unit, aberrations in acid-base balance, reflecting the summation of physiological abnormalities that may produce metabolic and/or respiratory acidosis or alkalosis, are also encountered. A marked fall in cardiac output immediately promotes metabolic acidosis by decreasing tissue perfusion and oxygenation, leading to progressively more severe lactic acid acidosis. Concurrently, marked reduction in glomerular filtration rate and renal plasma flow lead to impaired renal capacity to correct metabolic acidosis by distal tubular ammonia and hydrogen ion exchange. For example, when large doses of ammonium chloride are administered to patients in severe congestive failure to correct chloride depletion, the severely ischemic kidney cannot increase ammonia pro-

duction sufficiently to achieve full compensation and serious acidosis results. At times, but not frequently, respiratory acidosis may also result either from severe pulmonary congestion or from over-sedation from the analgesic drugs, given to counteract the severe pain of myocardial infarction. Although generally not severe, when superimposed on metabolic acidosis, respiratory acidosis may significantly lower body pH.

Metabolic alkalosis is rare in the previously untreated patient with acute myocardial infarction, but commonly occurs as a result of long-term diuretic therapy in the previously chronically ill patient. As discussed above, it may result from either intracellular potassium depletion *per se,* from chloride depletion produced by prolonged administration of diuretics without chloride replacement, or from attempted potassium repletion with salts such as Kaon or potassium Triplex without supplying chloride to patients on low sodium diets. Finally, respiratory alkalosis, resulting from hyperventilation due to acute pulmonary congestion, pain or anxiety, may occur at times.

The clinical significance of these acid-base abnormalities in the patient on the acute coronary care unit has received a good deal of attention recently. Metabolic alkalosis is of prognostic significance as an index of potential potassium depletion that, if uncorrected, may lead to dangerous arrhythmias in the digitalized myocardium. Of much greater significance is the question of how severe metabolic acidosis affects prognosis in myocardial infarctions, which has been much disputed since Mackenzie, *et al.*[21] first suggested that it was associated with a high mortality rate. In 58 per cent of 123 patients with myocardial infarction, Kirby and McNichol[22] observed a fall of plasma bicarbonate, which usually was compensated by a decrease in carbon dioxide content, so that the pH was reduced in only 22 per cent of these patients. The inverse rise in serum lactic acid levels suggested that the decrease in plasma bicarbonate was secondary to tissue hypoxia. In the patients with both hypotension and left ventricular failure, there was a fall in plasma bicarbonate and severe acidosis, which was associated with a very high mortality rate. Whether this association is causal or coincidental is not established as yet.

Acidosis is known to have marked cardiovascular effects. However, because neither correcting the hypoxia nor attempting to correct metabolic acidosis with sodium bicarbonate or THAM infusions had any effect on mortality, Kirby and McNichol concluded that the acidosis is only another aspect of the severe circulatory impairment but in itself does not affect mortality. From his own clinical experience and a review of the available clinical and experimental literature, Neaverson[23] drew the same conclusions. He felt that since correcting the acidosis failed to influence mortality, both acidosis and the associated higher mortality are independent reflections of the greater myocardial damage occurring with more massive infarctions. Nonetheless, it is my feeling that conventional methods of correcting acidosis solely by infusing alkalinizing solutions lead to further circulatory embarrassment and adversely affect survival.

The answer will not be known until more vigorous efforts are made to correct acidosis completely by combining peritoneal dialysis with the rapid administration of the required large amounts of concentrated bicarbonate, which can be safely given intravenously as fluid is being rapidly removed by dialysis without the danger of producing pulmonary edema or circulatory overload. In our myocardial infarction research unit at the Cedars of Lebanon Hospital, we plan to investigate this approach further.

HYPONATREMIA

The final fluid and electrolyte problem to be considered is hyponatremia. Generally, this is uncommon in patients previously not in congestive failure, unless excessive amounts of sodium-free fluids are given. However, many patients suffering acute myocardial infarction have long histories of pre-existing heart failure, which may have led to development of one or more of the factors that promote hyponatremia summarized in Table 3.

First, acute and chronic hyponatremia must be differentiated. The acute hyponatremia of congestive failure is largely dilutional, resulting from excessive water intake in a patient unable to dilute his urine despite the fall in serum osmolarity, which normally should lead to decreased release of posterior pituitary antidiuretic hormone and, consequently, to water diuresis. As discussed above, the sustained release of antidiuretic hormone, in response to either an increased disproportion between cardiac output and the body's metabolic needs or to some aberration in the volume-circulatory regulating mechanism in congestive failure, probably plays an important role in this phenomenon.[6] In addition, the profound reduction in the sodium load delivered to the diluting segments of the renal tubules also leads to continued elaboration of concentrated urine despite hyponatremia.

However, occasionally a patient in congestive failure may also develop sodium depletion as

TABLE 3
Hyponatremia in Congestive Heart Failure

Etiology
Acute
Dilutional
Sustained ADH Release
Decreased Tubular Na Load
Chronic
Sick Cell Syndrome
Osmoreceptor Reset
Intracellular Cation Depletion
Treatment
Restrict Water Intake
Administer Mannitol
Diuretics ? ? ? ?
Peritoneal Dialysis

well. For example, vomiting and/or diarrhea may actually lead to loss of sodium and hyponatremia in a patient on a low sodium intake who continues to ingest water. True depletional hyponatremia rarely occurs in congestive failure as a result of conventional diuretic therapy, since contraction of the extracellular fluid greatly reduces diuretic response, so that little or no sodium is removed. However, with the very potent newer diuretics like ethacrynic acid and furosemide, if fluid intake is not restricted between diuretic periods, retention of water after diuresis subsides may produce dilutional hyponatremia.

Chronic asymptomatic hyponatremia may reflect a number of pathogenetic mechanisms.[6] The first is the so-called sick cell syndrome that results from alterations in cellular and membrane metabolism, preventing maintenance of the normal electrolyte concentration gradients and extracellular fluid, with a consequent lowering of body osmolarity, in a variety of chronic illnesses. Secondly, an osmoreceptor reset may occur as a consequence of either the "sick cell" syndrome or of a third factor, intracellular potassium depletion, that may lower intracellular osmolarity, including that of the osmoreceptors which then become set at a somewhat lower level.

Usually, the patient with chronic hyponatremia is well adjusted to the gradual change in body tonicity which does not contribute to his cardiovascular or other symptoms. However, acute hyponatremia may have significant central nervous and cardiovascular consequences. Therefore, prophylactic treatment of acute hyponatremia in patients in acute congestive failure is mandatory. Water intake should be restricted until the patient's ability to dilute the urine and to excrete water *per se* is established. If acute severe hyponatremia is causing C.N.S. symptoms, active treatment may be necessary. Water diuresis may be induced by cautiously infusing 20 per cent solutions of the osmotic diuretic, Mannitol.

Since Mannitol must be excreted as an essentially isotonic concentration, each 250 ml. of 20 per cent Mannitol administered will lead, ultimately, to excretion of 1000 ml. of urine, containing Mannitol in a 5 per cent concentration plus a very low concentration of electrolytes, thereby correcting the hypotonicity and hyponatremia. It should be emphasized that Mannitol expands the extracellular fluid and, therefore if given too rapidly or in excess, may produce serious pulmonary congestion.

It has been suggested that the diuretics may perhaps help to correct hyponatremia because in salt retainers, sodium is excreted at a concentration less than that of plasma. However, the correction of hyponatremia following successful use of diuretics usually results from the improvement in the patient's cardiovascular status. The increased cardiac output is associated with a secondary shutting off of the antidiuretic mechanism, leading to a spontaneous water diuresis and to an increase in serum sodium concentration.

If acute hyponatremia is severe and symptomatic and water must be removed, particularly in an edematous patient to whom infusion of concentrated Mannitol is contraindicated because of the danger of pulmonary congestion, the safest method for quickly correcting hyponatremia is peritoneal dialysis. As discussed above, this procedure permits carefully controlled simultaneous correction of all the fluid, electrolyte and acid-base abnormalities, without danger to the patient. Moreover, while hyponatremia is being corrected, the excess intracellular fluid that entered cells due to the previous hypotonicity of the extracellular fluid can be continuously removed by dialyzing with solutions containing higher concentrations of dextrose or sorbitol. Thus, normal body tonicity and serum sodium concentration can promptly be restored without the dangers inherent in infusing either concentrated Mannitol or sodium solution.

SUMMARY

The fluid and electrolyte problems occurring in patients on the acute coronary unit reflect the effects of mechanisms activated whenever the cardiac output is inadequate for the body's metabolic needs. Often the acute effects are modified by or superimposed on the consequences of chronic congestive heart failure and various therapeutic agents. Fortunately, for management of these problems, there are new methods now available that permit life to be prolonged in what was once considered to be intractable congestive failure, giving time for the damaged myocardium to heal.

REFERENCES

1. Weston, R. E.: Pathogenesis and treatment of edema. *In* Clinical Disorders of Fluid and Electrolyte Metabolism. Ed. by Maxwell, M.H., and Kleeman, C. R. New York, McGraw-Hill, 1962.
2. Weston, R. E., Escher, D. J. W., Grossman, J., and Leiter, L.: Mechanisms contributing to unresponsiveness to mercurial diuretics in congestive heart failure. J. Clin Invest. *31*:901, 1952.
3. Barger, A. C.: Renal hemodynamic factors in congestive heart failure. Ann. New York Acad. Sci., *139*:276, 1966.
4. Bartter, F. C.: The role of aldosterone in normal homeostasis and in certain disease states. Metabolism, *5*:369, 1956.
5. Earley, L. E., and Daugharty, T. M.: Sodium Metabolism. New Eng. J. Med., *281*:72, 1969.
6. Weston, R. E., Grossman, J., Borun, E. R., and Hanenson, I. B.: The pathogenesis and treatment of hyponatremia in congestive heart failure. Am. J. Med., *25*:558, 1958.
7. Scribner, B. H., and Burnell, J. M.: Interpretation of the serum potassium concentration. Metabolism, *5*:468, 1966.
8. Schwartz, W. B.: Pathogenesis and replacement of diuretic induced potassium and chloride loss. Ann. New York Acad. Sci., *139*:506, 1966.
9. Morgenstern, L., Freilich, M., and Panish, J. F.: The circumferential small bowel ulcer. Clinical aspects in 17 patients. J.A.M.A., *191*:101. 1965.
10. Liddle, G. W.: Aldosterone antagonists. A.M.A. Arch. Int. Med., *102*:998, 1958.
11. Crosley, A. D., Jr., Ronquillo, L. M., Strickland, W. H., and Alexander, F.: Triamterine, a natriuretic agent. Ann. Int. Med., *56*:241, 1962.
12. Scribner, B. H., Bogardus, G. M., Fremont-Smith, and Burnell, J. M.: Potassium intoxication during and immediately following respiratory acidosis. J. Clin. Invest., *33*:965, 1954.
13. Greenstein, S., Goldburgh, W. P., Guzman, S. V., and Bellet, S. A.: Comparative analysis of molar sodium lactate and other agents in the treatment of induced hyperkalemia in nephrectomized dogs. Circulat. Res., *8*:223, 1960.
14. Foltz, E. L.: Preliminary clinical observations with an aryloxycetic acid diuretic. Fed. Proc., *22*:598, 1963.
15. Reubi, F. C.: Clinical Use of Furosemide. Ann. New York Acad. Sci., *139*:433, 1966.
16. Maxwell, M. H., Rockney, R. E., Kleeman, C. R. and Twiss, M. R.: Peritoneal dialysis I. technique and application. J.A.M.A., *170*:917, 1959.
17. Weston, R. E., and Roberts, M.: Clinical use of stylet-catheter for peritoneal dialysis. A.M.A. Arch. Int. Med., *115*:659, 1965.
18. Maillous, L. U., Swartz, C. D., Onesti, G., Heider, J., Ramirex, O., and Brest, A. M.: Peritoneal dialysis for refractory congestive heart failure. J.A.M.A., *199*:123, 1967.
19. Allen, H. N., Danzig, R., and Swan, H. J. C.: Incidence and significance of relative hypovolemia as a cause of shock associated with acute myocardial infarction. Circulation, *36*:Suppl. 2, 50, 1967.
20. Mclean, L. D., Duff, J. H., Scott, H. M., and Peretz,

D. I.: Treatment of shock in man based on hemodynamic changes. Surg. Gynec. & Obst., *120:*
1, 1965.

21. Mackenzie, G. J., Taylor, S. H., Flenley, D. C.,
McDonald, A. H., Stauton, H. P., and Donald,
K. W.: Circulatory and respiratory studies in myocardial infarction and cardiogenic shock. Lancet,
2:825, 1964

22. Kirby, B. J., and McNichol: Acid-base status in
acute myocardial infarction. Lancet, *2:*1054, 1966.

23. Neaverson, M. D.: Metabolic acidosis in acute
myocardial infarction. Brit. Med. J., *2:*383, 1966.

Management of Heart Block Complicating Acute Myocardial Infarction

Simon Dack and Ephraim Donoso

The widespread availability of the coronary care unit, with its improved facilities for constant electrocardiographic monitoring, cardiac pacing, and other emergency measures, has led to changes in the management of atrioventricular block, a serious complication of myocardial infarction. In this presentation, we shall summarize the current data on incidence, pathologic anatomy, hemodynamic effects, indications for and effects of cardiac pacing and comparison of the results of cardiac pacing with those of medical treatment.

INCIDENCE AND PROGNOSIS OF HEART BLOCK

Prior to electrocardiographic monitoring, the incidence of partial A-V block ranged from 1 to 12 per cent and that of complete block from 1.3 to 3.3 per cent of cases of acute myocardial infarction (Table 1).[1-4] Since 1964, the incidence in several series of monitored cases has ranged from 6 to 13 per cent for first degree block, 3.5 to 10 per cent for second degree block, and 4.2 to 8 per cent for complete block.[5-8] It is evident that, as in the case of other arrhythmias, the observed incidence of heart block rises as more cases of infarction are continuously monitored by electrocardiogram.

The mortality rate in the monitored series of myocardial infarction complicated by heart block (a total of 266 cases) [5,7,9-12] ranged from 10 to 30 per cent in cases of partial block and 27 to 53 per cent in cases of complete block (Table 2). Both medical treatment and cardiac pacing were used in these cases. The serious prognosis of complete heart block

TABLE 1
Incidence of Heart Block in Myocardial Infarction

	No. Cases	Incidence (Per Cent)		
		1° Block	2° Block	3° Block
Nonmonitored Cases				
Master et al.[1]	300		1	1.7
Imperial et al.[2]	153		3.3	3.3
Hurwitz and Eliot[3]	500	5.8	2	1.8
Pick[4]	3174	1–12%		1.3
Monitored Cases				
Lawrie et al.[5]	400	6	5	7
Day[6]	273	6	8	8
Julian et al.[7]	100	13	10	8
Meltzer and Kitchell[8]	141	8.5	3.5	4.2

TABLE 2
Mortality in Acute Myocardial Infarction Complicated by Heart Block (Monitored Series)

	No. Cases	1° Block (%)	2° Block (%)	3° Block (%)
Sutton et al[9]	55		11.6	47.8
Restiaux et al.[10]	9			33
Lawrie et al.[5]	70	14	10	27
Scott et al.[11]	50			48
Lassers and Julian[12]	51			47
Julian[7]	31	46	30	37

is evident from these mortality figures. It is still not clear whether cardiac pacing has improved the prognosis.

ANATOMIC BASIS FOR HEART BLOCK

In the great majority of cases, heart block in myocardial infarction results from acute occlusion of the right coronary artery from which the nutrient vessel of the A-V node arises.[13] However, the occlusion is generally distal to this branch and the A-V block is caused by impaired flow through the septal branches, producing ischemia of the A-V bundle and its branches. Occasionally (10% of cases) this septal vessel arises from the left circumflex artery. For this reason, heart block is generally associated with inferior or posterior wall infarction. Recently, heart block as a result of occlusion of the left anterior descending coronary artery and anteroseptal infarction has been observed with increased frequency. These cases must be recognized promptly because of the poor prognosis and high mortality as compared to posteroinferior wall infarction.

The pathologic involvement of the A-V conduction system differs in these two groups.[14-18] In inferior wall infarction, the A-V node and bundle of His are edematous and congested but rarely completely infarcted. In addition, there are localized lesions in the main bundle and its bifurcation and initial parts of the bundle branches. The damage and resulting conduction disturbance are therefore generally reversible. In anteroseptal infarction, on the other hand, the septal lesions are generally more extensive, producing necrosis and partial destruction of the left bundle branch and total destruction of the right branch. The bundle of His and the A-V node are not involved. Bilateral bundle branch block is usually the cause of the complete A-V block. In this type, the block may be irreversible, resulting in early death or permanent block.

It is evident that the difference in pathologic involvement of the conduction system in inferior and anterior infarction determines the difference in type and prognosis of resultant A-V block.[14-18] In posteroinferior infarction, the block is often first degree or partial, with a normal duration of QRS, reflecting a higher location of the conduction system damage. The ventricular rate may be normal or only moderately slowed (generally above 45/min.) and Wenckebach periods with dropped beats are common (Mobitz type I block). In most cases, the block is temporary and reverts to normal in several hours or days; permanent block is rare. Mortality rate is relatively low. In anterior infarction, there may be a sudden complete A-V block with asystole. The electrocardiogram shows advanced or complete block, or Mobitz type II partial block. The QRS is widened and the ventricular rate slow (below 45/min.). Stokes-Adams syndrome due to ventricular asystole or fibrillation is frequent, resulting in high mortality. In some cases, the appearance of bilateral bundle branch block, manifested by left axis deviation, right bundle branch block, and prolonged P-R interval may herald the development of complete A-V block. In our experience, clear-cut discrimination between these two types cannot always be made. Complete block with Stokes-Adams syndrome may develop in inferior infarction with type I Mobitz or Wenckebach block. Even sudden asystole has been observed in such cases.

HEMODYNAMIC EFFECTS OF HEART BLOCK

Heart block and bradycardia due to any type of arrhythmia cause significant hemodynamic alterations. These include increased stroke volume; reduced cardiac output when the increased stroke volume cannot compensate for the slow heart rate and maintain normal minute volume; increased intracardiac pressures (right atrial, right ventricular end-diastolic) and pulmonary artery wedge pressures; reduced arteriovenous oxygen difference; increased central venous pressure; and elevated systolic and reduced diastolic arterial pressure. In the presence of acute myocardial infarction and impaired ventricular performance these hemodynamic consequences of heart block attain even greater clinical importance. The acutely infarcted ventricular myocardium may be unable to increase the stroke output, resulting in severe diminution of cardiac output. The systolic pressure is low, the pulse pressure is small rather than increased, and arterial hypotension, shock, and heart failure may develop. For these reasons, bradycardia during the early stage of myocardial infarction constitutes an indication for urgent treatment to increase ventricular rate even in the absence of shock or Stokes-Adams syndrome.

The hemodynamic effects of artificial pacing in complete heart block complicating acute myocardial infarction have recently been studied in 13 patients.[19] The results of increasing the ventricular rate by cardiac pacing were as follows:

1. With two exceptions, cardiac output increased. A pacing rate of 100/min. or more was required to produce maximal cardiac output response, but an adequate response was obtained with a pacing rate of 80 to 90 per minute.

2. Stroke volume fell in most cases as the ventricular rate increased, but it rose in some cases, suggest-

ing improved myocardial performance.

3. Arterial blood pressure increased and the change paralleled fairly closely the changes in cardiac output as the pacing rate increased.

4. Systemic vascular resistance was high in most cases with low cardiac output and fell as the cardiac output rose during pacing.

5. There were no consistent changes in right atrial or pulmonary artery pressure during cardiac pacing.

6. Tension-time index was low during heart block and increased considerably during pacing, implying a corresponding increase in myocardial oxygen requirements. In the normal heart such a rise in oxygen demand is met by increased coronary flow. However, the restricted coronary flow in myocardial infarction may limit the increase in myocardial oxygen uptake.

7. Clinically, cardiac pacing improved the signs of depressed mental function and poor skin circulation, which were invariably associated with a severe reduction in cardiac output. However, it was emphasized that in clinical practice the value of improving the systemic circulation by cardiac pacing must be balanced against the increased work and oxygen requirements produced by increasing the ventricular rate. These factors must be considered in deciding which patients should be paced and the optimum rate of pacing.

MEDICAL MANAGEMENT OF HEART BLOCK

Drug therapy includes atropine, isoproterenol, and corticosteroids,[20,21] In mild degrees of A-V block, first or second degree, small intermittent doses of atropine (0.5 mg.) given intramuscularly or intravenously may be helpful in improving A-V conduction and increasing ventricular rate. However, it must be remembered that not infrequently the increased atrial rate produced by atropine may increase the degree of A-V block and actually slow the ventricular rate.[22] In more advanced block or when ventricular asystole or fibrillation occurs, prompt intravenous infusion or isoproterenol (2 mg./500 cc. of dextrose in water) is indicated, given at a sufficient rate to eliminate asystole and maintain a ventricular rate of 40 to 50 beats per minute. The electrocardiogram is monitored constantly during the infusion to detect signs of ventricular irritability. A slow infusion is maintained until a transvenous pacemaker can be inserted for cardiac pacing.

Corticosteroid therapy may be helpful by reducing edema and inflammatory reaction in the A-V node and bundle and enhancing A-V conduction.[20] Large doses are necessary, equivalent to 60–80 mg. of

prednisone orally or 40–80 mg. methyl prednisolone parenterally, or 250–500 mg. hydrocortisone intravenously daily. Such therapy may be helpful in cases in which facilities for prompt pacemaker therapy are not available.

CARDIAC PACING

One of the unique advantages of the coronary care unit is the facility for emergency cardiac pacing.[11,12, 16,23] This can be instituted to treat severe bradycardia and Stokes-Adams syndrome without the necessity of moving the patient from the unit. A pacing electrode wire can be inserted transvenously into the right ventricle either percutaneously or by venous cutdown. In an emergency, a thin unipolar or bipolar electrode wire (Elecath) is inserted percutaneously into an antebrachial or subclavian vein and the wire is guided into the right ventricle with the aid of the electrocardiogram.[24] The configuration of the P wave and QRS helps localize the tip of the wire when it enters the right atrium and right ventricle. This procedure can be done at the patient's bedside and can be completed in 5 to 20 minutes by a skilled resident or attending physician. This method is now the procedure of choice when rapid institution of cardiac pacing is required.

When the situation is less urgent and time permits, especially after an isoproterenol infusion has been started, the transvenous pacing wire can be inserted under fluoroscopic control. With the availability of portable image intensifier equipment, it is not necessary to move the patient to the cardiac catheterization or x-ray department to insert the transvenous pacemaker, but he is moved in a special bed into an adjacent treatment room in the coronary care unit. Under fluoroscopic control, a bipolar catheter electrode is inserted into the right ventricle through a cutdown over an external jugular or antebrachial vein. A battery-powered portable pacemaker generator is used, preferably a demand type. The rate is set at 70 to 90 per minute.

Another method which may be lifesaving in an emergency is the transthoracic insertion of a unipolar pacing wire through a needle inserted by puncture of the precordium into the cavity of the right ventricle.[25] This can be accomplished in a few seconds during ventricular asystole or fibrillation and temporary cardiac pacing may be accomplished until one of the above mentioned methods can be carried out.

Indications for Cardiac Pacing

The indications for pacing patients in the coronary care unit are based on the following considerations:

(1) Facilities and personnel for prompt attachment of a transvenous pacemaker are available; (2) Advanced A-V block or Stokes-Adams syndrome may occur without warning in myocardial infarction, even in apparently benign types of heart block (Mobitz type I) with inferior wall infarction; (3) Anterior wall infarction with Mobitz type II block or bilateral bundle branch block is associated with high mortality and when asystole occurs, it may not respond to drugs.[16-19]

The indications for insertion of a cardiac pacemaker in patients with myocardial infarction are:

1. First degree block if the P-R interval exceeds 0.30 second. The pacemaker is kept on standby or demand mode and is not activated unless the ventricular rate is 60 or less.

2. Second degree A-V block, including the Wenckebach type. The demand type pacemaker generator is set at 70 per minute to prevent bradycardia and periods of asystole.

3. Cardiac arrest due to ventricular asystole, tachycardia, or fibrillation.

4. Bilateral bundle branch block, even with normal sinus rhythm. In these patients, the generator is kept at standby unless the rate is slow.

In urgent situations where great speed is required (Stokes-Adams syndrome), percutaneous insertion of an Elecath electrode wire into a subclavian vein is the method of choice.[26] In less urgent situations (first and second degree block), a bipolar electrode catheter is inserted through a peripheral vein with the aid of portable image-intensifier fluoroscopic equipment. In such cases, the early insertion of a transvenous pacemaker when the patient's condition is relatively stable may prevent cardiac arrest and Stokes-Adams syndrome, when there may be insufficient time to insert a pacemaker before irreversible shock and death occur.[27] When the pacemaker is inserted prophylactically, the decision for pacing and the pacing rate depend on the cardiac mechanism and the heart rate. If the ventricular rate is adequate (70 or above), the pacemaker is turned off but kept on stand-by, or switched into the demand mode at a rate of 70 per minute to prevent asystole. When asystole or severe bradycardia has already occurred, or if cardiac output appears inadequate (hypotension, cerebral ischemia, shock), then the pacing is set at a faster rate, 80–90 per minute, or higher if necessary.

Careful monitoring of the electrocardiogram is necessary during cardiac pacing because of the increased ventricular irritability in myocardial infarction. Ventricular extrasystoles, tachycardia, and even fibrillation may be precipitated by the mechanical irritation of the pacing catheter in the right ventricle and also by the hyperirritability of the adjacent infarcted septum or left ventricle.[28] Also, the pacemaker electrical discharges may augment ventricular irritability particularly if the pacing rate is over 90 per minute. The pacing electrode is left in place until all signs of A-V block have disappeared. Ideally, it should be left in place for at least a week or two longer if possible, because of the danger of sudden recurrence of heart block and cardiac arrest in the first three weeks of the attack.

Pacing in Other Types of Bradycardia

Because of the ease of instituting cardiac pacing in a coronary care unit, the indications for pacing have been expanded to include bradycardia associated with other arrhythmias.[23] These include sinus or nodal bradycardia, sinoauricular block with nodal escape, atrial fibrillation with slow ventricular rate, and A-V dissociation with bradycardia. These arrhythmias have the common effect of diminishing cardiac output and cerebral blood flow and may result in hypotension, shock, and cerebral ischemia. When therapy with atropine and isoproterenol is ineffective in increasing the heart rate, cardiac pacing should be started promptly to improve the cardiac output and blood pressure.[23]

Complications of Cardiac Pacing

The following complications of pacemaker therapy have been observed:[28,29]

During electrode insertion
1. Difficulty in passing catheter
2. Anomalies of external jugular and other intrathoracic veins
3. Serious arrhythmias (ventricular tachycardia, ventricular fibrillation)
   a. Mechanically induced
   b. Induced by electrical pacing
   c. Induced by competition (idioventricular or paced beats occurring during vulnerable period)
4. Angina pectoris induced by pacing
5. Perforation of heart
6. Pneumothorax

During electrode use
1. Local infection
2. Septicemia (catheter induced)
3. Local phlebitis
4. Thromboembolism-pulmonary infarction
5. Displacement of catheter and need for repositioning
6. Perforation of right ventricle
7. Mechanical pacemaker failure

a. Defective catheter
b. Faulty catheter-pacemaker connection
c. Generator failure

Clinical Results of Cardiac Pacing

Recent experience has confirmed that the prompt institution of cardiac pacing abolishes severe bradycardia and Stokes-Adams syndrome in patients with myocardial infarction complicated by advanced heart block.[27] Immediate death from ventricular asystole or fibrillation is prevented. However, the ultimate proof of the effectiveness of cardiac pacing must be demonstrated by its effect on overall mortality—that is, on the number of patients surviving their hospital stay. The latter proof is difficult to obtain because of the nature of the underlying disease; namely, the acute myocardial infarction. It has already been emphasized that patients with heart block have extensive infarction involving not only the left ventricular wall, but also the septum and the intraventricular conduction system. In particular, when heart block occurs in anterior wall infarction, extensive septal damage may result in shock and congestive failure despite control of the A-V block. Also, cardiac pacing in such cases may produce very ineffective ventricular contraction with severely impaired cardiac output. Therefore, the results of cardiac pacing must be evaluated in the light of these prognostic factors present in each case; namely the presence or absence of shock or congestive failure, the occurrence of Stokes-Adams syndrome and the location of the infarction.

Shock and Heart Failure. In the series of Sutton *et al.*[9] (55 cases), there were 25 deaths; 13 of these (5

fibrillation was primary, the prognosis for resuscitation was better than when it occurred as a complication of shock or heart failure, and it was worse if there was massive myocardial infarction, when death from ventricular fibrillation was inevitable.

Scott *et al.*[11] reported on 50 patients, 26 (52%) of whom survived to leave the hospital. The influence of immediate cardiac pacing on mortality rate was related to clinical severity of the heart block. In 11 mild cases (severe shock or heart failure not evident whether or not pacing was used), there were no deaths in 26 moderately severe cases (either severe failure or shock present), mortality was 29 per cent in paced cases and 67 per cent in nonpaced cases; and in the 13 very severe cases (both shock and severe failure present), mortality was 86 per cent in 7 paced cases and 100 per cent in 6 nonpaced cases.

In the 51 cases of Lassers and Julian[12] there were 24 deaths (21 during cardiac pacing); 20 of these occurred within the first 72 hours. A common cause of death was cardiogenic shock in 11 cases, despite cardiac pacing in 9 of these.

Stokes-Adams Syndrome. The presence of Stokes-Adams attacks had a variable effect on the mortality rate. In the series of 50 patients of Scott *et al.*,[11] 11 of 21 with, and 15 of 29 patients without Stokes-Adams syndrome died, an incidence of 52 per cent in each group. In the series of 55 patients of Sutton *et al.*,[9] the mortality rate was 65.5 per cent when Stokes-Adams was present and 31 per cent when it was absent, a significant difference.

Location of the Infarction. This factor is probably the most important determinant of survival in patients with myocardial infarction complicated by heart block.[9,11,19,28,30,31] Table 3 indicates the much higher mortality rate in anterior infarction as com-

TABLE 3
Location of Infarction and Mortality of Heart Block

	Anterior			Posteroinferior					Combined Anterior and Inferior	
	No.	Died		No.	Died				No.	Died
		No.	%	No.	%	No.	%			
Scott et al.[11]	17	10	59	30	11	37				
Parsonet et al.[30]	4	4	100	9	1	11				
Lassers et al.[19]	11	10	9	27	9	33			7	5 (71%)
Paulk & Hurst[28]	3	2	67	32	19	60			8	4 (50%)
Friedberg et al.[31]	8	7	87.5	16	7	44			1	1 (100%)
Sutton et al.[9]	11	11	100	43	13	30				
Totals	54	42	78	157	60	38			16	10 (62.5%)

in patients with fixed-rate and 8 with demand pacemakers) were caused by cardiac failure. All hearts were being paced at the time of death, but there was no effective cardiac output. The other 12 deaths were caused by ventricular fibrillation during the pacing period. These authors concluded that if ventricular

pared to posteroinferior infarction. (78 vs. 38%).

Duration of QRS. The duration of the QRS was an accurate indication of the severity of the septal damage and was an important prognostic factor, particularly in those patients with posteroinferior infarction.[9,12,31] This is well demonstrated in Table 4.

TABLE 4
Duration of QRS and Mortality of Heart Block

	Lassers & Julian[12]		Friedberg et al.[31]		Sutton et al.[9]		Total	
	No.	Died	No.	Died	No.	Died	No.	Died
Posterior Infarction								
Wide QRS	6	5	7	5			13	10
Narrow QRS	26	3	9	2			35	5
Anterior Infarction								
Wide QRS	13	11	7	6			20	17
Narrow QRS	5	4	1	1			6	5
Infarction not Localized								
Wide QRS					20	15	20	15
Narrow QRS					33	8	33	8
Total Cases								
Wide QRS	19	16	14	11	20	15	53	42 (80%)
Narrow QRS	31	7	10	3	33	8	74	18 (24%)

The mortality rate in 53 patients with a wide QRS was 80 per cent compared to only 24 per cent in 74 patients with a narrow QRS. In anterior infarction, however, the mortality was the same whether the QRS was wide (85%) or narrow (83%).

SUMMARY

The indications for cardiac pacing in a coronary care unit are based on the considerations that: (1) adequate facilities and personnel for prompt insertion of a transvenous pacemaker are available; (2) advanced A-V block or Stokes-Adams syndrome may occur without warning in myocardial infarction, even in the benign type of A-V block with inferior wall infarction (Mobitz type I); and (3) anterior wall infarction with A-V block is generally associated with extensive septal damage and high mortality; when asystole occurs, it may not respond to drugs.

The present indications for cardiac pacing are: (1) first degree block if the P-R interval exceeds 0.30 sec. The pacemaker is left on stand-by or demand mode. (2) Second degree block, including Wenckebach type. The pacemaker is kept on demand mode at 60–70/min. to prevent bradycardia or asystole. (3) Cardiac arrest due to ventricular asystole, tachycardia, or fibrillation. (4) Bilateral bundle branch block, even with normal sinus rhythm. The pacemaker is kept on stand-by or demand mode.

The immediate effects of cardiac pacing on survival are excellent. The over-all figures for mortality during the hospital stay are dependent on the following prognostic factors: (1) shock and heart failure; (2) Stokes-Adams syndrome; and (3) location of infarction.

REFERENCES

1. Master, A. M., Dack, S., and Jaffe, L.: Disturbances of rate and rhythm in acute coronary artery thrombosis, Ann. Int. Med. *11*:735, 1937.

2. Imperial, E. S., Carballo, R., and Zimmerman, H. A.: Disturbances of rate, rhythm, and conduction in acute myocardial infarction. A statistical study of 153 cases, Am. J. Cardiol. *5*:24, 1960.

3. Hurwitz, M., and Eliot, R. S.: Arrhythmias in acute myocardial infarction, Dis. Chest *45*:616, 1964.

4. Pick, A. Cardiac arrhythmias associated with recent myocardial infarction, *in* Likoff, W., and Moyer, J. (eds.), Coronary Heart Disease. New York, Grune and Stratton, 1963.

5. Lawrie, D. M., Greenwood, T. W., Goddard, M., Harvey, A. C., Donald, K. W., Julian, D. G., and Oliver, M. F.: A coronary care unit in the routine management of acute myocardial infarction, Lancet *2*:111, 1967.

6. Day, H. W.: Acute coronary care—a five year report, Am. J. Cardiol. *21*:252, 1968.

7. Julian, D. G., Valentine, P. A., and Miller, G. G.: Disturbances of rate, rhythm, and conduction in acute myocardial infarction. A prospective study of 100 consecutive unselected patients with the aid of electrocardiographic monitoring, Am. J. Med. *37*: 915, 1964.

8. Meltzer, L. E., and Kitchell, J. R.: The incidence of arrhythmias associated with acute myocardial infarction, Progr. Cardiovas. Dis. *9*:50, 1966.

9. Sutton, R., Chatterjee, K., and Leatham, A.: Heart block following acute myocardial infarction, Lancet *2*:645, 1968.

10. Restiaux, N., Bray, C., Bullard, H., Murray, M., Robinson, J., Brigden, W., and McDonald, L.: 150 patients with cardiac infarction treated in a coronary unit, Lancet *1*:1286, 1967.

11. Scott, M. G., Geddes, J. S., Patterson, G. C., Adgey, A. A. J., and Pantridge, J. F.: Management of complete heart block complicating acute myocardial infarction, Lancet *2*:1382, 1967.

12. Lassers, B. W., and Julian, D. G.: Artificial pacing in management of complete heart block complicating acute myocardial infarction, Brit. M. J. *2*:142, 1968.

13. James, T. N.: Anatomic relationships of a coronary occlusion to the blood supply of the sinus node and atrioventricular node, *in* The Etiology of Myocardial Infarction, Henry Ford Hospital International Symposium, Boston, Little, Brown & Co. 1961, pp. 341–357.

14. Blondeau, M., Rizzon, P., and Lenegre, J.: Les troubles de la conduction auriculoventriculaire dans

l'infarctus myocardique recent. I. Etude clinique, Arch. Mal. Coeur *54*:1092, 1961. II. Etude anatomique, Arch. Ma. Coeur *54*:1104, 1961.

15. Sutton, R., and Davis, M.: The conduction system in acute myocardial infarction complicated by heart block, Circulation *38*:987, 1968.

16. McNally, E. M., and Benchimol, A.: Medical and physiological considerations in the use of artificia pacing. Part I, Am. Heart J. *75*:380, 1968.

17. Stock, R. J., and Macken, D. L.: Observations on heart block during continuous electrocardiographic monitoring in myocardial infarction, Circulation *38*:993, 1968.

18. Langendorf, R., and Pick, A.: Atrioventricular block, Type II (Mobitz). Its nature and clinical significance (Edit.), Circulation *38*:819, 1968.

19. Lassers, B. W., Anderton, J. L., Muir, A. L., and Julian, D. G.: Hemodynamic effects of artificial pacing in complete heart block complicating acute myocardial infarction, Circulation *38*:308, 1968.

20. Dack, S. Management of the Stokes-Adams syndrome, Am. Heart J. *66*:579–583, 1963.

21. Dack, S., and Donoso, E.: Heart block with Stokes-Adams syndrome, Ann. New York Acad. Sc. In Press.

22. Lister, J. W., Stein, E., Kosowsky, B. D., Lau, S. H., and Damato, A. N.: Atrioventricular conduction in man. Effect of rate, exercise, isoproterenol and atropine on the P-R interval, Am. J. Cardiol. *16*:516, 1965.

23. Kimball, J. T., Kline, S. W., and Killip, T.: Cardiac pacing in acute myocardial infarction, Am. J. Cardiol. *19*:162, 1967.

24. Kimball, J. T., and Killip, T. III.: A simple bedside method of intracardiac pacing, Am. Heart J. *70*:35, 1965.

25. Lillehei, C. W., Levy, J., Bonnebeau, R. C., Long, D. M., Jr., and Sellers, R. D.: Direct wire electrical stimulation for acute postsurgical and postinfarction complete heart block, Ann. New York Acad. Sc. *111*:938, 1964.

26. Escher, D. J. W.: Transvenous emergency cardiac pacing. Presented at Conference on Advances in Cardiac Pacemakers, New York Acad. Sci., Nov. *17*, 1968.

27. Beregovich, J., Fenig, S., Lasser, J., and Allen, D.: Management of acute myocardial infarction complicated by advanced atrioventricular block. Role of artificial pacing, Am. J. Cardiol. *23*:54, 1969.

28. Paulk, E. A., and Hurst, J. W.: Complete heart block in acute myocardial infarction. A clinical evaluation of the intracardiac bipolar catheter pacemaker, Am. J. Cardiol. *17*:695, 1966.

29. Furman, S., Escher, D. J. W., and Solomon, N.: Experiences with myocardial and transvenous implanted cardiac pacemakers, Am. J. Cardiol. *23*:66, 1969.

30. Parsonnet, V., Zucker, I. R., Gilbert, L., Rothfeld, E., Brief, D. K., and Alpert, J.: Evaluation of transvenous pacing of the heart in complete heart block following acute myocardial infarction, Israel J. M. Sc. *3*:206, 1967.

31. Friedberg, C. K., Cohen, H., and Donoso, E.: Heart block as a complication of acute myocardial infarction. Role of pacemaker therapy, Prog. Cardiovasc. Dis. *10*:466, 1968.

Clinical Experience With Phase-Shift Pumping in Medically Refractory Cardiogenic Shock After Myocardial Infarction

Adrian Kantrowitz, Joseph S. Krakauer, Steinar Tjonneland, and Alfred N. Butner

The successful use of cardiopulmonary bypass in open-heart repair of many congenital and acquired lesions provides evidence that a mechanical substitute for the heart can effectively support the circulation for limited periods. A corollary proposition, that mechanically assisted circulation is of benefit in clinical conditions in which the heart's pumping capability is compromised, has been studied in considerable depth during the last 15-20 years.

Mechanical methods for ventricular support now under investigation were recently reviewed by Cooper and Dempsey.[1] Among these is intra-aortic balloon pumping, suggested and studied in the laboratory by Moulopoulos and co-workers,[2] and by Clauss and his associates,[3] in 1962. In this technic, a flexible pumping chamber is passed into the thoracic aorta and inflated so as to displace blood during diastole of the cardiac cycle.

An early investigation of the hemodynamic effects produced by causing peak arterial pressures to occur during the diastolic phase of the cardiac cycle was reported by Kantrowitz and Kantrowitz[4] in 1953. Using an experimental preparation in which blood emerging from the aortic valve was routed through a length of tubing so as to arrive in the central arterial tree during diastole, they observed increased coronary artery flow and reduced left ventricular work with maintenance of systemic perfusion.

Thereafter, a number of investigators studied the hemodynamic effects of what was variously termed arterioarterial pumping, diastolic augmentation, counterpulsation, postsystolic augmentation, or, as we prefer, phase-shift pumping. Summaries of some of these studies are presented in reports by Kantrowitz[5] and also by Nachlas and Siedband.[6]

The latter workers found that increasing coronary artery perfusion during diastole and reducing left ventricular work decreased the size of experimental myocardial infarctions in dogs. Kantrowitz and colleagues, working first with autogenous muscle and subsequently with permanently implantable prostheses, also reported beneficial hemodynamic effects in a variety of experimental preparations and also in two patients with irreversible impairment of myocardial contractility.[5,7,8]

The problem of improving the therapeutic outcome in cardiogenic shock due to acute myocardial infarction offered an opportunity to determine if assisted circulation by means of phase-shift pumping has a place in the clinical armamentarium. Although major advances have been made in the medical management of acute myocardial infarction in recent years, the treatment of cardiogenic shock remains unsatisfactory. Despite the availability of powerful inotropic and pressor substances such as isoproterenol hydrochloride and levarterenol bitartrate, potent diuretics such as ethacrynic acid, improved respirators and monitoring facilities, the mortality rate continues to range from 70 to 90 per cent in various series.[9,10] If the primary pathophysiologic defect in this syndrome is low cardiac output due to ischemic failure of the heart as a pump, then it is reasonable to consider mechanically assisted circulation as a possible treatment, as suggested by Friedberg[9] and Ross,[11] among others.

It is widely agreed that a temporary cardiac assist method should require minimal surgery, reduce myocardial work while maintaining coronary and peripheral circulation, and be capable of intermittent or continuous use for days or weeks. In addition, the technic should be suitable for use by professional personnel without prolonged specialized training. Of the various mechanical methods under development, intra-aortic balloon pumping most nearly appeared to meet these criteria.

The investigations described in this paper were supported by United States Public Health Service Grant HE-11173.

LABORATORY STUDIES

Studies to evaluate the method in animals were begun in our laboratory in 1966. For these studies, a cigar-shaped polyurethane pumping chamber joined to a catheter was passed through a femoral arteriotomy into the descending thoracic aorta just below the origin of the subclavian artery. Fully expanded, the pumping chamber displaced 14 ml. of blood. The extracorporeal end of the catheter was connected through a solenoid valve controlled by a modified Tektronix Model 565 oscilloscope to a helium source. To activate the solenoid valve, signals from the subject's ECG were used to trigger the driving system. The balloon was expanded shortly after the beginning of left ventricular diastole and vented to atmosphere just before systole.

In the initial series of experiments,[12] hemodynamic responses to phase-shift pumping in control animals (29 dogs and 2 calves) included immediate falls in left ventricular peak and end-diastolic pressures, ranging from 7.3 to 13.3 per cent and from 15 to 20 per cent, respectively; 6.7–22 per cent decrease in central aortic systolic peak pressure; and 10–19 per cent reduction of the myocardial tension-time index (8 dogs).

In a subsequent study, pumping produced a 9 per cent average increase in peripheral blood flow and a 32 per cent average reduction of the myocardial tension-time index in 30 normal dogs. In 6 dogs a cardiogenic shock syndrome was induced by ligation of the circumflex or anterior descending branch of the left coronary artery, and in 13, by microsphere embolization. In all hemodynamic parameters studied, significant improvement as a result of phase-shift pumping was observed.[12]

In the next series of experiments, severe left ventricular failure was established in 6 control dogs by simultaneous ligation of the coronary artery branches supplying the left ventricle. All animals died within 132 minutes. In 6 other dogs prepared in the same manner, balloon pumping was started within 1 minute after coronary ligation and continued for 20 minutes. Survival times ranged from 18 to 42 hours.

More recently, the effect of pumping on hemodynamic parameters in a cardiogenic shock syndrome also produced by coronary ligation was evaluated. With 20–40 minutes pumping in 20 dogs, cardiac output increased from 52 per cent ($\pm$ 13.8 per cent) to 79 per cent ($\pm$ 15.4 per cent) of the preligation base line value. Coronary flow rose from 42 ml./min. ($\pm$ 23 ml./min.) to 84 ml./min. ($\pm$ 27 ml./min.). Left ventricular end-diastolic pressure fell from 17 mm. Hg ($\pm$ 10.8 mm. Hg) to 10 mm. Hg ($\pm$ 3.6 mm. Hg). Peripheral resistance decreased by 38 per cent, and the left ventricular tension-time index was lowered by 25 per cent. At the same time, the peak of the first derivative of the left ventricular pressure curve improved by 25 per cent.[13]

The experimental studies established the safe operation of all components of the balloon pumping system, as did exhaustive *in vitro* testing. The pumping chamber, in particular, can withstand a 300 mm. Hg transmembrane pressure without elastic deformation and a substantially higher pressure—about 600 mm. Hg—before bursting. The transmembrane pressure does not exceed 100 mm. Hg in experimental or in clinical use. Significantly elevated free plasma hemoglobin levels or other indications of significant deleterious effects on the blood have not been observed. The laboratory studies also showed that pumping could be initiated rapidly. The pumping equipment was fully mobile.

CLINICAL OBSERVATIONS

The experimental studies progressed to the point that a clinical trial was indicated early in 1967. The pumping procedure in patients, described more fully elsewhere,[14–16] was similar to that used in the laboratory, except that the pumping chamber displaced approximately 32 ml. of blood and that a Dacron side-arm arterial graft was sutured to the arteriotomy site so that blood flow to the leg could be restored during pumping. When possible, medications were discontinued at the onset of pumping. Heparin, 50–75 mg., was given as the pumping chamber and catheter were introduced and at 4-hour intervals thereafter. To patients manifesting vasoconstrictive phenomena, chlorpromazine was given in small doses (0.2 mg./Kg. body weight) to produce peripheral vasodilation and thereby to enhance the effectiveness of pumping. Cardiac arrhythmias were treated pharmacologically or by means of a transvenous pacemaker. Correction of blood volume, tonicity, red cell mass, and pH, mechanically assisted ventilation and cardiotonic drugs were given as indicated.

Peripheral arterial and central venous pressures were monitored, as was the ECG; where possible, central aortic pressure was also monitored. The urine output was recorded. The arteriovenous O_2 difference and other blood gas and chemical parameters were periodically determined.

Balloon pumping was temporarily discontinued when the patient's cardiogenic shock appeared clinically resolved. If the patient's circulation was maintained at adequate levels for several hours, the balloon was removed. If there were any indications of relapse into cardiogenic shock, however, pumping was resumed until stabilization was regained. At this point, pumping was again interrupted for a trial period.

As reported previously,[14],[15] candidates for phase-shift pumping were restricted to those in whom medical therapy for cardiogenic shock due to acute myocardial infarction had failed. Of the patients treated to date, all had myocardial infarction documented by history, clinical findings, electrocardiographic changes, and elevations of serum enzyme levels. The clinical management of these patients provided in the medical intensive care unit comprised bed rest, heavy sedation, heparinization, diuretics, oxygen, and digitalization when indicated. When the patients became hypotensive, isoproterenol hydrochloride was usually given, followed by levarterenol bitartrate or metaraminol bitartrate. The patients were transferred to the cardiac assistance team when the cardiologists attending them agreed that the shock was refractory to therapy and that the prognosis was extremely guarded. At the time of transfer (Table 1), the patients were hypotensive, despite maximal pharmacologic therapy. They manifested generalized sympathetic hyperactivity, persistent oliguria, and cloudy sensorium or coma. In addition, all but one had gross pulmonary edema.

To date, 21 patients have undergone balloon pumping. In 16 of the patients, the interval from onset of myocardial infarction to development of intractable shock was 36 hours or less. These patients are provisionally classified as having "early" circulatory failure. In 5 patients, this interval exceeded 36 hours; these patients are considered to have "delayed" circulatory failure.

The results of balloon pumping in the early

TABLE 1
Age, Sex and Clinical Condition of 21 Patients Immediately Prior to Phase-Shift Balloon Pumping

Case	Age & Sex	ECG	BP* mm. Hg	CVP cm. H₂O	Sympathetic Reaction	Oliguria	Arrhythmias	Pulmonary Edema	Mental Confusion or Coma	Previous MI
1	45,F	Posterior wall MI*	U*	14	+*	+	+	−	+	−
2	58,M	Anterolat. wall MI	U	H*	+	+	+	+	+	+
3	66,F	Anterior wall MI	50/30	14	+	−	+	+	+	−
4	76,F	Anterolat. wall MI	U	5	+	+	+	+	+	−
5	48,M	Anterolat. wall MI	80/50	14	+	+	−	+	+	+
6	79,F	Anterolat. wall MI	50/30	20	+	+	+	+	+	−
7	57,M	Posterior wall MI	60/−	14	+	+	+	+	−	−
8	72,M	Posterolat. Wall	30	30	+	+	A*	+	+	−
9	50,M	Anterior and posterior wall MIs	U	H	+	+	−	+	+	−
10	64,M	Anterosept. MI	80/54	15	+	+	+ A	+	−	+
11	76,M	Anterolat. wall MI*	75/40	26	+	+	+ A	+	+	−
12	76,M	Posterior wall MI	70/40	23	+	+	+	+	+	+
13	60,F	Anterosept. wall MI	U	40	+	+	+	+	+	+
14	54,M	Anterosept. wall MI	50/−	6	+	+	+	+	+	−
15	65,M	Anterosept. and lat. MI	97/71	20	+	+	+	+	−	+
16	61,M	Diaphragmat. MI	70/?	23	+	+	+	−	+	−

MI=myocardial infarction; +=present; −=absent; U=blood pressure unobtainable; H=distended jugular vein, no exact CVP available; A=prior cardiac arrest.
*During (levarterenol) infusion.

TABLE 1, *(Continued)*

Case	Age & Sex	BCG	BP* mm. Hg	CVP cm. H₂O	Sympathetic Reaction	Oliguria	Arrhythmias	Pulmonary Edema	Mental Confusion or Coma	Previous MI
17	73,F	Anterosept. wall MI* (later extension laterally)	80/50	16	+	+	+	+	+	−
18	66,M	Inferior wall MI	80/?	20	+	+	+	+	+	−
19	53,M	Anterolat. and inferior wall MI	100/?	26	+	+	−	+	+	+
20	63,F	Anterosept. MI	70/?	12	+	+	A	+	+	−
21	62,M	Diaphragmat. MI	100/?	22	+	+	+	+	+	−

MI=myocardial infarction; +=present; −=absent; U=blood pressure unobtainable; H=distended jugular vein, no exact CVP available; A=prior cardiac arrest.
*During (levarterenol) infusion.

TABLE 2

Results of Phase-Shift Balloon Pumping in Refractory Cardiogenic Shock: Early Circulatory Failure Group

Case	Duration of Pumping*	Interval of Time from MI to shock	Interval from Shock to Assist	Status
Long-term Survivors				
1	4 hrs. 20 min.	Immediately	6 hrs.	Alive and well after 17 months
4	15 hrs. 37 min.	Immediately	48 hrs.	Alive and well after 13 months
7	5 hrs.	Immediately	16 hrs.	Alive and well after 12 months
9	10 hrs. 30 min.	Immediately after arrest	20 min.	Alive and well after 11 months
10	3 hrs. 30 min.	Immediately after extension of MI	24 hrs.	Alive and well after 11 months
14	14 hrs.	Immediately after extension of MI	24 hrs.	Alive and well after 8½ months
16	3 hrs. 45 min.	12 hrs.	10 hrs.	Alive and well after 7 months
Short-term Survivors				
3	1 hr. 25 min.	Immediately	7 hrs.	Died 3 days later of CVA
5	10 hrs.	Immediately	>48 hrs.	Died 7 days later of pneumonia and renal failure
8	55 hrs.	24–30 hrs.	15 hrs.	Died 3 days later from sudden rupture of mitral papillary muscle with acute ventricular failure
11	28 hrs. 30 min.	Immediately	12 hrs.	Died 8 hours later of cardiac arrest during sudden exertion
12	11 hrs.	12 hrs.	12½ hrs.	Died 5 days later; no autopsy obtained
15	8 hrs.	Immediately	12 hrs.	Died 5 days later; no autopsy obtained
Immediate Deaths Due to Procedural Causes				
2	1 hr. 26 min.	Immediately	8 hrs.	Died during interruption of Pumping
6	3 hrs.	Immediately	?	Died during interruption of Pumping
13	25 hrs.	Immediately	3½ hrs.	Died of fibrillation due to demand pacing during interruption of pumping

*Cumulative totals of periods of intermittent pumping.

circulatory failure group are presented in Table 2. The duration of mechanical assistance varied from 85 minutes to more than 55 hours. During pumping the circulation was supported at physiologic levels and the patients were clinically no longer in shock in all but one patient (Case 6). Thirteen patients went on to recover from cardiogenic shock. The pumping chamber was removed from the vascular system in these cases, and thereafter the circulation was maintained without recourse to vasoactive preparations.

Six of these patients died within 7 days after discontinuation of pumping. Eight hours after pumping, one patient suddenly became agitated, struggled to get out of bed, and had a cardiac arrest from which he could not be resuscitated. Another patient succumbed from sudden rupture of a mitral valve papillary muscle, followed by acute ventricular failure. The other deaths in this group were primarily due to noncardiac causes.

Seven patients were well 7 to 17 months after their recovery from medically refractory cardiogenic shock.

The results in the delayed circulatory failure group are presented in Table 3. In these 5 patients,

and by the clinical course, in the other, accounted for the fatal outcome. In the third case, extensive necrosis of the interventricular septum with perforation led to the patient's death.

COMMENT

In our initial clinical experience with phase-shift balloon pumping, our primary emphasis has been on development of the technic, and full evaluation must await acquisition and analysis of additional data. The evidence already at hand, however, strongly indicates that balloon pumping is an effective and safe treatment for refractory cardiogenic shock.

As noted above, in the early circulatory failure group signs of shock were not present in 15 of the 16 patients during pumping. Both the short-term survival (81 per cent) and the long-term survival (44 per cent) in a group of patients considered unresponsive to any medical therapy by their attending physicians appear to compare favorably with the exceedingly limited survival in refractory shock treated conventionally.[9,10]

The experience in the delayed circulatory failure group to date does not appear to be as clear-cut.

TABLE 3

Results of Phase-Shift Ballon Pumping in Refractory Cardiogenic Shock: Delayed Circulatory Failure Group

Case	Duration of Pumping*	Interval of Time from MI to Shock	Interval from Shock to Assist	Status
17	122 hrs.	72 hrs.	96 hrs.	Died after 8 days' intermittent pumping; ruptured ventricle through infarct
18	65 hrs.	36 hrs.	5 hrs.	Died during pumping; rupture of interventricular septum
19	51 hrs.	43 hrs.	8 hrs.	Died 12 days after pumping; autopsy refused; clinical evidence of pulmonary infarct
20	12 hrs.	72 hrs.	12 hrs.	Died 24 hrs. after pumping from ruptured ventricle through infarct
21	31 hrs.	33 hrs.	12 hrs.	Died during pumping and levarterenol infusion; autopsy refused; clinical evidence of ruptured ventricle through infarct

*Cumulative totals of periods of intermittent pumping.

the duration of circulatory assistance varied from 12 to 122 hours. Shock was clinically reversed in 2 of these 5 cases. One patient died 48 hours after termination of pumping in shock and with clinical evidence of pulmonary infarction. The other patient died 24 hours after pumping from cardiac tamponade secondary to rupture of the ventricle.

In the remaining three cases, it was not possible to discontinue pumping, although circulatory stabilization was achieved during pumping. In 2 cases, ventricular rupture, proved at autopsy in one,

We do not believe that the ventricular rupture occurring in these patients was the result of balloon pumping. Rather, we feel, necrosis with perforation developed in patients who without mechanical assistance would not have survived long enough to allow these complications of their myocardial infarctions to arise. Further study is needed to establish or refute this impression, and also to indicate whether the shock in these patients reflected solely acute myocardial infarction, or, in addition, preexisting chronic circulatory failure.

The experience to date indicates that balloon pumping is safe as well as effective. There have been no significant failures of the driving apparatus or the intracorporeal components of the system. Evidence of trauma to the formed elements of the blood has not been indicated in hematologic studies. Analysis of blood specimens taken during pumping in 5 cases disclosed no elevation of plasma hemoglobin, no exhaustion of haptoglobin, no significant fragmentation of erythrocytes, and no significant coagulopathies.

The complications of the assist procedure, moreover, have been minimal. In the first patient, signs of arterial insufficiency were noted while the balloon and catheter were *in situ*, and sequelae developed which responded to treatment during the patient's convalescence. The Dacron side-arm graft has been used in all subsequent cases, and no distal circulatory embarrassment has occurred. However, wound infections at the arteriotomy site in two other patients necessitated performance of a femoral-popliteal artery bypass procedure in one (Case 9) and of a vein patch in the other (Case 16). A clinically insignificant subadventitial hematoma was noted in the aorta adjacent to the pumping chamber in a short-term survivor (Case 8). In other cases in which necropsy has been performed, no evidence of damage due to pumping has been reported.

SUMMARY

The successful use of the pump-oxygenator in open-heart surgery suggested the possibility of mechanically assisting the circulation in conditions associated with impairment of the heart's pumping capability. Cardiogenic shock after acute myocardial infarction is refractory to medical therapy in a significant percentage of cases and thus offers a clinical model for evaluating the effectiveness of assisted circulation. Of various mechanical methods of circulatory support, intra-aortic phase-shift balloon pumping, a form of arterioarterial pumping in which the only surgical procedure required is femoral arteriotomy, appeared promising for the treatment of cardiogenic shock. Experiments in our laboratory provided substantial indications of the method's effectiveness and safety, and a clinical trial was undertaken. Candidates for balloon pumping were restricted to patients with acute myocardial infarction in whom cardiogenic shock became intractable despite maximal pharmacologic therapy. Pumping was attempted only when the physicians attending the patients had agreed that medical therapy had been exhausted and that the prognosis was extremely poor.

To date, 21 patients have been treated. The cumulative experience suggests that the interval from the onset of myocardial infarction to the development of shock may have a bearing on the outcome of the assist procedure. In 16 patients, this interval was less than 36 hours. During pumping, signs of shock were no longer present in 15 of these 16 patients. Thirteen recovered from cardiogenic shock and were returned to their referring physicians for postinfarction care. Six of these patients died 8 hours to one week after pumping, for the most part, of noncardiac causes. The remaining 7 patients were well at the time of writing, 5 to 17 months after balloon pumping.

In 5 patients the interval from infarct to shock exceeded 36 hours. Only two of these patients recovered from shock. In the other three patients in this group, it was not possible to discontinue mechanical assistance, although hemodynamic stabilization was achieved during pumping.

Although many questions remain open and more data must be analyzed before the technic can be fully evaluated, the evidence already at hand suggests that phase-shift balloon pumping is an effective treatment in medically refractory cardiogenic shock.

REFERENCES

1. Cooper, T., and Dempsey, P. J.: Assisted circulation, Mod. Concepts Cardiovas. Dis. *37*:95, *37*:101, 1968.
2. Moulopoulos, S. D., Topaz, S., and Kolff, W. J.: Diastolic balloon pumping (with carbon dioxide) in the aorta–A mechanical assistance to the failing circulation, Am. Heart J. *63*:669, 1962.
3. Clauss, R. H., Missier, P., Reed, G. E., and Tice, D.: Assisted circulation by counterpulsation with an intra-aortic balloon. Methods and effects (abstract), Dig. Am. Conf. Eng. Med. & Biol., 15th, 1962, p. 44.
4. Kantrowitz, A., and Kantrowitz A. R.: Experimental augmentation of coronary flow by retardation of the arterial pressure pulse, Surgery *34*:678, 1953.
5. Kantrowitz, A.: An intracorporeal auxiliary ventricle, *in* Advances in Biomedical Engineering and Medical Physics, edited by Levine, New York, John Wiley and Sons, 1968.
6. Nachlas, M. M., and Siedband, M. P.: The influence of diastolic augmentation on infarct size following coronary artery ligation, J. Thorac. & Cardiovas. Surg. *53*:698, 1967.
7. Kantrowitz, A., Sherman, J. L., Jr., and Krakauer, J.: Clinical experience with permanent mechanical circulatory assistance. Prog. Cardiovas. Dis. *10*:134, 1967.
8. Kantrowitz, A., Krakauer, J., and Sherman, J. L., Jr.: A permanent mechanical auxiliary ventricle: Experimental and clinical experience, J. Cardiovas. Surg. *9*:1, 1968.
9. Friedberg, C. K.: Editorial, Cardiogenic shock in acute myocardial infarction, Circulation *23*:325, 1961.

10. Eichna, L. W.: The treatment of cardiogenic shock. III. The use of isoproterenol in cardiogenic shock, Am. Heart J. *74*:848, 1967.

11. Ross, J., Jr.: Editorial, Left ventricular contraction and the therapy of cardiogenic shock, Circulation *35*:611, 1967.

12. Schilt, W., Freed, P. S., Khalil, G., and Kantrowitz, A.: Temporary non-surgical intraarterial cardiac assistance, Tr. Am. Soc. Artif. Internal Organs *13*:322, 1967.

13. Yahr, W. Z., Butner, A. N., Krakauer, J., Tomecek, J., Tjonneland, S., and Kantrowitz, A.: Cardiogenic shock: Dynamics of coronary blood flow with intraaortic phase-shift balloon pumping, Surg. Forum *19*:142, 1968.

14. Kantrowitz, A., Tjonneland, S., Freed, P. S., Phillips, S. J., Butner, A. N., and Sherman, J. L., Jr.: Initial clinical experience with intraaortic balloon pumping in cardiogenic shock, J. A. M. A. *203*:113, 1968.

15. Kantrowitz, A., Tjonneland, S., Krakauer, J., Butner, A. N., Phillips, S. J., Yahr, W. Z., Shapiro, M., Freed, P. S., Jaron, D., and Sherman, J. L., Jr.: Clinical experience with cardiac assistance by means of intraaortic phase-shift balloon pumping, Tr. Am. Soc. Artif. Internal Organs *14*:344, 1968.

16. Kantrowitz, A., Phillips, S. J., Butner, A. N., Tjonneland, S., and Haller, J. D.: Technique of femoral artery cannulation for phase-shift balloon pumping, J. Thorac. & Cardiovas. Surg. *56*:219, 1968.

Surgical Treatment for Coronary Artery Disease

Chairman

Charles P. Bailey, M.D.

Surgical Treatment of Complications of Coronary Occlusive Disease

C. Walton Lillehei, M.D.

Criteria of Selection of Patients and Operations for Myocardial Revascularization

Arthur Vineberg, M.D.

Myocardial Revascularization by Direct Coronary Artery Surgery

F. Mason Sones, Jr., M.D.

Selective Revascularization of the Myocardium

Charles P. Bailey, M.D.
Teruo Hirose, M.D.
Cesar Vera, M.D.
Elliot J. Howard, M.D.
Daniel Larson, M.D.
Frank S. Folk, M.D.

Objective Evaluation of Revascularization Procedures

F. Mason Sones, Jr., M.D.

The Cardiologist Evaluates Myocardial Revascularization

Charles K. Friedberg, M.D.

A Surgeon Evaluates Myocardial Revascularization

John J. Collins, Jr., M.D.

Panel Discussion: Status of Myocardial Revascularization

Moderator: C. Walton Lillehei, M.D.
Panelists: Charles K. Friedberg, M.D.
F. Mason Sones, Jr., M.D.
Arthur Vineburg, M.D.
Henry Russek, M.D.

Where Next? A Look Into the Future

E. Grey Dimond, M.D.

Surgical Treatment of Complications of Coronary Occlusive Disease

C. Walton Lillehei

Surgery for the complications of myocardial infarction has become an active and on the whole quite successful endeavor because a good deal can be accomplished for these complications through appropriate surgical treatment. In addition to angina and chronic left heart failure requiring revascularization, there are surgical approaches to correct papillary muscle disease, the dyskinesias or akinesias, abnormalities of ventricular function, and aneurysms. These days, of course, for far advanced cases there is even heart replacement.

In the time available, I would like to direct my attention principally to the disorders of contractility of the left ventricular wall, for two reasons. First, because these are reasonably common and second, because they quite often present a diagnostic problem unless their existence is recognized or clinical manifestations are evident.

I think that most of you are quite aware that ventricular aneurysms occur in 10 to 20 per cent of myocardial infarctions and that they, by and large, do not present any problem of recognition or of treatment. There has been a satisfactory operation available since about 1956 for these conditions. It consists of bicardial pulmonary by-pass, emptying the heart of blood, opening the lesion, resecting the lesion back to the reasonably normal wall and enclosing the ventriculostomy.

I think that the reasons the dyskinesias have presented a diagnostic problem in many instances are two-fold. One reason is that it is rather surprising how large the lesion can get in the ventricle without distorting the x-ray configuration appreciably. A patient who died some 10 years ago in the University of Minnesota Medical Service illustrates this point. The Medical Service is not mentioned because of any reflection on diagnostic acumen; We have all learned a lot in the past 10 years. At any rate, a diagnosis of chronic heart failure due to diffuse myocardiopathy was made. But at autopsy an amazingly large aneurysm of the left ventricle was found characteristically filled with clot. Now this was, of course, a myopathy, but it was not a diffuse one and was certainly quite remediable, even at that time, by surgery. Yet the condition was not recognized because it was not appreciated at that time. Many other instances observed even today illustrate how large a lesion can get before it is obvious on the ordinary roentgenogram.

The dyskinesias, or akinesias, depending upon the degree or extent of involvement, develop when there is an infarction which causes full thickness scarring of the ventricular wall. The patient survives and recovers, and the scar tissue remains firm and thick enough so that no aneurysmal outpouching develops. However, the effect on ventricular contractility is just as devastating as if there was a large saccular aneurysm, because the problem with the contractility relates to the size of this area of noncontractility. In correlating angiographic studies with what we have seen in surgery, if this scar approximates more than 20 per cent of the interior cross sectional area of the left ventricle, the patient will remain in chronic left heart failure. But often there will be no distortion whatsoever in the cardiac silhouette on the roentgenogram.

The reason, of course, that these lesions produce left heart failure is that during systole, when the myocardium should contract, the area without muscle does not contract and acts exactly as though there was a regurgitation through the mitral valve. This failure to contract reduces the stroke volume by a significant amount and produces decreased output and chronic left heart failure.

Now I shall describe one of the 20 patients with this condition whom we have treated surgically during the last two years. This man was 44 years of age and had been incapacitated for 2 years since a myocardial infarction. Yet, looking at his roentgenogram which was taken shortly before the evaluation that I will describe in a moment, he was found to have a heart size within normal limits.

Perhaps there was a little fullness in the left base, but nothing very spectacular, and on the lateral one would likewise have to agree that the film was essentially normal. However, the patient remained incapacitated with left heart failure. His chief manifestation was a lack of physical exercise tolerance. His angina was not particularly severe although he had some. Such a patient needs objective evaluation because it is about the only way that one can recognize certain abnormalities and choose an appropriate form of treatment. Coronary arteriography in this 44-year-old man showed that the right coronary artery was very severely and diffusely diseased, while the left coronary main trunk was diseased, but patent; the anterior descending was essentially totally obstructed and very severe disease was observed in the circumflex artery. This is the usual picture seen in patients with dyskinesia and is one of the important reasons for combining resectional therapy with revascularization, as I will bring out in a moment.

All patients who have coronary arteriography, as I and those who deal with these problems fairly frequently think, need left ventriculography. It is an integral and essential part of the evaluation. A left ventriculogram in this man immediately showed the filling of the left ventricle but with a complete lack of contractility in an area of heart muscle. This gave rise to a large double shadow as the ventricle emptied. In other words, an opaqueness was superimposed upon that portion of the left ventricle which had partially emptied. A large area was therefore observed in the anterior lateral left ventricle, which was not contracting. The dye retained in the left ventricle was actually more dense than in the aorta. This patient, who had a rather severe left heart failure, was treated surgically. Although the ordinary roentgenogram was within normal limits, the extent of the lesion was quite surprising.

As I have mentioned, all of these patients on arteriography have severe diffuse coronary disease or they would not have these large areas of non-contractility. Consequently, we always combine resection of the lesion with myocardial revascularization by the Vineberg operation, namely, mammary artery implantation. So, the first thing done on entering the chest, before we even open the pericardium (and that is important because often when the pericardium is open the heart function deteriorates rather rapidly since the pericardium is a supporting mechanism), is freeing up the left internal mammary artery.

In this patient, we planned to implant only one mammary artery because the entire anterior-lateral left ventricle was to be excised. Thus, we prepared to place the internal mammary artery into the diaphragmatic posterior portion to provide some protection during the late postoperative interval. After freeing up the internal mammary, the pericardium was opened and a large area of non-contractility was observed, as expected from his previous ventriculogram. Of course, there was also evidence of diffuse coronary artery disease. After putting the patient on cardiopulmonary by-pass, the heart was arrested with 3 volts of 60 cycle current to get a quiet field. This procedure, of course, obviates any need for cross clamping the aorta, which seems very unwise in patients who have already diffuse myocardial ischemia.

When the pericardium was freed up over the apex of the left ventricle, we were quite surprised by the size of the area of involvement. It then became quite understandable why the patient had had a left ventricular end-diastolic pressure of 25 mm. and had remained these 2 years in chronic left heart failure. In the entire area of the lesion there was nothing but full-thickness scar tissue. It was firm and thus had not developed the characteristic aneurysmal outpouching. As I already mentioned, it is not the size of the sac that is important to the cardiac function, but the area of absence of muscle or non-contractility. These lesions never have clot inside of them as do the characteristic aneurysms.

The first step after freeing the pericardium was to incise it over the apex to see the full extent of the lesion. In this way we got a good idea of the lack of any muscular tissue remaining in this wall. Although the aorta was not cross clamped, the tissue was completely avascular, as is characteristic of scar tissue. We incised the lesion down to where we saw some reasonably normal cardiac muscle. This excision could, of course, have tremendous immediate benefit on the left ventricular function, because this large area of akinesia acts as a severe parasitic burden on the left ventricle and its removal considerably improves left ventricular function immediately.

We observed that the papillary muscles were not involved. If they had been, the mitral valve would have had to be replaced. There was considerable scarring on the ventricular septum, but we resected the scar tissue back to definite and obvious myocardial muscle, which, of course, showed some bleeding. The area of the excised lesion was about 8 by 10 centimeters. The internal mammary artery was then put into a posterior lateral tunnel. If we thought it was necessary, we would have put in both mammary arteries. At the conclusion of surgery, the entire anterior lateral ventricle had been excised and the posterior diaphragmatic surface had been revascularized.

So in summary, the key to success in the accurate evaluation of some of the complications of myocardial ischemia is a degree of suspicion and awareness combined with objective studies, usually angiography and certain hemodynamic measurements. With the objective information one can choose an appropriate treatment that, in most instances, will benefit the patient greatly.

In the 20 individuals who have had resection of this lesion together with myocardial revascularization, 18 have survived the operation and have left the hospital. Thank you.

Criteria of Selection of Patients and Operations for Myocardial Revascularization

Arthur Vineberg

Before discussing selection of patients and the type of operations to be used for revascularization, there are certain principles that I would like to draw to the attention of the reader. From the beginning,[1-4] I have attempted to introduce extracardiac blood into the left ventricular myocardial wall, through an implanted internal mammary artery (Fig. 1). The purpose of this operation is to pour extracardiac

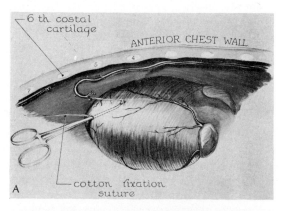

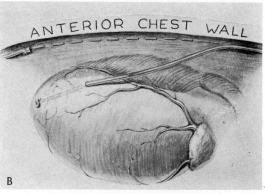

FIG. 1. (*A*) Method of implanting internal mammary artery into left ventricular myocardium. (*B*) Artery in position with its branches joining the surrounding vessels, via intramyocardial arterioles.

oxygenated blood into the arteriolar system of the left ventricle. In so doing, the diseased surface coronary arteries are bypassed. The arterioles within the myocardium are disease free except in patients with severe diabetes and hypertension. The coronary arteries, in their epicardial courses, show diffuse disease, which is progressive. This principle of a bypass operation has been used by me on patients since 1950, and well over 400 patients, followed up to $17\frac{1}{2}$ years, have undergone various modifications and supplements to the original internal mammary artery implantation.

Revascularization of Entire Heart

With experience, it was learned that one internal mammary artery implanted in the left ventricle, would supply the arteriolar zone into which it was implanted,[14] and that epicardiectomy and free omental graft were necessary for this artery to supply the circumflex and right coronary arteriolar zones, unless there were pre-existing collateral channels (Fig. 2). With the addition of epicardiectomy and free omental graft,[15] patients with large left ventricles and with ventricles in chronic failure have been successfully treated; in fact, 25 per cent of our patients in the past six years have had chronic left ventricular failure, which has been successfully reversed in 61 per cent. It was learned that multiple, previous myocardial infarctions were not contraindications to revascularization surgery. At least 75 per cent of our patients have had from 1 to 6 previous myocardial infarctions. The point of no return is still not clear-cut. It has gradually diminished as we developed new operative procedures which have widened the spectrum of patients so that it is possible to operate upon them with a low operative mortality and a high chance of successful relief from their symptoms.[16-18]

It is important not to compare our series with those reported in which a single internal mammary artery has been implanted, or in which double

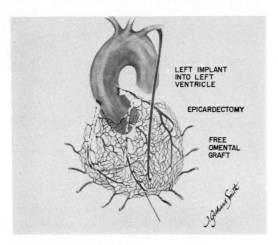

FIG. 2. A left internal mammary artery implanted into the left ventricular wall with its branches joining the arterioles within the myocardium. When placed between the heart and pericardium the omentum, after epicardiectomy and seropericardiectomy, forms its own anastomoses with the heart vessels and the vessels of the pericardium. Thus arterial oxygenated blood is distributed from one part of the heart to the other.

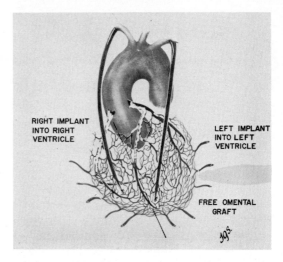

FIG. 3. A right internal mammary artery implanted into the anterior right ventricular myocardium, with its branches joining the branches of the right coronary artery. The left internal mammary artery is implanted into the left ventricular myocardium with its branches joining the arteriolar system of the left myocardium. The omental graft lies between the seropericardium, which has been removed, and the epicardium, forming arteriolar communications between the mediastinal vessels and the heart arterioles. Thus oxygenated blood is distributed from one part of the heart to the other.

implants have been carried out in the left ventricular wall in patients with no sizable infarction or enlargement of the left ventricle or ventricular failure.

In the past two years, we have added a fourth procedure, the right internal mammary artery implant, into the right ventricular wall,[19] (Fig. 3) and in the past year have found three areas in the left ventricle where an implanted internal mammary artery is capable of revascularizing the entire heart. The three areas referred to are arteriolar zones which are supplied by the terminations of the right marginal artery, the right posterior descending and the right coronary artery itself, as well as by the anterior descending, the circumflex and the left marginal. Injection studies with Schlesinger mass and by digestion cast studies have shown the terminations of these arteries, beyond which are the arteriolar zones supplied by them.[20] It is into the arteriolar zones that the internal mammary artery is implanted. The first zone is in the region of the apex between the anterior descending and its last oblique branch. The right marginal reaches the apex in 92 per cent of human hearts, the anterior descending in 100 per cent, and the left marginal in 72 per cent. Therefore, in this region, an artery has the opportunity of anastomosing with branches of both right and left coronary systems in 88 per cent of all human hearts. The second triarteriolar zone lies roughly 4 cm. superior and lateral to the apex on the left

margin of the heart, at the junction of the lateral and diaphragmatic surfaces of the left ventricle. Here, by cast and injection studies, it has been shown that the left marginal reaches this area in 72 per cent, the right coronary artery in 81 per cent, and the termination of the branches of the anterior descending in 100 per cent of cases when the intramyocardial tunnel includes an area on the anterolateral surface of the left ventricle. The third triarteriolar zone lies higher up on the diaphragmatic surface of the left ventricle and will not be described in this article. In view of our frequently published proof that the internal mammary artery, when implanted in the middle third of the left ventricle, sends out branches which connect with the surrounding arterioles, arteries implanted into the two aforementioned triarteriolar zones have an opportunity, in over 80 per cent of hearts, of anastomosing with the branches of both right and left circulations. Thus, in selecting patients for revascularization surgery, it is necessary to know a great deal about the patient; in particular, the condition of his left ventricle, and also to know what operative procedure or procedures are contemplated.

Indications for Surgery in Treatment of Coronary Artery Insufficiency

In spite of good medical treatment, well documented anginal pain of at least a year's duration is our major and only indication for revascularization surgery. It is because of pain that the patient consults his physician. The problem is to ascertain that the pain, whether it be in the chest, arm, neck, back, or upper part of the abdomen, is truly due to coronary artery insufficiency. Our cardiologists have always accepted positive electrocardiographic evidence of myocardial ischemia and, in particular, documented evidence of one or more myocardial infarctions. Proven electrocardiographic evidence of myocardial infarction has been correlated by Proudfit and others[21] with cinearteriographic evidence of coronary artery occlusion, and the correlation has been found to be correct in 99 per cent of cases. In the diagnosis of true anginal pain, we have made use of the patient's history and electrocardiographic evidence of one or more myocardial infarctions, and finally, the more recent cinearteriographic evidence of occlusion of one or more main stem coronary arteries.

Classification of Patients with Anginal Pain Caused by Coronary Artery Insufficiency

We have divided our patients into two groups: Grade 1, those with no pain while resting, and Grade 2, those with pain without cause while resting. This simple classification, based upon clinical anginal pain, has been used since 1950. Quite early in our experience, the Grade 2 patients were found to have more coronary artery disease at autopsy than the Grade 1 patients; thus, they presented higher operative risk.

Condition of Left Ventricle

The crux of myocardial revascularization rests with the condition of the left ventricle at the time of surgery. There are still no tests to quantitate the amount of myocardial fiber mass present and, what is more important, how such fibers may react to the improved circulation. Fluid retention, inability to lie flat in bed without shortness of breath, and elevated diastolic left ventricular pressures are still the best indicators of left ventricular failure. In attempting to assess patients, we have combined anginal pain with left ventricular status, particularly with regard to size and efficiency, and with regard to the scope of the operative procedure to be used.

Cinearteriography

Today, and prior to the development of cinearteriography, radiologic visualization of main stem coronary artery disease was carried out in our hospital, beginning in 1960, with the two-plane, six-plate per second, cassette changer, and aortic root filling, to outline the main stems of the coronary arteries. In the succeeding years, individual coronary artery catheterization has been carried out, with cinearteriography, as recommended by Proudfit et al.[21]

Objective of Coronary Artery Visualization

We have considered the condition of the main stem coronary arteries to be all-important; that is, the origins of the right coronary artery and of the anterior descending and circumflex coronary arteries, as well as those of the main left coronary artery. These are the main arteries that supply the heart. When they are obstructed at their origins, there is no room for collateral vessels to form, which might eventually bypass the sites of obstruction. Thus, proof of coronary artery occlusion is not enough. It must involve the main stem of one or more coronary arteries. In our center, evidence of diseased coronary arteries alone has not been an indication for revascularization surgery. It has been used as confirmatory evidence. In 1956, ameroid constrictors were placed on the origins of the anterior descending and circumflex coronary arteries of dogs in our laboratory to determine the degree of coronary artery occlusion compatible with active life.[22] It was found that when two major coronary arteries were narrowed 50 per cent or more at their main stems, the animals died.[23,24] This and subsequent studies have greatly influenced our thinking with regard to coronary artery arteriography. We have seen patients with a history and electrocardiographic evidence of myocardial infarction, in whom a coronary artery narrowing or occlusion was a considerable distance from the origin of the vessels. Such patients have been discharged for further medical treatment, because we believe that when the main stem coronary arteries are fully patent, and the obstruction is distally placed, collateral arteries will develop within the heart to bypass the point of coronary artery occlusion.

Cinearteriographic evidence of coronary artery occlusion itself has not been accepted as an indication for surgery. The patient must have true anginal pain. In only one instance has this rule been broken. A doctor had had two previous myocardial infarctions and there was cineangiographic evidence of triple main stem coronary artery disease. Because of a bad family medical history, he was operated upon at his own request. He is still alive. This point of view should be changed. The excellent work of Sones, which so clearly outlines the coronary arteries along their epicardial courses, in conjunction with our studies of coronary artery occlusion with ameroid constrictors in dogs, suggest that coronary artery occlusion of the main stems of two major coronary arteries with or without pain calls for revascularization surgery.

Therapeutic Aims

From the beginning, all our efforts have been directed towards (1) survival of the patient, (2) relief of anginal pain, (3) return to work, and (4) prolongation of life expectancy.

Relief of anginal pain has always been difficult to evaluate because of the possible psychologic benefit that may follow any operation. After consultation with members of the Department of Psychiatry, our cardiologist decided not to evaluate any patient less than six months after surgery. It was considered that psychologic benefits from the operation were not likely to endure longer than this. Our patients were divided into (1) those with no pain or slight pain postoperatively, (2) those with less pain (groups 1 and 2 are classified improved), and (3) those in whom the pain was the same or worse (these are listed as unimproved). Hill, in a study of 31 consecutive patients followed for five years, showed that only 2 patients (7%) with left internal mammary artery implants were pain free at the end of nine months, whereas 10 patients (31%) were pain free at the end of five years, and 12 patients (38%) had slight or less pain. A total of 22 patients (69%) were improved (Fig. 4). Hill's clinical analysis of pain relief following single internal mammary

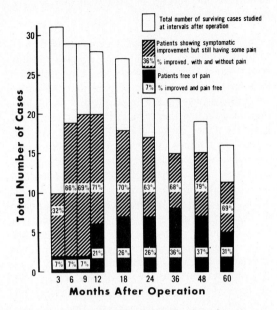

FIG. 4. Record of symptomatic improvement in 31 consecutive patients followed for five years after internal mammary artery implantation.

artery implantation and epicardiectomy was confirmed by the experimental evidence of Duschesne and Vineberg.[14] They showed that a left internal mammary artery, implanted into the anterior wall of the left ventricle, requires nine months before it revascularizes the entire left ventricle. Many years later, the clinical observations of Hill and the experimental findings of Duschesne and Vineberg[14] were confirmed by Sones,[25] who, with cineangiography, showed that an internal mammary artery implanted into the left ventricle forms anastomoses with the surface vessels between six and nine months postoperatively.

Return to Work

In order to make the work record meaningful, we have recorded those patients who were working part-time or at a secondary job, prior to surgery, as not working. After surgery, if the patient has not returned to work at his own job, he is not considered to be working.

The results of left internal mammary artery implantation and epicardiectomy in 126 patients, followed up to 12 years, are shown in Table 1. It will be noted that the Grade 1 patients with no angina while resting had a low operative mortality rate (2 or 1.9%); 77 (76%) followed up to 4 years had improved, while 56 (55%) were similarly

TABLE 1

Implantation of Left Internal Mammary Artery into Left Ventricle and Epicardiectomy

	No. of Cases	Postoperative Mortality	% Improved
Grade 1			
No angina at rest 1950–1962	102	2 (1.9%)	76 up to 4 yr. 55 up to 12 yr.
Grade 2			
Angina at rest without cause 1950–1956*	24	10 (41%)	20 up to 2 yr.

*Implant surgery discontinued on this type of case until development of bloodless omental graft in 1962.

classified after 12 years. The 24 patients with angina decubitus had a 41% operative mortality (10 patients) and only 5 (20%) showed improvement when followed up to two years.

Evolution of Revasculation Surgery for Relief of Myocardial Ischemia

During the past 18 years, our concept of the treatment of coronary artery insufficiency by a single arterial implant has progressed to multiple arterial implants combined with epicardiectomy and free omental graft. Selection of a patient for myocardial revascularization is influenced not only by the type of anginal pain suffered and the condition of the left ventricle, but by the type of operation that is to be performed. Thus, from 1950 to 1962, all patients underwent a single internal mammary artery implantation, into either the anterior descending or the circumflex coronary arteriolar zone. It became clear that such an implant supplied the arterial zone into which it was implanted. To open the collateral arteries between all parts of the left ventricle, epicardiectomy was performed. This allowed implantation of an internal mammary artery into the left ventricle to supply the entire left ventricle but not the right ventricle. However, this took nine months, so that the conditions of patients with angina decubitus and those with hypertrophied ventricles and left ventricular failure remained poor. However, our first surviving patient, operated upon on October 22, 1950, was a patient with left ventricular failure and left ventricular hypertrophy. The patient lived and was free of failure for ten years after the operation. He was active as a mining oil prospector in western Canada until his death. A few of our patients with hypertrophied hearts who died three and four years postoperatively were examined at autopsy. The deeply placed internal mammary artery lying in the thick left ventricular muscle wall, even though it was fully patent, appeared quite small compared with the size of the muscle mass revascularized. Looking at these fully patent internal mammary arteries, it was evident that for hypertrophied hearts, internal mammary artery implantation needed to be supplemented by other, extracoronary sources of blood.

Continuous experimental research for a more rapid method of revascularization for such patients was carried out. Finally, it was found that the bloodless omental graft formed arteriolar connections within eight days. When the bloodless omental graft was wrapped around the heart after epicardiectomy and seropericardiectomy, and the left internal mammary artery was implanted into the left ventricle, it was possible to revascularize the entire heart within 18.8 days very effectively. In the experimental animal, all three major coronary arteries were occluded and both the animal and the myocardium survived, whereas there was 100 per cent mortality in the control animals and 95 per cent extensive infarction of both ventricles.[26] This combined operation, after many years of experimental testing, was then used in the treatment of patients with triple coronary artery disease, starting in December 1962. All types of cases have thus been treated, including patients with angina decubitus and those with hypertrophied hearts, as well as hearts in a state of chronic left ventricular failure.

A total of well over 200 patients have undergone this combined operation. The clinical data of 171 such patients is outlined in Table 2. These patients have been followed for up to $4\frac{3}{4}$ years postoperatively. It will be seen that 75 per cent of this group had from one to six previous myocardial infarctions, 28 per cent had left ventricular hypertrophy, and 21 per cent had left ventricular failure.

The preoperative cinearteriographic studies on 124 patients is shown in Table 3. It is interesting to note that there were 2.9 main stem coronary artery occlusions per heart in Grade 1 patients and 3.1 diseased main stem coronary arteries in Grade 2 patients. It was clear that cinearteriography in itself cannot determine the severity of the disease from a clinical point of view, as there is no statistical significance between 2.9 and 3.1, whereas there is a great difference in the operative mortality and the results between patients in Grade 1 and Grade 2 categories. Of 133 Grade 1 patients with triple main stem coronary artery occlusion followed up to $4\frac{3}{4}$ years, there was 77 per cent improvement in the whole group and 94 per cent improvement for those who were followed (108). The operative mortality figure was 7 (5.3%), and if those without left ventricular enlargement and failure were excluded, it was 4.3 per cent for 92 patients. There were 14 (11%) deaths later. All but one patient had preoperative anginal pain. Of the 102 patients whose condition improved after surgery, 75 had either slight or no anginal pain, 27 had less pain, and in 6 it was the same as before. Fifty-three patients (40%) were working full time prior to surgery and after surgery, 77 (58%) were employed full time. There was no follow-up on four (3%) of the patients.

The combined operation was performed on 38 Grade 2 patients who were followed up to $4\frac{3}{4}$ years. The operative mortality figure for patients with angina decubitus was reduced to nine (24%), com-

TABLE 2
Preoperative History and Physical Findings in Patients with Main Stem Coronary Artery Disease*

	Grade 1, No Angina at Rest	Grade 2, Angina at Rest Without Cause	Total
No. of patients	133	38	171
Age (yrs.)			
25–50	71 (54%)	15 (40%)	
51–60	54 (40%)	21 (55%)	
61 and over	8	2	
Duration of symptoms (yrs.)			
Under 2	32	4	
2–10	87 (65%)	28 (74%)	115 (67%)
11–20	14	6	
No. of infarctions			
1	53	21	129 (75%)
2–6	42	13	
Left ventricular hypertrophy	33	14	47 (28%)
Left ventricular failure	19	17	36 (21%)

*Treated by implantation of left internal mammary artery, epicardiectomy, and free omental graft.

TABLE 3
Preoperative Patency of Coronary Arteries as Shown by Cineangiogram in 124 of 171 Patients Operated On (73%)

	Right Coronary Artery	Left Coronary Artery	Anterior Descending	Circumflex	Total
Grade 1 (98 cases):	2.9 diseased main stem coronary arteries per heart.				
Blocked	30	0	40	3	73
Narrowed (50%–95%)	31	52	52	75	210
Total	61 (62%)	52 (53%)	92 (94%)	78 (80%)	283
Grade 2 (26 cases):	3.1 diseased main stem coronary arteries per heart.				
Blocked	9	2	14	2	27
Narrowed (50%–95%)	12	11	11	20	54
Total	21 (80%)	13 (50%)	25 (97%)	22 (84%)	81

pared with 41% mortality which had prevailed when only a single implant was performed. Excluding patients with left ventricular failure, the operative mortality rate was only 15%. Of 20 patients followed, 18 (90%) improved; 47% of the original group improved. There were seven deaths later (18%) and two patients (5%) were not followed up. There was either slight or no anginal pain in 11 of the 20 patients followed postoperatively; 7 had less pain; and in 2 it was the same as before. Two patients were working before surgery and ten were working after surgery. A survey was made of this entire series to evaluate the condition of the left ventricle immediately after surgery and after follow-up. A study of Table 4 shows that patients in Grade 1 with normal-sized left ventricles with or without failure did well, as did patients with hypertrophied left ventricles. Those with hypertrophied left ventricles in failure have had poor follow-up results. Grade 2 patients (Table 5) with normal-sized left ventricles, with or without failure, did very well. However, in those with hypertrophied left ventricles there was a high operative risk and high follow-up mortality rate, as there was with patients with hypertrophy and left ventricular failure.[27]

Effect of Combined Operation on Left Ventricular Failure

The most objective evidence of value has been the reversal of chronic left ventricular failure when the combined operation was used. In our series, there were 35 patients who had left ventricular failure. Twenty of these had no failure or slight failure when followed up to 4¾ years after surgery. Patients who have a condition of chronic left ventricular failure and who have this condition at the time of surgery in spite of extensive diuresis, form a very good base line for evaluation of the effect of revascularization on ischemic myocardium. The reduction or abolition of diuretics, the disappearance of dyspnea, and the ability of such patients to lie flat in bed cannot be considered as true psychologic benefit.[27]

Implantation of the right internal mammary artery into the right ventricle, in addition to the combined operation, in 15 patients resulted in no deaths immediately after surgery and no later deaths

TABLE 4

Postoperative Mortality and Later Deaths†
in 133 Grade 1 Patients After Combined
Operation for Triple Main Stem Coronary
Artery Occlusion*

	No. of Cases	Mortality Post-operative	Later
Good Risk			
Normal-sized left ventricle without failure	92	4 (4.3%)	7†
Normal-sized left ventricle with failure	10	0	2
Left ventricular hypertrophy	23	3	0
Poor Risk			
Left ventricular hypertrophy with failure	8	0	5
Total	133	7 (5.3%)	14 (11%)

*Within 28 days
†Up to 43/4 years later (duration of follow-up)
††One from lung cancer, one stroke, one ruptured spleen, eight cardiac.

TABLE 5

*Postoperative Mortality and Later Deaths in 38
Grade 2 Patients After Combined Operation for
Triple Main Stem Coronary Artery Occlusion**

	No. of Cases	Mortality Postoperative	Later
Good Risk			
Normal-sized left ventricle without failure	16	3	3#
Normal-sized left ventricle and left ventricle failure	8	1	1
Poor Risk			
Left ventricular hypertrophy	7	3	1
Left ventricular hypertrophy and failure	7	3	2
Total	38(18%)	10(26%)	7(20%)

*Patients followed 4¾ years.
#One case of meningitis 4½ years postoperatively.

up to 1 to 2½ years later (Table 6). Eleven patients had no pain, two had less, and two were the same as before. Seven patients were in the Grade 2 category. Apparently, implantation of the right internal mammary artery into the right ventricular wall reduced our original operative mortality rate for patients with angina decubitus from 41 to 0 per cent in this small series.[28]

Selection of Patients

Thus, from our experience, selection of patients for revascularization should be based on the type of anginal pain, the degree of main stem coronary artery obstruction, and the condition of the left ventricle. It is also influenced by the type and scope of the revascularization operation. Thus, in Grade 1 patients, a single implant may be useful for obstruction in one artery, where not more than 80 per cent effective mammary-coronary artery anastomoses can be expected. In our experience, no patients have had revascularization surgery for only one diseased artery. Prior to cineangiography, the need for revascularization surgery depended on the locations of ischemia and/or infarctions indicated by electrocardiogram confirmed at operation. Since 1950, it has been routine to examine the entire coronary artery tree by palpation at the time of surgery, as well as to record locations and extent of myocardial infarctions, which usually are clearly visible. Patients accepted for revascularization surgery at present are in the Grade 1 category, with small left ventricles and small left ventricles in failure, as well as hypertrophied left ventricles. Those with hypertrophied left ventricles can be operated on, but the long-term results are only fair. It is hoped that the use of the intramyocardial omental strip graft implantation, which acts so rapidly in revascularizing the myocar-

TABLE 6

*Bilateral Internal Mammary Artery Implantation into
Right and Left Ventricular Myocardium, Epicardiectomy, and Free Omental Graft**

	No. of Cases	Mortality Post-operative	Later	Pain None	Less	Same	Working Before, Full-time	After, Full-time
Grade 1 (Vineberg) No pain at rest	8	..	..	6 88% improved	1	1	4	8
Grade 2 (Vineberg) Pain at rest without cause	7	..	..	5 86% improved	1	1	3	6
Angina decubitus Total	15	..	..	87%			7	14

*Patients followed six months to two years.

dium and in blood distribution, may improve these results.[29]

For patients in the Grade 2 category (those with small left ventricles and small left ventricles in failure), the results have been excellent, but patients with hypertrophied left ventricles in failure have had poor results from the combined operation.

Selection of Operation For Revascularization of Entire Heart

Throughout the years, it has become clear to us that the correction of one, or even two perfusion deficits in different arteriolar zones of the left ventricle, in themselves, are not sufficient. It is necessary to revascularize both the right and left coronary arteriolar systems, and join all three arteriolar areas together by collaterals whenever possible; that is, to revascularize the entire heart.

The operations capable of revascularizing the entire heart are the following:

1. Implantation of a single internal mammary artery into one of three triarteriolar zones of the left ventricle, which are present at (a) the apical region of the left ventricle, (b) the inferior-lateral region of the left ventricle, and (c) an area in the diaphragmatic portion of the left ventricle in its inner one third, midway between base and apex.

2. Implantation of two internal mammary arteries into the right and left ventricular walls respectively, the latter into one of the three arteriolar zones of the left ventricle.

3. Epicardiectomy and seropericardiectomy plus free omental graft applied to both ventricles.

4. Single or double implant operations, with epicardiectomy and free omental graft. The ideal operation in our hands is the combination of 2 and 3 (see Fig. 3).

Single internal mammary artery implantations into the apical region of the left ventricle have been performed in our clinic in over 200 patients, 126 of whom have been followed up to 12 years with an over-all improvement of 54–76 per cent. In this series, cine or pathologic studies, or both, have shown an average mammary-coronary anastomoses patency of 84 per cent, when studied up to $17\frac{1}{2}$ years. Seven of our patients have been shown to have nothing else open in their hearts except the internal mammary artery. Two examples of these are the following:

1. A motorcar salesman underwent internal mammary artery implantation on July 12, 1954. Six months after the operation, he was completely pain-free and returned to work.

In November 1961, $7\frac{1}{2}$ years after his surgery, I

sent the patient to Sones of the Cleveland Clinic, for visualization of the internal mammary artery implant. Sones showed that the right coronary artery was narrowed at its origin as were the left coronary artery and circumflex vessels. The anterior descending was blocked. Visualization of the left internal mammary artery showed it to be fully patent, perfusing the left ventricular myocardium down to the apex (Fig. 5). In November 1966, the patient report-

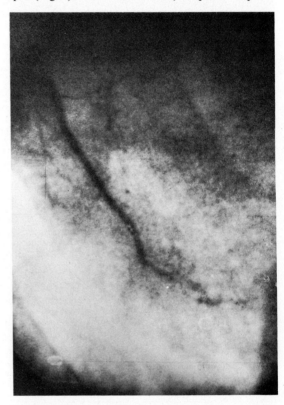

FIG. 5. Roentgenogram from cineangiogram made by Sones (November 1961) of left internal mammary artery implanted by Dr. Vineberg into Montreal salesman (July 1954). Note full patency of implanted artery with many intramyocardial mammary-coronary anastomoses $7\frac{1}{2}$ years after implantation.

ed recurrence of anginal pain. Cineangiography in our hospital showed that the only artery open in his heart was the implanted left internal mammary artery which I had placed there over 12 years before. In January 1967, the patient underwent right internal mammary artery implantation in the anterior wall of the right ventricle, at The Royal Victoria Hospital, Montreal. He died of bilateral pneumonia.

At the autopsy, the author attempted to inject the right and left coronary arteries unsuccessfully. The left internal mammary artery, however, accepted Schlesinger mass which filled the entire right and left coronary systems up to their points of occlusion (Fig. 6). The implanted internal mammary artery lying in the myocardium and outside the myocardium, 12 years after implantation, was fully patent,

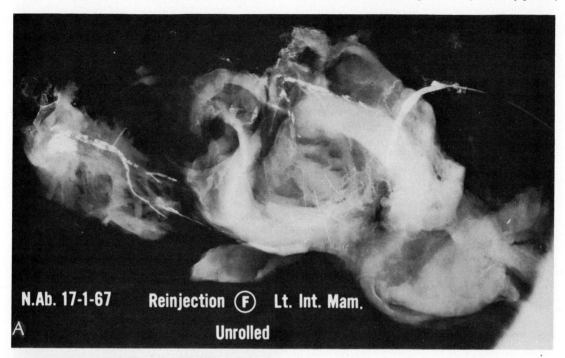

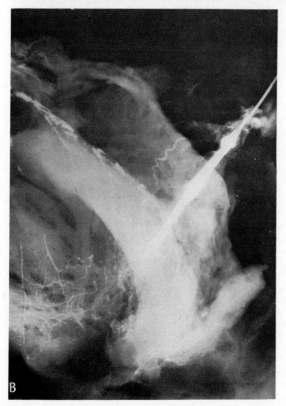

FIG. 6. Autopsy injection study of implanted internal mammary artery of the patient in Figure 5, $12\frac{1}{2}$ years after implantation. (*A*) Left internal mammary artery filled with Schlesinger mass after injection. Mass filled right and left coronary artery systems as far as completely blocked, calcified main stem coronary arteries (unrolled heart). (*B*) Close-up of site of internal mammary artery implantation.

showing no evidence of intimal proliferation (Fig. 7). It was the only artery open in this patient's heart. The origins of both right and left coronary arteries by histologic section were shown to be completely occluded (Fig. 8).

2. A second patient underwent left internal mammary artery implantation in March, 1961. At the operation, a scar was found occupying the space between the anterior descending and its 2nd branch, in the apical region, thus preventing the introduction of the left internal mammary artery into the myocardium between the anterior descending and its second branch, as has been the custom in our implants, both in the animal and in man. Lateral to the scar, there was good muscle, and the internal mammary artery was therefore placed into the lateral inferior portion of the left ventricle, in an area which we have designated as the second triarteriolar zone in the left ventricular wall (Fig. 9). This patient returned home and remained perfectly well for 14 years, when he had a stroke, from which he recovered. He had no anginal pain, except when lifting heavy machinery at night, after his evening meal. At the age of 74, 17½ years after implantation, the patient underwent

prostatectomy and died from pneumonia.

The heart was shipped to The Royal Victoria Hospital. The internal mammary artery had been carefully dissected out and was found to be soft outside the heart and of normal thickness. Before injecting Schlesinger mass, the right coronary artery was sectioned near its origin and found to be completely occluded. It was necessary to make multiple sections until an area of 3 to 4 cm. down the right coronary artery was cut and a definite lumen found. The same procedure was carried out for the left anterior descending and for the circumflex. Both of these arteries showed no lumen in their first 3–4 cm. Once visible lumens were identified in the distal cut ends of all three arteries, Schlesinger mass was injected into the cannulated internal mammary artery. It promptly appeared at the distal openings of all three coronary arteries (Fig. 10). Histologic sections taken through the right, anterior descending and circumflex coronary arteries showed them to be completely blocked. The internal mammary artery itself was normal, showing no evidence of atherosclerosis or intimal proliferation (Fig. 11).

The decision as to the type of operation for revas-

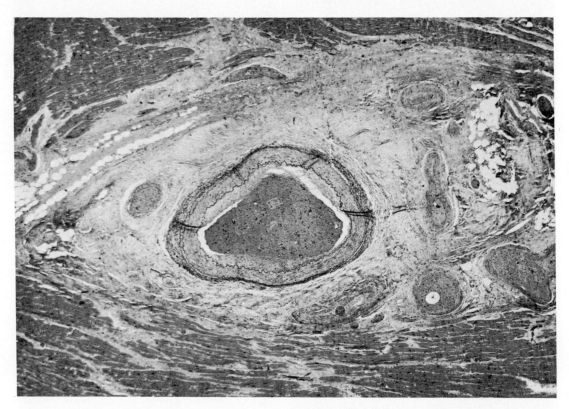

FIG. 7.   Same patient as Figures 5 and 6. Section through middle of myocardial tunnel. Fully patent internal mammary artery without intimal proliferation filled with Schlesinger mass, which has filled surrounding arteries. Implant was only artery open in heart.

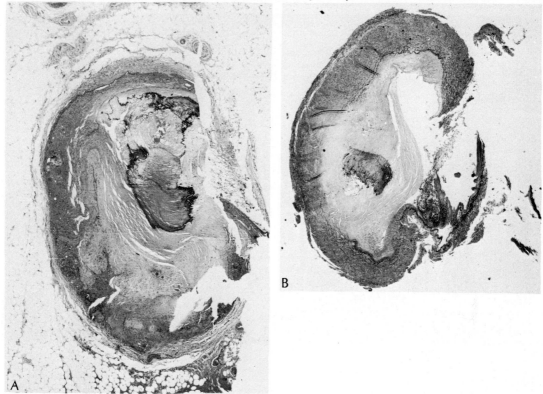

FIG. 8.   Same patient as Figures 5, 6, and 7. Histologic sections from origins of right and left coronary arteries. (*A*) Right coronary artery completely blocked at origin. (*B*) Left coronary artery completely blocked at origin.

Both open on cineangiography (November, 1961). Progressive disease over 5 years closed both major coronary arteries at their origins.

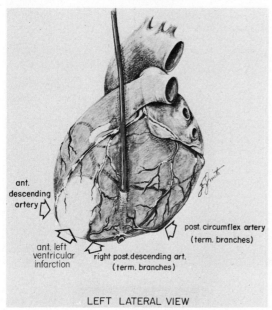

FIG. 9.   New tricoronary internal mammary artery implant, arterial zonal (Vineberg).

cularization surgery is influenced by (1) main stem coronary artery occlusion, (2) collateral channels, and (3) location of myocardial infarctions.

An infarction in the anterior wall of the left ventricle permits only a single left internal mammary artery implant. However, it permits a right internal mammary artery implant into the right ventricular wall, epicardiectomy, and free omental graft. An infarction in the posterior wall of the left ventricle prohibits two implants into the left ventricle, but permits one in each ventricle in addition to epicardiectomy and free omental graft. The same is true when there is an infarction in the anterior and posterior wall of the left ventricle. The only time double internal mammary artery implantations into the left ventricle (Effler type) can be carried out effectively is when there is no major infarction in this ventricle; this is also true of the Effler anterior-posterior wall implantations.

When the anterior wall of the right ventricle is thin, fatty, or infarcted, it is not possible to implant the right internal mammary artery into the right ventricular wall. However, a left internal mammary

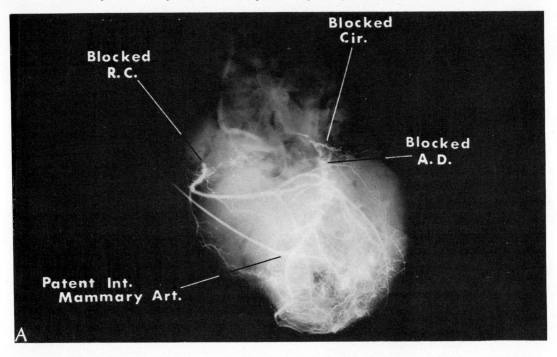

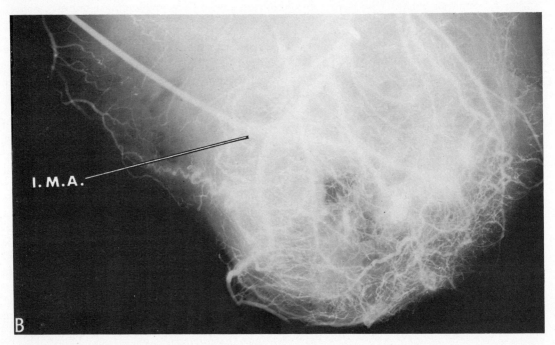

FIG. 10.   Roentgenogram taken after the right anterior descending and circumflex coronary arteries were cut until an opening was found in the vessels and the internal mammary artery, which had been implanted $17\frac{1}{2}$ years earlier, was injected with Schlesinger mass. (*A*) Internal mammary artery filling all vessels retrograde to their points of occlusion. (*B*) A close-up of the injected internal mammary artery and its surrounding communications.(*Continued on facing page*)

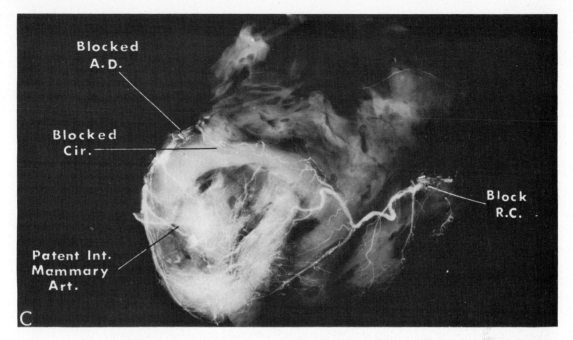

FIG. 10. (Continued). (*C*) The unrolled heart, showing how a single internal mammary artery, injected with Schlesinger mass, filled all coronary arteries before points of occlusion. It was the only artery open in this human heart, $17\frac{1}{2}$ years after implantation.

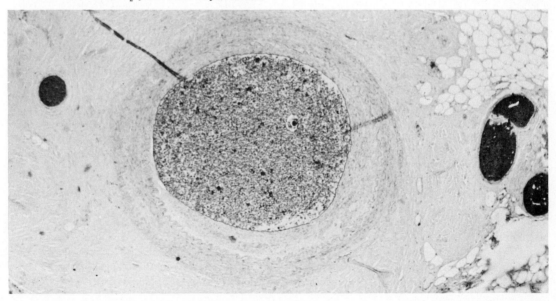

FIG. 11. Histologic section through the internal mammary artery shown in Figure 10, $17\frac{1}{2}$ years after it had been implanted into a human myocardium. This patient was completely asymptomatic for 14 years.

artery implant can be carried out in addition to epicardiectomy and free omental graft.

General contraindications to revascularization surgery are (1) recent myocardial infarction (surgery must be postponed for six months), (2) preinfarction syndrome (stabilization must occur), (3) severe hypertension or diabetes, (4) diminution in lung function, (5) impending stroke, and (6) recent stroke (patient must recover).

Specific contraindications are (1) angina decubitus, (2) left ventricular hypertrophy, and (3) left ventricular failure with small ventricle (true for 1 through 3, unless epicardiectomy and free omental graft are used with arterial implant), (4) previous pericardial poudrage, (5) bilateral internal mammary artery ligation, and (6) large thin-walled ventricles in a state of failure. (For 4 through 6, refer to Intramyocardial Omental Strip Implantations.)

For coronary artery insufficiency, revascularization surgery is the major answer. The sooner it is performed, the more heart muscle the patient will retain.

Influence of Operative Technic on Results of Revascularization Surgery

Many variations of the original internal mammary artery implant operation have been described but the majority of these have not been based on firm experimental evidence. These variations, which are listed below, will tend to lower the percentage of effective mammary-coronary anastomoses, regardless of whether the artery is placed in ischemic or non-ischemic heart muscle.

Making Tunnel. The long and thin tunnel affords no advantages and does not open up the same number of myocardial sinusoids necessary for effective run-off as does a shorter, broader tunnel. Flow studies have been carried out in comparative tunnels by Zamora, working in my laboratory at McGill University, and are shown in Table 7.

Location of Tunnel. It was shown by Niloff[30] in 1950 that the greatest number of mammary-coronary anastomoses occurred when the internal mammary artery was implanted in the middle third of the left ventricular wall. It has subsequently been shown by Kato[31] that there is a reversal of flow with elevated pressure during systole (Fig. 12). Arteries placed superficially did not receive the benefit of the to and fro action of a contracting left ventricular myocardium. In addition, arteries placed in the mid-ventricular zone are lying surrounded by myocardial arterioles, which have lower pressures than the diastolic pressure present in the internal mammary artery. Thus, arteries placed in such a zone will remain open for many years in a normal heart.[32] The pressure relationships of an artery lying beneath

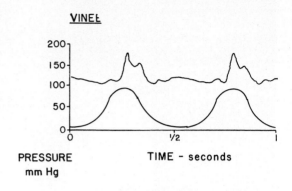

VINEŁ

PRESSURE
mm Hg

TIME - seconds

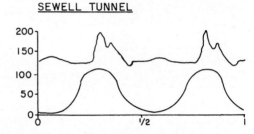

SEWELL TUNNEL

FIG. 12. A pressure recording made by Kato inside an anterior wall of a left ventricular tunnel. Studied through implanted internal mammary artery or a balloon catheter implanted in the tunnel, it showed no difference in pressures whether the tunnel was made with an artery forceps or with a knife. The recording demonstrates clearly the long period of low pressure during diastole in the ventricular tunnel, during which time the blood in the opened side branches of the implanted internal mammary artery is able to flow into the myocardial sinusoidal spaces.

the surface arteries, as compared with a deeply placed artery, are shown in Fig. 13. However, as we have stated earlier, our objective has always been to connect extracardiac oxygenated blood sources with the intramyocardial arteriolar system, which never becomes diseased except in severe diabetes and hypertension, rather than having the implanted vessels communicate with the coronary arteries in

TABLE 7
Technic of Making Intramyocardial Tunnel Influence Flow Through Implant

	No. Animals	Tunnel Made by	Average Flow/Min.	Range Min./cc.
Right ventricle	20	Vineberg (Forceps widely spread)	7.05	4.5–12
	9	Effler forceps	4.0	2.5–6
	11	Groove Direction	3.5	1.2–5
Left ventricle	20	Vineberg	6.8	4–13
	9	Effler	4.4	3.5–5.5
	11	Groove Direction	3.04	1–5

Flow studies made by Dr. Ben Zamora.

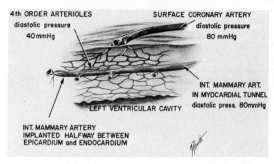

4th ORDER ARTERIOLES
diastolic pressure
40 mmHg

SURFACE CORONARY ARTERY
diastolic pressure
80 mmHg

INT. MAMMARY ART.
IN MYOCARDIAL TUNNEL
diastolic press. 80mmHg

LEFT VENTRICULAR CAVITY

INT. MAMMARY ARTERY
IMPLANTED HALFWAY BETWEEN
EPICARDIUM and ENDOCARDIUM

FIG. 13. Diagram shows why an internal mammary artery remains open when implanted in normal ventricular myocardium (Vineberg).

their epicardial courses, which progressively become diseased.

There Is a Maximum Effective Length of Artery Which Should Be Freed. The action of the contracting ventricle on an implanted internal mammary artery in moving a column of blood within the artery to and fro is diminished when the column of blood is too long, as occurs when the artery is freed too high and when the artery, after implantation, is too loose.

Angulation. The point of entrance in the left ventricular myocardium, or in the right ventricular myocardium, should be in a straight line with the point of take-off from the chest wall. Failure to heed this technical point results in narrowing of the artery at its point of entrance into the myocardium.

Epicardiectomy and Free Omental Graft

The epicardium must be removed as efficiently as possible between coronary vessels to have the development of intracoronary anastomoses and to permit the free omental graft to join its vessels with those of the heart. Likewise, the omental graft must be properly prepared so that it is not too thick. The serous layer of the pericardium must be completely removed for the omental graft to obtain a mediastinal blood supply and the ascending aorta must be properly cleared of its pleural-pericardial reflection in order for the graft to obtain a blood supply from the ascending aorta. The graft must be fixed to the heart with multiple sutures, and to the diaphragm and the pericardium. Failure to properly prepare the graft and failure to do a proper epicardiectomy and seropericardiectomy will result in a fibrotic, useless piece of omentum, as has been reported by others. We have examined now four human omental grafts, after being placed in human hearts, 6 months, 8 months, 4 years and 4¾ years after surgery, in patients who have died from different causes, primarily strokes, and who had shown marked improvement of left ventricular

failure and anginal pain. In these patients, the internal mammary artery was injected with Schlesinger mass and in each case, the intramyocardial arterioles were completely filled, as well as the vascular network in the omental graft, which had been placed on the surface of the heart. The injection mass likewise filled the larger vessels of the omentum and the pericardium, as well as the mediastinal vessels outside the pericardium. By gross examination and histologic study, the omentum was found to be healthy in each case and obviously was transporting oxygenated blood from the mediastinal vessels into the coronary arteriolar system.

One of the best examples of the value of the combined operation of left internal mammary artery implantation, epicardiectomy, seropericardiectomy and free omental graft was supplied by a patient who was operated on, on June 27, 1963, at which time he had already suffered six previous myocardial infarctions, was in chronic left ventricular failure and had not worked for a number of years. Prior to the operation, the cineangiogram showed that there was nothing open except a sausage-shaped left coronary, emptying into a markedly narrowed circumflex artery (Fig. 14). Following the combined operation, this patient required vaso-pressors for over a month to maintain his blood pressure. He eventually returned to work, using no nitroglycerin at the end of six months, but still in left ventricular failure. In Figure 15 it is clear that the patient is still in left ventricular failure 11 months after surgery, but he is working. Twenty-two months after the roentgenogram makes it clear that he is out of failure. Four and three-quarter years after surgery, the patient died from what appeared to be a stroke. The internal mammary artery was injected with Schelsinger mass and it will be seen from Figure 16 that the entire coronary arteriolar network plus the vessels outside the heart, were filled. Histologic sections showed that the omentum was healthy, containing Schlesinger mass, which extended beyond the pericardium, filling vessels in the mediastinum. The artery itself was fully patent, showing no intimal proliferation in the vessel lying within the myocardium. Thus, if one is to get good results with internal mammary artery implantation and the omental graft procedure, the technics which have been carefully worked out over a great number of years must be followed through. This is no different from other forms of surgery in which there are established methods of performing for example, a gastrectomy or a pneumonectomy. Failure to heed certain fundamental principles with these procedures results in peritonitis or blown bronchial stumps

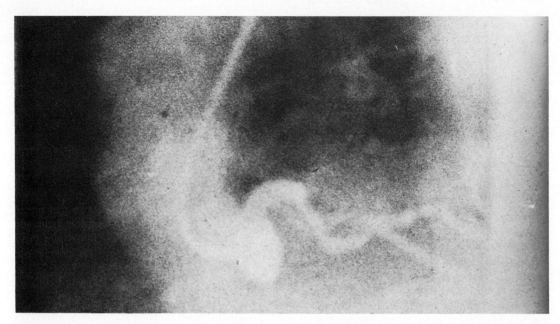

FIG. 14.   Coronary arteriogram of a patient operated upon on the June 27, 1963, in chronic left ventricular failure, with severe angina decubitus. The only artery open in the heart was a sausage-shaped main left coronary which fed into a markedly narrowed circumflex.

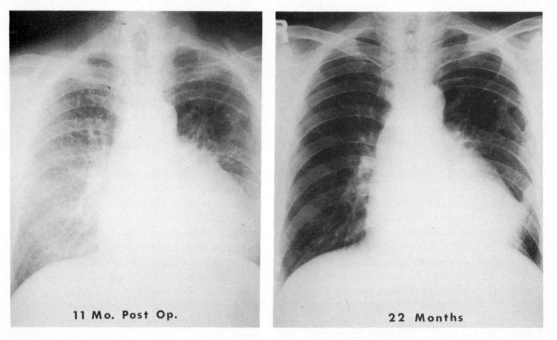

FIG 15. Roentgenogram of chest of patient shown in Fjgure 14, 11 months postoperatively, still in left ventricular failure, but without anginal pain and working. Twenty-two months postoperatively, the heart is smaller. There is no longer failure. The patient is working eight hours daily without pain. Prior to surgery, this patient was taking 120 nitroglycerin tablets per day. At the time of the last roentgenogram, he was taking none.

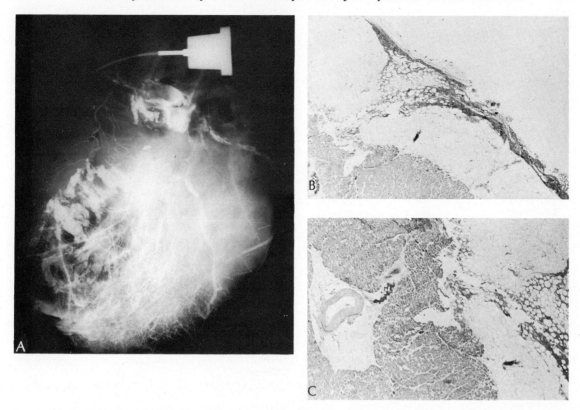

FIG. 16. (*A*) Roentgenogram of heart of patient who underwent left implantation, epicardiectomy, seropericardiectomy and free omental graft $4\frac{3}{4}$ years before death. This patient was taking 120 nitroglycerin tablets per day, had had six previous myocardial infarctions and had not worked for six years. He had an enlarged left ventricle in failure. His coronary arteriogram showed nothing patent except for a pin-point communication between a dilated left coronary and the circumflex. Surgery was performed in July, 1962. Patient required vasopressors for one month postoperatively. He returned to work and was still in chronic left ventricular failure at the end of 11 months. He was completely free of failure at the end of 22 months and in good health up to 4 years postoperatively. He died suddenly $4\frac{3}{4}$ years after surgery. The roentgenogram shows filling of the entire coronary circulation after the implanted internal mammary artery was injected. It was the only artery injected. In addition, numerous vessels in the pericardium and in the omental network of vessels, lying on the surface of the heart, were filled with the Schlesinger injection mass. Note left of film are calcium deposits in the interventricular septum. (*B*) Microphotograph of heart of the same patient showing the internal mammary artery lying within the myocardium, fully patent towards the end of the tunnel. To the right of the photograph, healthy omentum is seen on heart muscle with vessels which have been filled with Schlesinger mass after injection of the implanted internal mammary artery. (*C*) Same as (*B*), showing Schlesinger mass filling the vessels of the omentum at the junction with the pericardium.

Revascularization Surgery by Direct Attack on Surface Vessels

It is my opinion that this type of surgery is bound to give poor long-range results. Placement of a patch graft to widen a segmentally obstructed coronary artery results in turbulence in this area, and can only result in the occlusion of the area with progress of time. Likewise, the replacement of a segment of an artery by a vein graft will only last as long as the distal branches of the artery to which it is anastomosed remain open. Since the disease of coronary atherosclerosis is progressive, this type of operation, as well as the operations which anastomose an internal mammary artery to the distal end of a right coronary, with time appear doomed to failure. Thus, the new channels are most likely destined to close off because of occlusion of the surface vessels beyond the points of grafting or anastomosis.

BIBLIOGRAPHY

1. Vineberg, A.: Development of an anastomosis between the coronary vessels and a transplanted internal mammary artery, Canad. M. A. J. *55*:117, 1946.

2. _____and Jewett, B. L.: Development of an anastomosis between the coronary vessels and a transplanted internal mammary artery, Canad. M. A. J. *56*:609, 1947.

3. _____: Development of anastomosis between the coronary vessels and a transplanted internal mammary artery, J. Thoracic Surg. *18*:839, 1949.

4. _____and Miller, D.: An experimental study of the physiological role of an anastomosis between the left coronary circulation and the left internal mammary artery implanted in the left ventricular myocardium, Surgical Forum (1950), p. 294, 1951.

5. _____and Miller, G.: Internal mammary coronary anastomosis in the surgical treatment of coronary artery insufficiency, Canad. M. A. J. *64*:204, 1951.

6. _____and Miller, D.: Functional evaluation of an internal mammary coronary artery anastomosis, Am. Heart J. *45*:873, 1953.

7. _____: Internal mammary artery implant in the treatment of angina pectoris: A three year follow-up. Canad. M. A. J. *70*:367, 1954.

8. _____Munro, D. D., Cohen, H., and Buller, W. K.: Four years' clinical experience with internal mammary artery implantation in the treatment of human coronary insufficiency including additional experimental studies, J. Thoracic Surg. *29*:1, 1955.

9. _____and Buller, W. K.: A study of the amount of blood and oyxgen delivered to the myocardium through the implanted mammary artery, Surgical Forum (1954) *5*:78, 1955.

10. _____and Walker, J.: Six months to six years experience with coronary artery insufficiency treated by internal mammary artery implantation. Am. Heart J. *54*:851, 1957.

11. _____: Internal mammary artery implantation: Survey of fifteen years of experimental study and ten years experience with human cases, Ohio State M. J. *58*:1139, 1962.

12. _____and Walker, J.: The surgical treatment of coronary artery heart disease by internal mammary artery implantation. Report of 140 cases followed up to thirteen years, Dis. Chest *45*:190, 1964.

13. _____: Experimental background of myocardial revascularization by internal mammary artery implantation and supplementary technics, with its clinical application in 125 patients: A review and critical appraisal, Ann. Surg. *159*:185, 1964.

14. _____ and Duschesne, E. R.: An experimental study of the effect of mechanically induced ischemia upon the mammary coronary anastomoses, Surgery *43*:837, 1958.

15. _____ Pifarre, R., and Kato, Y.: The treatment of multiple coronary occlusions by internal mammary artery implantation and free omental graft: Report on two human cases, Canad. M. A. J. *88*:499, 1963.

16. _____ Shanks, J., Pifarre, R., Criollos, R., and Kato, Y.: Combined internal mammary artery implantation and free omental graft operation: A highly effective revascularization procedure (a study of 17 cases), Canad. M. A. J. *90*:717, 1964.

17. _____ and Baichwal, K. S.: Myocardial revascularization by omental graft without pedicle: Experimental background and report on 25 cases followed 6 to 16 months, J. Thorac Cardiovas. Surg. *49*:103, 1965.

18. _____: Results of fourteen years experience in the surgical treatment of human coronary artery insufficiency, Canad. M. A. J. *92*:325, 1965.

19. _____ and Zamora, B. O.: Right internal mammary implantation into right ventricular myocardium for revascularization of the entire heart, Canad. M. A. J. *95*:570, 1966.

20. _____ Baroldi, G., and Scomazzoni, G.: Coronary Circulation in the Normal and the Pathologic Heart, Armed Forces Institute of Pathology, General Department of the Army, Washington, D. C., 1967.

21. _____ Proudfit, W. L., Shirey, E. K., and Sones, M.: Selective cine coronary arteriography correlation with clinical findings in 1000 patients, Circulation *33*:901, 1966.

22. _____ Litvak, J., and Siderides, L.: The experimental production of coronary artery insufficiency and occlusion, Am. Heart J. *53*:505, 1957.

23. _____ Mahanti, B. C., and Litvak, J.: Experimental gradual coronary artery constriction by ameroid constrictors, Surgery *47*:765, 1960.

24. _____: Evaluation of experimental revascularization operations by ameroid coronary artery constriction, Surgery *47*:748, 1960.

25. _____ Favaloro, E. D. B., Grooves, L. K., and Sones, M.: Myocardial revascularization by internal mammary artery implant procedures: Clinical experience, J. Thorac. Cardiovas. Surg. *54*:359, 1967.

26. _____ Kato, Y., and Pirozynski, W. J.: Experimental revascularization of the entire heart: Evaluation of epicardiectomy, omental graft, and or implantation of the internal mammary artery in preventing myocardial necrosis and death of the animal, Am. Heart J. *72*:79, 1966.

27. _____: Revascularization of the right and left coronary arterial systems: Internal mammary artery implantation, epicardiectomy and free omental graft operation, Am. J. Cardiol. *19*:344, 1967.

28. _____ and Zamora, B.: Revascularization of the right ventricular myocardium via right coronary arterial system by right internal mammary artery implantation, Am. J. Cardiol. *22*:218, 1968.

29. _____ and Syed, A. K.: Arterial vascular pathways from subclavian arteries to coronary arterioles created by free omental myocardial implants, Canad. M. A. J. *97*:399, 1967.

30. _____and Niloff, P.: The value of surgical treatment of coronary artery occlusion by implantation of the internal mammary artery into the ventricular myocardium, Surg. Gynec. & Obst. *91*:551, 1950.

31. Kato, Y.: Development of Triple Ameroid Coronary Artery Occlusion—A 100% Lethal Test, Value of Epicardiectomy, Omental Graft and/or Internal Mammary Artery Implant Operation in Preventing Death of the Animal-Myocardia, Thesis submitted for Ph. D., McGill University, April 1, 1955, granted June 1965.

32. Vineberg, A., and McMillan, G. C.: The fate of the internal mammary artery implant in the ischemic human heart, Dis. Chest *33*:64, 1958.

Myocardial Revascularization by Direct Coronary Artery Surgery

F. Mason Sones, Jr.

As of the first of December 1968, Dr. Effler and his colleagues, Dr. Favaloro and Dr. Groves, have performed 2,900 procedures designed to improve the natural history of patients afflicted with degenerative heart disease. Of these, 2,530 were internal mammary artery implants. For single implants, the operative mortality, with all cases considered, was 3.2 per cent; for double implants, it was 5.6 per cent. In Cleveland, we are much more excited, at this stage, with some of the direct technics that have been developed by Dr. Favaloro and Dr. Effler for dealing with significant isolated obstructions.

There have now been over 200 pericardial patch grafts or vein grafts used to correct severe segmental obstructions in major trunks. There have been 155 saphenous vein replacements. Most of these have been interposed segments of saphenous vein replacing segmental obstructions. Fifteen of the 155 have been by-pass grafts from the aortic root to the proximal anterior descending-circumflex bifurcation, or to middle or distal thirds of dominant right coronary arteries. Overall mortality in that group, to date, has been 6 per cent.

The first left main trunk coronary artery obstruction that Dr. Effler approached surgically was so severely narrowed near its orifice that it was impossible to catheterize it. We have become particularly fearful of this type of lesion because, in more than 13,000 patients studied, we have seen only 31 survivors of total occlusion of the left main coronary artery. In this first case, restudy six months after a vein patch was placed above the obstructed segment showed excellent filling of the previously narrowed trunk. The patient returned to work, and has been working without interruption now for longer than 6 years. He has never had a recurrence of anginal pain, despite the fact that angiography, 6 months after operation, did show evidence of diffuse but relatively minor distal obstructive lesions. He has worked continuously since he recovered from the operative procedure, doing heavy farm labor in the summer time and driving a snow plow in the winter in weather as low as 20° below zero for the Ohio State Road Commission. Cine-angiography, performed again $5\frac{1}{2}$ years after operation, revealed that patency had been maintained without aneurysmal dilatation at the site of the vein patch, and the patient remains asymptomatic. He is one of the fortunate people in whom progression of obstructive lesions has occurred at a relatively slow pace. The diagonal branch of his left coronary artery has developed progressive obstruction, while his right coronary artery also shows diffuse but not mechanically severe obstructive lesions—$5\frac{1}{2}$ years after direct intervention.

In another patient, we observed extremely severe obstructive disease of the left coronary artery, the major lesion occurring in the proximal anterior descending trunk. In this area the vessel was almost completely obstructed and its distal segment actually filled in retrograde fashion by way of a diagonal branch from the circumflex trunk. It was clearly evident that the extremely severe obstructive disease in his left anterior descending system was producing a major perfusion deficit in the area of distribution of the anterior descending coronary artery. Study of his right coronary artery revealed that it was the dominant vessel and the site of diffuse disease. The little collaterals seen communicating with the distal circumflex appeared to be jeopardized by the horrendous obstruction in the upper third of the right main trunk.

After a large pericardial patch was placed at the point of obstruction in the right coronary artery, very effective collateral channels to distal radicals of the anterior descending system developed, as well as much more effective collateralization to the distal circumflex system. So, even though we were dealing with a patient with very severe diffuse obstructive changes, a direct attack on a single, key lesion provided not only protection for the distal right coronary, but also collateral channels to the severely diseased left coronary artery.

Incidentally, in over 13,000 patients, we have as yet to see normal or naturally occurring inter-coronary collateral channels develop to a vessel which is not obstructed at least 90 per cent. If there is more than a 10 per cent residual lumen diameter, effective collaterals are virtually never seen. This bears on the previous discussion in that we do not think one should operate on people with 50 per cent obstruction.

The next case is relatively rare and is one of 31 instances of left main trunk occlusion with survival. Despite total occlusion of this vessel, the patient managed to survive because his huge right coronary artery was providing effective collateralization to both the anterior descending system and the circumflex system. The mechanism permitted survival of myocardial tissue but, in the middle third of the right main trunk, his collateral circulation was severely jeopardized by the presence of a large atheromatous plaque causing about 85 to 90 per cent obstruction. If he lost that he was certainly going to lose the whole ball game. So, in the face of such diffuse disease, a direct attack on the localized segmental obstruction permitted more effective development of pre-existing collaterals to the anterior descending and circumflex systems. It also eliminated the potential lethal injury which would result if that obstruction progressed to total occlusion.

This patient, incidentally, was a command airline pilot, who was flying regularly until 6 months prior to the time the initial study was performed. He now plays golf, 18 holes, three times a week, but does not fly airplanes any more. However, two years after surgery, this patient developed a posterolateral infarct of relatively small extent; he recovered well and his electrocardiogram returned to normal. We wondered if the lesion he had in his right coronary artery had progressed to complete obstruction. Angiographic study showed this was not the case. Instead, complete obstruction was observed in the circumflex trunk and this, of course, was the reason for the development of his posterolateral infarct two years later. His right coronary artery had been reconstructed but it now showed evidence of progressive disease. Nevertheless, the right coronary was still providing quite effective collateral channels to distal radicals of the left circumflex trunk. This minimized the magnitude of his injury and modified the natural history of his disease.

Selective Revascularization of the Myocardium

Charles P. Bailey, Teruo Hirose, Cesar Vera, Elliott J. Howard, Daniel Larson, and Frank S. Folk

Over the past three and one-half years the authors have been carrying out procedures designed to accomplish "selective and comprehensive" revascularization of the ischemic myocardium in clinical patients, using several different surgical technics. Two methods, revascularization of the posterior (diaphragmatic) wall of the ventricle by intramyocardial implantation of the right gastroepiploic artery[1,2,3,4] and direct mammary-coronary arterial anastomosis by a "minivascular suturing technic,"[5] were developed in our own experimental laboratory during the course of a still ongoing animal research program.

IMPLANT REVASCULARIZATION

Many experimental and clinical articles in medical literature [6-16,18] attest to the soundness of the practice of revascularizing the heart by intramyocardial implantation of a systemic artery. Most of the procedures reported have involved use of the left internal mammary artery as the systemic vessel, with implantation into a tunnel created within the anterior or lateral wall of the left ventricle, as first proposed by Vineberg[6] in 1946.

Modifications of this technic have been introduced by others. Bloomer[19,20] has advocated use of the splenic artery and Pearce and Creech[21] have used the intercostal arteries. Bailey and Hirose[1,2,3,4] have mobilized the right, and sometimes the left gastroepiploic artery, especially for ischemia of the posterior wall of the left ventricle. More recently, Vineberg[22] has implanted the right internal mammary artery anteriorly within the thickness of the right ventricular wall.

While no one has clearly demonstrated the mechanism by which implant revascularization takes place, the authors offer the following hypothesis. Anatomically, the structure of the left ventricular myocardium resembles somewhat a "hemangioma extensively infiltrated by muscle fibers."[2] Terminal arterial tributaries and venous radicles communicate with this system of interlocking endothelially lined spaces which vary from the size of capillaries to macroscopic sinusoids.

In the event of central obstruction of the regional coronary trunk to a given area of the ventricular wall, the arterial perfusion pressure is reduced and the rate of ingress of arterial blood is significantly slowed. There may be sufficient perfusion for the aerobic metabolic needs of the myocardium under conditions of rest, but several studies[23,24,25] suggest that even at rest anaerobic metabolism may be the prevalent pattern in severely ischemic regions of the affected myocardium.

In coronary artery disease the normally minute interocoronary arterial communications, which connect the branches of each of the three major trunks, may gradually enlarge to provide a collateral blood supply to ischemic areas of the myocardium. In the patient who experiences angina pectoris on exertion presumably the rate of development of collateral circulation has not kept pace with the increasing perfusion deficit in one or more of the major myocardial irrigation beds, at least it is insufficient with respect to conditions of increased metabolic demand.

The ligated end of a mobilized systemic artery, bearing several lateral bleeding openings, is implanted within a tunnel made surgically in the presumably structurally intact, though functionally ischemic myocardial "irrigation bed" of the affected coronary trunk. The integrity of the system of interlocking endothelially lined spaces will have been interrupted at literally thousands of points by the surgical creation of the myocardial tunnel. Into this tunnel now flows richly oxygenated nutrient bearing arterial blood at a normal systemic arterial pressure. Since direct anatomic communication must exist from the very beginning with at least a large number of lacerated myocardial sinusoids, these become distended and rapidly "bleed off" into their directly communicating draining venous radicles. That this, in fact, does take place has been demonstrated by injection technic by Neptune,[26] and by cineangiography by Lillehei and associates[27] and by Ferlic *et al.*[28]

Blood from the newly introduced arterial implant does not, however, enter by the usual route of arterial and arteriolar vessels of progressively diminishing caliber. Consequently the minute venous draining components of this system are exposed directly to the systemic arterial pressure introduced by the implant. The late obliteration of the venous microvasculature reported by Hahn[29,30] in follow-up of surgically created aortico-coronary sinus anastomoses (Beck II operation), in which a similar high arterial pressure is imposed upon minor coronary venous elements, leads us to believe that the presence of such unnaturally high pressure tends to induce obliterative sclerosis of the draining venous capillaries and venules. The pressure head within the still communicating tributaries of the centrally obstructed coronary arterial trunk, which are quite capable of tolerating systemic arterial pressures, is abnormally low owing to this very occlusive process. Hence, the higher pressure of the implant artery, once the option of venous run-off has been denied, will tend to overcome the former. Thus, retrograde

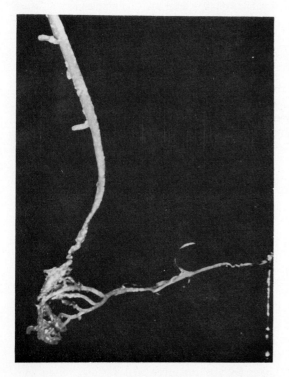

FIG. 1. Retrograde perfusion of the distal portion of the centrally obstructed anterior descending branch (horizontal) of the left coronary artery taking place by way of collaterals from the implant (vertical vessel) to distal branches (*corto-sion* specimen). Courtesy of Arthur Vineberg.

perfusion of the distal portion of the natural (but diseased) coronary artery will take place by way of its distal branches (Fig. 1).

Clinical Material

This inferred course of events fits well with all of our available knowledge derived both from experimental studies and from clinical observation of cases in which intramyocardial implantation has been carried out.

Because others have written extensively of their experiences with single implant revascularization, presumably for single coronary trunk obstruction, and since the vast majority of our clinical patients have suffered from critical obstruction of two or more of the main coronary trunks, we will present here only the results we have obtained with concomitant anterior and posterior implant, revascularization procedures.

Usually this has meant implantation of the left internal mammary artery within the anterior wall of the left ventricle, in close proximity to the course of the anterior descending branch of the left coronary artery, and the simultaneous implantation of the mobilized right gastroepiploic artery within a myocardial tunnel made obliquely beneath the posterior descending coronary branch respectively, for critical obstruction of the anterior descending and the right coronary artery. Occasionally, because of severe central obstructive disease of the circumflex branch of the left coronary artery, the left internal mammary artery has been implanted more laterally. In two instances, because of occlusion of a previous left internal mammary implant, the right internal mammary has been mobilized extensively and brought into a tunnel made diagonally beneath the course of the anterior descending branch of the left coronary.

Results

Since it has been established that elapse of a certain time period is necessary for the development of effective implant revascularization, we have restricted our follow-up evaluation to those patients who had been submitted to surgery at least one year previously. The results attained in 43 such patients are presented in Tables 1, 2, 3, 4 and 5. It is now realized that our initial enthusiasm for the possible benefit to be obtained from this procedure led us to apply it in certain excessively ill patients who would be excluded from surgical consideration today.

Careful pre- and postoperative examination by

the usual clinical and laboratory modalities has been the basis for evaluation of operative benefit in this series. A precise anatomic and functional diagnosis was first established by selective coronary cineangiography,[31] by ventriculography[32] and in some cases by performance of metabolic studies.[23–25] Postoperative clinical evaluation in doubtful cases has been weighed in the light of these more objective parameters.

In the course of our work we have had two bitter experiences after postoperative visualization of a widely patent mammary artery implant on check-up cineangiography. In both instances there was a sudden return of untoward symptoms shortly after the procedure. Subsequent cineangiographic studies revealed occlusion of the implant.

We believe that the adverse angle at which an internal mammary artery must be approached by the angiographic catheter tends to produce localized trauma which may sometimes result in thrombotic obliteration of the lumen. More recently, we have refrained from the routine performance of check-up cineangiograms in patients who have been doing well clinically, reserving these studies for patients with an unsatisfactory or doubtful course. For this reason reliable postoperative cineangiographic data was accumulated only in the less favorable portion of our total series (Table 5) In this group, by visualization of the implanted vessels, major coronary communication has been demonstrated in approximately one third while minor coronary communication was evident in another third.

TABLE 1
Double Implant Revascularization

Total	Operative Mortality	Late Mortality
43	9 (21%)	3 (7%)

TABLE 2
Postoperative Infarction

Total	Early Postoperative	Late
43	5 (11.5%)	1 (2%)

TABLE 3
Causes of Death

	Early	Late
Myocardial Infarction	4	1 (8 mos.)
Shock (falling B.P.)	1	0
Pulmonary Embolism	1	1
Arrhythmia	1	1
Mediastinal Infection	1	0
Technical Error	1	0
Total	9 (21%)	3 (7%)

TABLE 4

Total	Excellent (Full activity, no angina)	Good (Full activity, rare angina)	Fair (Less angina)	Poor (No better)
31	18 (58%)	8 (26%)	2 (6%)	3 (10%)

TABLE 5
12 Month Cineangiography, 23 Patients

	Internal Mammary	Gastroepiploic
Major coronary communications	7	4
Minor coronary communications	9	6
Patent but no demonstrable coronary communications	3	8
Arterial fistula with visible coronary communications	1	0
No postoperative study of vessel (technical difficulty)	1	3
Closed	2	2
Total	23	23

Discussion

In the performance of implant revascularization in the past[6–16,18–22] certain currently accepted parameters of investigation were not practiced in the selection of patients for these revascularization procedures. Unfortunately our series is partially vulnerable to criticism on similar grounds.

It should be obvious that revascularization of a frankly aneurysmal portion of the ventricular wall cannot be achieved by arterial implantation or by any other surgical or medical mode of treatment. Similarly, areas of severe through-and-through fibrosis or scarring of the ventricular wall which do not bulge out the cardiac outline cannot be revascularized (Fig. 2). The work of Herman and associates[32] in delineating areas of myocardial asynergy by multipositional cineventriculography has proved to be of inestimable value more recently in recognition and rejection of such patients.

Sometimes unusual resistance is encountered during surgical passage of tunneling forceps through the ventricular wall, presumably due to fibrous infiltration of the myocardium. In cases in which enough of the original spongy myocardial structure is retained, implant revascularization can, no doubt, be of significant benefit even when some fibrous infiltration is present. However, when very little muscle tissue remains, the endothelially lined interlocking blood containing spaces largely having been obliterated or replaced by fibrous connective tissue, any attempt at surgical revascularization would seem to be but an exercise in futility.

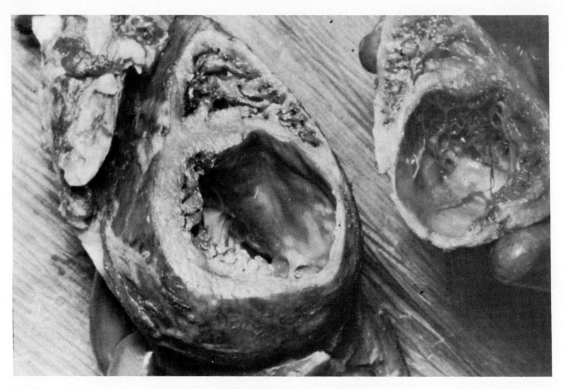

FIG. 2.   Areas of through-and-through fibrosis and scarring of the ventricular wall. Whether they bulge out the cardiac outline or not, they cannot be effectively revascularized.

Subjective benefit reported early after implant revascularization is suspect as functional or spurious unless it persists for at least six to eight months. If there is doubt of its validity, confirmation may be obtained by cineangiographic demonstration of communication between the implant and the regional coronary branches after the elapse of ten to twelve months. Localized transient myocardial "blushing" alone following injection of contrast medium into an implanted artery would seem at best to indicate only a very limited degree of re-vascularization. At worst, it may signify the direct passage of contrast material from the implant vessel through purely venous channels, indicating no "revascularization" at all. Moreover, one may postulate the possibility of surgical production of a direct systemic artery—coronary venous fistula due to inadvertent perforation of a coronary vein by the tunneling forceps. Similarly, demonstration of patency of an implant vessel down to, or even within, the myocardial tunnel would seem to mean nothing unless some coronary communication can be shown to exist.

We gladly concede high level effectiveness to implant revascularization when later it can be shown cineangiographically that major communica-tion with the regional coronary branches of an exclusively centrally obstructed trunk has developed. When, however, the atherosclerotic process has involved the trunk and its major branches more extensively, demonstration of major communication with one or more of its isolated branches does not necessarily imply direct revascularization of the entire myocardial irrigation bed normally supplied by that trunk.

Minor communications with the regional coronary branches are somewhat less convincing than more major communications, even when the trunk vessel is centrally obstructed. Presumably the lesser flow so permitted affords correspondingly less benefit. Although many patients with an "excellent" clinical response have only such communications, one must remember that "excellent" responses have sometimes followed frankly "sham" operations and those in which the implant vessel has become occluded. It is our belief that minor communication with the regional coronary branches represents a lower level of effective revascularization.

With this in mind, it would be amiss to ignore other methods of myocardial revascularization which, in properly selected cases, may provide a much greater degree of benefit.

BYPASS-CORONARY ARTERIAL ANASTOMOSIS

In 1941 Schlesinger and Zoll demonstrated pathologically that in 69 per cent of 125 hearts of patients who had died of myocardial infarction, the obstructive arterial lesion was limited to the first four centimeters of one or more of the main coronary trunks.[17] Sones's [31,33] introduction of selective coronary cineangiography now provides a method for precise diagnosis during life of the extent and location of many coronary lesions.

In 1961 Goetz[34] first attempted poststenotic bypass anastomosis of the coronary artery by joining the right internal mammary to the right coronary artery, using a nonsuture tantalum ring technic of anastomosis. Kolessov,[35] more recently, has accomplished direct surgical union by an interesting four stitch end-to-side anastomotic technic, connecting the left internal mammary artery to the "interventricular coronary artery" (anterior descending branch of the left). Nearly simultaneously with our own work, Tice and Green[36] have used the high power operating microscope, cold cardiac arrest and extracorporeal circulation to anastomose the left internal mammary to the anterior descending branch of the left coronary artery.

On the other hand, Favaloro[37] and Effler[38] have interposed saphenous vein segments into the continuity of the right coronary artery after resecting an area of segmental disease.

Urschel[39] and associates and Johnson *et al.*[40] have preferred to use arterialized saphenous vein segments to surgically bypass areas of segmental coronary obstruction. A limited experience with this latter technic in our hands has confirmed the somewhat greater technical facility with which such bypasses can be established.

Clinical Material and Methods

On February 8, 1968 the authors[5] undertook to perform a direct anastomosis of the right internal mammary artery to the right coronary artery, distal to an area of central obstruction (Fig. 3). The patient, a 46-year-old taxicab driver, had been submitted to posterior implantation of the right gastroepiploic artery 14 months earlier but had not experienced either immediate or later relief of his angina pectoris. Although the implant vessel had remained patent, no communication with the regional coronary arterial branches could be demonstrated on check-up angiography.

The anastomotic operation was performed at

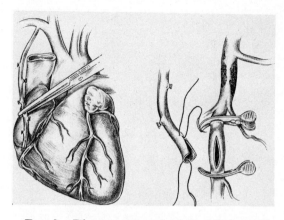

FIG. 3. Direct anastomosis of the right internal mammary artery to the right coronary artery, distal to an area of central obstruction.

normothermic temperatures with the aid of $2\frac{1}{2}$ power ophthalmological "loupes," without extracorporeal bypass. The steps of the surgical procedure are shown in Figure 4.

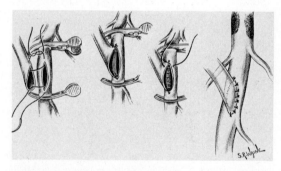

FIG. 4. The steps involved in performance of the direct anastomosis procedure.

Ten additional patients have been operated on by the same general technic. A method for continuous perfusion of the distal portion of the temporarily obstructed coronary artery has been added (Fig. 5). Anticoagulation with heparin was used during the performance of the surgery and for three days postoperatively, followed by subsequent coumadin control.

Among such bypass anastomotic operations included in this series, left internal mammary-coronary anastomosis was performed for central obstruction of the left circumflex branch in one patient and for obstruction of the anterior descending branch of the left coronary artery in another patient. Nine patients with exclusive or preponderant central right coronary artery obstruction were submitted to right internal mammary-

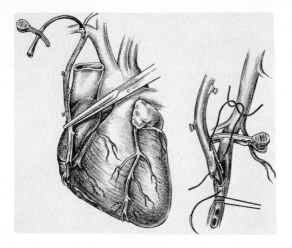

FIG. 5. A method for continuous perfusion of the distal portion of the temporarily obstructed coronary artery in performance of a direct mammary-coronary anastomosis.

right coronary anastomosis, using either a right posterolateral or a mid-line sternum splitting thoracic incision. When untoward electrocardio-

graphic or clinical change has followed test-cross-clamping of the dissected coronary artery trans-anastomotic perfusion of the distal portion of the artery has been practiced (Fig. 5).

Results

The original patient has done well postoperatively and has had no further anginal distress. Post-operative cineangiography after six and one-half weeks showed that the affected portion of the coronary artery had now become completely obstructed (Fig. 6, A and B). At that time the distal portion was being perfused entirely by way of the mammary-coronary anastomosis (Fig. 6, C).

There were two deaths in this series, one un-questionably due to inept management of the program of anticoagulation and one due to late development of an antibiotically refractory pneu-monia. Both deaths occurred among the cases with right coronary obstruction.

In view of the much better survival rate currently being reported with direct procedures such as vein graft bypass of the right coronary artery,[37-40] we

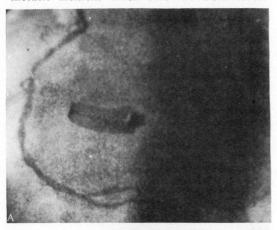

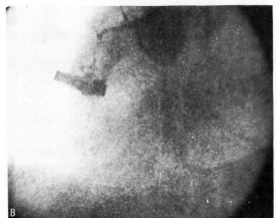

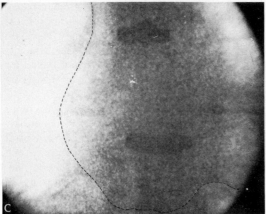

FIG. 6. (*A*) Preoperative cineangiogram of right coronary of M.B. showing central obstructive lesions. (*B*) Postoperative cineangiogram obtained after $6\frac{1}{2}$ weeks, showing that the affected portion of the coronary artery had become fully obstructed since the time of surgery. (*C*) The distal portion of the right coronary artery was now being perfused entirely by way of the mammary-coronary anas-tomosis.

believe that this unexpectedly high early operative mortality will prove unrepresentative and misleading. The immediate general condition and the subsequent postoperative course of the survivors were distinctly better than we have come to expect from patients with double implant operations. However, postoperative cineangiographic studies in our series have disclosed that in two patients the anastomosis has become occluded. In one of them, the procedure unavoidably had been performed in an area of significant arterial disease.

SUMMARY AND CONCLUSIONS

Experience accumulated to date suggests that the ideal patient for implant revascularization is one with obstructive lesions limited to the central portion of one or more of the main coronary trunks in conjunction with the presence of a widely patent distal arterial lumen and structurally undamaged myocardium. Since this pathology also conforms best to the requirements for a direct mammary-coronary or arterialized vein-coronary bypass procedure, the authors submit that in many cases this may be the preferable type of operative intervention. If operative mortality levels can be kept as low as those reported for other types of direct coronary surgery, direct mammary-coronary anastomosis should provide a nearly ideal and, most importantly, an immediate surgical solution to the problem of coronary obstruction in well selected cases.

When conditions are not ideal for implant revascularization, usually direct bypass anastomosis also will not be feasible. In such cases arterial implantation sometimes may, nevertheless, be attempted in the hope that developing collaterals might prove to be unusually beneficial. But this must be done with expectancy of a lower level of ultimate clinical success and at the risk of a higher operative mortality. The final agonizing decision can best be made after measurement of the end-diastolic pressure within the left ventricle and performance of multipositional ventriculography.

Successful selective myocardial revascularization implies not only choice of the most probably beneficial procedure for that individual but also a continued awareness that surgery may not be indicated or even possible in every patient with atherosclerotic coronary artery disease.

REFERENCES

1. Bailey, C. P., Hirose, T., Brancato, R., Aventura, A., and Yamamoto, N.: Revascularization of the posterior (diaphragmatic) portion of the heart, Ann.

Thorac. Surg. *2*: No. 6, November, 1966.
2. Bailey, C. P., and Hirose, T.: Surgical treatment of coronary artery disease, Current Med. Dig. *34*: 1967.
3. Bailey, C. P., Gollub, S., and Shapiro, A. G. (eds.): Revascularization of the Ischemic Posterior Myocardium. First Symposium of the St. Barnabas Hospital on Rheumatic and Coronary Heart Disease, Philadelphia, J. B. Lippincott Co., 1967.
4. Bailey, C. P., Hirose, T., Aventura, A., Yamamoto, N., Brancato, R., Vera, C., and O'Connor, R.: Revascularization of the ischemic posterior myocardium, Dis. Chest *52*: 1967.
5. Bailey, C. P., and Hirose, T.: Successful internal mammary-coronary arterial anastomosis using a "minivascular" suturing technique, Int. Surg. *49*: 416, 1968.
6. Vineberg, A. M.: Development of an anastomosis between the coronary vessels and a transplanted internal mammary artery, Canad. M. J. *55*:117, 1946.
7. Vineberg, A. M., and Jewett, B. L.: Anastomosis between coronary vessels and internal mammary artery, Canad. M. A. J. *56*:609, 1947.
8. Vineberg, A. M.: Development of anastomosis between the coronary vessels and a transplanted internal mammary artery, J. Thoracic Surg. *18*:835 1949.
9. Vineberg, A. M., and Niloff, P.: The value of surgical treatment of coronary artery occlusion by implantation of the internal mammary artery into the ventricular myocardium, Surg. Gynec. & Obst. *91*:551, 1950.
10. Vineberg, A. M., Munro, D. D., Cohen, H., and Buller, W. C.: Four years' clinical experience with internal mammary artery implantation in the treatment of human coronary artery insufficiency including additional experimental studies, J. Thoracic Surg. *29*:1, 1955.
11. Bakst, A., Maniglia, R., Adams, A., and Bailey, C. P.: The physiological and pathological evaluation of the implantation of the internal mammary artery into the left ventricular myocardium for the treatment of coronary artery disease, Surgery *29*:188, 1955
12. Sabiston, D., and Blalock, A.: An experimental study of the fate of arterial implants in the left ventricular myocardium, Ann. Surg. *145*:927, 1959.
13. Vineberg, A. M., Pifarre, R., and Kato, Y.: The treatment of multiple coronary occlusion by internal mammary artery implantation and omental graft, Canad. M. A. J. *88*:499, 1963.
14. Sewell, W. H.: Basic physiologic approach to myocardial revascularization, Conn. Med. *27*:76, 1963.
15. Effler, D. B., Groves, L. K., Sones, F. M., Jr., and Shirey, E. K.: Increased myocardial perfusion by internal mammary artery implant. Vineberg's operation, Ann. Surg. *158*:526, 1963.
16. Vineberg, A. M.: Experimental background of myocardial revascularization by internal mammary implantation and supplementary techniques with its clinical application in 125 patients, Ann. Surg. *159*:185, 1964.
17. Schlesinger, M. J., and Zoll, P. M.: Incidence and Localization of Coronary Artery Occlusions, Arch. Path. *32*:178, 1941.
18. Sewell, W. T.: Results of 122 mammary pedicle implantations for angina pectoris, Ann. Thorac.

Surg. *2*:17, 1966.

19. Bloomer, W. E., and Vidone, P.: Implantation of the splenic artery into the myocardium as the source of collateral circulation; quoted by Vansant, J. H., and Muller, W. H., Jr.: Surgical procedures to revascularize the heart, Am. J. Surg. *100*:572, 1960.

20. Bloomer, W. E., Beland, A. J., and Cope, J.: Clinical use of the splenic artery for myocardial revascularization, Ann. Thoracic Surg. *5*:419, 1968.

21. Pearce, C. W., Hyman, A. L., Brewer, P., Smith, P. E., and Creech, O., Jr.: Myocardial revascularization: Implantation of intercostal artery, J. Thorac. Cardiovas. Surg. *52*:809, 1966.

22. Vineberg, A. M., and Kato, Y.: Implantation of the right and left internal mammary arteries with epicardiectomy and free omental graft, Canad. M. A. J. *93*:709, 1965.

23. Herman, M. V., Klein, M. D., Elliott, W. C., and Gorlin, R.: Electrocardiographic, metabolic and anatomic predictions of zonal myocardial ischemia in coronary artery disease, Circulation 32 (Suppl. 2): 111, 1965.

24. Gorlin, R., and Taylor, W. S.: Selective revascularization of the myocardium by internal mammary artery implant, New England J. Med. *275*:283, 1966.

25. Taylor, W. S., and Gorlin, R.: Clinical, anatomic and physiologic assessment following internal mammary implantation: The Second St. Barnabas Hospital Symposium on Therapeutic Advances in the Practice of Cardiology. To be published.

26. Neptune, W.: Work carried out in the laboratories of Hahnemann Medical College, 1951 and 1952.

27. Lillehei, C. W., Ferlic, R. M., and Quattlebaum, F. W.: Myocardial Revascularization by Autogenous Vein Graft between Aorta and Myocardium. Presented at Meeting of the American College of Cardiology, Chicago, Ill., February 4, 1966.

28. Ferlic, R. M., Quattlebaum, F. W., and Lillehei, C. W.: Experimental and clinical results of myo-cardial revascularization with "arterialized" autogenous vein grafts, J. Thorac. Cardiovas. Surg. *52*:813, 1966.

29. Hahn, R. S., Kim, M., and Beck, C. S.: Revascularization of the heart: Observations on the circulation following arterialization of the coronary sinus, Am. Heart J. *44*:810, 1952.

30. Hahn, R. S., and Kim, M.: Revascularization of the heart: Histological changes after arterialization of the coronary sinus, Circulation *5*:801, 1952.

31. Sones, F. M., Jr., and Shirey, E. K. Cinecoronary arteriography, Mod. Concepts Cardiovas. Dis. *31*: 735, 1962.

32. Herman, M. V., Heinle, R. A., Klein, M. D., and Gorlin, R.: Localized disorders in myocardial contraction, New England J. Med. *277*:222, 1967.

33. Sones, F. M., Jr: Cinecoronary arteriography, Ohio M. J., *58*:1018, 1962.

34. Goetz, R. H., Rohman, J., Haller, J. D., Dee, R., and Rosenak, S. S.: Internal mammary—coronary artery anastomosis. A non-suture method employing tantalum rings, J. Thorac. Cardiovas. Surg. *41*: 1961.

35. Kolessov, V. I.: Mammary artery—coronary artery anastomosis as method of treatment for angina pectoris, J. Thorac. Cardiovas. Surg. *54*:435, 1967.

36. Tice, D. A., Green, G. E., Paul, R. S., Wallsh, E.: Coronary artery bypass grafting, Surgical Forum *19*:159, 1968.

37. Favaloro, R.: Saphenous vein autograft. Replacement of severe segmental coronary artery occlusion, Ann. Thorac. Surg. *5*:334, 1968.

38. Effler, D. B.: A New Approach to Localized Coronary Artery Obstruction using Arterialized Autologous Vein Grafts. Second St. Barnabas Hospital Symposium, New York, December 16, 1967. To be published.

39. Urschel, H. C., Jr: Presented at Society of Thoracic Surgeons Meeting, San Diego, January 1969.

40. Johnson, W. D., Personal communication to C. P. Bailey.

Objective Evaluation of Revascularization Procedures

F. Mason Sones, Jr.

I would like to begin by making 3 points:

1. In our opinion, there is no such entity as a triarteriolar zone that one can use specifically to put in an implant and then anticipate that this implant will perfuse all three major systems of the coronary tree.

2. You can take a normal coronary circulation and begin to inject thin Schlesinger mass and you can always perfuse the entire coronary tree in a post-mortem specimen.

3. This does not represent what actually happens in the living human.

It is essential not only to define the specific areas of obstruction but also to implant vessels beneath the distal radicals of those obstructed vessels. These procedures will not work unless they are applied in instances of proximal obstruction causing more than a 90 per cent reduction in lumen diameters. *Nature has taught us this and we had best learn the lesson.*

I will present a few cases to illustrate some of these points. In one patient, the right coronary artery showed diffuse obstructive changes of varied minor degree. He had sustained an antero-lateral myocardial infarct 6 months previously. He recovered from the infarction but continued to have anginal pain. His pain was not due to ischemia in any area of the myocardium perfused by his right coronary artery. The circumflex trunk showed minor changes, similar to those observed in the right coronary artery, but his left anterior descending trunk was completely obstructed at a point in its upper third. There was also a 50 per cent obstruction higher up in the anterior descending vessel. If he had occluded at that point he probably would not have survived. We have seen fewer than 150 survivors of anterior descending obstruction above the first perforating trunk. Survival is rare unless there is very extensive pre-existing collateral. In this patient, no pre-existing collateral from the right coronary was observed, although he did have a little collateralization to the distal radicals of the anterior descending coronary from his circumflex trunk. It was apparent that he had only one ischemic zone in his myo-cardium and that specifically was the area to which the surgeon's attention was directed.

This, then, was an ideal patient for anterior internal mammary artery implantation. The one thing anticipated was re-perfusion of distal radicals of the anterior descending coronary artery beyond its point of total obstruction, and this is what actually happened. It would not have occurred so predictably however, if we had been dealing with 50, 60 or 70 per cent obstructions; it only occurs with any degree of dependability if you are dealing with more than 90 per cent lumenal obstruction in the proximal trunk.

In this case, the internal mammary artery, studied about 11 months later, was found to be connected up to distal radicals of the anterior descending system which were now filling completely. This overcame the specific localized perfusion deficit in this individual.

Now, during the past $2\frac{1}{2}$ years, it has been possible to extend very significantly technics utilizing both internal mammary arteries; it is preferable to use the right internal mammary artery to get to the distal distribution of the anterior descending system and the left internal mammary artery for the distal distribution of the left circumflex and right coronary trees. *You cannot stick an implant in one area and perfuse all three segments of the coronary tree.* When Dr. Vineberg is able to show us evidence, in the living human, that he has accomplished this in one single instance, I will publicly give him 500 to 1 odds. It cannot be done!

In another patient, we noted total occlusion of the right coronary artery with collaterals to the totally occluded left anterior descending trunk. A Sewell implant had been done many years before, in an era when there was only one area that could be effectively implanted, namely, the area of distribution of the distal anterior descending coronary artery. The implant observed a year later was found to be filling the diagonal branch of the anterior descending trunk and very faintly filling the main anterior descending trunk. This was followed by

469

filling of the anterior ventricular vein and the great cardiac vein in perfectly normal time sequence. The perfusion noted was not due to arteriovenous fistulae. I have never seen an arteriovenous fistula produced by implantation of a systemic artery into an intact myocardium. I have seen, in a very few instances, implantation of the end of an internal mammary artery directly into the left ventricular chamber, producing an internal mammary artery-left ventricular fistula. If you want to grow an internal mammary artery, this is a great way to do it in a hurry. You can clinically recognize this quite readily because it produces a continuous murmur that begins in systole and continues into diastole over the precordium. You can then send the surgeon a congratulatory note without even looking at the artery.

When the same internal mammary artery was visualized after administration of a potent coronary vasodilator, the characteristics and morphologic size of the internal mammary artery was completely *unchanged,* but the distal radicals of the anterior descending coronary artery perfused by the implant were markedly *dilated.* The entire anterior descending trunk became opacified, by exactly the same type of mechanical injection, all the way back up to its point of obstruction. The point I am trying to emphasize is that these drugs effectively modify resistance in vessels that have a visceral distribution. They do not do this in vessels that are systemically distributed.

We use the right internal mammary artery to specifically handle the anterior descending system. To try further to clarify this, I present the following case. In this patient, there was more than 95 per cent obstruction in the proximal portion of the anterior descending coronary artery, at one point. The circumflex trunk was not significantly involved. The patient had not had an infarct but he was disabled by severe and frequently occurring anginal pain. His angiogram, as stated, showed the anterior descending vessel to be almost completely obstructed, but fortunately below the first perforating branch. Perfusion deficit was present in a large area of the myocardium but he still had a good ventricle. All segments of the ventricle contracted effectively so that fortunately, there had been no replacement by scar tissue of functioning myocardium. An internal mammary artery implant was performed.

He was restudied a year later. He never had an infarct or a clinical episode of prolonged pain. His angina had disappeared but the left coronary artery had now progressed to total occlusion. This patient did not get an infarct because his internal mammary artery had effectively taken over the entire distal anterior descending coronary function. This was so effective that neither he nor any of us who were observing his progress ever realized that he had progressed to total occlusion. However, he was one of the lucky ones. The operation had nothing to do with the progress of the basic pathology—it progressed to total occlusion. Fortunately, the implant had been in long enough to compensate for the severe obstruction. In addition, his left ventricle still demonstrated perfectly normal left ventricular function even after he completely obstructed his anterior descending trunk. Now this can happen if you are lucky, but if total occlusion develops before the implant is able to take over, you are in trouble.

The next case demonstrates the use of the left internal mammary artery to compensate for total obstruction of the left circumflex trunk. The patient had enough naturally occurring collateral to protect the myocardium from irreversible injury. He had severe anginal pain. Angiographic study showed that the circumflex branch was completely obstructed near its origin but that the anterior descending system was perfectly all right; the right coronary showed no significant obstructions. Fortunately he, too, still had a good ventricle. The diaphragmatic surface in the apical area was well perfused, so he had had no irreversible scar tissue replacement. He was considered a good candidate for implantation of the left internal mammary artery beneath distal circumflex branches. This was performed successfully and the patient was again studied one year later. His left internal mammary artery was visualized going way across but not communicating with the anterior descending system. It was, however, effectively perfusing distal branches of the left circumflex trunk.

This is such a simple thing that I fail to see why there is any reason for continued argumentation, except that we persist in promising too many people too much. The response is readily achieved using double internal mammary artery implants if there is diffuse disease. You can join distal radicals of the anterior descending trunk with the right internal mammary artery and distal radicals of the right or circumflex trunk, or both, with the left internal mammary artery. For example, in a patient with total occlusion of both the anterior descending and circumflex trunks, double internal mammary artery implants were performed. Subsequently, it was found that the right internal mammary artery of this patient was filling the entire right anterior descending system while the left internal mammary artery was quite effectively filling distal radicals of the left circumflex trunk.

Now we cannot possibly get to both of these vessels with one implant. We have done over 150 so-called AP-implants. We have managed to get effective communications to two vessels directly in only 3 of the patients studied postoperatively so far. I hope this helps to clarify some of the mystery surrounding this area of medical study. Thank you very much.

The Cardiologist Evaluates Myocardial Revascularization

Charles K. Friedberg

First may I take note of the distinguished cardiological surgeons who have appeared, and in one single morning, on this stage. And may I express my homage to them for pioneering in a field which, of course, is the most important field in cardiology.

However, I hope you realize that it shouldn't detract one iota from my regard for them as to say that I have more than a little skepticism. And while I admire the enthusiasm of surgeons, which in fact is essential to their success, I urge the medical men at least to use a little restraint and to temper the enthusiasm of the surgeons.

I come here with some timidity, sort of a lamb in the den of surgeons. I think I see six surgeons on the Panel with one medical man. Originally I thought there were two, but after Dr. Sones gave a surgical presentation the best I can do is to classify him as being of the neuter gender.

I am including Table 1 because I would I like to simplify the problem. I do not take issue with most of the things that have been said by the surgeons, certainly not with most of the things that Dr. Sones says. I just think they are irrelevant to our problem.

We have a patient who is ill, who has complaints, who has more or less disability. And we have to decide what is the best way of treating him. And if surgery is one of the modalities available, we simply go through the same process of balancing the advantages and disadvantages that we do in any surgical procedure. Obviously, some procedures are better established than others.

Table 1 shows some of the things that are promised by the surgeon. If true, we certainly can take no issue with the procedure. We also must decide whether the patient has been refractory to the measures we have utilized. Symptoms have to be very severe, disability has to be great, and the prognosis must be poor.

There are always, of course, reasons that make us hesitate. Certainly the surgical risk is said to be very small. It's not the same risk in all clinics. And I don't have to tell a sophisticated audience like this that sometimes there is flexibility in the way surgical mortality statistics are stated in a report. And if you talk to the resident, sometimes even the assistant resident, then you find out. So we have to be very careful.

Furthermore, we can't send everybody to the Cleveland Clinic. Nor can we always send them to be included in their last hundred cases; i.e., those with their lowest mortality. Some physicians had to send their patients to be included in the first hundred and the second hundred, and so forth. And the question is, was it justified?

And so, opposition to surgery is always based on the same problem, that there is a mortality, early and late. And do not forget the late, because some of the late is indirectly, if not directly, due to the surgery. One must always say: "Would that pneumonia have occurred if he wasn't operated?" Think of it! You're dealing with severely ill patients with advanced coronary disease (otherwise surgery would not be indicated), and a thoracotomy is being performed. And do you really think that that can be done innocuously to such a patient? So the risks are mortality and morbidity (Table 2). In addition to the patient's morbidity, you must also count the morbidity for the family doctor. That is often great even when the patient recovers. Consider also the increased disability that sometimes occurs. And finally, and perhaps this is the most important,

TABLE 1
Myocardial Revascularization: Balance of Forces

Favoring Surgery	Opposing Surgery
Surgical Promise	*Surgical Risk*
Relief of Symptoms	Mortality
Increased Funct.	Early—Late
Capacity	Morbidity
Increased Longevity	Increased
Infarct Protection	Disability
Medical Refractoriness	*Medical Promise*
Severity of	Favorable
Symptoms	Natural History
Severity of	New Drugs, etc.
Disability	
Poor Prognosis	*Better Surgery*
	Later

whenever you see your patient you must say: "What is likely to happen without surgery?" Are we so certain when we are told that the patient will not survive 3 months or 6 months that it is indeed true? Remember, that with the revascularization procedures, great emphasis is laid on the fact that you must wait 3 months or 6 months before benefit is obtained because this is the time the heart requires to develop an adequate collateral circulation.

But this is also the time necessary for most patients with intractable angina to become nonintractable, either because an artery closes off or because a collateral circulation develops without the surgery.

We really do not know enough about the natural history or we do not pay enough attention to it. Remember also that so long as the patient is alive there is always hope of a new drug. Or even if this surgical procedure is of value, it may be performed with less risk and with more effectiveness at a later date. If you have listened, and especially if you have listened over the past two years, you will notice that the same surgeons who were enthusiastic one year ago are more enthusiastic now about some other

TABLE 2
Myocardial Revascularization by Internal Mammary Artery Implant. Complications (675 Cases, Effler)

Acute Myocardial Infarction	10%
Cardiac Arrhythmias (Atrial Fibrill.)	8%
Hemorrhage (May Require Re-exploration)	3%
Congestive Heart Failure	2%
Postcardiotomy Syndrome	1%
Thrombophlebitis	1%

procedure or some improvement in the old procedure. Perhaps the patient you sent last year should have waited until this year. Perhaps you would have discovered that this patient did not have a good indication. Perhaps he had a thickened scar that needed removal rather than revascularization.

Dr. Vineberg presented certain indications for his revascularization operation. Actually Dr. Vineberg's indications would include every patient with angina pectoris since almost all patients with angina pectoris continue to experience it, at least occasionally, despite medical therapy. You will be in trouble if you try to promise the patient that his angina will disappear. That may happen on and off for brief periods of time, especially if he cuts down on his activity. Angina may actually disappear in perhaps 10 per cent of the cases. But most patients continue to have angina. In fact, one of the reasons for difficulty with the term intractable angina is that

some physicians define angina as intractable if it continues to occur, regardless of frequency, severity or circumstance. But although most patients continue to experience angina it is easy to live with and it is safer than some of the procedures.

Usually if a patient is operated upon it should be because the angina pectoris is of such severity that it is intolerable and because his functional capacity is greatly impaired. He should be aware of the surgical risks and should be willing to take these risks. In some cases I have seen patients who were recommended for surgery because of objective findings (Table 3). Occasionally I have seen a young patient in whom coronary angiography showed 2 occlusions. He was told that if revascularization was performed he would be protected in case there was a further occlusion.

TABLE 3
Indications for Myocardial Revascularization by Internal Mammary Artery Implant

A. Angina pectoris
   1. Severity of symptoms
   2. Functional incapacity
B. Advanced coronary stenosis or single or multiple occlusion by coronary arteriography
   1. With severe angina pectoris
   2. With heart failure (?)
   3. With risk of dangerous additional occlusion (prophylaxis)
C. History of 2 coronary occlusions in young person (prophylactic surgery)

Table 4 shows in general the procedure I go through in deciding whether a patient ought to be considered for surgical revascularization. How great is his distress? What is it he can't do? Have I really given medical treatment a fair trial? This is where deficiency is most likely to occur. Perhaps the most important; have I been sufficiently patient? The patient is very patient after he gets into the surgeon's hands. Long periods elapse before he says he is well. Has he given himself an equal chance medically? Very often it is the physician who cannot face the patient when the patient says "Doctor, I still have angina." Somehow he finds it easier to face the patient who has migraine headache and to tell her that she has to live with it. And he manages her by various medical technics. It is very easy for most patients to live with their angina, if you can encourage them, and tell them how to handle each episode or how to avoid most of them.

Effectiveness of surgery is next considered. This has not been demonstrated in my opinion. The natural history of angina pectoris is much more favorable than the surgeons tell you. Consider the surgical versus medical risk. I used to be told that

TABLE 4
Clinical Evaluation for Myocardial
Revascularization

1. Symptomatic distress
2. Functional disability
3. Adequacy of treatment
4. Adequacy of patience
5. Effectiveness of surgery
6. Natural history of angina pectoris
7. Surgical versus medical risk
8. Therapeutic advances versus clinical deterioration

every year 20 per cent died after a myocardial infarct. Then it was 10 per cent, then it was 5. Today I heard it was only 2 per cent. We must also consider therapeutic advances versus clinical deterioration. These are hard to estimate. If you practice medicine for many years, you will find that the clinical deterioration of the great majority of patients with angina pectoris is not rapid. And certainly not as rapid as I hope the advances in coronary surgery will be.

Some of the criteria that the surgeons have presented are shown in Table 5. They include relief of the patient, the development of anastomoses,

and myocardial lactate extraction. I hope you will not be misled by these objective findings, especially reports of improvement in myocardial metabolism. The studies are relatively sparse. There may be problems in methodology. I have not seen confirmation of the results by multiple groups of investigators. Much of this may be irrelevant. Essentially you must consider why you have sent your patient and whether the operation accomplishes what it is supposed to do. As far as you are concerned, that is enough evidence.

There is a mortality, as shown in Table 6. Perhaps it is low. Remember that in some series the late mortality is relatively high. The procedure is not innocuous. If you decide to refer a patient for surgical myocardial revascularization, you should ask, "Will he be alive in six months? What are his chances of dying?" You decide on some number. Then you should say to yourself: "What are the chances that he will die without operation in the next six months?" For this too estimate a percentage. You will find that the surgical mortality is much higher than that in the natural course of the disease.

TABLE 5
Myocardial Revascularization Internal Mammary Artery Implant Criteria of Benefit

	Relief of Angina		Patient Implant		Anastomoses With Coronaries		Incr. Blood Flow	Myo. Lactate Extraction	Longevity
	Cases		Cases		Cases				
	No.	%	No.	%	No.	%			
Vineberg	197	84							
Bigelow	48	54 +25	30	93	30	63			
Effler	249	78	127	92	127	54			
Sewell	94	64	94		43 +35				
Gorlin-Taylor	100	75	40	95	24	60	+	6/9	

TABLE 6
Internal Mammary Artery Implant Mortality

	Total Operations	Deaths			
		Number		Per Cent	
		Early	Late	Early	Late
Vineberg	140	7	24	5	17
	100	8	9		
Bigelow	77	13	11	17	14
	95	3		3.3	
Effler	249	16		6.4	8.8
Sewell	94	6		6.3	
Gorlin-Taylor	40	2	2	5	5

Six months from now you can sit down again and take stock of this patient. And only when you begin to find: (1) that the surgical procedure is indeed effective, and (2) that the risk is less with surgery than otherwise, should you be ready to consider surgery in that patient.

In the last paper I saw there were 675 cases. This report impressed me with the high incidence of acute myocardial infarction (10%). That incidence is much higher than would be expected to occur in patients with angina between the time they are referred for operation and the postoperative period. Perhaps some of these patients were brewing an infarction when they underwent surgery.

I only want to point out how fast the new operations are being introduced. I am way behind. Table 7 indicates the reasons for my skepticism of the procedure. You must realize that there have been many recommended revascularizing procedures. And what is more important, all of these procedures were said to be very effective.

I must read one little comment because it is representative of all the statements in all the papers whenever any of these procedures was reported. I have chosen a comment from this procedure, internal mammary ligation, because all of us now agree that it was totally ineffective. And this is what this surgeon said: "The patient is certainly not to blame if he feels better" [this is said sarcastically referring to the doubting physician], "is more productive in society, and is

TABLE 7
Revascularization of Myocardium

Phenolization of epicardium
Epicardial abrasion with silica (talc)
Ligation of internal mammary artery
Ligation of coronary vein or coronary sinus
Arterialization of coronary sinus
Grafting vascularized tissues to epicardium
    cardio-omentopexy
    cardio-pneumopexy
    implanted intestinal loop
Implantation internal mammary artery
Coronary autogenous vascular grafts
Coronary endarterectomy or resection
Mammary artery-coronary artery anastomosis

enjoying improved health to the consternation of the physician who just will not believe it. . . . As a conservative clinical evaluation, 68 per cent lost their symptoms of pain or were immeasurably relieved of their discomfort." These are almost exactly the words that we hear today about the newer revascularization procedures.

I do not deny that internal mammary implantation is a better procedure. I merely point out that claims of great benefit have been made over 20-odd years

with operation after operation for revascularization and then abandoned. I also ask why we needed all these newer studies to prove that Dr. Vineberg's operation was effective. It would seem to me that an operation which was capable of taking patients with intractable angina and making them well would have brought thousands to his doorstep, without requiring the evidence of coronary arteriography.

Table 8 is from the Metropolitan Life Insurance Company and shows the standard life risk of a patient at age 55 who has had no infarction. He would be expected to survive an additional 19 to 24 years. This means that he would live to between 74 and 79 years of age. And patients who had suffered a single myocardial infarct and applied for life insurance had a longevity of 16 to 18 years, not very much less, i.e., they survived to between 71 and 73 years. Only those who were completely disabled after an infarct at age 55 lived as little as 9 to 14 years. Their outlook for survival was the achievement of an age between 64 and 69.

In conclusion I would like to say first that most patients with angina pectoris who are being considered for surgical procedures are not sick enough

TABLE 8
Duration of Life After First Myocardial Infarct

Group	Duration of life after onset	
	Age 45 at onset	Age 55 at onset
Std. Life Ins. Risks	28–32 yrs.	19–24 yrs.
Men/1st myo. infarct:		
Applicants-life ins.	17–19 yrs.	16–18 yrs.
Disabled policyholders	11–15 yrs.	9–14 yrs.
Insurance company employees	16–19 yrs.	11–16 yrs.
Employees in industry	*	10–13 yrs.
Hospital, clinic & private patients	12–14 yrs.	7–11 yrs.

*Not available.
From Metropolitan Life Insurance Company.

to warrant it. With patience and confidence, and knowledge as to how to handle these patients, you are able to carry them along until they get past the acute phase of their symptoms (Table 9).

Secondly, the coronary surgical procedures are

TABLE 9
Treatment of Intractable Angina Pectoris

1. General approach to patient	7. Oxygen therapy
2. The natural history of angina pectoris	8. Sedation
3. Reassurance and patience	9. Avoidance of opiates
4. Elimination of contributing or precipitating factors	10. Antidepressant drugs
5. Use of nitroglycerin	11. Propranolol
6. Placebo value of long-acting nitrates	12. Radioiodine

very promising but I expect them to undergo considerable improvement. I have more optimism for the procedures that are direct approaches to the artery than the revascularization procedure, about which I have continued skepticism. But if I am wrong, time will indicate that. Only very infrequently should you be compelled to send a patient for surgery at this time. Those patients who feel that life is not worth living as they exist now, or that they are incapable of working as they are now, and who knowingly are willing to undertake the risk of a procedure, and knowingly recognize that this is an experimental procedure may be subjected to the operation.

As for other patients, let the other fellow do it first and we shall see. At the appropriate time we will take advantage of the contribution of the surgeons which has indeed been great.

A Surgeon Evaluates Myocardial Revascularization

John J. Collins, Jr.

Operations designed to achieve myocardial revascularization may be considered in three categories: local coronary reconstruction, enhancement of collateral circulation and introduction of an extra cardiac vascular pedicle. Coronary artery reconstruction is applicable only to local obstruction in a limited portion of the right coronary artery and for that reason will not be discussed in detail. Enhancement of collateral circulation by arterio-arterial or phase-shift balloon counterpulsation has not yet been widely used clinically and there are little data available concerning the effect of counterpulsation upon myocardial blood flow, metabolism or the relief of angina pectoris. This discussion, then, will be focused primarily upon the effects of introduction of an extra cardiac vascular pedicle, specifically internal mammary artery implantation.

The criteria by which one may evaluate myocardial revascularization are similar to those for evaluation of any operation. (1) Is the operation well conceived? (2) Is it technically feasible? (3) Are the experimental results favorable? (4) Is the risk reasonable? (5) Are the objectives realized?

Because of peculiarities in the capillary network in the myocardium, a bleeding vascular pedicle introduced into the myocardium will find a run-off sufficient to preserve patency of the implant in most instances. We are indebted to the persistent fervor of Dr. Arthur Vineberg for the now widespread acceptance of this fact which may be demonstrated by selective angiography. Mammary artery implantation is now an established concept after a stormy early history.

Technical feasibility of mammary artery implantation is proven by the fact that a high rate of patency can be obtained in a large series of patients who have demonstrated obstructive coronary artery disease and incapacitating angina pectoris. Nearly 90 per cent of pedicles implanted at the Peter Bent Brigham Hospital have remained patent.

Studies of mammary artery implantation in the laboratory have demonstrated prolonged patency, collateral formation proportional to the degree of ischemia in the surrounding muscle, flow comparable to the native coronary artery in some instances and a normal distribution of blood flow. So the experimental results are favorable.

The question of operative risk is being resolved. The risk at the Peter Bent Brigham Hospital is 4 per cent for a single pedicle and 6 per cent for bilateral mammary artery implantation in well over 100 patients.

The question of whether this well conceived, technically feasible, experimentally supported operation of moderate risk actually achieves its intended objective is obviously of vital importance. Four points must be resolved. (1) Is angina relieved? (2) Is myocardial perfusion improved? (3) Is life prolonged? (4) Is myocardial infarction prevented?

In our experience 80 per cent of patients achieve good to excellent relief of angina. Relief generally occurs only after three to six months, suggesting that time is required to establish improved perfusion. The evidence that improved myocardial perfusion does actually occur is indirect. Angiography demonstrates patency and formation of collateral circulation communicating with the native coronary circulation but flow rate is difficult to establish with certainty. The rate of disappearance of Kr[85] injected into the mammary artery is similar to that observed with injection into the native coronary orifice demonstrating that large arteriovenous fistulas are not present. Studies of lactate levels in the coronary sinus before and after implantation show a tendency for clinical improvement and angiographic patency to parallel reversal of lactate production. These data have been carefully gathered by Doctors Richard Gorlin and Warren J. Taylor and, while not unassailable, strongly suggest that myocardial metabolism is improved.

The questions of prolongation of life and prevention of myocardial infarction are not yet clear. Sufficient time has not elapsed. However, the surgical mortality seems compensated in about 18 months and perhaps this suggests that life may be prolonged.

479

These questions will eventually be resolved. Meanwhile, it seems reasonable to continue mammary implantation and to pursue studies to prove its physiologic efficacy. But we should not neglect, for example, counterpulsation, with its solid experimental support, or even de-epicardialization and puodrage which has relieved angina in 75 per cent of some series. With a better understanding of angina pectoris and myocardial ischemia, better operations will be devised.

Panel Discussion: Status of Myocardial Revascularization

CHAIRMAN LILLEHEI: I think that we might begin on a somewhat lower-keyed level and direct several of the questions that have come in to Dr. Friedberg and Dr. Sones. There are three or four that are quite similar. Would you comment, Dr. Friedberg, on what effect exercise has in stimulating the development of collaterals and if it has any real value at all in ischemic heart disease.

DR. FRIEDBERG: I can't say that I know what it does. I'm familiar with studies that purport to show that collateral circulation is improved and we know from some of the older experiments that myocardial anoxia is the best stimulant to collateral circulation. So, to the extent that exercise, at least transiently, produces myocardial ischemia, one would expect that collaterals would be increased. Dr. Sones could probably give better information on that. As you know, Dr. Hellerstein of Cleveland has had a study going with patients who've had myocardial infarction and in whom, with the aid of coronary arteriographic studies, there has been evidence of improved collaterals. I'm a little disturbed about the lack of controls and what happens in these patients even without exercise.

DR. LILLEHEI: Dr. Sones, there is also a question not only related to exercise, but also to the effect of vasodilators on the coronary circulation.

DR. SONES: With regard to the first question, there is absolutely no objective evidence that an exercise program specifically improves in any sense the rapidity of development or effectiveness of intercoronary collateral channels. The timely development of intercoronary collateral channels is a major reason why people survive coronary occlusion. This means you've got to have these channels before total occlusion of major trunks occur, and they've got to be adequate enough to protect the myocardium and to preserve its viability. If they are not already there, the myocardium dies, and it either dies transmurally or interstitially. Most of these occlusive events result in some degree of interstitial fibrosis, if you are dealing with surviving patients.

The biggest slobs I have ever seen, and I have seen hundreds of them with fantastic collateral flow, testify eloquently to the fact that an exercise program is by no means essential to the development of intercoronary collateral channels. And I can show you thousands of patients who've never done any exercise of any more magnitude than pushing themselves away from the table too late, who also testify eloquently to this fact. There is not the remotest doubt that a properly controlled exercise program will improve the functional capability of the whole human. But this has nothing to do specifically with the development of intercoronary collateral channels.

DR. LILLEHEI: Do any members of the panel have any comment on that subject?

DR. VINEBERG: I'd like to question Dr. Friedberg and Dr. Sones concerning this exercise program, particularly for people with coronary heart disease. Before they are put on this program, hadn't we better see if they have coronary arteries which may develop collaterals by locating the points of occlusion? Isn't it a bit dangerous if a man has major occlusions of two main trunks to have him jogging up and down Central Park? I'd like to get your views on that.

DR. FRIEDBERG: I don't want to pretend to be scientific about it because I don't think I know. Let's say this: patients in general, as Dr. Sones indicated, feel better and have greater capacity for activity if they keep in good physical trim by exercise; to the extent that that can be done with progressive, moderated control, I encourage it. I try to discourage patients who've had myocardial infarction or other clinical evidence of serious coronary disease from engaging in competitive sports that involve endurance and speed. Otherwise, I depend on common sense in the clinical response of the patient as he tries to increase his activity. But I do believe that exercise is good for the general well being of a person, to the extent that he doesn't do it without some use of common sense and with due regard for the symptoms that may occur as he increases his activity.

CHAIRMAN LILLEHEI: Dr. Vineberg, Dr. Sones (the Quasimodo of the Cleveland Clinic) is really a pediatrician and he apparently doesn't understand your triarterial zone. Do you have any comments on that?

DR. VINEBERG: No further comments. He can read about it in the printed paper.

DR. SONES: We use our imagination in print, as well as in public.

CHAIRMAN LILLEHEI: Dr. Friedberg, in regard to indications for surgery, I guess it is fair to say that you are not enthusiastic about the accomplishments of surgery.

DR. FRIEDBERG: Oh, that's not true, Dr. Lillehei. I'm very aware of the accomplishments; I've always said that in the modern era, the surgeons have certainly done more to forward cardiology than the medical men. Maybe the electricians have done a little, too. But I do agree that, with respect to individual patients, I stand off as to the indications for surgery. In other words, procedure may be effective, but I believe that fewer patients have an indication for the procedure than the surgeon thinks.

CHAIRMAN LILLEHEI: I imagine it would be fair to say that you think about a third, at least, are too good to need surgery for this condition and perhaps as many as a fourth or a third are too bad, and there are perhaps another third who need it, but you'd like to wait. So that sums up the indications for surgery—is that correct?

DR. FRIEDBERG: Those are your statements, Dr. Lillehei.

DR. SONES: I really think that Dr. Friedberg should be proposed for next year's president of the American Thoracic.

DR. FRIEDBERG: I knew I was in trouble in this "Den of Surgeons."

CHAIRMAN LILLEHEI: There are several questions related to propranolol. I think our propranolol expert is over there. Dr. Russek, do you want to comment on a question asking specifically, "Do you use propranolol in the medical treatment of ischemic heart disease?"

DR. HENRY RUSSEK: Very definitely, we use propranolol in conjunction with the nitrates, particularly isosorbide dinitrate, for patients with forms of angina that do not respond to the nitrates alone and to the conventional modes of therapy. And, we have found this to be a highly promising mode of therapy for these severe cases of angina pectoris. In fact, we feel that the improvement in symptoms and exercise tolerance obtained from the use of these drugs is far greater than that achieved through surgical revascularization. In addition, complications and mortality appear far less frequent on medical therapy.

CHAIRMAN LILLEHEI: In the remote event that surgery would become necessary in such a patient, one question asks, would you continue propranolol or would you discontinue it prior to surgery, and if so, how long before?

DR. RUSSEK: Prior to revascularization surgery I definitely would discontinue propranolol because of fear that congestive heart failure might be precipitated. But once the patient has gone through the procedure, should tachycardia develop postoperatively which cannot be controlled, I would not hesitate to use the drug. Certainly for the patient who postoperatively continues to have angina, particularly for the first six months, propranolol plus nitrate therapy has proved distinctly valuable. Obviously we must continue to treat our patients until surgery has had its full effect, and this may take a number of months. Similarly, in patients who do not have symptomatic benefit or who have only minor degrees of symptomatic benefit after surgery, such therapy is often clearly beneficial. These drugs, therefore, can convert a poor postoperative clinical result to a far better one, so they do provide valuable adjuvant therapy after revascularization procedures.

CHAIRMAN LILLEHEI: Another question directed to the surgeons of the panel: "Would any of the surgeons recommend arteriography and a revascularization procedure in a patient showing only an abnormal Master two-step test on routine examination without symptoms?"

DR. BAILEY: Yes.

DR. VINEBERG: Well, if he has no symptoms I don't think we'd be seeing him at all. I see no reason why he should have it.

DR. SONES: It is established that 30 to 40 per cent of the people who die of this disease, die before a doctor ever recognizes the symptoms. If you find something that points toward the probability of myocardial ischemia, *look*—if you've got somebody around who can look effectively. A bad study is a whole lot worse than no study at all. What we've got to do is improve the quality of arteriography.

DR. FRIEDBERG: Dr. Sones, may I ask you, won't they die if they have the operation?

DR. SONES: Well some do die. The question really is "would you look?" Depending on what you find, that is what will decide whether or not you are going to intervene surgically. I've seen people with 95 per cent obstructions of a right coronary artery who had only occasional bouts of anginal pain and who certainly constituted no major threat to the physician's sleep. But a 95 per cent obstruction in the dominant right coronary artery, even though it is not producing much in the way of symptoms in a sedentary individual, is certainly a threat to his myocardium and to his life. If I found this as a result of diagnostic study, most certainly we would try to convince him to eradicate the obstruction.

DR. FRIEDBERG: Oh, well that's a different story.

DR. SONES: You don't find it unless you look.

DR. FRIEDBERG: But do you have evidence that revascularization means that there will no longer be a threat to his life?

DR. SONES: Of course not. You can only compensate for lesions which already exist. You cannot compensate for lesions that are yet to occur. Now, Dr. Vineberg may promise you that, but I don't believe it.

DR. FRIEDBERG: I'm glad the surgeons are on to each other.

DR. VINEBERG: I don't think there is any difference in the point of view at all between Dr. Sones and myself. It is a matter of semantics and terminology and I want to bury that part right now. But I would like to discuss survival a little more—there has been a suspicion around here of a high operative mortality. With regard to this, revascularization of one zonal area, as Dr. Mason Sones has just so ably shown (one implanted artery in a patient who has no angina at rest) cannot have an operative mortality, in good hands, of more than 1.9 per cent. Now, I don't believe anybody will deny the fact that people do die from angina pectoris in spite of the figures that seem to come up in Dr. Friedberg's books. It is a fact, as the U. S. Public Health Service has indicated, that we still are losing more people per year from this disease than in any other way. Now I don't understand how, on the one hand, we can have such a high mortality from medical treatment, and then be told on the other hand, that if you have angina the risk is small and if you have an infarction it doesn't mean anything. It stands to reason that if a whole area is blocked off suddenly, as Dr. Sones has just said, this isn't very good for the heart and it's not good for the patient.

The implantation of two arteries has just been shown to carry a mortality of about 4 per cent. And the reason some patients have to have two arteries is because they have more disease. And, of course, they've got double the chance of dying from one or the other arteries, if we accept the fact that they may infarct on us. I don't care where you put the arteries, as long as you get some more revascularization. Whether the direct approach is going to be more valuable or not, time will tell. Maybe it is an adjunct that has to be used; I question whether it is. But to say that there is a high operative mortality from revascularization surgery, doesn't make any sense.

I would like to ask Dr. Friedberg if he could give me a documented case, other than the two cases of Learn's reported in 1929 and 1930, of any patient that has been living without coronary arteries. The 7 patients that I have documented, are living or have lived on nothing but internal mammary artery and are either very well or have died for one reason or another. One lived up to $17\frac{1}{2}$ years on one artery, the only artery open in the heart. Now don't tell me the heart was taking blood up the artery and sending it back to the aorta. How else does this heart live?

Will you answer this question then: Is there any other documented evidence, anywhere, except for those two cases of Learn and his associate, O'Leary, in which a patient has been shown to be living with all his coronary arteries blocked?

DR. FRIEDBERG: Dr. Vineberg, you've said so many things that require a reply that I'm not going to be pinned into a "yes" or "no." It's well known that a patient may have every vessel apparently blocked and yet he survives for some time. For example, there are syphilitic arteries as in the case to which you made reference. It's nonsense to say that the mammary artery is what kept them alive. We don't have enough understanding of the collateral circulation nor do we know what makes people live to the day they die, sometimes without symptoms and often suddenly.

But the confusion in this situation lies in the following. First, you talk about the high mortality from coronary disease. You're referring to sudden death, to deaths from acute myocardial infarction. That's not what we're talking about when we consider a patient who walks into our office with angina pectoris. When we decide that a patient is to be sent for an operation, we have to consider what is going to happen to him between now and say three months after operation; what are his chances of dying from the operation in that 3 or 6 months' period; and what are the chances of this patient with angina dying without having an operation. And I tell you that it is higher with the operation.

DR. VINEBERG: I'm sorry to take up the time, but this is an extremely important point. You say there are hundreds of cases

DR. FRIEDBERG: I didn't say hundreds of cases.

DR. VINEBERG: Well, you said there are many documented cases

DR. FRIEDBERG: I didn't say many documented cases.

DR. VINEBERG: Would you give me, except for the two that have been published by Learn and O'Leary, one other publication?

DR. FRIEDBERG: That isn't the point. I'm not familiar with everything.

CHAIRMAN LILLEHEI: Gentlemen, I think Dr. Sones has some objective evidence and this is derived from hundreds of arteriograms.

DR. SONES: I'm going to repeat some operative mortality statistics, and this means death in hospital. And regardless of anybody's insinuations, these figures are "by God" true.

In 2530 implants, the total mortality for single implants in the hospital was 3.2 per cent; the total mortality for double implants was 5.6 per cent. Now, I'll tell you something else. I've got a list of about 750 patients at the moment waiting to get into the Cleveland Clinic because somebody was convinced that they might be benefited by at least a "look." An average of 3 to 4 of those patients are dying every month. Now, maybe it's because they are afraid of the trip to Cleveland—I don't know. But God knows they are all on medical management and that is not a minor degree of mortality. A larger number are having myocardial infarction between the time their doctor asks for an implantment and the time set for admission to the hospital. We are not dealing with an itch. This is a lethal disease and I think we had better consider it so.

The next thing is that there has never been in our total series evidence of regression of an obstructive lesion, due to atheromatous plaque, in a single instance on repetitive study. We've seen two or three patients in whom thrombotic emboli have completely lysed following myocardial infarction, leaving completely clean vessels. But that is the only kind of coronary artery obstruction that I've ever seen clear up!

Finally, and then I'm going to be quiet, there has as yet been no definitive evidence of any capacity to bring in a new source of extra-coronary flow or to eradicate significant, potentially lethal obstructions in major branches of the coronary tree by any measure of medical management that I'm aware of— not one. What we do have here is not something that's perfect, but it is a whole lot better than what we had. And if we evolve and develop as we should, with increasing experience and increasing understanding, we will be in a position to add to those measures of medical management which have been available to us. This silly business of saying you exclude medical management simply by the utilization of available surgical technics, is childishly absurd.

CHAIRMAN LILLEHEI: Have you seen any patients in all your series where there were no coronary arteries open at the main stems so that they were living on manna from heaven and so-called collaterals?

DR. SONES: I've seen a number of patients in whom all three coronary arteries were obstructed. But I've never seen a patient in whom both main trunks were obstructed at the orifice. This glib statement of total occlusion of all three vessels is frequently made, but the thing that people forget is that these obstructions are in main trunks but they lie below vessels that provide incredible collaterals.

CHAIRMAN LILLEHEI: Well, I think the fact that coronary artery disease is often referred to at the present time as the "Black Death" or the plague of the twentieth century, shows that there is probably plenty of work both for the internist and for the cardiac surgeon. Certainly with a million and a half people incapacitated at the present time in the United States, there is a great deal that the younger generation has left to accomplish. Thank you very much.

Where Next? A Look Into the Future

E. Grey Dimond

This book has dealt with a disease which surely possesses all of its readers, coronary artery disease. It we are even moderately realistic, surely one fourth of us will die from it, not aged, full in years, but unexpectedly, swiftly; almost an impertinent death.

Coronary artery disease is thoroughly an epidemic and is far more threatening to our generation than automobiles, guns, or drugs. Must we lose that man who is trained, contributing in his prime years, needed by his children, his family, by his immediate society, needed by his government, even needed as a taxpayer? For a man to lose 20 years of his prime productive time is surely a sufficient tragedy to make it a national emergency.

This symposium has been both a success story and a failure. It has been successful because it showed the resourceful, new approaches to the diagnosis and care of the patient with this disease.

However, I suggest that even more this conference has reminded us of the basic fault of medicine as a career. We physicians glean the heaviest of disease. We concern ourselves with this thing called atherosclerosis 20 or 30 years after the disease began. Only a few lonely voices through the years, Raab in Vermont, White in Boston, have seen the need for preventive cardiology. Most of us, clinicians, surgeons, radiologists, have become immensely skillful in "placing labels," correcting or, more often, accommodating to the end results of atherosclerosis.

During these past few months I have been living in Washington, D. C., and my route to the office takes me by the Shoreham Hotel each morning. The Shoreham Hotel is familiar to all of us as a popular site for meetings and especially medical meetings. On many mornings there are clusters of men gathered in front of the hotel, getting a breath of air before the day's sessions. I have found it stimulating to my diagnostic skills to try and form an opinion of the particular groups' profession from my rapid automobile view: their height, weight, age, dress and demeanor. Later in the day, I make it a point to cross check my opinion. One's success is remarkable! Sporty attire, jackets, open shirts, hush puppies

on their feet, bare headed, rather skinny and semiprofessional looking? Anesthesiologists! Of course!

A group of mesomorphic, bold men. Talking animatedly *at* each other, with gestures. Prosperous yet somewhat rumpled? Surgeons, of course.

A group of disheveled men. Perhaps unconventional in dress and hair and demeanor. A few whiskers. Ankle length, droopy sox. Some furtive, some expansive, all intelligent. Why they are psychiatrists, of course!

A group of lean, taciturn, smokeless men. Some striding vigorously, an occasional one doggedly trotting. Calm men, quiet men, men who appear accustomed to listening, not doing. Thinking men, pale men, neatly tailored, buttoned-down men? Clinicians? Yes. Internists? Yes. Cardiologists? Of course!

Now there is a reason why I have made these touring Rorshach comments. My point is that we are all of us *victims* of our careers, more perhaps than we care to identify. A process of selectivity has brought us to this narrowed perch and, while we may suggest that chance had little to do with it and that we had arrived at this point by making the necessary decisions, surely we are all too analytical to accept this as a full answer.

I find it useful to think of life as a giant sieve with holes of many shapes and sizes. We all tumble into this sieve because we finished high school; the shaking continues and we find holes which fit us and we become college students, pre-medical students, medical students—and then the shape of the holes becomes increasingly critical. We are separated out by a choice of internship, then residency, the subspecialty, then the Boards—and by this time 15 years have passed and it is obvious that no simple random design has brought us into a common field of work or a common "life-style."

The computer of life itself has sought us out, even as we thought we were in control. Like it or not, we are similar, and we tend to think similarly, and act similarly, and when in front of the Shoreham Hotel, we look similar.

This similarity would identify us if we were each asked to do that which I am attempting to do, to predict the future in our chosen field. We would each prepare a quite similar list: Successful heart transplants; a major role for pump assist devices; an increasing effort in getting rapid assistance to the coronary occlusion patient; including mobile resuscitation teams; new medications for arrhythmias, ischemia and failure; increased enthusiasm for full physical rehabilitation after an occlusion; and finally, safe suggestions that electronics, computers and atomic energy would undoubtedly have an important role.

However, when one makes such a list it is useful to look back and think of the incredible events of the past years. The greatest hazard of all is to underestimate, isn't it? And the danger of underestimating the rate of change is made so clear to me when I consider where we are now and where we were a very short time ago.

First, think of the entire field of medicine. Do you remember the syphilologist with his little vial of plasmodium vivax, provoking malaria in his patient with CNS lues? Tabes? Paresis? Almost forgotten diseases here in the U.S.A. And, ominous reminder of obsolescence, the now extinct syphilologist?

Do you remember the Drinker respirators in a row with the season's poliomyelitis victims? Do you remember bulbar polio?

Do you remember the frightening isolation ward with scarlet fever, meningitis, erysipelas, whooping cough, diphtheria?

Do you remember the vast isolated tuberculosis hospitals? Hospitals which had become a complete way of life for the victims? Of years of rest, of collapse therapy, of drainage, of arrest and activation and arrest and activation.

Do you remember the brutality of the mastoidectomy and of the surgical treatment of osteomyelitis?

To change my orientation, do you remember uremic frost, the uremic pericardial rub? And the absolute inevitability of death? And now renal dialysis can be done at home by the patient, with a return to health.

Do you remember the entire ward of acute rheumatic fever patients? The jumping, flicking motion of Sydenham's chorea?

I won't attempt to exhaust you with this almost endless narration, which would prove how little we are able to see ahead and how what will happen is always beyond our expectations.

In our own field there are the following: Total correction of Tetralogy of Fallot; replacement of the entire arch of the aorta; destroyed mitral, tricuspid, and aortic valves all replaced by plastic ones; Ebstein's Disease treated with a plastic tricuspid valve; the ischemic limb, the ischemic brain and now the ischemic myocardium treated by conduits; the acute myocardial infarction with ventricular fibrillation treated by "laudable electrocution;" the deadly Stokes-Adams syndrome solved by connecting the heart to a battery; total cure of patent ductus arteriosus, coarctation of the aorta, ostium secundum.

Do you remember when it was considered only necessary to identify the problem as congenital heart disease, blue or not blue?

Do you remember when an internist was considered a cardiologist if he knew how to interpret a chest lead? When your diagnostic tools consisted of your stethoscope, blood pressure cuff and a three lead electrocardiogram and a crackling fluoroscope?

And would you have predicted the ultimate of science fiction: a young boy dying in Illinois, flown by jet airplane to Houston, Texas, and his heart given as a replacement to a middle age-man who had outlived his own myocardium?

I need not go on to make myself realize how impossible it is to predict in an exponential era such as this.

Yet in this listing of the future successes, I have reaffirmed the restrictions of our professions. Replacing the heart? New plastic valves? Pump assistance? Vasodilators? Anti-arrhythmia treatment? Our thinking is conditioned upon the *presence* of disease, not upon the elimination.

We are all physicians and we are trained to give our attention to a single individual, the familiar one-to-one ratio which is the essence of our pride and ethics, the doctor-patient relationship.

Within this ethic, we have found our careers and our reason for being. We have found the hole in the sieve which was ready for us.

Yet one suspects that a different kind of man will fit the future template. One agrees that our kind of a physician will continue to be an essential part of the social fabric. Disease will not go away and people will continue to need private, personal counsel.

However, the larger sieve of medicine will change and it is here that I wish to make my own prediction.

I believe another kind of man will come into the medical school and he will come out of it differently constructed. He will be oriented towards a broader definition of responsibility. Community, team, group, region, prevention, total health care, will be comfortable terms for him. Still he will be a physician and he will continue to bear the burden and the privileges of our profession.

I respectfully suggest that, different from the experience of these past many years, the *social system of delivery of health care* will be altered and that this will be for good, not bad, I believe the concept of personal dedicated service will be strengthened, not lessened, in these years to come. Our often expressed professional concern over the hazards of socialized medicine will prove unneeded and a career in medicine will continue to be one of the few truly satisfying ways to serve man.

Index

Numerals in italics indicate a figure, "t" following a page number indicates a table concerning the subject mentioned.